Micronutrients in Health and Disease

Micronutrients in Health and Disease

Kedar N. Prasad, Ph.D.

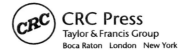

CRC Press
Taylor & Francis Group
Boca Raton   London   New York

CRC Press is an imprint of the
Taylor & Francis Group, an **informa** business

CRC Press
Taylor & Francis Group
6000 Broken Sound Parkway NW, Suite 300
Boca Raton, FL 33487-2742

© 2011 by Taylor and Francis Group, LLC
CRC Press is an imprint of Taylor & Francis Group, an Informa business

No claim to original U.S. Government works

International Standard Book Number: 978-1-4398-2106-0 (Hardback)

This book contains information obtained from authentic and highly regarded sources. Reasonable efforts have been made to publish reliable data and information, but the author and publisher cannot assume responsibility for the validity of all materials or the consequences of their use. The authors and publishers have attempted to trace the copyright holders of all material reproduced in this publication and apologize to copyright holders if permission to publish in this form has not been obtained. If any copyright material has not been acknowledged please write and let us know so we may rectify in any future reprint.

Except as permitted under U.S. Copyright Law, no part of this book may be reprinted, reproduced, transmitted, or utilized in any form by any electronic, mechanical, or other means, now known or hereafter invented, including photocopying, microfilming, and recording, or in any information storage or retrieval system, without written permission from the publishers.

For permission to photocopy or use material electronically from this work, please access www.copyright.com (http://www.copyright.com/) or contact the Copyright Clearance Center, Inc. (CCC), 222 Rosewood Drive, Danvers, MA 01923, 978-750-8400. CCC is a not-for-profit organization that provides licenses and registration for a variety of users. For organizations that have been granted a photocopy license by the CCC, a separate system of payment has been arranged.

Trademark Notice: Product or corporate names may be trademarks or registered trademarks, and are used only for identification and explanation without intent to infringe.

Library of Congress Cataloging-in-Publication Data

Prasad, Kedar N.
  Micronutrients in health and disease / by Kedar N. Prasad.
    p. ; cm.
  Includes bibliographical references and index.
  ISBN 978-1-4398-2106-0 (alk. paper)
  1. Antioxidants--Health aspects. 2. Active oxygen--Pathophysiology. 3. Trace elements in nutrition. 4. Dietary supplements. I. Title.
  [DNLM: 1. Micronutrients--therapeutic use. 2. Antioxidants--therapeutic use. 3. Dietary Supplements. QU 130.5 P911m 2011]
  RB170.P737 2011
  613.2'86--dc22
                                                                                    2010010721

Visit the Taylor & Francis Web site at
http://www.taylorandfrancis.com

and the CRC Press Web site at
http://www.crcpress.com

Dedication

This book is dedicated to my family for their encouragement.

Contents

Preface xxi
Acknowledgment xxiii
Author xxv

Chapter 1 Basic Facts about Antioxidants 1

    Introduction 1
    Evolution of the Antioxidant System 1
    History of the Discovery of Antioxidants 1
    Sources and Forms of Vitamins 2
    Solubility of Antioxidants 3
    Distribution of Antioxidants in the Body 3
    Storage of Antioxidants 5
    Can Antioxidants Be Degraded during Cooking? 5
    Absorption of Antioxidants and Its Significance 6
    Functions of Individual Antioxidants 6
    Antioxidant Defense Systems 7
        Group A Antioxidants 7
        Group B Antioxidants 7
        Group C Antioxidants 8
    Known Functions of Antioxidants 8
    Current Controversies about Antioxidants 8
    Misuse of Antioxidants in Clinical Studies 8
    Conclusions 11
    References 11

Chapter 2 Basic Facts about Oxidative Stress, Inflammation, and the Immune System 13

    Introduction 13
    Oxidative Stress 14
        What Are Free Radicals? 14
        Types of Free Radicals 14
        Formation of Free Radicals Derived from Oxygen and Nitrogen 14
    Oxidation and Reduction Processes 16
    What Is Inflammation? 16
        Types of Inflammatory Reactions 17
    Products of Inflammatory Reactions 17
        Cytokines 17
        Complement Proteins 18
        AA Metabolites 18
        Endothelial/Leukocyte Adhesion Molecules 18
    Immune System 18
    What Is the Immune System? 19
    Innate Immunity 19
    Adaptive Immunity 20
    Conclusions 20
    References 21

Chapter 3 Scientific Rationale of Current Trends in Clinical Studies of Micronutrients for Prevention of Chronic Diseases 23

    Introduction 23
    Levels of Oxidative Stress and Chronic Inflammation in High-Risk Populations 24
        High-Risk Populations for Cancer... 24
        High-Risk Populations of CAD 24
        High-Risk Populations of AD and PD 24
    Biology of Antioxidants 24
    Results of Clinical Trials with a Single Antioxidant... 26
        Cancer... 26
        Coronary Artery Disease 26
        Alzheimer's Disease and Parkinson's Disease 27
    Reasons the Use of a Single Antioxidant Produced Inconsistent Results 28
    Results of Clinical Studies with Multiple Dietary Antioxidants in Cancer 28
    Results of Clinical Studies with Fat and Fiber.. 29
    Using Multiple Micronutrients with a Low-Fat, High-Fiber Diet to Reduce the Risk and Progression of Chronic Diseases 30
    Recommended Micronutrients for Reducing the Risk and Progression of Chronic Diseases.. 30
    Conclusions 31
    References 31

Chapter 4 Micronutrients in Healthy Aging 35

    Introduction 35
    Oxidative Stress during Aging 36
        Sources of Oxidative Stress... 36
        Influence of Environmental, Dietary, Metabolic, and Lifestyle-Related Stressors on Oxidative Stress 36
        Oxidative Stress Influences Mitochondria, Lysosome, and Proteasome Function during Aging 37
            Mitochondrial Dysfunction 37
            Impairment of Proteasome and Lysosomal-Mediated Proteolytic Activities 38
        Oxidative Stress Influences the Length of Telomere during Aging 38
    Chronic Inflammation during Aging 39
    Aging Influences Immune Function... 39
    Aging Influencing Antioxidant Defense Systems 40
        Antioxidant Enzymes 40
            Changes in Antioxidant Enzyme Activities in Animals 40
            Changes in Antioxidant Enzyme Activities in Humans 40
        Dietary and Endogenous Antioxidants Levels 41
            Vitamin C 42
            Glutathione 42
            Vitamin E 42
            Coenzyme Q_{10} 42
    Antioxidant Supplementation Influences Age-Related Functional Deficits............... 43
        Vitamin E 43
        Coenzyme Q_{10}.. 43

Contents

    Carotenoids 44
    Melatonin 44
    Flavonoids 44
    Glutathione and *N*-Acetylcysteine 44
    Alpha-Lipoic Acid 44
    Multiple Dietary Antioxidants 44
Rationale for Not Using a Single Dietary Antioxidant to Reduce Age-Related Functional Deficits 45
Rationale for Recommending Multiple Micronutrients to Reduce the Rate of Aging 45
Recommended Micronutrients for Adults and Children 46
Changes in Diet and Lifestyle 46
Conclusions 47
References 47

Chapter 5 Role of Micronutrients in the Prevention of Coronary Artery Disease and Improvement of the Standard Therapy 55

Introduction 55
Incidence and Cost 55
Primary Risk Factors and Involvement of Oxidative Stress and Inflammation in CAD 56
Consequences of Increased Oxidative Stress and Chronic Inflammation 56
Low-Dose Aspirin in CAD 57
Role of Antioxidants in CAD 57
    Animal Studies after Treatment with Antioxidants 57
    Epidemiologic Studies with Antioxidants 57
Intervention Human Studies after Treatment with One or More Dietary Antioxidants 58
    Vitamin E Alone Producing Beneficial Effects 59
    Vitamin C Alone Producing Beneficial Effects 60
    Dietary Antioxidants Producing No Effects or Adverse Effects 60
    Endogenous Antioxidants Producing No Effect or Beneficial Effects 62
    Dietary and Endogenous Antioxidants with Cholesterol-Lowering Drugs 63
    Multiple Dietary Antioxidants with Cholesterol-Lowering Drugs 63
    Resveratrol and Omega-3 Fatty Acids 65
        Resveratrol 65
        Omega-3 Fatty Acids 65
Intervention Studies with B-Vitamins to Lower Homocysteine Levels 66
Scientific Rationale for Using Multiple Micronutrients Including Dietary and Endogenous Antioxidants in Prevention and Improved Treatment of CAD 67
Proposed Multiple Micronutrient Preparation 68
Importance of Dose Schedule 68
Antioxidants and Aspirin Resistance 69
Scientific Rationale for Using Multiple Micronutrient Preparations in Combination with Cholesterol-Lowering Drugs and Aspirin for Reducing the Progression of CAD 69
Modifications in Diet and Lifestyle 69
Conclusions 69
References 70

Chapter 6 Micronutrients for the Prevention of Diabetes and Improvement of the Standard Therapy 77

Introduction 77
Incidence and Cost 77
Types of Diabetes 78
    Type 1 Diabetes 78
    Type 2 Diabetes 78
    Gestational Diabetes 78
    Other Types of Diabetes 78
    Prediabetes and Metabolic Syndrome 78
Complications of Diabetes 79
Evidence for Increased Oxidative Stress in Diabetes 79
    Type 1 Diabetes 79
    Type 2 Diabetes 80
    Metabolic Syndrome 80
Evidence for Increased Chronic Inflammation in Diabetes 80
Beneficial Effects of Antioxidants and Other Nutrients in Diabetes 81
    Vitamin A 81
    Vitamin C 81
    Vitamin D 82
    Vitamin E 82
    Alpha-Lipoic Acid 83
    N-Acetylcysteine 83
    L-Carnitine 84
    Coenzyme Q_{10} 85
    Antioxidant Mixtures 86
    Vitamin A and Insulin 86
Folic Acid and Thiamine 86
Chromium 87
Antioxidants in Combination with Diabetic/Cardiovascular Drugs and/or Insulin 87
Omega-3 Fatty Acids 88
    Animal Studies 88
    Human Epidemiologic Studies with Omega-3 Fatty Acids 88
    Human Intervention Studies with Omega-3 Fatty Acids Alone 88
    Human Studies with Omega-3 Fatty Acids, Antidiabetic Drugs and Heart Medications 89
Treatments of Diabetes 89
    Standard Treatments 89
    Aspirin 90
    Aspirin Resistance 90
    Animal Studies with Aspirin 90
Problems Associated with Using a Single Agent in Diabetic Patients 91
Rationale for Using Multiple Micronutrients in Diabetic Patients 91
Recommended Micronutrient Supplement for the Prevention of Diabetes in High-Risk Populations 92
Recommended Micronutrient Supplement in Combination with Standard Therapy in Diabetic Patients 93
Diet and Lifestyle Recommendations for Prediabetic Individuals and Diabetic Patients 93

	Conclusions	93
	References	94
Chapter 7	Micronutrients in Cancer Prevention	103
	Introduction	103
	Cancer Incidence, Mortality, and Cost	103
	Proposed Stages of Human Carcinogenesis	104
	Diagrammatic Representation of the Proposed Stages of Human Carcinogenesis	105
	Some Examples of Tumor Initiators and Tumor Promoters	106
	Contribution of Environmental, Dietary, and Lifestyle-Related Factors	106
	Some Examples of Lifestyle-Related Carcinogens	107
	Some Examples of Environment-Related Carcinogens	108
	Some Examples of Diet-Related Carcinogens	108
	Some Examples of Diet-Related Cancer Protective Agents	109
	Functions of Antioxidants Relevant to Cancer Prevention	109
	Analysis of Cell Cultures after Treatment with Antioxidants	110
	Analysis of Cancer Prevention Studies in Animals after Treatment with Antioxidants	110
	Analysis of Epidemiologic Studies on Antioxidants and Cancer Prevention	112
	Analysis of Intervention Studies on Antioxidants and Cancer Prevention	114
	Cancer Risk in Heavy Tobacco Smokers after Treatment with a Single Dietary Antioxidant	114
	Other Cancer Risks after Treatment with a Single Dietary Antioxidant	115
	Cancer Risk after Treatment with Multiple Dietary Antioxidants	116
	Cancer Risk after Treatment with Vitamin D and Calcium	117
	Cancer Risk after Treatment with Folate and B-Vitamins	117
	Cancer Risk after Treatment with Fat and Fiber	118
	Cancer Risk after Treatment with NSAIDs	119
	Proposed Cancer Prevention Strategies	119
	Recommendations for Cancer-Free Normal Individuals	119
	Recommendations for Cancer-Free High-Risk Individuals	120
	Recommendations for Cancer Survivors	121
	Diet and Lifestyle Recommendations for Individuals of High-Risk Populations	121
	Rationale for Using Multiple Micronutrients in Proposed Cancer Preventive Strategy	121
	Unique Features of Proposed Micronutrient Formulation	122
	Toxicity of Micronutrients	123
	Conclusions	123
	References	123
Chapter 8	Micronutrients for Improvement of the Standard Therapy in Cancer	133
	Introduction	133
	Preventive and Therapeutic Dose Ranges of Antioxidants	134
	Recommendation by Oncologists and Use of Antioxidants by Their Patients	135
	Effects of Therapeutic Doses of Individual Antioxidants on Growth of Cancer and Normal Cells	136
	Vitamin E and Its Derivatives	136

    Vitamin C 137
    Combination of Vitamin C or Vitamin E with Other Agents 138
    Vitamin A and Carotenoids 138
    Selenium 138
    Mixture of Dietary Antioxidants 139
    NAC and Alpha-Lipoic Acid 139
    Coenzyme Q_{10} 140
    Antioxidant Enzymes 140
Treatment Schedules 140
Effects of Therapeutic Doses of Individual Antioxidants on Gene Expression
Profiles in Cancer Cells 140
Effects of Preventive Doses of Individual Antioxidants on Cancer
Cell Growth 141
Effects of Therapeutic Doses of Individual Antioxidants on Radiation-Induced
Damage in Cancer Cells and Normal Cells 141
    Cell Culture Studies 141
    Animal Studies 142
    Clinical Studies 144
Effects of Therapeutic Doses of Individual Antioxidants on Chemotherapeutic
Agent-Induced Damage in Cancer Cells and Normal Cells 144
    Cell Culture Studies 144
    Animal Studies 147
    Clinical Studies 147
        Glutathione-Elevating Agents (NAC and Alpha-Lipoic Acid) 148
        Coenzyme Q_{10} 148
        Vitamin E 149
        Selenium 149
        Glutamine 149
Mechanisms of Enhancing the Efficacy of Standard Therapy on Cancer Cells
by Therapeutic Doses of Individual Antioxidants 150
Clinical Studies with Multiple Dietary Antioxidants 150
Rational for Using Multiple Micronutrients 151
Rationale for Not Recommending Antioxidant Supplements during Standard
Therapy 152
    Preventive Doses of Individual Antioxidants Reduce the Efficacy of Cancer
    Therapeutic Agents 152
    Utilization of Data Obtained from the Use of Preventive Doses of
    Individual Antioxidants in High-Risk Populations 152
    Utilization of Data Obtained from the Use of Antioxidant Deficiency in
    Combination with Therapeutic Agents on Cancer Cells 153
Effects of Therapeutic Doses of Individual Antioxidants in Combination with
Experimental Cancer Therapies on Cancer Cells 154
    Hyperthermia 154
    Sodium Butyrate and Interferon-Alpha2b 155
    Cellular Vaccine 156
    Gene Therapy 156
Proposed Micronutrient Protocols 156
    AMTP Using Therapeutic Doses of Multiple Antioxidants 156
    Preventive Micronutrient Protocol Using Preventive Doses of Multiple
    Antioxidants 157
Recommendations for Diet and Lifestyle Modifications 157

Contents   xiii

          Conclusions 157
          References 158

Chapter 9   Micronutrients in the Prevention and Improvement of the Standard Therapy
                for Alzheimer's Disease 167

          Introduction 167
          Incidence and Cost 168
          Etiology of AD 168
          Neuropathology of AD 168
          Increased Oxidative Stress in AD 168
                Sources of Free Radicals in Normal Brain.. 168
                Formation of Free Radicals Derived from Oxygen and Nitrogen 169
                Oxidative Stress–Induced Mitochondrial Damage in AD 171
                Beta-Amyloid Mediates Its Neurotoxic Effects through Free Radicals in AD... 172
          Cholesterol-Induced Generation of Beta-Amyloid.. 172
          Proteasome Inhibition Induced Neurodegeneration in AD........................... 173
          Genetic Defects in Idiopathic AD 173
          Mutated Genes Mediate their Effects through Increased Production of
          Beta-Amyloid in Familial AD 174
          Increased Levels of Markers of Chronic Inflammation in AD 174
          Neuroglobin in AD 176
          Current Treatments of AD 176
          Laboratory and Clinical Studies with Antioxidants in AD 176
                Alpha-Lipoic Acid 177
                Coenzyme Q_{10} and Melatonin 177
                Nicotinamide, Nicotinamide Adenine Dinucleotide (NAD+), and
                Nicotinamide Adenine Dinucleotide Dehydrogenase (NADH) 178
                Vitamin A, Vitamin E, and Vitamin C 178
                Serum Levels of Dietary Antioxidants... 179
                B-Vitamins.. 179
                Resveratrol.. 179
                Ginkgo biloba and Omega-3 Fatty Acids 180
                Green Tea Epigallocatechin-3-Gallate and Caffeine 180
          Problems with Using a Single Nutrient in AD 180
          Rationale for Using Multiple Micronutrients in AD 181
          Rationale for Using NSAIDs in AD Prevention... 182
          Recommended Micronutrients in Combination with Low-Doses of NSAIDs
          for Prevention of AD in High-Risk Populations 183
          Rationale for Using Acetylcholinesterase Inhibitors in the Treatment of AD 183
          Recommended Micronutrients and Low-Dose NSAIDs with Standard Therapy
          in Patients with Dementia 183
          Diet and Lifestyle Recommendations for AD 184
          Conclusions 184
          References 184

Chapter 10 Micronutrients for the Prevention and Improvement of the Standard Therapy
                for Parkinson's Disease 197

          Introduction 197
          Incidence and Cost 198

Etiology 198
Neuropathology and Symptoms 198
Genetics of PD... 199
    DJ-1 Gene 199
    Alpha-Synuclein Gene.. 200
    PTEN-Induced Putative Kinase 1 201
Increased Oxidative Stress in PD 201
Increased Inflammation in PD 203
Mitochondrial Dysfunction in PD.. 203
Laboratory and Human Studies in PD with Antioxidants 204
    In Vitro Studies... 204
    Studies in Animal Models of PD.. 204
    Studies in Human PD 205
Problems of Using a Single Antioxidant in PD... 207
Rationale for Using Multiple Micronutrients in PD.. 207
Rationale for Using an NSAID in PD Prevention 209
Recommended Micronutrient Supplement for Use in Combination with
a Low-Dose NSAID for the Prevention of PD in High-Risk Populations 209
Recommended Micronutrient Supplement for Use in Combination with
a Low-Dose NSAID for Reducing the Rate of Progression of PD in
Early-Stage Patients... 209
Current Treatments of PD 210
Rationale for Using a Micronutrient Supplement and an NSAID in
Combination with Standard Therapy in PD Patients 210
Recommended Micronutrient Supplement and Low-Dose NSAID in
Combination with Standard Therapy in PD Patients 210
Diet and Lifestyle Recommendations for PD.. 211
Conclusions 211
References 211

Chapter 11 Micronutrients in Prevention and Improvement of the Standard Therapy
in Hearing Disorders 221

Introduction 221
Incidence and Cost 221
Types of Hearing Disorders 222
    Conductive Hearing Loss 222
    Sensorineural Hearing Loss 222
    Tinnitus... 222
    Meniere's Disease 222
Agents or Conditions Causing Hearing Disorders 223
Measurements of Hearing Loss... 223
Current Prevention and Treatment Strategies 223
Involvement of Oxidative Stress in Hearing Disorders.. 224
Involvement of Inflammation in Hearing Disorders 225
Beneficial Effects of Antioxidants in Hearing Disorders 225
    Animal Studies 225
    Human Studies 226
Rationale for Using Multiple Micronutrients in Hearing Disorders 226
Proposed Micronutrient Recommendation for Prevention and Improved
Treatment of Hearing Disorders.. 229

Contents

	Conclusions	229
	References	230
Chapter 12	Micronutrients in Improvement of the Standard Therapy in Posttraumatic Stress Disorder	235
	Introduction	235
	Incidence and Cost of PTSD	235
	Symptoms of PTSD	236
	Biochemical Events in PTSD	236
	Increased Oxidative Stress in PTSD	237
	Chronic Inflammation in PTSD	237
	Release of Glutamate in PTSD	238
	Standard Therapy in PTSD	238
	Rationale for Using Micronutrients in PTSD	239
	Problems of Using a Single Micronutrient in PTSD	240
	Rationale for Recommending Multiple Micronutrients Including Dietary and Endogenous Antioxidants in PTSD	240
	Recommended Micronutrients for Reducing the Risk of PTSD in High-Risk Populations	242
	Recommended Micronutrients in Combination with Standard Therapy in PTSD	243
	Diet and Lifestyle Recommendations for PTSD	243
	Conclusions	243
	References	244
Chapter 13	Micronutrients in Improvement of the Standard Therapy in Traumatic Brain Injury	249
	Introduction	249
	Causes of TBI	249
	Incidence and Cost of TBI	250
	U.S. Troops	250
	U.S. Civilians	250
	Symptoms and Consequences of TBI	250
	Symptoms and Consequences of Concussive Injury	250
	Risk of Posttraumatic Disorder Associated with TBI	251
	Biochemical Events that Contribute to the Progression of Damage Following TBI	251
	Evidence for Increased Oxidative Stress in TBI	251
	Mitochondrial Dysfunction in TBI	252
	Evidence for Increased Levels of Markers of Inflammation in TBI	253
	Evidence for Increased Release of Glutamate in TBI	254
	Role of Matrix Metalloproteinases in TBI	255
	Treatments of TBI	255
	Treatments of Sports-Related Concussive Injury	255
	Treatments of TBI with Antioxidants	256
	Antioxidants Reduce Glutamate Release	256
	Problems of Using a Single Agent in TBI	257
	Rationale for Using Multiple Micronutrients in TBI	257

Recommended Micronutrients for Reducing the Late Adverse Effects in
High-Risk Populations 259
Recommended Micronutrient Supplement in Combination with Standard
Therapy in TBI Patients with Penetrating Head Injury 260
Diet and Lifestyle Recommendations for TBI 260
Conclusions 260
References 261

Chapter 14 Micronutrients in Prevention and Improvement of the Standard Therapy
in HIV/AIDS 269

Introduction 269
History, Incidence, and Cost of HIV/AIDS 270
Role of Immune Function in HIV Infection 270
    Micronutrient Deficiency Impairs Immune Function 270
    Illicit Drugs Impair Immune Function 271
Increased Oxidative Stress and Inflammation Enhance the Risk and
Progression of HIV Infection 271
Current and Proposed Prevention Strategies for HIV Infection 272
    Primary Prevention 272
    Secondary Prevention 273
Evidence for Micronutrients Reducing Progression of HIV Infection 273
Current Treatments of HIV/AIDS 274
Role of Micronutrients in Combination with Antiviral Drugs 275
Rationale for Using Multiple Micronutrients in Primary and Secondary
Prevention of HIV Infection 275
Recommended Micronutrients for Primary and Secondary Prevention of HIV
Infection 277
Recommended Micronutrients for Improving the Efficacy of Antiviral
Therapy 277
Diet and Lifestyle Recommendations 278
Conclusions 278
References 278

Chapter 15 Micronutrients in Protecting Against Late Adverse Health Effects
of Diagnostic Radiation Doses 285

Introduction 285
Probable Biochemical and Genetic Steps Involved in Radiation-Induced
Carcinogenesis 286
Interactions between Radiation and Chemical and Biological Carcinogens
and Tumor Promoters 287
Risk Estimates of Radiation-Induced Cancer 287
Risk of Low-Dose Radiation-Induced Non-Neoplastic Diseases 289
Current Recommendations for Radiation Protection 290
Evidence for a Micronutrient Strategy for Biological Protection against
Radiation Damage 290
    Radioprotective Studies with Antioxidants in Cell Culture 290
    Radioprotective Studies with Antioxidants in Animals 290
    Radioprotective Studies with Antioxidants in Humans 291

Contents   xvii

        Recommended Micronutrient Preparations for Biological Protection against
        Low Doses of Radiation 291
            Individuals Receiving Diagnostic Radiation Procedures and
            Frequent Flyers 292
            Radiation Workers, and Pilots and Flight Attendants 292
        Toxicity of Antioxidants 293
        Conclusions 293
        References 293

Chapter 16 Micronutrients in Protecting Against Lethal Doses of Ionizing Radiation 297

        Introduction 297
        Radiation Damage Caused by High Doses of Ionizing Radiation 298
            Bone Marrow Syndrome 298
            GI Syndrome 299
            CNS Syndrome 299
            High-Dose Radiation-Induced Damage to Organs 300
            Late Effects of High Doses of Radiation on Cancer Incidence 300
            Late Effects of High Doses of Radiation on the Risk of Non-Neoplastic
            Diseases 300
        Brief History and Description of Radiation Protection Studies 301
            Radiation Protection Studies with Antioxidants in Cell Culture Models 301
            Radiation Protection Studies with Antioxidants in Animal Models 302
            Radiation Protection Studies with Antioxidants in Humans 303
        Scientific Rationale for Using Multiple Antioxidants in Radiation
        Protection 303
        Scientific Basis for Using Antioxidants Orally before and after Irradiation for
        an Optimal Radioprotective Efficacy 304
            Radiation Protection Study with a Mixture of Multiple Antioxidants
            Administered Orally before and after Irradiation in Sheep 304
            Radiation Protection Study with a Mixture of Multiple Antioxidants
            Administered Orally before and after Irradiation in Rabbits 305
            Radiation Protection Study with a Mixture of Multiple Antioxidants
            Administered Orally before Irradiation in Mice 305
            Radiation Protection Study with a Mixture of Multiple
            Antioxidants Administered Orally before and after Irradiation in
            Drosophila melanogaster 307
        Studies with Radiation Therapeutic Agents or Procedures 307
            Chemical Agents 308
            Biological Agents 309
        Recommended Multiple Micronutrients for Radiation Protection in Humans 310
        Combination of a Multiple-Micronutrient Preparation with Replacement
        Therapy 311
        Conclusions 311
        References 312

Chapter 17 Micronutrients in Prevention and Improvement of the Standard Therapy
        in Arthritis 319

        Introduction 319
        Incidence and Cost 319

  Types of Arthritis 320
    Rheumatoid Arthritis 320
    Osteoarthritis 320
    Juvenile Rheumatoid Arthritis 321
  Evidence for the Role of Oxidative Stress...321
  Evidence for the Role of Inflammation 322
  Role of Antioxidants in Arthritis 323
    Animal Studies 323
    Human Studies 324
  Current Prevention Strategies...325
  Current Treatment Strategies 325
    Low-Dose MTX 325
    Anticytokines Therapy 326
    Toxicity of Standard Therapy 327
    Glucosamine and Chondroitin 327
    Nonsteroidal Anti-Inflammatory Drugs 328
    Complementary Medicine 328
  Proposed Micronutrient Strategies for Prevention in High-Risk Populations 328
  Problems of Using a Single Agent...328
  Rationale for Using Multiple Micronutrients 329
  Recommended Micronutrient Supplement for High-Risk Populations.....................330
  Recommended Micronutrient Supplement in Combination with Standard
  Therapy for RA Patients...330
  Diet and Lifestyle Recommendations for High-Risk Populations and RA
  Patients 331
  Conclusions 331
  References 331

Chapter 18 Myths and Misconceptions about Antioxidants and Health 339

  Introduction 339
  Misconception 1 339
  Misconception 2 339
  Misconception 3 339
  Misconception 4 340
  Misconception 5 340
  Misconception 6 340
  Misconception 7 340
  Misconception 8 340
  Misconception 9 341
  Misconception 10 341
  Misconception 11 341
  Misconception 12 341
  Misconception 13 341
  Misconception 14 342
  Misconception 15 342
  Misconception 16 342
  Conclusions 342

Contents

Chapter 19 Dietary Reference Intakes of Selected Micronutrients 343
  Introduction 343
  DRI (Dietary Reference Intakes) 343
  Adequate Intake (AI) 343
  Tolerable Upper Intake Level (UL) 343
  DRI Values for Antioxidants, Vitamins, Micronutrients, and Minerals 344
  Conclusions 355

Index 357

Preface

The growing sentiments against the use of micronutrient supplements for improving human health, preventing disease, and improving treatment outcomes among most academic and practicing physicians, and many health professionals, have created confusion and uncertainties in the minds of many consumers and health professionals. These sentiments are primarily based on a few clinical trials in which supplementation with a single dietary antioxidant, primarily vitamin E and beta-carotene, increased the levels of risk factors and/or incidence of the disease in high-risk populations, such as heavy tobacco smokers, patients with coronary artery disease, and cancer survivors. Without critically examining the experimental designs of the trial with respect to the selection of antioxidants, recommendations are being made not to take any micronutrient supplements for health benefits. Such recommendations are alarming from the public health point of view. The adverse health effects of a single antioxidant in high-risk populations were expected, because such populations have high internal oxidative environments in which the individual antioxidants are oxidized and then act as pro-oxidants.

A few clinical trials with vitamin E alone produced no adverse health effects in normal populations with low internal oxidative environments, whereas others revealed beneficial effects in high-risk populations. Unfortunately, these clinical trials never receive as much publicity as those with negative results. I and others have published several reviews in peer-reviewed journals challenging the current trends of using single antioxidants in high-risk populations for preventing the risk of disease or improving treatment. I have also proposed that multiple micronutrients, including standard dietary and endogenous antioxidants, may be more useful in prevention and management of disease than single antioxidants. These articles failed to have any significant impact on the design of clinical trials, and the inconsistent results on the effect of a single antioxidant continued to be published. The growing antimicronutrient views promoted by most academic and practicing physicians and science writers of the major news media have alarmed me enough to write this book.

Many books and conference proceedings on the value of individual micronutrients in health and disease are available. I myself have coedited 12 conference proceedings, primarily on nutrition and cancer. These books provide an adequate summary of the history, properties, functions, and value of individual micronutrients, including dietary and endogenous antioxidants, herbal antioxidants, and antioxidants from fruits and vegetables in human health and disease. These books provide both the positive and negative effects of antioxidants on human health and disease. None of the these books have critically analyzed the published data on antioxidants and health, and never questioned whether the experimental designs of the study on which the conclusions are based are scientifically valid, whether the results obtained from the use of a single antioxidant in high-risk populations can be extrapolated to the effect of the same antioxidant in a multiple antioxidant preparation for the same population, and whether they could be extrapolated to normal populations. Furthermore, a comprehensive micronutrient program that has a sound scientific rationale and evidence for improving health, preventing disease, and improving treatment outcomes was never proposed.

In this book, I propose the unified hypothesis that increased oxidative stress and chronic inflammation are primarily responsible for the initiation and progression of most chronic human diseases as well as accelerated aging. Additionally, I contend that the glutamate release that occurs in certain chronic human diseases such as post-traumatic stress disorder (PTSD) and other anxiety disorders also plays a role in the maintenance and progression of the disease. Antioxidants represent a group of compounds that are nontoxic in humans, neutralize free radicals, and reduce inflammation. They can also block the release and neurotoxicity of glutamate. Thus, they represent a good candidate to help maintain good health and may reduce the risk of chronic diseases and improve the efficacy of current treatment modalities. Based on the specific health conditions, I have developed a series of formulations of multiple micronutrients containing dietary and endogenous antioxidants. I have included only standard micronutrients that have been used by consumers for decades without reported toxicity. I have not included any herbs, herbal antioxidants, or antioxidants from fruits and vegetables in these formulations, because none of them produced any unique effect that can not be produced by standard antioxidants present in the formulation. The rationale for these formulations is discussed with respect to each specific health or disease condition.

In this book, I also propose a clinical study design for each disease that can be used to test the efficacy of these micronutrient formulations in healthy aging and prevention and improved treatment of certain common human diseases. Those who are taking daily supplements will be comforted by the information provided in this book, those who are on the sidelines may decide to take a micronutrient supplement daily, and some who are currently opposed to recommending micronutrient supplements will find this book challenging and may decide to test the proposed idea clinically or continue to believe that micronutrient supplements may be harmful. In the latter case, they should provide scientific reasons for their recommendations.

I hope this book will arouse enough passion for and against taking multiple micronutrient supplements to lead to comprehensive, randomized, double-blind, and placebo-controlled clinical studies in high-risk and normal populations. Only then can we make a conclusive recommendation whether or not micronutrient supplements are useful for human health and disease. Meanwhile, I recommend that individuals continue to take appropriately prepared multiple micronutrients in consultation with their physicians and health professionals for healthy aging, reduced risk of chronic diseases, and improved current treatment outcomes.

I hope that this book will serve as a reference book for graduate students in nutrition, instructors teaching courses in nutrition and health, researchers involved in prevention and improving treatments of diseases using micronutrients, primary care and academic physicians interested in complimentary medicine, and health professionals in complimentary medicine and the nutrition industry.

Kedar N. Prasad, PhD

Acknowledgment

I thank my colleague Dr. William C. Cole for valuable discussions on various issues during the writing of this book.

Author

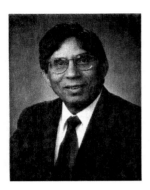

Dr. Kedar N. Prasad obtained a masters degree in zoology from the University of Bihar, Ranchi, India, and a PhD in radiation biology from the University of Iowa, Iowa City, Iowa, in 1963. He received postdoctoral training at the Brookhaven National Laboratory, Long Island, New York, and joined the Department of Radiology at the University of Colorado Health Sciences Center, where he became professor and director for the Center for Vitamins and Cancer Research. He has published more than 200 articles in peer-reviewed journals, and authored and edited 15 books in the area of radiation biology, nutrition and cancer, and nutrition and neurological diseases, particularly Alzheimer's disease and Parkinson's disease. These articles were published in such prestigious journals as *Science*, *Nature*, and the *Proceedings of the National Academy of Sciences*. Dr. Prasad has received several honors, which include an invitation by the Nobel Prize Committee to nominate a candidate for the Nobel Prize in medicine for 1982, the 1999 Harold Harper Lecture at the meeting of the American College of Advancement in Medicine, an award for the best review of 1998–1999 on antioxidants and cancer, and an award in 1999–2000 for a review on antioxidants and Parkinson's disease by the American College of Nutrition. He is a fellow of the American College of Nutrition, and has served as president of the International Society of Nutrition and Cancer, 1992–2000. Currently, he is chief scientific officer of the Premier Micronutrient Corporation.

1 Basic Facts about Antioxidants

INTRODUCTION

Micronutrients include dietary and endogenous antioxidants, B-vitamins, and certain minerals, whereas macronutrients primarily include fats, carbohydrates, and proteins. Although all micronutrients are essential for growth and development, antioxidants in particular have been the subject of extensive laboratory research and clinical studies because of their potential importance in reducing oxidative stress and inflammation, which contribute to health and disease. Before describing the role of micronutrients in healthy aging and in prevention and improved management of diseases, it is essential to understand certain basic facts about antioxidants.

This chapter briefly surveys the evolution of the antioxidant system; provides a historical perspective on some antioxidants; describes the sources, solubility, distribution, storage, absorption, and functions of dietary and endogenous antioxidants; explains antioxidant defense systems and current controversies about antioxidants; and observes the misuse of antioxidants in clinical studies. In Chapters 4 to 18 of this volume, the detailed role of antioxidants in health and disease is discussed with respect to aging and specific diseases. There are several books that have been published on this topic, and a few of them are referenced at the end of this chapter.[1-9]

EVOLUTION OF THE ANTIOXIDANT SYSTEM

Antioxidants are essential for the growth and survival of all organisms that depend on oxygen, which includes humans. In its early stage, Earth's atmosphere had no oxygen. Anaerobic organisms, which can live without oxygen, thrived in the oceans and rivers. About 2.5 billion years ago, blue-green algae in the oceans acquired the ability to split water (H_2O) into hydrogen (H) and oxygen (O_2). This chemical reaction initiated the release of oxygen into the atmosphere, leading to the extinction of many anaerobic organisms due to the toxicity of oxygen. Those organisms that developed antioxidant defense systems survived—an important biological event that led to the rapid evolution of multicellular organisms that use oxygen for survival. Today, the amount of oxygen in dry air is about 21%, and in water it is about 34%.

HISTORY OF THE DISCOVERY OF ANTIOXIDANTS

Vitamin A. Night blindness, which we now know is caused by vitamin A deficiency, existed for centuries before the discovery of vitamin A. As early as about 1500 B.C., the Egyptians knew how to cure this disease. Roman soldiers suffering from night blindness traveled to Egypt where they would receive liver extract for treatment. It is now well established that liver is the richest source of vitamin A. The treatment of night blindness with liver extract was not performed outside Egypt for centuries; the medical establishment during that period must not have accepted this treatment. It was not until 1912 when Dr. McCollum of the University of Wisconsin discovered vitamin A in butter, and therefore it was initially called "fat-soluble A." The structure of vitamin A was determined in 1930, and this vitamin was synthesized in the laboratory in 1947.

Carotenoids. In 1919, carotenoid pigments were isolated from yellow plants, and in 1930, it was found that some of the ingested carotene was converted to vitamin A. This carotene was referred to as beta-carotene.

Vitamin C. Scurvy is caused by vitamin C deficiency. The symptoms of this disease were known to Egyptians as early as 1500 B.C. In the 5th century B.C., Hippocrates described the symptoms of scurvy, which included bleeding gums, hemorrhage, and death. Native North Americans knew the cure for this disease, but knowledge of the treatment remained limited to this population. During the sea voyages of European explorers between the twelfth and sixteenth centuries, the epidemic of scurvy among sailors forced some to land in Canada where the native people gave them extract of pine bark and pine needles (prepared like tea). This treatment completely cured scurvy in these sailors. In 1536, Jacques Cartier, a French explorer, brought this formulation for curing scurvy to France, but the medical establishment rejected it as a fraud because it came from Native Americans, who were referred to as savages. In 1593, Sir Richard Hawkins recommended that his sailors take sour oranges and lemons. In 1770, the British Navy began recommending that ships carry sufficient lime juice for all personnel aboard. In 1928, Albert Szent-Gyorgyi, a Hungarian scientist, isolated a substance from the adrenal gland that was called hexuronic acid. This substance was vitamin C, and in 1932 it was the first vitamin to be synthesized in the laboratory.

Vitamin D. Although rickets, a bone disease, may have existed in the human population for centuries, it was not until 1645 when Dr. Daniel Whistler described the symptoms of rickets, which we now know is due to vitamin D deficiency. In 1922, Sir Edward Mellanby discovered vitamin D while working toward a cure for rickets. This vitamin was later found to require sunlight for its formation. The chemical structure of vitamin D was determined by a German scientist, Dr. Windaus, in 1930. Vitamin D_3 was chemically characterized in 1936 and was considered a steroid that was effective in the treatment of rickets.

Vitamin E. In 1922, Dr. Herbert Evans of the University of California, Berkeley, observed that rats reared exclusively on whole milk grew normally but were not fertile. Their fertility was restored when they were additionally fed wheat germ. However, it took another 14 years (i.e., 1936) before the active substance responsible for restoring fertility was isolated. Dr. Evans named it *tocopherol* from the Greek word meaning "to bear offspring" with the ending "ol" signifying its chemical status as an alcohol.

B vitamins. All B vitamins were discovered in the period 1912–1934. In 1912, the Polish-born biochemist Dr. Casimir Funk isolated active substances from the rice husks of unpolished rice that prevented the disease beriberi. He named the substances "vitamines," because he thought they were amines, which are derived from ammonia. In 1920, the "e" was dropped when it became clear that not all vitamins are amines.

SOURCES AND FORMS OF VITAMINS

Vitamin A. The richest sources of vitamin A are liver (6.5 mg per 100 g liver) from beef, pork, chicken, turkey, and fish, carrot (0.8 mg per 100 g), broccoli leaves (0.8 mg per 100 g), sweet potatoes (0.7 mg per 100 g), kale (0.7 mg per 100 g), butter (0.7 mg per 100 g), spinach (0.5 mg per 100 g), and pumpkin (0.4 mg per 100 g). Other minor sources include cantaloupe, eggs, apricots, papaya, and mango (40–170 µg per 100 g). Fruits and vegetables (yellow and red) are very rich sources of beta-carotene. One molecule of beta-carotene is converted to 2 molecules of retinol in the intestinal tract.

Vitamin A exists as retinyl palmitate or retinyl acetate, which is converted into the retinol form in the body. Vitamin A can also exist as a retinoic acid in the cells. It was determined that 1 international unit (IU) equals 0.3 µg retinol or 0.6 µg beta-carotene. The activity of vitamin A is also expressed as retinol activity equivalent (RAE). It was determined that 1 µg RAE corresponds with 1 µg retinol and 2 µg beta-carotene in oil. Vitamin A and beta-carotene and the synthetic retinoids are also available commercially.

Carotenoids. The richest sources of carotenoids are sweet potatoes, carrots, spinach, mango, cantaloupe, apricot, kale, broccoli, parsley, cilantro, pumpkins, winter squash, and fresh thyme. There are two main forms of carotenoids found in nature: alpha-carotene and beta-carotene. Beta-carotene is the more common form of carotenoids. Other carotenes include lutein and lycopene.

Vitamin C. The richest sources of vitamin C are fruits and vegetables. These include rose hip (2000 mg per 100 g rose hip), red pepper (2000 mg per 100 g), parsley (2000 mg per 100 g), guava (2000 mg per 100 g), kiwi fruit (2000 mg per 100 g), broccoli (2000 mg per 100 g), lychee (2000 mg per 100 g), papaya (2000 mg per 100 g), and strawberry (2000 mg per 100 g). Other sources of vitamin C include orange, lemon, melon, garlic, cauliflower, grapefruit, raspberry, tangerine, passion fruit, spinach, and lime, and these contain about 30–50 mg per 100 g fruit or vegetable. Vitamin C is sold commercially as L-ascorbic acid, calcium ascorbate, sodium ascorbate, or potassium ascorbate.

Vitamin E. The richest sources of vitamin E include wheat germ oil (215 mg per 100 g oil), sunflower oil (56 mg per 100 g oil), olive oil (12 mg per 100 g oil), almond oil (39 mg per 100 g oil), hazelnut oil (26 mg per 100 g oil), walnut oil (20 mg per 100 g oil), and peanut oil (17 mg per 100 g oil). The sources for small amounts of vitamin E (0.1–2 mg per 100 g) include kiwi fruit, fish, leafy vegetables, and whole grains. In the United States, the fortified breakfast cereals are important sources of vitamin E. At present, most of the natural form of vitamin E is extracted from vegetable oils, primarily soybean oil.

Vitamin E exists in eight different forms: four tocopherols (alpha-, beta-, gamma-, and delta-tocopherol) and four tocotrienols (alpha-, beta-, gamma-, and delta-tocotrienol). Alpha-tocopherol has the most biological activity. Vitamin E can exist in the natural form commonly indicated as *d*, whereas the synthetic form is referred to as *dl*. The stable esterified form of vitamin E is available as alpha-tocopheryl acetate, alpha-tocopheryl succinate, and alpha-tocopheryl nicotinate. The activity of vitamin E is generally expressed in international units. It is determined that 1 IU equals 0.66 mg *d*-alpha-tocopherol, and 1 IU racemic mixture (*dl*-form) equals 0.45 mg *d*-tocopherol.

Glutathione. Glutathione is synthesized from three amino acids (L-cysteine, L-glutamic acid, and glycine) and is present in all cells; however, the liver contains the highest amount, up to 5 mM. Glutathione exists in the cells in reduced form or oxidized form. In healthy cells, more than 90% of glutathione is present in the reduced form. The oxidized form of glutathione can be converted to the reduced form by the enzyme glutathione reductase. The reduced form of glutathione acts as an antioxidant.

Coenzyme Q_{10}. In 1957, Dr. Fredrick Crane isolated coenzyme Q_{10}, and in 1958, Dr. Wolf, working under Dr. Karl Folkers, determined the structure of coenzyme Q_{10}.

L-Carnitine. L-Carnitine is synthesized from the amino acids lysine and methionine and was originally discovered as a growth factor for mealworms. It is primarily synthesized in the liver and kidneys. Vitamin C is necessary for the synthesis of L-carnitine. It exists as L-carnitine, a biologically active form, and as D-carnitine, a biologically inactive form.

SOLUBILITY OF ANTIOXIDANTS

The lipid-soluble antioxidants include vitamin A, vitamin E, carotenoids, coenzyme Q_{10}, and L-carnitine, and the water-soluble antioxidants include vitamin C, glutathione, and alpha-lipoic acid. Fat-soluble vitamins should be taken with meals so that they are more readily absorbed.

DISTRIBUTION OF ANTIOXIDANTS IN THE BODY

Carotenoids. Beta-carotene is one of the more than 600 carotenoids found in fruits, vegetables, and plants. It is commercially available in natural or synthetic forms. The natural form of beta-carotene is more effective than the synthetic form. Preparations of natural carotenoids primarily contain beta-carotene; however, the other types of carotenoids are also present. A portion of ingested beta-carotene is converted to retinol (vitamin A) in the intestinal tract before absorption, and the remainder is distributed in the blood and tissues of the body. One molecule of beta-carotene forms 2 molecules of vitamin A. In humans, the conversion of beta-carotene to vitamin A does not occur if the body has sufficient amounts of vitamin A. Beta-carotene is primarily stored in the eyes and in fatty tissues. Other carotenoids such as lycopene accumulate in the prostate more than in other organs, whereas lutein accumulates in the eyes more than in other organs.

Vitamin A. Vitamin A is commercially sold as retinyl palmitate, retinyl acetate, and retinoic acid and its analogues. Retinyl acetate or retinyl palmitate is converted to retinol in the intestine before absorption. Retinol is converted to retinoic acid in the cells. Retinoic acid performs all functions of vitamin A except for maintaining good vision. Retinol is stored in the liver as retinyl palmitate. Vitamin A exists as a protein-bound molecule. The level of retinol can be determined in the plasma.

Vitamin C. Vitamin C is commercially sold as ascorbic acid, sodium ascorbate, magnesium ascorbate, calcium ascorbate, and time-release capsules containing ascorbic acid and vitamin C ester. Vitamin C is present in all cells. Ascorbic acid is converted to dehydroascorbic acid, which can be reduced to form vitamin C. It is interesting to note that dehydroascorbic acid can cross the blood–brain barrier, but vitamin C cannot. All mammals make vitamin C except guinea pigs. An adult goat makes about 13 g vitamin C every day. The plasma level of vitamin C may not reflect the tissue levels of vitamin C, but in humans, it is difficult to obtain tissues for determining vitamin C. Vitamin C can recycle oxidized vitamin E to its reduced form, which acts as an antioxidant.

Vitamin E. Among vitamin E isomers, alpha-tocopherol is biologically more active than others. In recent years, research on tocotrienols has revealed some important biological functions. Synthetic vitamin E is referred to as the *dl*-form; the natural form is termed the *d*-form. Vitamin E is commercially sold as *d*- or *dl*-tocopherol, alpha-tocopheryl acetate (alpha-TA), or alpha-tocopheryl succinate (alpha-TS). The esterified forms of vitamin E (alpha-TA and alpha-TS) are more stable than alpha-tocopherol. Alpha-TA has been widely used in basic research and clinical studies. It has been presumed that alpha-TA or alpha-TS is converted to alpha-tocopherol before absorption. This assumption may be true as long as the stores of alpha-tocopherol in the body are not saturated; however, if the body stores of alpha-tocopherol are saturated, alpha-TS can be absorbed as alpha-TS. Alpha-TS enters the cells more easily than alpha-tocopherol because of its greater solubility. Alpha-TS has some unique functions that cannot be produced by alpha-tocopherol. Alpha-TS is now considered the most effective form of vitamin E, but it cannot act as an antioxidant until converted to alpha-tocopherol. Alpha-tocopherol is located primarily in the membranous structures of the cells. The level of vitamin E can be determined in the plasma.

Glutathione and alpha-lipoic acid. Glutathione is the most important antioxidant within the cells. Glutathione is sold commercially for oral consumption; however, the molecule is degraded totally in the intestine. Therefore, oral administration of glutathione does not increase the cellular levels of glutathione. *N*-Acetylcysteine (NAC) increases the cellular levels of glutathione. In the body, *N*-acetyl is removed from NAC by the enzyme esterase, and then cysteine is used to synthesize glutathione. Alpha-lipoic acid also increases the cellular levels of glutathione by a mechanism different than that of NAC and is present in all cells.

Coenzyme Q_{10}. About 95% of energy is generated from the use of coenzyme Q_{10} by the mitochondria. Therefore, organs such as the heart and liver that require high energy have the highest concentrations of coenzyme Q_{10}. Other organelles inside the cells that contain coenzyme Q_{10} include endoplasmic reticulum, peroxisomes, lysosomes, and Golgi apparatus.

L-Carnitine. L-Carnitine is made in the human body, but it can also be obtained from the diet. The highest concentration of L-carnitine is found in red meat (95 mg per 3.0 oz). In contrast, chicken breast has only 3.9 mg per 3.5 oz. L-Carnitine is present in all cells of the body.

NADH (reduced form of nicotinamide adenine dinucleotide). Nicotinamide adenine dinucleotide (NAD+) and NADH are present in all cells of the body. NAD+ is an oxidizing agent; therefore, it can act as a pro-oxidant, whereas NADH can act as an antioxidant. NAD+ accepts an electron from other molecules and is reduced to form NADH. It can recycle oxidized vitamin E to the reduced form, which can act as an antioxidant. NADH is essential for mitochondria to generate energy.

Polyphenols. Polyphenols are a group of chemical substances found in plants. They include tannins, lignins, and flavonoids. The largest and best studied polyphenols are flavonoids, which include quercetin, epicatechin, and oligomeric proanthocyanidins. The major sources of flavonoids include all citrus fruits, berries, ginkgo biloba, onions, parsley, tea, red wine, and dark chocolate. More than 5000 naturally occurring flavonoids have been characterized from various plants. Flavonoids are poorly absorbed by the intestinal tract in humans. All flavonoids possess varying degrees of antioxidant activity.

Melatonin. Melatonin is a naturally occurring hormone produced primarily by the pineal gland in the brain. It is also produced by the retina, the lens, and the gastrointestinal tract. Melatonin is synthesized from the amino acid tryptophan. Melatonin is also produced by various plants, such as rice. It is readily absorbed from the intestinal tract; however, 50% of melatonin is removed from the plasma in 35 to 50 min. Melatonin has several biological functions including antioxidant activity and is necessary for sleep.

STORAGE OF ANTIOXIDANTS

Carotenoids. Most commercially sold carotenoids in solid form can be stored at room temperature away from light for a few years. Beta-carotene in solution, however, degrades within a few days even when stored cold and away from light.

Vitamin A. Crystal forms of retinol, retinoic acid, retinyl acetate, and retinal palmitate can be stored at 4°C for several months. A solution of retinoic acid is stable at 4°C, stored away from light, for several weeks.

Vitamin C. Vitamin C should not be stored in solution form because the molecule is easily degraded within a few days. Crystal or tablet forms of vitamin C can be kept at room temperature, stored away from light, for a few years.

Vitamin E. Alpha-tocopherol is relatively unstable at room temperature in comparison with alpha-TA or alpha-TS. Alpha-tocopherol can be stored at 4°C for several weeks, whereas alpha-TA or alpha-TS can be stored at room temperature for a few years. A solution of alpha-TS is stable for several months at 4°C if stored away from light.

Glutathione, NAC, and alpha-lipoic acid. Solid forms of glutathione, NAC, and alpha-lipoic acid are stable at room temperature, stored away from light, for a few years. The solutions of these antioxidants are stable at 4°C, stored away from light, for several months.

Coenzyme Q_{10} and NADH. These antioxidants in solid form are stable at room temperature, stored away from light, for a few years. The solutions of these antioxidants are stable at 4°C, stored away from light, for several months.

Polyphenols. Polyphenols are very stable at room temperature, stored away from light, for a few years.

Melatonin. The powder form of melatonin is stable at 4°C for a year or more.

CAN ANTIOXIDANTS BE DEGRADED DURING COOKING?

Carotenoids. Most carotenes, especially lutein and lycopene, are not degraded during cooking. In fact, their bioavailability improves when they are derived from a cooked or extracted preparation (e.g., lycopene from tomato sauce).

Vitamin A. Routine cooking does not degrade vitamin A, but slow heating for a long period may reduce its potency. Canning and prolonged cold storage may also diminish the activity of vitamin A. The vitamin A content of fortified milk powder substantially declines after 2 years.

Vitamin E. Food processing, frying, and freezing degrade vitamin E. The vitamin E content of fortified milk powder is unaffected over a 2-year period.

Glutathione, NAC, and alpha-lipoic acid. These compounds can be partially degraded during cooking.

Polyphenols. Polyphenols are not degraded during cooking.

Coenzyme Q_{10} and NADH. These compounds can be partially degraded during cooking.

ABSORPTION OF ANTIOXIDANTS AND ITS SIGNIFICANCE

Antioxidants are absorbed from the intestinal tract and then distributed to various organs of the body. The highest levels of vitamins A, C, and E are present in the liver, and the lowest levels of these antioxidants are present in the brain. Heart and liver have the highest levels of coenzyme Q_{10}. Only about 10% of ingested water-soluble or fat-soluble antioxidants are absorbed from the intestinal tract. It has been argued by some that 90% of antioxidants are therefore wasted. This argument has no scientific merit. During digestion processes, many toxic substances including mutagens and carcinogens are formed. Meat eaters form such toxic substances more than do vegetarians. The consumption of organic food will make no difference in amounts of toxins formed during the digestion of food. A portion of these toxins are absorbed from the gut and could increase the risk of chronic diseases over a long period. The presence of excessive amounts of antioxidants markedly reduced the levels of toxins formed during digestion and thereby reduced the risk of these toxins on health and the incidence of chronic diseases. Thus, unabsorbed antioxidants perform a very useful function in reducing the levels of mutagens and carcinogens during digestion of food.

FUNCTIONS OF INDIVIDUAL ANTIOXIDANTS

The functions of antioxidants are varied and complex. Most believe that antioxidants have only one function, that is, to neutralize free radicals. In view of recent advances in antioxidant research, this belief is incorrect. In addition to neutralizing free radicals, antioxidants reduce inflammation, stimulate immune function, act as cofactors for several biological reactions, and regulate expressions of genes involved in proliferation, growth, differentiation, and immune function. Each antioxidant has some unique function that cannot be produced by others.

Vitamin A. In addition to quenching free radicals, vitamin A plays an important role in maintenance of vision, stimulation of immune function, regulation of gene activity, in embryonic development and reproduction, bone metabolism, in inhibition of precancer and cancer cell proliferation, and in skin health.

Carotenoids. Beta-carotene is a precursor of vitamin A. Carotenes are also known to protect against ultraviolet light–induced damage. Beta-carotene increases the expression of the connexin gene, which codes for gap junction protein, which holds two normal cells together, whereas vitamin A cannot produce such an effect. Beta-carotene is a more effective quencher of free radicals in high atmospheric pressure than vitamin A or vitamin E.

Vitamin D. Vitamin D is essential for bone formation and regulates calcium and phosphorus levels in the blood. Vitamin D inhibits parathyroid hormone secretion from the parathyroid glands. It stimulates immune function by promoting phagocytosis and also exhibits antitumor activity.

Vitamin C. Vitamin C acts as an antioxidant and participates as a cofactor of enzymes that are involved in the formation of many vital compounds in the body. Vitamin C helps in the formation of collagen, and it also takes part in formation of interferon, a naturally occurring antiviral agent. Vitamin C regenerates oxidized vitamin E.

Vitamin E. Vitamin E acts as an antioxidant and regulates gene expression and translocation of certain proteins from one compartment to another. It helps to maintain good skin texture, reduces scarring, and acts as an anticoagulant. Vitamin E reduces inflammation and stimulates immune function. Its derivative vitamin E succinate exhibits a potent anticancer activity.

Alpha-lipoic acid. Alpha-lipoic acid is a more potent antioxidant than vitamin C or vitamin E because it is easily oxidized or reduced. Alpha-lipoic acid is soluble in both water and lipid; therefore, it protects cellular membranes as well as water-soluble compounds. It regenerates tissue levels of vitamin C and vitamin E and markedly elevates glutathione levels in cells. Alpha-lipoic acid acts as a cofactor for multienzyme dehydrogenase complexes.

N-Acetylcysteine. NAC increases glutathione levels in cells. This function is important because orally administered glutathione is totally degraded in the small intestine. At high doses, NAC binds with metals and removes them from the body.

Glutathione. Glutathione is one of the most important antioxidants and protects cellular components inside the cells. It is needed for detoxification of toxins that are produced as by-products of normal metabolism or for detoxification of certain exogenous toxins. Glutathione also acts as a substrate for several enzymes and reduces inflammation.

Coenzyme Q_{10}. This is a weak antioxidant, but it recycles vitamin E. Coenzyme Q_{10} is essential for energy generation by the mitochondria.

Nicotinamide adenine dinucleotide. NAD+ also acts as an antioxidant and is essential for energy generation by the mitochondria. NADH has been shown to increase the formation and release of acetylcholine in cholinergic nerve cells responsible for storage of memory.

Polyphenols. Flavonoids are one of the polyphenols that have been studied extensively. They exhibit antioxidant activity and reduce inflammation. They also regulate the expression of certain genes.

Melatonin. Melatonin is important in regulating circadian rhythms through its receptor. It also acts as an antioxidant and reduces inflammation. Unlike other antioxidants, the oxidation of melatonin is irreversible, and thus it cannot be regenerated by other antioxidants. It also stimulates immune function. Melatonin prevents the toxicity of beta-amyloid fragments and hyperphosphorylation of tau protein. Beta-amyloid (fragment of amyloid precursor protein) and hyperphosphorylation of tau protein are involved in Alzheimer's disease (AD). (Details of the value of antioxidants in aging and diseases is discussed in subsequent chapters of this volume dealing with the specific health conditions.)

ANTIOXIDANT DEFENSE SYSTEMS

What are antioxidants? Generally speaking, antioxidants are defined as chemical substances that donate an electron to a free radical and convert it into a harmless molecule. The antioxidant defense system in humans can be divided into three groups: group A antioxidants, group B antioxidants, and group C antioxidants.

GROUP A ANTIOXIDANTS

Group A antioxidants are antioxidants not made in the body and obtained principally through the diet. They include vitamin A, carotenoids, vitamin C, vitamin E, flavonoids and other polyphenols, and other plant antioxidants.

GROUP B ANTIOXIDANTS

Group B antioxidants are antioxidant enzymes made in the body, such as superoxide dismutase (SOD), catalase, and glutathione peroxidase. SOD requires manganese (Mn) or copper–zinc (Cu–Zn) for its biological activity. Manganese SOD is present in the mitochondria, whereas Cu–Zn SOD is present in the cytoplasm. They can destroy free radicals and hydrogen peroxide. Catalase requires iron (Fe) for its biological activity; it, too, destroys hydrogen peroxide in the cell. Selenium itself is not an antioxidant, but glutathione peroxidase, an antioxidant enzyme, requires selenium for its biological activity.

Group C Antioxidants

Group C antioxidants are antioxidant chemicals primarily made in the body but also obtained through the diet (primarily through meat and eggs) and in the form of supplements. They include glutathione, coenzyme Q_{10}, NADH, alpha-lipoic acid, and L-carnitine.

KNOWN FUNCTIONS OF ANTIOXIDANTS

1. They scavenge free radicals.
2. They decrease markers of proinflammatory cytokines.
3. They alter gene expression profiles.
4. They alter protein kinase activity.
5. They prevent release and toxicity of excessive amounts of glutamate.
6. They act as cofactors for several biological reactions.
7. They induce cell differentiation and apoptosis in cancer cells.
8. They induce cell differentiation in normal cells but not apoptosis.
9. They increase immune functions.

The functions of antioxidants with respect to aging and each specific disease are discussed in detail in Chapters 4 to 18 of this volume.

CURRENT CONTROVERSIES ABOUT ANTIOXIDANTS

Although antioxidants are essential for human survival and growth, they remain the most misunderstood and misused molecules by most public and health professionals. The reasons for this include inaccurate claims by many in the nutrition industry, inconsistent human data (stemming from epidemiologic studies), and the results of poorly designed clinical studies in which one or sometimes two or more dietary antioxidants in high-risk populations were administered. Therefore, it is essential to understand antioxidant types, forms, sources, and functions to appreciate how they can potentially be used to improve health and reduce the risk of chronic diseases.

Humans consume some antioxidants such as vitamin A, carotenoids, vitamin C, and vitamin E from the diet, whereas the human body makes some antioxidants such as glutathione, alpha-lipoic acid, coenzyme Q_{10}, and L-carnitine. Despite basic scientific evidence for the role of antioxidants in disease prevention and as an adjunct to standard therapy in the treatment of diseases, the medical establishment has refused to acknowledge their importance. This is not the first time that the medical establishment has resisted the application of novel agents in the treatment of diseases. As a matter of fact, the history of discovery of the antioxidants illustrates some examples of such resistance by the medical establishment. The current controversies regarding the use of micronutrient supplements will be discussed in detail in Chapter 3 and Chapters 5–17.

MISUSE OF ANTIOXIDANTS IN CLINICAL STUDIES

Humans need dietary antioxidants (vitamins A, C, and E and carotenoids, especially beta-carotene) as well as endogenous antioxidants made by the body such as antioxidant enzymes, glutathione, coenzyme Q_{10}, (R)-alpha-lipoic acid, L-carnitine, NADH, B-vitamins, and certain minerals for growth and survival. The distribution of these antioxidants markedly varies from one organ to another, and even within the same cell. Their subcellular distribution markedly differs from one cellular compartment to another within the same cell.

The human body generates different types of inorganic and organic free radicals derived from oxygen and nitrogen in response to the use of oxygen. The exposure to various environmental stressors, such as ozone, dust particles, smoke, toxic fumes, toxic chemicals, and ionizing radiation (x-rays or gamma rays), also produces excessive amounts of free radicals. Free radical–induced damage is called oxidative damage, which also occurs during the normal aging process and during the initiation and progression of certain diseases. Both dietary and endogenous antioxidants neutralize free radicals, but their affinities to specific types of free radicals differ, and their efficacy in reducing oxidative damage may also differ. In addition, increased oxidative damage and chronic inflammation are associated with most chronic diseases. Some antioxidants also reduce the levels of chronic inflammation.

These observations make it clear that supplementation with one or two dietary or endogenous antioxidants is not useful in maintaining healthy aging or in reducing the rate of progression of diseases. Instead, these studies suggest that supplementation with multiple micronutrients including dietary and endogenous antioxidants may be essential for improving human health and for disease prevention. Unfortunately, nearly all previous clinical studies have used just one or two dietary antioxidants in populations at high risk of developing certain chronic diseases, yielding inconsistent results.

In addition to the above considerations, selection of the type of antioxidant is equally important for any human clinical studies. For example, it has been reported that natural beta-carotene prevented x-ray–induced transformation of normal-like murine fibroblasts in culture, whereas synthetic beta-carotene did not. An animal study showed that various organs accumulated the natural form of vitamin E (d-alpha-tocopherol) more than the synthetic form (dl-alpha-tocopherol). Furthermore, it has been reported that vitamin E in the form of d-alpha-TS is more effective than other forms of vitamin E. The published human studies on antioxidants have not taken into consideration these important issues in the design of experiments; therefore, the results regarding the efficacy of antioxidants have been contradictory.

The doses of antioxidants are very important to produce optimal health benefits or disease prevention. Low doses (around Recommended Dietary Allowance values) may be useful in reducing some oxidative damage and preventing deficiency; however, they may not be sufficient in reducing inflammation or optimizing immune function. The differences in changes in the expression of gene profiles between low and high doses of an antioxidant are marked. In commercially sold multivitamin preparations, the doses of antioxidants and other micronutrients markedly vary. The selection of appropriate doses of various micronutrients including dietary and endogenous antioxidants that are safe and standardized is essential for health benefits and disease prevention.

The dose schedule of antioxidant micronutrients is critical for achieving the desired health benefits. Most people take once-a-day micronutrient supplements that may not produce optimal health benefits. This is due to a high degree of fluctuation in the levels of antioxidants in the body because of variation in the plasma half-lives of various micronutrients. In addition, the gene expression profiles of cells markedly differ depending on the level of antioxidants in the body; therefore, cells have to readjust their genetic activity all the time, which can stress cells over a long period. It is interesting to note that all previous human studies with antioxidants have used the once-a-day dose schedule in spite of scientific evidence to the contrary.

In all human studies with antioxidants, the selection of the target population and the statistical analysis have been appropriate, but the selection of antioxidants, their doses and dose schedule have been without any scientific rationale. This can be demonstrated by a few widely publicized results of antioxidant studies in humans. In the first two clinical studies, the synthetic form of beta-carotene was administered orally once a day to male, heavy tobacco users to reduce the incidence of lung cancer. The results showed that the incidence of lung cancer in beta-carotene–treated smokers increased by about 17%, prompting one of the studies to be stopped before the completion of the investigation. Federal agencies then promoted the idea that supplementation with beta-carotene may be harmful to one's health and recommended that consumers not take beta-carotene in any form or in any other multiple-vitamin preparation. These erroneous conclusions and recommendations were without any scientific merit for the following reasons: It had been known before the start of the above human studies that individual antioxidants such as beta-carotene can be oxidized in a high oxidative environment to become pro-oxidants. Heavy tobacco smokers have a high internal oxidative environment. Therefore, when beta-carotene is administered to smokers, it is oxidized and acts as a pro-oxidant rather than as an antioxidant. This would then be expected to increase the incidence of cancer in tobacco smokers.

Knowing the above facts about beta-carotene and heavy tobacco smokers, one could have predicted that beta-carotene would increase the risk of lung cancer in smokers. Indeed, the results of the trials confirmed this prediction. In contrast with the adverse effects of beta-carotene in heavy tobacco smokers, the same dose and type of beta-carotene did not increase the risk of cancer among doctors and nurses who were nonsmokers during a 5-year follow-up. Again, this result was also expected because populations of nonsmokers do not have a high internal oxidative environment.

The synthetic form of vitamin E has produced inconsistent results in patients with a high risk of cardiovascular disease who have an increased internal oxidative environment. Some studies showed beneficial effects, whereas others showed no effect or even adverse effects in some cases. Harmful effects of vitamin E alone in cardiovascular disease can be attributed to the same biological events as those observed with beta-carotene. At this time, cardiologists do not recommend vitamin E to their patients. There are no human data (intervention studies) to show that the same dose of vitamin E or beta-carotene, when present in an appropriately prepared multiple-micronutrient supplement including dietary and endogenous antioxidants, produces adverse health effects among normal or high-risk populations.

The human studies featuring a single antioxidant have also produced inconsistent results in neurologic diseases such as Parkinson's disease (PD) and AD. In both studies, high doses of the synthetic form of vitamin E at a dose of 800 IU/day in PD and 2000 IU/day in AD were used. No beneficial effects of vitamin E were observed in PD, but some beneficial effects were observed in AD. These studies were started without careful consideration of the biochemical factors involved in the disease processes and of antioxidant status in the patients. It has been reported that deficiency of the antioxidant glutathione rather than vitamin E is found in both AD and PD patients. In addition, dysfunction of the mitochondria is consistently observed in autopsied samples of brains of patients with PD or AD. Furthermore, evidence of high oxidative damage and chronic inflammation are also found in these brains. Therefore, the idea of supplementation with antioxidants for prevention and for reduction in the rate of progression of disease is a very good one. Supplementation with a multiple-micronutrient preparation that contains appropriate doses of dietary and endogenous antioxidants including glutathione-elevating agents, as well as antioxidants that improve the function of mitochondria to generate energy, would have provided better health outcomes than those obtained by vitamin E alone.

It is unfortunate that the harmful results obtained with use of primarily one antioxidant in high-risk populations are often extrapolated to all multiple antioxidant preparations and to all populations. This erroneous extrapolation of data regarding the harmful effects of beta-carotene or vitamin E alone is further propagated by the publication of meta-analyses of published data on the same vitamins with the same conclusion. A meta-analysis publication is often misinterpreted as an original study. In my opinion, a meta-analysis should critically examine an experiment's design instead of just summarizing the results of previous studies. These types of experiments and extrapolations have created a wide disconnect between the public and most health professionals—especially physicians—regarding the health benefits of micronutrients. To avoid these problems, the subsequent chapters in this book discuss the scientific basis for using multiple micronutrients including dietary and endogenous antioxidants in healthy aging and in reducing the risk of chronic diseases. In addition, the role of these micronutrients in improving the efficacy of standard therapy for various chronic diseases is discussed.

CONCLUSIONS

Micronutrients include antioxidants, vitamin D, B-vitamins, and selenium and other minerals, whereas macronutrients include fats, carbohydrates, and proteins. However, only the properties and function of antioxidants are described in this chapter. Certain antioxidants are obtained through the diet, and others are made in the body. Both groups of antioxidants are necessary for optimal health and disease prevention. Antioxidants exhibit complex mechanisms of action, and their capacity to neutralize free radicals represents only one of these mechanisms. High but nontoxic doses of micronutrients including dietary and endogenous antioxidants are essential for healthy aging and disease prevention. In addition, the combination of some of these micronutrients when used as an adjunct may improve the efficacy of standard therapy in the treatment of chronic diseases. Unfortunately, the clinical studies with antioxidants in populations at high risk of developing chronic diseases have used a single antioxidant. The results of these studies have been inconsistent. Therefore, any strategy for optimal health or disease prevention should use multiple micronutrients including dietary and endogenous antioxidants.

REFERENCES

1. Sen, C. K. P., H. Lester, and P. A. Baeuerle. 1999. *Antioxidants and Redox Regulation of Genes*. New York, NY: Academic Press.
2. Shils, M. S., M. Shine, J. Olson, and C. Ross. 2005. *Modern Nutrition in Health and Disease*, 10th ed. Philadelphia, PA: Lippincott Williams & Wilkins.
3. Anderson, J. J. B. 2005. *Nutrition & Health: An Introduction.* Durham, NC: Carolina Academic Press.
4. The Development of DRIs 1994–2004: Lessons Learned and New Challenges. Workshop. 2008. Washington, DC: The National Academic Press. Sources: Dietary Reference Intakes for Calcium, Phosphorus, Magnesium, Vitamin D, and Fluoride (1997); Dietary Reference Intakes for Thiamine, Riboflavin, Niacin, Vitamin B_6, Folate, Vitamin B_{12}, Pantothenic Acid, Biotin, and Choline (1998); Dietary Reference Intakes for Vitamin C, Vitamin E, Selenium, and Carotenoids (2000); and Dietary Reference Intakes for Vitamin A, Vitamin K, Arsenic, Boron, Chromium, Copper, Iodine, Iron, Manganese, Molybdenum, Nickel, Silicon, Vanadium, and Zinc (2001).
5. Packer, L. H., M. Hiramatsu, and T. Yoshikawa. 1999. *Antioxidant Food Supplements in Human Health.* New York, NY: Academic Press/Elsevier.
6. Combs, G. F., Jr. 1998. *The Vitamins: Fundamental Aspects in Nutrition & Health*, 2nd ed. San Diego, CA: Academic Press.
7. Caballero, B. A., L. Allen, and A. Prentice. 2005. *Encyclopedia of Human Nutrition*. Boston, MA: Academic Press/Elsevier.
8. Cadenas, E. P., and L. Packer. 1996. *Handbook of Antioxidants*. New York, NY: Marcel Dekker.
9. Frei, B. 1994. *Natural Antioxidants in Human Health and Disease*. New York, NY: Academic Press.

2 Basic Facts about Oxidative Stress, Inflammation, and the Immune System

INTRODUCTION

Increased oxidative stress due to the production of excessive amounts of free radicals derived from oxygen and nitrogen plays a central role in the initiation and progression of damage associated with acute and chronic diseases; therefore, a basic understanding of this process is essential for the development of any preventive or improved treatment strategies. The mechanisms of generating different types of free radicals in the body are very complex; therefore, they are discussed here in general terms. The significance of increased oxidative stress in aging, various diseases, and injuries is discussed in Chapters 4 through 18.

Cell injury initiates an important biological event called inflammation, which is considered a protective response following infection with pathogenic organisms or antigens or cellular damage. Inflammation is considered a double-edged sword. It is necessary to kill invading pathogenic organisms and to remove cellular debris in order to facilitate the recovery process. However, it can also damage normal tissue by releasing a number of toxic chemicals. The chronic inflammatory responses are more relevant to chronic diseases than the acute inflammatory reactions. This is a highly complex biological response that is tightly regulated. Therefore, only a brief discussion of this process in general and simple terms is included in this section. The significance of chronic inflammation in aging and various chronic diseases is discussed in Chapters 4 through 18.

The immune system is an important defense system against invading foreign pathogenic microorganisms, and is essential for the healing of injured tissues. Foreign antigens or cell injury evokes an immune response that, through the complex processes of acute inflammation, removes pathogenic microbes and cellular debris. It is a highly regulated system, and is turned off when the invading organisms are killed or injured tissues are healed. Chronic inflammation in response to chronic infection or cellular injury is not turned off; therefore, through its toxic products, it is one of the major factors that contribute to chronic diseases. The immune cells cannot distinguish endogenous antigens from foreign antigens and, consequently, these activated immune cells start damaging the body's own tissues, which produce these antigens causing autoimmune disease. The importance of acute immune response is relevant to HIV infection and cancer prevention, and is discussed in Chapters 7 and 14.

This chapter briefly describes the basic concepts of oxidative stress, inflammation, and the immune system in simple and general terms. These issues are huge and complex. This chapter has attempted to describe them in a few pages for a basic understanding of the oxidative stress, inflammation, and immune functions. For further study of these topics, the references and books that have been used are listed at the end of the chapter.[1–10]

OXIDATIVE STRESS

Increased oxidative stress is caused by excessive production of free radicals derived from oxygen and nitrogen. It is linked with most chronic human diseases such as arthritis, heart disease, Alzheimer's disease, and diabetes.

WHAT ARE FREE RADICALS?

The radicals referred to as free radicals are atoms, molecules, or ions with unpaired electrons. These unpaired electrons are highly reactive and play an important role in several chemical reactions such as combustion, atmospheric chemistry, and polymerization. In living organisms, including humans, they play an important role in several biochemical reactions and gene expressions. In 1900, the first organic free radical, triphenylmethyl radical, was identified by Moses Gomberg of the University of Michigan in the United States. Free radicals can be derived from oxygen or nitrogen and are symbolized by a dot ($^\bullet$).

In the beginning, the Earth's atmosphere had no oxygen and anaerobic organisms, which can live without oxygen, thrived. About 2.5 billion years ago, blue-green algae in the ocean acquired the ability to split water (H_2O) into hydrogen (H) and oxygen (O_2). This chemical reaction initiated the release of oxygen into the atmosphere. The increased levels of atmospheric oxygen led to the extinction of many anaerobic organisms from oxygen's toxicity, probably due to the generation of free radicals. This important atmospheric chemical event forced the organisms to acquire antioxidant systems to quench these free radicals. Those that succeeded in developing antioxidant protective systems survived, and ultimately led to the evolution of multicellular organisms, including humans, who utilize oxygen for survival and have a comprehensive antioxidant system to defend against damage produced by free radicals.

TYPES OF FREE RADICALS

There are several different types of free radicals derived from oxygen and nitrogen that are generated in the body. The oxygen-derived free radicals include hydroxyl radical ($OH^\bullet$), peroxyl radical ($ROO^\bullet$), alkoxyl radical ($RO^\bullet$), phenoxyl and semiquinone radicals ($ArO^\bullet$, $HO-Ar-O^\bullet$) and superoxide radical ($O_2^{\bullet-}$). The nitrogen-derived free radicals include $NO^\bullet$, $ONOO^-$ (peroxynitrite), and $^\bullet NO_2$.

FORMATION OF FREE RADICALS DERIVED FROM OXYGEN AND NITROGEN

The formation of some of the reactive oxygen species (ROS) is described below.

When molecular oxygen (O_2) acquires an electron, the superoxide anion ($O_2^{\bullet-}$) is formed when $O_2 + e^- = O_2^{\bullet-}$.

Superoxide dismutase (SOD) and H^+ can react with $O_2^{\bullet-}$ to form hydrogen peroxide, H_2O_2:

$$2O_2^{\bullet-} + 2H^+ + SOD \rightarrow H_2O_2 + O_2$$

$$O_2^{\bullet-} + H^+ \rightarrow HO_2^\bullet \text{ (hydroperoxy radical)}$$

$$2HO_2^\bullet \rightarrow H_2O_2 + O_2$$

Ferric and ferrous forms of iron can react with superoxide anion and hydrogen peroxide to produce molecular oxygen and hydroxyl radical ($OH^\bullet$), respectively:

$$Fe^{3+} + O_2^{\bullet-} \rightarrow Fe^{2+} + O_2$$

$$Fe^{2+} + H_2O_2 \rightarrow Fe^{3+} + OH^{\bullet} + OH^- \text{ (Fenton reaction)}$$

The hydroxyl radical can also be formed from a superoxide anion by the Haber–Weiss reaction:

$$O_2^{\bullet-} + H_2O_2 \rightarrow O_2 + OH^- + OH^{\bullet}$$

Both the Fenton and Haber–Weiss reactions require a transition metal such as copper or iron. Among ROS, $OH^{\bullet}$ is the most damaging free radical and is very short-lived.

The hydroxyl radical is very reactive with a variety of organic compounds, leading to production of more radical compounds:

$$RH \text{ (organic compound)} + OH^{\bullet} \rightarrow R^{\bullet} \text{ (organic radical)} + H_2O$$

$$R^{\bullet} + O_2 \rightarrow RO_2^{\bullet} \text{ (peroxyl radical)}$$

For example, the DNA radical can be generated by a reaction with a hydroxyl radical, and this can lead to strand lesions.

Catalase detoxifies hydrogen peroxide to form water and molecular oxygen:

$$H_2O_2 + \text{catalase} \rightarrow H_2O \text{ and } O_2$$

Reactive nitrogen species (RNS) are represented by nitric oxide ($NO^{\bullet}$). NO is synthesized by the enzyme nitric oxide synthase from L-arginine. $NO^{\bullet}$ can combine with a superoxide anion to form peroxynitrite, a powerful oxidant.

$$NO^{\bullet} + O2^{\bullet-} \rightarrow ONOO^- \text{ (peroxynitrite)}$$

When protonated (likely at physiological pH), peroxynitrite spontaneously decomposes to reactive nitric dioxide and hydroxyl radicals:

$$ONOO^- + H^+ \rightarrow {}^{\bullet}NO_2 + OH^{\bullet}$$

SOD can also enhance the peroxynitrite-mediated nitration of tyrosine residues on critical proteins, presumably via species similar to the nitronium cation (NO_2^+):

$$ONOO^- + SOD \rightarrow NO_2^+ \rightarrow \text{Nitration of tyrosine}$$

There are several oxidizing agents that are formed in the body, in addition to free radicals. They include peroxynitrite, hydrogen peroxide, and lipid peroxide and are very damaging to the cells. Many other radical species can be formed by biological reactions inside the body. For example, phenolic and other aromatic species can be formed during metabolism of xenobiotic agents. Furthermore, any antioxidant, when oxidized, can act as a free radical.

Oxidative stress occurs when the generation of ROS exceeds the ability of the body's antioxidant defense system to neutralize them. Similarly, nitrosylative stress occurs when the generation of RNS exceeds the ability of the body's antioxidant defense system to neutralize them. Chronic increases in oxidative and nitrosylative stresses have been implicated in the initiation and progression of most human chronic diseases. However, a short-term increase in oxidative stress, such as seen during viral or bacterial infections, may be important in killing invading organisms although they can also damage normal tissue. ROS are also used in cell signaling systems that regulate growth, differentiation, and apoptosis. Free radicals can damage DNA (deoxyribonucleic acid), RNA (ribonucleic acid), proteins, carbohydrates, and membranes. The half-lives of various free radicals vary from

10^{-9} seconds to days. This means that most are quickly destroyed after causing damage. For example, the half-life of hydroxyl free radicals is 10^{-9} seconds, whereas that of a superoxide anion is 10^{-5} seconds, and the lipid peroxyl free radical has a half-life of 7 seconds. The semiquinone free radical half-life is in days while nitric oxide's is about 1 second and hydrogen peroxide's is in minutes.

Normally, free radicals are generated in the body during the use of oxygen in the metabolism of certain compounds. Mitochondria—elongated membranous structures present in all cells in varying numbers—use oxygen to produce energy. During this process of generating energy, superoxide anions, hydroxyl radicals, and hydrogen peroxide are produced as byproducts. It is estimated that about 2% of the oxygen consumed by mitochondria remains partially used, and this unused oxygen leaks out of the mitochondria, making about 20 billion molecules of superoxide anions and hydrogen peroxide per cell per day.

During bacterial or viral infection, phagocytic cells are activated and generate high levels of nitric oxide, superoxide anions, and hydrogen peroxide within the infected cells to kill the infective agents. Excessive production of free radicals by phagocytes can also damage normal cells and, thereby, increase the risk of acute and/or chronic diseases. During the oxidative metabolism of fatty acids and other molecules in the body, free radicals are produced. Certain habits, such as tobacco smoking, and some trace minerals, such as free iron, copper, and manganese, can also increase the rate of production of free radicals in the body. Thus, the human body is exposed daily to different types and varying levels of free radicals.

OXIDATION AND REDUCTION PROCESSES

To understand the role of free radicals and antioxidants in the human body, it is important to grasp the relationship between the oxidation and reduction processes, which are constantly taking place in the body. Oxidation is a process in which an atom or molecule gains oxygen, loses hydrogen, or loses an electron. For example, carbon gains oxygen during oxidation and becomes carbon dioxide. A superoxide radical loses an electron during oxidation and becomes oxygen. Thus, an oxidizing agent is a molecule or atom that changes another chemical by adding oxygen to it or by removing an electron or hydrogen from it. Examples of oxidizing agents are free radicals, ozone, and ionizing radiation.

Reduction is a process in which an atom or molecule loses oxygen, gains hydrogen, or gains an electron. For example, carbon dioxide loses oxygen and becomes carbon monoxide, carbon gains hydrogen and becomes methane, and oxygen gains an electron and becomes superoxide anion. Thus, a reducing agent is a molecule or atom that changes another chemical by removing oxygen from it or by adding electrons or hydrogen to it. All antioxidants can be considered reducing agents. The balanced processes of oxidation and reduction maintain cells in a healthy state. Increased oxidation processes over reduction processes can lead to cellular injury, and eventually chronic diseases or cell death. The role of oxidative stress in various diseases is discussed in Chapters 4 through 18.

WHAT IS INFLAMMATION?

Inflammation in Latin is referred to as *inflammation*, which means *a setting on fire*. The primary features of inflammation at the affected sites include redness, swelling, warmth upon touch, and varying degrees of pain. These characteristics of inflammation were first recognized by a Roman physician, Dr. Cornelius, who lived from about 30 B.C. to A.D. 45. Inflammation is the complex biological response by which the body removes infective agents such as bacteria, viruses, and damaged cells caused by physical agents (such as ionizing radiation, traumatic bodily injuries, or chemical or biological agents). The inflammatory reactions involve the movement of plasma and white blood cells (leukocytes, macrophages, monocytes, lymphocytes, and plasma cells) from the blood to the injured sites. It is a protective response by which the body removes the injurious infective microorganisms, as well as initiates the healing process in the damaged tissue. During the healing process, the injured tissue is replaced by regeneration of native parenchymal cells, by filling of the injured site with fibroblastic tissue (scarring), or, most commonly, by a combination of both processes.

TYPES OF INFLAMMATORY REACTIONS

Inflammation is divided into two categories: acute and chronic inflammatory reactions. Acute inflammation occurs following cellular injury or infection with microorganisms. The period of acute inflammation is relatively short, lasting from a few minutes to a few days. The main features of acute inflammations are edema (accumulation of exudation of fluid and plasma in extracellular spaces) and the migration of leukocytes, primarily neutrophils, to the site of injury. Chronic inflammation also occurs following persistent cellular injury and infection. The period of chronic inflammation is relatively long and can last as long as injury or infection exists. The main features of chronic inflammation are the presence of lymphocytes and macrophages and the proliferation of blood vessels, fibrosis, and tissue necrosis.

Acute inflammation. Acute inflammation causes marked alterations in the blood vessels that allow plasma protein and leukocytes to leave the circulation. Subsequently, the leukocytes migrate to the site of injury by a process called chemotaxis. Leukocytes engulf pathogenic organisms by phagocytosis and kill them by generating bursts of ROS and other toxins. They can also engulf cellular debris and foreign antigens by a similar process and then degrade them by lysosomal proteolytic enzymes. On the other hand, leukocytes may release excessive amounts of ROS, proinflammatory cytokines, prostaglandins, adhesion molecules, and complement proteins that can damage normal tissues. An acute inflammatory reaction is tightly regulated and turned off soon after the injured sites are healed or invading microbes removed. It is absolutely an important process for removing both pathogens and cellular debris from the damaged site, thus allowing healing to occur.

Acute inflammation is effective only when the injurious stimuli or tissue are relatively mild. If the tissue damage is extensive, or the levels of infective organisms are high, acute inflammatory reactions are not tuned off, and consequently, the toxic products of these reactions can enhance the rate of progression of damage that may cause organ failure and eventually even death.

Chronic inflammation. Persistence of low-grade cellular injury, exposure to exogenous agents such as particulate silica, or infection can initiate chronic inflammation. In addition, production of endogenous antigens can sometimes evoke a self-perpetuating immune response that causes autoimmune diseases such as rheumatoid arthritis and lupus. Chronic inflammation is often associated with chronic human diseases such as heart disease, Alzheimer's disease, arthritis, diabetes, and HIV/AIDS.

In contrast to acute inflammation, which is characterized by vascular changes, edema, and primarily neutrophilic infiltration, chronic inflammation is characterized by the presence of mononuclear cells, which include macrophages, lymphocytes, and plasma cells, and also tissue damage caused by the inflammatory cells. During chronic inflammation, the presence of angiogenesis and fibrosis can be observed at the site of injury.

PRODUCTS OF INFLAMMATORY REACTIONS

During inflammation, several highly reactive agents are released, including cytokines, complement proteins, arachidonic acid (AA) metabolites, and endothelial/leukocyte adhesion molecules. They are briefly described below.

CYTOKINES

Cytokines are proteins released during both acute and chronic inflammation. They are produced primarily by activated lymphocytes and macrophages, but also by many cell types such as endothelium, epithelium, and connective tissue cells. Cytokines play an important role in modulating the function of many other cell types. They are multifunctional and individual cytokines may have both positive and negative regulatory actions. Cytokines mediate their action by binding to specific receptors on target cells. These receptors are regulated by exogenous and endogenous signals.

Cytokines that regulate lymphocyte activation, growth, and differentiation include interleukin-2 (IL-2), interleukin-4 (IL-4, favors growth), and interleukin-10 (IL-10), as well as transforming growth factor-beta (TGF-beta). These are negative regulators of immune responses. Cytokines involved with natural immunity include inflammatory cytokines, tumor necrosis factor-alpha (TNF-alpha), IL-1beta, type I interferons (IFN-alpha and IFN-beta), and interleukin-6 (IL-6). Cytokines that activate inflammatory cells such as macrophages include IFN-gamma, TNF-alpha, TNF-beta, IL-5, IL-10, and IL-12. Cytokines that stimulate hematopoiesis (growth and differentiation of immature leukocytes) include IL-3, IL-7, c-kit ligand, granulocyte-macrophage colony-stimulating factor (G-M-CSF), macrophage colony-stimulating factor (M-CSF), granulocyte CSF, and stem cell factor.

Chemokines are also cytokines that stimulate leukocyte movement and direct them to the site of injury during inflammation. Many classical growth factors may also act as cytokines, and, conversely, many cytokines exhibit activities of growth factors.

COMPLEMENT PROTEINS

During inflammation, 20 complement proteins, including their cleavage products, are released into the plasma. When activated, they can cause cell lysis and can exhibit proteolytic activity. They participate in both innate and adaptive immunity for protection against pathogenic organisms. Complement proteins are numbered C1 through C9, each of which has complex mechanisms of action on cells. Some of the complement proteins are also neurotoxic.

AA METABOLITES

The AA metabolites include prostaglandins, leukotrienes, and lipoxins. AA is a 20-carbon fatty acid that is derived from dietary sources or is formed from the essential fatty acid linoleic acid. During inflammation, AA metabolites, also called eicosanoids, are released. These eicosanoids have diverse biological actions, depending upon the cell type. The eicosanoids are synthesized by two major classes of enzymes: Cyclooxygenase (COX) for the synthesis of prostaglandins and thromboxanes and lipoxygenase for the synthesis of leukotrienes and lipoxins. There are two isoforms of cyclooxygenase, COX1 and COX2.

ENDOTHELIAL/LEUKOCYTE ADHESION MOLECULES

The immunoglobulin family molecules include two endothelial adhesion molecules: intracellular adhesion molecule-1 (ICAM-1) and vascular adhesion molecule-1 (VCAM-1). These adhesion molecules bind with leukocyte receptor integrins. They are induced by IL-1 and TNF-alpha. Both ICAM-1 and VCAM-1 are released during inflammatory reactions and have diverse mechanisms of action on cells.

IMMUNE SYSTEM

The immune system plays an important role in the defense of the organisms against invading pathogens and is essential for the survival of the organism. Under certain conditions, the immune system can produce toxic chemicals that play an important role in the initiation and progression of chronic diseases, as well as causing autoimmune diseases.

WHAT IS THE IMMUNE SYSTEM?

The immune system is a highly complex and tightly regulated organ and represents a double-edged sword. On one hand, it defends the body against foreign invading pathogenic microorganisms and antigenic molecules or particles. On the other hand, it has ability to produce toxic chemicals, such as ROS, proinflammatory cytokines, complement proteins, adhesion molecules, and prostaglandins, that are toxic to tissues and that can increase the risk of chronic diseases such as arthritis, heart disease, Alzheimer's disease, and diabetes. Furthermore, the presence of endogenous antigens can initiate an immune response that damages the body's own tissue, as seen in rheumatoid arthritis. The immune system, once exposed to an antigen and successful in removing it, stores the recognition factor of this antigen in its memory. Thus, during the lifetime of an individual, the immune system stores recognition factors of millions of different antigens; and thus, protects the body from these antigens all the time. This process of exposure to an antigen and successfully removing is generally referred to as acquired immunity, which is the basis of vaccination.

The immune system is a network of cells, tissues, and organs that works together in a highly coordinated manner to defend the body against foreign invading organisms or antigenic molecules or particles. The organs of the immune system are located throughout the body. They are the lymphoid organs that contain lymphocytes and bone marrow that contains all blood cells, including lymphocytes. Thymus-derived lymphocytes are referred to as T lymphocytes (T cells). In blood, T cells represent about 60% to 70% of peripheral lymphocytes. Bone marrow-derived lymphocytes are referred to as B lymphocytes (B cells). They constitute about 10–20% of peripheral lymphocytes in the blood. B cells mature to plasma cells that secrete specific antibodies in response to a particular antigen. Macrophages are derived from monocytes of bone marrow, and are a part of the mononuclear phagocyte system. They exhibit phagocytic activity and play important roles in both the induction and the effector phase of immune responses. A specialized form of cells with numerous fine dendritic cytoplasmic processes, called dendritic cells, do not exhibit phagocytic activity. They play an important role in presenting antigens to the T cells. Natural killer (NK) cells represent about 10% to 15% of the peripheral blood lymphocytes and lack T-cell receptors. They can kill tumor cells.

The major components of the immune system are innate immunity and adaptive immunity. The innate immune defenses are nonspecific, but it is the dominant system of the host's defense.[11] The innate immune response is activated when microorganisms are identified by pattern recognition receptors or when damaged cells send signals to the immune system for a defensive response.[12,13] The innate immune responses do not confer long-lasting immunity against pathogenic organisms. The innate immune system responds to infection by inducing inflammation, releasing complement proteins, and recruiting leukocytes. It can also activate the adaptive immunity.

INNATE IMMUNITY

The components of innate immunity include inflammation, complement proteins, and leukocytes.

Inflammation. Inflammation is one of the first responses of the immune system to infection with microorganisms. The injured or infected cells release eicosanoids and cytokines, as well as growth factors and cytotoxic factors. These cytokines and other chemicals recruit immune cells to the site of infection for the elimination of the invading organisms or promotion of healing of the injured tissue.[14]

Complement proteins. There are more than 20 complement proteins released from the activated immune cells in response to infection or injury. These proteins are the major humoral components of the innate immune response.[15] They complement the killing of pathogenic microorganisms by antibodies through a complex mechanism. Complement proteins can also be directly toxic to organisms and cells.

Leukocytes. Leukocytes are also important components of innate immunity. They include the phagocytes (primarily macrophages and neutrophils) and dendritic cells, mast cells, eosinophils, basophils, and NK cells. These cells identify and kill microorganisms by phagocytosis. Phagocytosis is an important feature of cellular innate immunity. Neutrophils and macrophages are the most active in phagocytosis following infection with microorganisms. These cells engulf pathogens that are trapped in an intracellular vesicle called phagosomes, which fuse with lysosomes to form phagolysosomes. The pathogens are killed by proteolytic enzymes of the lysosomes, aided by a burst of ROS released by the phagocytes. NK cells can kill tumor cells or cells infected with viruses.

ADAPTIVE IMMUNITY

The adaptive response to an antigen is strong and is responsible for storing and recalling immunologic memories for recognizing and eliminating a specific antigen all the time. The lymphocytes (T cells and B cells) are responsible for the adaptive immune response. Both T cells and B cells carry receptors that recognize specific targets. T cells can recognize only membrane-bound antigens. The cell surface major histocompatibility complex (MHC) molecules bind peptide fragments of foreign proteins for presentation to appropriate antigen-specific T cells. There are two major subtypes of T cells: the killer T cells and the helper T cells. The killer T cells can recognize antigens bound to Class I MHC molecules, whereas the helper cells recognize antigens bound to Class II MHC molecules. A minor subtype of T cells is $\gamma\delta$ T cells, which recognize intact antigens that are not bound to MHC receptors

In contrast to the T cells, the surface of a B cell has an antibody molecule for a specific antigen. The antibody molecules recognize whole pathogens and do not need any antigen presenting mechanism for their action. Each lineage of a B cell expresses a different antibody. A B cell first identifies pathogens when an antibody on its surface binds to a specific foreign antigen. This antibody/antigen complex is engulfed by the B cell where it is converted into peptides by proteolytic enzymes. The B cells then display on their surface antigenic peptides and Class II MHC molecules that attract matching T helper cells that release lymphokines and activate B cells. The activated B cells proliferate and differentiate to plasma cells that secrete millions of copies of the antibody that recognize this antigen. These antibodies circulate in the blood and the lymph, and bind to pathogens expressing this particular antigen. These antibody/antigen-bound pathogens are destroyed by complement activation or by phagocytes. Antibodies can also neutralize bacterial toxins by directly binding to them and kill bacteria or viruses by interfering with their receptors that are used to infect cells.

CONCLUSIONS

Increased oxidative stress is caused by excessive production of free radicals derived from oxygen and nitrogen. The cell injury initiates an important biological event, called inflammation, which is considered a protective response following infection with pathogenic organisms or antigens or cellular damage. It is needed to kill invading pathogenic organisms, and for the removal of cellular debris in order to facilitate the recovery process. However, it can also damage normal tissues by releasing a number of toxic chemicals. This is a highly complex biological response that is tightly regulated. The immune system plays an important role in the defense of organisms against invading pathogens. Under certain conditions, the immune system can produce toxic chemicals that play an important role in the initiation and progression of chronic diseases as well as cause autoimmune diseases. Increased oxidative stress and chronic inflammation are associated with the initiation and progression of most chronic human diseases such as cancer, heart disease, arthritis, diabetes, Alzheimer's disease, and Parkinson's disease. Therefore, attenuation of these two biological processes may reduce the risk of these diseases.

REFERENCES

1. Cotran, R. S. K., V. Kumar, and T. Collins. 1999. Disease of immunity. In *Pathologic Basis of Disease*, 188–259. New York, NY: W. B. Saunders Company.
2. Ryter, A. 1985. Relationship between ultrastructure and specific functions of macrophages. *Comp Immunol Microbiol Infect Dis* 8 (2): 119–133.
3. Langermans, J. A., W. L. Hazenbos, and R. van Furth. 1994. Antimicrobial functions of mononuclear phagocytes, *J Immunol Methods* 174 (1–2): 185–194.
4. Holtmeier, W., and D. Kabelitz. 2005. Gammadelta T cells link innate and adaptive immune responses. *Chem Immunol Allergy* 86: 151–183.
5. Sproul, T. W., P. C. Cheng, M. L. Dykstra, and S. K. Pierce. 2000. A role for MHC class II antigen processing in B cell development. *Int Rev Immunol* 19 (2–3): 139–155.
6. Kehry, M. R., and P. D. Hodgkin. 1994. B-cell activation by helper T-cell membranes. *Crit Rev Immunol* 14 (3–4): 221–238.
7. Asmus, K.-D., and M. Bonifacio. 1994. Free radical chemistry. In *Excercise and Oxygen Toxicity*, ed. C. K. Sen, L. Packer, and O. Hanninen, 1–47. New York, NY: Elsevier.
8. Vaillancourt, F., H. Fahmi, Q. Shi, P. Lavigne, P. Ranger, J. C. Fernandes, and M. Benderdour. 2008. 4-Hydroxynonenal induces apoptosis in human osteoarthritic chondrocytes: The protective role of glutathione-S-transferase. *Arthritis Res Ther* 10 (5): R107.
9. Pryor, W. A. 1994. Oxidants and antioxidants. In *Natural Antioxidants in Human Health and Disease*, ed. B. Frei, 1–24. New York, NY: Academy Press, Inc.
10. Kehrer, J. P., and C. V. Smith. 1994. Free radicals in biology: Sources, reactives, and roles in the etiology of human diseases. In *Natural Antioxidants in Human Health and Disease*, ed. B. Frei, 25–62. New York, NY: Academy Press, Inc.
11. Litman, G. W., J. P. Cannon, and L. J. Dishaw. 2005. Reconstructing immune phylogeny: New perspectives. *Nat Rev Immunol* 5 (11): 866–879.
12. Medzhitov, R. 2007. Recognition of microorganisms and activation of the immune response. *Nature* 449 (7164): 819–826.
13. Matzinger, P. 2002. The danger model: A renewed sense of self. *Science* 296 (5566): 301–305.
14. Martin, P., and S. J. Leibovich. 2005. Inflammatory cells during wound repair: The good, the bad and the ugly. *Trends Cell Biol* 15 (11): 599–607.
15. Rus, H., C. Cudrici, and F. Niculescu. 2005. The role of the complement system in innate immunity. *Immunol Res* 33 (2): 103–112.

3 Scientific Rationale of Current Trends in Clinical Studies of Micronutrients for Prevention of Chronic Diseases

INTRODUCTION

In spite of extensive basic and clinical research in prevention and progression of chronic diseases such as cancer, heart disease, Alzheimer's disease (AD), and Parkinson's disease (PD) over the past two decades, the incidence of these diseases has not significantly changed. As a matter of fact, the incidence of cancer appears to have risen. For example, a decade ago, the annual incidence of cancer was 1.2 million new cases; in 2009, there were estimated to be about 1.5 million new cases. About 1.5 million new cases of coronary artery disease (CAD) are detected annually. The current estimate is that about 62 million Americans have one or more types of cardiovascular disease,[1] and about 14 million per year suffer a heart attack or angina. At present, about 5.3 million Americans suffer from dementia, with or without AD. The incidence of AD and other dementias doubles every 5 years beyond the age of 65 years or older and about 50% of individuals 80 years or older may have dementia, with or without AD. Currently, PD affects about 500,000 Americans,[2] with about 50,000 new cases diagnosed annually.

Despite several randomized, double-blind and placebo-controlled, and nonrandomized clinical studies primarily of individual antioxidants in high-risk populations, controversy still exists about the usefulness of micronutrient supplements in reducing the risk of chronic diseases. The results of these clinical trials have varied from no effect, beneficial effects, to harmful effects. Repeated reviews and meta-analyses of such clinical studies revealed the same conclusions and recommendations made by the original studies. Fundamental questions arise about whether these clinical trials took into consideration the status of oxidative stress and chronic inflammation that are elevated in high-risk populations, the biology of antioxidants, and the consequences of using a single antioxidant in such populations. After carefully reviewing these studies, I have concluded that the major clinical trials have been performed without the above considerations and, therefore, the conclusions and recommendations drawn from such clinical studies with respect to the efficacy of antioxidants should be considered inaccurate and misleading.

This chapter discusses the status of oxidative stress and chronic inflammation in high risk populations, the biology of antioxidants, and the consequences of using a single antioxidant in selected high-risk populations of chronic diseases such as cancer, heart disease, AD, and PD. This chapter describes an example of a clinical trial (randomized, double-blind, and placebo-controlled) with a single antioxidant for each disease in order to show that these studies were performed without a scientific rationale with respect to the antioxidant. The scientific rationale and its supporting evidence for making a shift in the current clinical trial paradigm from one or two micronutrients to multiple micronutrients, together with a high-fiber and low-fat diet, to reduce the risk of chronic diseases in high-risk populations are also presented.

LEVELS OF OXIDATIVE STRESS AND CHRONIC INFLAMMATION IN HIGH-RISK POPULATIONS

High levels of oxidative stress and chronic inflammation exist in high-risk populations of cancer, CAD, AD, and PD. However, the sources and mechanisms of inducing increased oxidative stress and chronic inflammations between these high-risk populations may, in part, be different.

HIGH-RISK POPULATIONS FOR CANCER

High-risk populations for cancer, which include heavy tobacco smokers and survivors of cancer treatment, have high levels of internal oxidative environment. This is because inhalation of smoke generates excessive amounts of free radicals that cause depletion of antioxidants and damage to cells and organs. Long-term survivors of cancer treatment may also have a high internal oxidative environment, because most treatment agents induce increased oxidative stress.[3-5] Markers of proinflammatory cytokines such as ineterleukin-6 (IL-6) and tumor necrosis factor-alpha are also elevated in these populations. These high-risk populations are very suitable models by which to evaluate the efficacy of micronutrients, including antioxidants, in reducing the risk of primary cancer (smokers) and second primary tumors, and recurrence of the primary tumor (cancer survivors) by well-designed, randomized, double-blind, placebo-controlled trials.

HIGH-RISK POPULATIONS OF CAD

This high-risk population includes individuals with high levels of cholesterol, homocysteine, and C-reactive protein (CRP), as well as individuals taking statins with or without any previous cardiac event. The sources of free radicals include cigarette smoking, homocysteine, high glucose in diabetes, an increased store of free iron, and a high-fat diet. In addition to high levels of oxidative stress, high levels of chronic inflammation, as evidenced by the presence of increased levels of CRP, exist in high-risk populations. These high-risk populations are very suitable models to evaluate the efficacy of micronutrients, including antioxidants, in reducing the risks and progression of CAD via well-designed, randomized, double-blind, placebo-controlled trials.

HIGH-RISK POPULATIONS OF AD AND PD

These high-risk populations include individuals older than 65 years, individuals with a family history of the diseases, and patients with an early stage disease. The sources of free radicals in the brains of high-risk populations of AD include partially utilized oxygen by the mitochondria, auto-oxidation of acetylcholine, increased production and processing of amyloid precursor proteins (APPs) to beta-amyloid fragments, impaired mitochondrial function, and mutations in APPs and presenilins I and II. Reactive microglia release proinflammatory cytokines that are toxic to cholinergic neurons. The sources of free radicals in the brains of high-risk populations of PD include partially utilized oxygen by the mitochondria, auto-oxidation of dopamine, impaired mitochondrial function, accumulation of free iron in the substantia nigra, and overexpression or mutations in alpha-synuclein, and mutations in *DJ-1*, *Parkin*, and *PINK1* genes, all of which impair mitochondrial function and generate free radicals. Reactive microglia release proinflammatory cytokines that are toxic to DA neurons. Thus, increased oxidative stress and chronic inflammation exist in both AD and PD. These high-risk populations are very suitable models to evaluate the efficacy of micronutrients, including antioxidants, in reducing the risk and progression of AD and PD by well-designed, randomized, double-blind, placebo-controlled trials.

BIOLOGY OF ANTIOXIDANTS

Although antioxidants are known to neutralize free radicals, they also inhibit the levels of chronic inflammation and markedly alter the gene expression profiles of several genes, protein kinase activities, and translocation of certain proteins from one subcellular compartment to another within the same cell. It is well established that an individual antioxidant, when oxidized, acts as a pro-oxidant. Therefore, administration of a single antioxidant in the high-risk populations for cancer, CAD, AD, or PD is expected to increase the risk of chronic diseases after prolonged consumption because of oxidation of the single antioxidant. Administration of the same single antioxidant with other multiple antioxidants in high-risk populations may produce beneficial effects, because oxidation of a single antioxidant could be counteracted by cooperative reduction by other antioxidants.

The natural forms of vitamin E and beta-carotene are more effective than their synthetic counterparts. For example, natural beta-carotene reduced radiation-induced transformation in mammalian cells in culture, but the synthetic beta-carotene did not.[6] Cells accumulate more of the natural form of vitamin E than the synthetic form,[7] and alpha-tocopheryl succinate is now considered the most effective form of vitamin E.[8,9] Low doses of vitamin C can stimulate the growth of cancer cells, whereas high doses of the same antioxidant can inhibit the growth of some cancer cells.[10] The results of these studies cannot be extrapolated to humans; however, in high-risk populations of cancer, the possibility of the presence of undetectable cancer cells exists. Therefore, administration of low doses of a single antioxidant could enhance the rate of growth of tumor cells, which would then become detectable earlier.

It is known that different types of free radicals are produced in the body that have multiple dietary and endogenous antioxidants. Each antioxidant has a different affinity for each of these free radicals, depending on the cellular environment. Antioxidants are distributed differently in organs and even within the same cells. The gradient of oxygen pressure varies within the cell and tissues. Vitamin E is more effective as a quencher of free radicals in reduced oxygen pressure, whereas beta-carotene and vitamin A are more effective in higher oxygen pressures.[11] Vitamin C is necessary to protect cellular components in aqueous environments, whereas carotenoids and vitamins A and E protect cellular components in nonaqueous environments. Vitamin C also plays an important role in maintaining cellular levels of vitamin E by recycling the vitamin E radical (oxidized) to the reduced (antioxidant) form.[12] Also, the DNA damage produced by oxidized vitamin C can be ameliorated by vitamin E. The form and type of vitamin E used are also important. It is known that various organs of rats selectively absorb the natural form of vitamin E.[7] It has been established that alpha tocopheryl-succinate (alpha-TS) is the most effective form of vitamin E.[8,9] We have reported that oral ingestion of alpha-TS (800 IU/day) for more than 6 months in humans increased plasma levels of not only alpha-tocopherol, but also of alpha-TS, suggesting that alpha-TS can be absorbed from the intestinal tract without hydrolysis to alpha-tocopherol, provided the pool of alpha-tocopherol in the body has become saturated.[8] Selenium, a cofactor of glutathione peroxidase, acts as an antioxidant; therefore, selenium supplementation together with other dietary and endogenous antioxidants is also essential.

The deficiency of glutathione, an important endogenous antioxidant present in millimolar levels in the cells, is consistently observed in autopsied samples of brains of both AD and PD patients. Glutathione represents a potent intracellular protective agent against oxidative damage. It catabolizes H_2O_2 and anions and is very effective (in the presence of glutathione peroxidase) in quenching peroxynitrite.[13] Therefore, increasing the intracellular levels of glutathione is essential for the protection of various organelles within the cells. Oral supplementation with glutathione failed to significantly increase plasma levels of glutathione in human subjects,[14] suggesting that this tripeptide is completely hydrolyzed in the gastrointestinal tract. N-acetylcysteine and alpha-lipoic acid increase the intracellular levels of glutathione and, therefore, they can also be used in combination with dietary antioxidants. Coenzyme Q_{10} is needed by the mitochondria to generate energy. It also scavenges peroxy radicals faster than alpha-tocopherol[15] and, like vitamin C, can regenerate vitamin E in a redox cycle.[16]

B-vitamins and vitamin D should be combined with multiple antioxidants because some studies have reported the value of vitamin D in cancer risk reduction. B-vitamins are also important for overall health.

RESULTS OF CLINICAL TRIALS WITH A SINGLE ANTIOXIDANT

The issues discussed in the above paragraphs were not considered while designing the clinical trials with antioxidants in high-risk populations of chronic diseases, and this could have contributed to the inconsistent results. Since all clinical studies are discussed in detail in the chapters on individual diseases, the results of only a few clinical trials, primarily with one dietary antioxidant, in a high-risk population of each chronic disease are discussed below. Some of these clinical trials were selected because they are often quoted as not recommending antioxidants for the prevention or reduction of the rate of progression of chronic diseases.

CANCER

In well-designed clinical studies, an oral administration of synthetic beta-carotene once a day at a dose of 20 mg/day increased the incidence of lung cancer, prostate cancer, and stomach cancer among male heavy tobacco smokers.[17–19] This increase in cancer incidence could have been predicted because beta-carotene in the high internal oxidative environments of heavy smokers would act as a pro-oxidant. In contrast, one would predict that the same dose of beta-carotene may not have a significant effect in normal populations who have lower internal oxidative environments. Indeed, the same dose of beta-carotene did not affect the incidence of cancer in healthy populations who have lower internal oxidative environments than the heavy tobacco smokers.[20] Consumption of vitamin E increased the incidence of secondary cancer after cancer therapy.[21] This observation also could have been predicted for the same reasons as discussed with beta-carotene.

CORONARY ARTERY DISEASE

A randomized, double blind, placebo-controlled international trial, Heart Outcomes Prevention Evaluation (HOPE), was conducted from December 21, 1993 to April 15, 1999. One of the objectives of this trial was to evaluate the efficacy of natural vitamin E (400 IU/day) on patients 55 years or older with vascular disease or diabetes, many of whom were heavy cigarette smokers, in reducing the risk of CAD. The analysis of data, published in five separate publications, has revealed inconsistent results.

In the analysis published in 2000, the primary end points were major cardiac events (myocardial infarction, stroke, and death due to coronary heart disease), and the secondary end points were unstable angina, heart failure, revascularization, amputation, or death due to coronary heart disease and complications of diabetes. No significant effect of vitamin E supplementation on primary or secondary end points was observed.[22]

In the analysis published in 2001, in a subset of the study population, the effect of vitamin E on carotid intimal medial thickness as measured by ultrasound was evaluated. The results showed that vitamin E supplementation had no effect on the progression of atherosclerosis.[23]

In the analysis published in 2002, the primary end points were the same as those in the analysis made in 2000, but the secondary end points included, as an additional criterion, nephropathy. The results showed that vitamin E had no effect on either the primary or the secondary end points.[24]

In the analysis published in 2004, the primary end points were the same as those in the analysis of 2000, but the secondary end points included an additional criterion, clinical proteinuria (renal insufficiency). The results showed that in people with mild to moderate renal insufficiency, vitamin E had no effect on primary or secondary end points.[25]

In the analysis published in 2005, the primary and secondary end points were the same as those in the analysis of 2000. The results showed that vitamin E supplementation had no effect on the primary or most secondary end points; however, it increased the risk of two secondary end points: heart failure by about 13% and hospitalization for heart failure by about 21%.[26] The analysis of the subpopulation of heavy tobacco smokers revealed that smoking increased the risk of morbidity and mortality among the high-risk patients despite the treatment with standard medications known to reduce cardiovascular disease.[27] This is consistent with another independent study (outside of the HOPE study) in which daily consumption of 800 IU of vitamin E increased the levels of oxidative stress markers in heavy smokers.[28] These studies suggest that smoking plays a dominant role in increasing morbidity and mortality. If these major cardiac events increased despite the gold standard medications that were given to reduce the risk of cardiovascular disease in this population, it is not surprising that administration of vitamin E alone either had no significant effect on all primary end points as well as most secondary end points or increased risk of some of the secondary end points (heart failure and hospitalization for heart failure) in one study. Individual antioxidants in high-risk populations such as heavy tobacco smokers and individuals with type 2 diabetes may be oxidized because of their high internal oxidative environment and, thereby, act as pro-oxidants rather than as antioxidants.

A recent analysis of the HOPE study population showed that the levels of markers of inflammation were significantly related to future cardiovascular risk; however, the combination of traditional risk factors and N-terminal pro-brain natriuretic (NTproBNP) provided the best clinical predictive for the secondary prevention population.[29]

ALZHEIMER'S DISEASE AND PARKINSON'S DISEASE

A recent analysis of clinical studies revealed that vitamin E may not be useful in the prevention or treatment of AD.[30] Treatment with vitamin E alone produced inconsistent results varying from no effect to some beneficial effects. However, a randomized, double-blind, placebo-controlled clinical trial with DL-alpha-tocopherol (synthetic form; 2000 IU/day) in patients with moderately severe impairment from AD showed some beneficial effects with respect to the rate of deterioration of cognitive function.[31] The dose of vitamin E used in this trial could produce clotting defects after long-term consumption. Such a high dose of vitamin E is not recommended for any clinical study or consumption by the consumers.

Most clinical trials in PD utilized a single antioxidant primarily vitamin E that may have contributed to the inconsistent results. Deprenyl and tocopherol antioxidative therapy of Parkinsonism (DATATOP), a double-blind, placebo-controlled, multicenter clinical trial, was initiated in 1989 to evaluate the efficacy of deprenyl (10 mg/day) and DL-tocopherol (2000 IU/day) individually and in combination in patients with early stage of PD when no therapy was required. The primary outcome was prolongation of the time needed for levodopa therapy. After a follow-up period of 8.2 years, deprenyl significantly delayed the time when levodopa therapy was needed, but alpha tocopherol was ineffective.[32,33] The use of a single dietary antioxidant, vitamin E, was a major flaw in this study design, in view of the fact that glutathione deficiency in the brain is a consistent finding in most neurodegenerative diseases including PD. The addition of a glutathione-elevating agent such as alpha-lipoic acid or N-acetylcysteine would have produced beneficial effects. Mitochondrial dysfunction is also commonly observed in PD and other neurodegenerative diseases; therefore, addition of coenzyme Q_{10} and L-carnitine, which improve the function of mitochondria, would have been useful. There was another flaw in the DATATOP study design with an antioxidant. A multiple vitamin preparation (One A Day®) was allowed for all participants who wished to take it. It was argued that the effect of 30 IU of vitamin E, which was present in the multiple vitamin preparation, would not significantly contribute to the effect of 2000 IU of vitamin E. This argument may not be valid since it has been shown that antioxidants when used individually had no effect on the growth of mammalian cancer cells in culture, but when they are combined at the same doses produced pronounced effect on the growth inhibition, suggesting antioxidants may interact with each other in a synergistic manner.[10,34] Therefore, the impact of 30 IU of vitamin E in a multiple vitamin preparation would be more pronounced than that produced by 30 IU of vitamin E alone. Hence, the consumption of a multiple vitamin preparation with a low dose of vitamin E is likely to create an unacceptable variable while evaluating the efficacy of high doses of vitamin E alone in early PD patients. The patients with PD have a high oxidative environment in the brain. It is known that the individual antioxidant, when oxidized, act as a pro-oxidant. Therefore, the conclusion of the DATATOP study that antioxidants are not useful in reducing the progression of PD is not valid. The extrapolation of data obtained from the use of a single antioxidant to the effects of a multiple antioxidant preparation has no scientific rational.

REASONS THE USE OF A SINGLE ANTIOXIDANT PRODUCED INCONSISTENT RESULTS

Most human epidemiologic studies with diet show that certain micronutrients such as antioxidants, along with a high-fiber and low-fat diet, may reduce the risk of chronic diseases, such as cancer and heart disease. However, from these studies it was not clear whether supplementation with antioxidants or low-fat and high-fiber diet can reduce the risk of these diseases. In vitro and animal models, supplementation with a single antioxidant reduced the levels of oxidative stress and chronic inflammation, and inhibited the risk of chemical-induced chronic diseases. This is in contrast to epidemiologic studies in which a diet containing multiple micronutrients including antioxidants was found to be necessary to reduce the risk of chronic diseases. Most clinical trials extrapolated the results of animal studies rather than of epidemiologic studies, and utilized a single antioxidant in order to evaluate the efficacy of a supplemented antioxidant in reducing the risk or progression of chronic diseases. The results of the clinical studies presented above suggest that this extrapolation was unfortunate, and future clinical trials should not utilize the results of animal studies in designing clinical trials with antioxidants. Both the biology of antioxidants and human epidemiologic studies suggest that the use of multiple micronutrients including both dietary and endogenous antioxidants may be necessary in order to have a full impact on the incidence and progression of chronic diseases.

The results obtained from the use of a single antioxidant should not be extrapolated to the effect of the same antioxidant present in multiple antioxidant preparations or to antioxidants in general. Nevertheless, many scientists, researchers, and physicians are promoting the idea that supplementation with antioxidants can be deleterious to your health, and should not be taken for healthy aging or reducing the risk of chronic diseases. The correct conclusion from these clinical studies with individual antioxidants should be that consumption of a single antioxidant in high-risk populations could be harmful and, therefore, should not be taken by individuals in high-risk or normal populations.

RESULTS OF CLINICAL STUDIES WITH MULTIPLE DIETARY ANTIOXIDANTS IN CANCER

The administration of multiple dietary antioxidants vitamin A (40,000 IU/day), vitamin C (2000 mg/day), vitamin E (400 IU/day), zinc (90 mg/day), and vitamin B_6 (100 mg/day) in combination with the BCG (Bacilli bilie de Calmette–Guerin) vaccine caused a 50% reduction in the incidence of recurrence of bladder cancer in 5 years, as compared to control patients who received multiple vitamins containing RDA levels of nutrients and BCG.[35]

Supplementation with antioxidants (vitamin A, 30,000 IU/day; vitamin C, 1000 mg/day; vitamin E, 70 mg/day) reduced the incidence of recurrence of colon polyps from 36% to 6%[36]; however, consumption of synthetic beta-carotene (25 mg/day), vitamin C (1000 mg/day), and vitamin E (400 mg/day) failed to show any beneficial effects on the recurrence of colon polyps.[37] In another study, daily supplementation with vitamin C (4000 mg/day) and vitamin E (400 mg/day) also failed to reduce the risk of colon polyps, but when they were combined with a high-fiber diet (more than 12 g/day) there was a significant reduction in the incidence of recurrence of polyps.[38] This study indicated the importance of a high-fiber diet in combination with antioxidants in cancer prevention in high-risk populations.

In the Linxian General Population Nutrition Interventional Trial, a preparation of multiple dietary antioxidants (beta-carotene, vitamin E, and selenium at doses 2 to 3 times that of the U.S. RDA) reduced mortality by 10%, and cancer incidence by 13%.[39] The beneficial effects of this supplementation on mortality were still evident up to 10 years after the cessation of supplementation, and were consistently greater in younger participants.[40]

The combination of vitamins A, C, and E, omega-3 fatty acids, and folic acid significantly reduced recurrence of adenoma in patients after a polypectomy.[41] In a randomized placebo-controlled trial involving 80 untreated patients with prostate cancer, daily supplementation with vitamin E, selenium, vitamin C, and coenzyme Q_{10} did not affect serum levels of prostate specific antigen (PSA).[42] In a randomized, placebo-controlled trial referred to as the Selenium and Vitamin E Cancer Prevention Trial (SELECT) involving 35,553 healthy men from 427 participating sites in the United States, Canada, and Puerto Rico, with a follow-up period of a minimum of 7 years and a maximum of 12 years, it was observed that selenium (200 μg/day) or vitamin E (400 IU/day), alone or in combination, did not reduce the risk of prostate cancer.[43]

It is interesting to note that none of the studies cited has utilized endogenous antioxidants such as alpha-lipoic acid, N-acetylcysteine, a glutathione-elevating agent, or coenzyme Q_{10} and L-carnitine. The addition of these antioxidants may have produced consistent beneficial effects in high-risk populations.

From the studies discussed above, it appears that supplementation with one or more dietary antioxidants alone may not be sufficient to produce beneficial and consistent effects on reducing the risk of cancer. Inclusion of endogenous antioxidants may be necessary in any experimental design to test the efficacy of antioxidants in cancer prevention. In recent years, there have been trends to perform meta-analysis of published data in which far reaching conclusions have been made. Since the total number of participating subjects in such analyses becomes huge, numbering in the hundred of thousands, the conclusions appear impressive and definitive. However, if the meta-analysis is performed on publications that have flawed experimental design, the conclusions would be the same that were made in the initial publications. The publications of such meta-analyses are of no scientific value except that they add to the existing misinformation about the value of antioxidants in cancer prevention.

RESULTS OF CLINICAL STUDIES WITH FAT AND FIBER

A review of published data on supplementation with high fiber showed no significant effects on recurrence of adenoma, although most epidemiological studies showed an inverse relationship between consumption of a high-fiber diet and cancer incidence. It should be pointed out that high-fiber diets contain other micronutrients such as multiple antioxidants; thus, the presence of other micronutrients in the diet may have aided to the protective effect of the high-fiber diet on cancer incidence. A few clinical studies on supplementation with high fiber alone have produced inconsistent results. These studies are described below.

An intervention study (The Women's Health Initiative Dietary Modification Trial) in which postmenopausal women received either a low-fat (40%) diet or a high-fat (60%) diet showed that a low-fat diet did not reduce the risk of colorectal cancer during the 8.1 years of follow-up.[44] I am not sure if a diet in which fat content represents 40% should be considered a low-fat diet. A difference of 20% in the fat amount may not be sufficient to exert any protective effect on cancer incidence. I would consider a low-fat diet that contains no more than 25% of calories from fat. The protective effect of low-fat alone may be minor; therefore, the cancer protective effect of a low-fat diet alone cannot be adequately assessed in any intervention trial.

In the Polyp-Prevention Trial, dietary intervention with reduced fat and increased consumption of fruits, vegetables, and fiber produced no effect on PSA or incidence of prostate cancer in men without prostate cancer.[45] A dietary supplement (13.5 vs. 2 g/day) with wheat-bran fiber did not protect against recurrence of colorectal adenomas.[46] Testing the effect of a high-fiber diet alone in which the difference between the control and experimental group is 2 vs. 13.5 g/day may not yield any significant reduction in cancer incidence, because the effect of an additional 10 g of fiber alone on the risk of cancer may be too small to be detected. Such an interventional trial does not appear to have any scientific rational.

In a multi-institutional randomized controlled trial involving 3088 women previously treated for early stage breast cancer, supplementation with a diet high in vegetables, fruits, and fiber and low in fat did not reduce additional breast cancer incidence or mortality during a 7.3-year follow-up period.[47]

The lack of additional micronutrients such as dietary and endogenous antioxidants, B-vitamins, and calcium with vitamin D may have contributed to the failure of detecting protective effects of a high-fiber, low-fat diet on cancer incidence in these studies. No studies have been performed on the role of a high-fiber, low-fat diet in reducing the risk of CAD, AD, and PD. This may be because no significant mechanistic studies exist to suggest that they may be important in affecting the incidence or progression of these diseases. However, a low-fat diet could be important for the heart, because a high-fat diet can increase the levels of cholesterol and triglycerides, a risk factor for CAD. A high-fat diet can also generate increased levels of prostaglandins that contribute to the aggregation of platelets, another risk factor in CAD. Therefore, a high-fiber, low-fat diet is recommended for all chronic diseases discussed in this chapter.

USING MULTIPLE MICRONUTRIENTS WITH A LOW-FAT, HIGH-FIBER DIET TO REDUCE THE RISK AND PROGRESSION OF CHRONIC DISEASES

The biology of antioxidants and the inconsistent results obtained by the use of one or more dietary or endogenous antioxidants alone, or fat and fiber alone, suggests that the use of multiple dietary and endogenous antioxidants may be necessary for optimal effect on the reduction of incidence and progression of chronic diseases. Most of the clinical studies have utilized a once-a-day dose schedule. Taking micronutrients once-a-day creates huge fluctuations in the levels of antioxidants in the body. This is because the biological half-lives (time needed to remove antioxidants from the body) of antioxidants vary markedly depending on their lipid or water solubility. A twofold difference in the levels of vitamin E succinate can produce marked alterations in the expression profiles of several genes in neuroblastoma cells in culture.[48] Therefore, taking micronutrients once-a-day can create genetic stress in the cells that may compromise the efficacy of the micronutrient supplementation after long-term consumption.

RECOMMENDED MICRONUTRIENTS FOR REDUCING THE RISK AND PROGRESSION OF CHRONIC DISEASES

Based on the limitations of the clinical studies discussed in this review, I propose that a shift in the clinical experimental paradigm from one or two micronutrients to multiple micronutrients together with a low-fat, high-fiber diet for testing the efficacy of multiple micronutrients, including dietary and endogenous antioxidants, in high-risk populations should be adopted. Since the micronutrient preparations have been described in each chapter on specific diseases, only one example of a micronutrient preparation for cancer prevention is stated here.

The preparation of multiple micronutrients contains dietary antioxidants such as vitamin A and natural mixed carotenoids (90% represent beta-carotene), two forms of vitamin E (D-alpha tocopheryl acetate and D-alpha tocopheryl succinate), vitamin C (calcium ascorbate), and endogenous antioxidants such as R-alpha-lipoic acid, N-acetylcysteine, coenzyme Q_{10} and L-carnitine, and vitamin D, all B-vitamins, and minerals such as selenium (selenomethionine), zinc, calcium magnesium, and chromium. It should be noted that both vitamin A and beta-carotene were added because beta-carotene, in addition to acting as a precursor of vitamin A, performs unique functions that cannot be produced by vitamin A, and vice versa. For example, beta-carotene increases the expression of the connexin gene, which codes for the gap junction proteins that hold two normal cells together,[49] whereas vitamin A does not produce such an effect. Vitamin A produced differentiation in normal and cancer cells, but beta-carotene did not.[50,51] Beta-carotene was more effective in quenching oxygen radicals than most other antioxidants.[52] Thus, the addition of both vitamin A and beta-carotene may enhance the efficacy of supplements in cancer prevention. The micronutrient preparation contains two forms. alpha-TS is now considered the most effective form of vitamin E.[48] Alpha-TS is more soluble than alpha tocopherol or alpha tocopheryl acetate and enters the cells easily, where it is converted to alpha-tocopherol and provides intracellular protection against oxidative damage. It has its own unique function as alpha-TS. Therefore, to increase the efficacy of vitamin E, the addition of both forms of vitamin E is essential. This micronutrient preparation contains no herbs or herbal antioxidants. This is because certain herbs may interact with the prescription and over-the-counter drugs in an adverse manner. Also, herbal antioxidants do not produce unique antioxidant effects that cannot be produced by antioxidants present in the proposed micronutrient preparations.

The proposed micronutrient formulation does not contain iron, copper, or manganese, because they are known to combine with vitamin C and produce free radicals that could reduce optimal effects of the formulation. In addition, these trace minerals in the presence of antioxidants are absorbed more efficiently and that could increase the body stores of free forms of these minerals. The increased body stores of iron and copper have been associated with the enhanced risk of most chronic human diseases.

The placebo group in the proposed experimental design should not have any dietary recommendation. Dietary compliances can be monitored by questionnaires, whereas the compliances for the micronutrient group can be monitored by measuring plasma levels of selected micronutrients every 6 months. The efficacy of a proposed multiple micronutrient preparation in a high-risk population of cancer is testable. One may argue that this experimental design is complicated, because at the end of the study we may not know for certain which particular micronutrient was responsible for the cancer risk reduction. This argument may not be valid, because the aim of any clinical study is to achieve success in reducing the risk of cancer. For a mechanistic study on micronutrients, animal and cell culture models are most suitable.

CONCLUSIONS

Despite nearly two decades of randomized, double-blind, placebo-controlled, and nonrandomized clinical trials primarily with a single dietary antioxidant in high-risk populations, controversy still exists about the usefulness of antioxidant supplements in reducing the risk and progression of chronic diseases such as cancer, CAD, AD, and PD. The results of these trials have varied from no effects, to beneficial effects, to harmful effects. This chapter has critically examined the results of these studies and concluded that the present trends in clinical research using a single antioxidant to evaluate the efficacy of antioxidants in reducing the risk and progression of chronic diseases lack a scientific rationale and, therefore, have not yielded consistent beneficial effects. This chapter has provided a rationale and evidence for a shift in the clinical study paradigm from using one dietary antioxidant or endogenous antioxidant alone to multiple micronutrients including both dietary and endogenous antioxidants together with a low-fat, high-fiber diet. The proposed micronutrient experimental design can be tested in high-risk populations of chronic diseases by well-designed randomized, double-blind, placebo-controlled trials in order to reduce their incidence.

REFERENCES

1. AHA, Heart and Stroke Statistical Update, American Heart Association, 2001.
2. NINDS. 2008. Parkinson's Disease: A Research Planning Workshop, National Instutute of Health, Bethesda, MD.

3. Rourke, M. T., W. L. Hobbie, L. Schwartz, and A. E. Kazak. 2007. Posttraumatic stress disorder (PTSD) in young adult survivors of childhood cancer. *Pediatr Blood Cancer* 49 (2): 177–182.
4. Thomson, C. A., N. R. Stendell-Hollis, C. L. Rock, E. C. Cussler, S. W. Flatt, and J. P. Pierce. 2007. Plasma and dietary carotenoids are associated with reduced oxidative stress in women previously treated for breast cancer. *Cancer Epidemiol Biomarkers Prev* 16 (10): 2008–2015.
5. Zhao, W., D. I. Diz, and M. E. Robbins. 2007. Oxidative damage pathways in relation to normal tissue injury. *Br J Radiol* 80 (Spec No 1): S23–S31.
6. Kennedy, A. R., and N. I. Krinsky. 1994. Effects of retinoids, beta-carotene, and canthaxanthin on UV- and X-ray-induced transformation of C3H10T1/2 cells in vitro. *Nutr Cancer* 22 (3): 219–232.
7. Ingold, K. U., G. W. Burton, D. O. Foster, L. Hughes, D. A. Lindsay, and A. Webb. 1987. Biokinetics of and discrimination between dietary *RRR*- and *SRR*-alpha-tocopherols in the male rat. *Lipids* 22 (3): 163–172.
8. Prasad, K. N., B. Kumar, X. D. Yan, A. J. Hanson, and W. C. Cole. 2003. alpha-Tocopheryl succinate, the most effective form of vitamin E for adjuvant cancer treatment: A review. *J Am Coll Nutr* 22 (2): 108–117.
9. Carini, R., G. Poli, M. U. Dianzani, S. P. Maddix, T. F. Slater, and K. H. Cheeseman. 1990. Comparative evaluation of the antioxidant activity of alpha-tocopherol, alpha-tocopherol polyethylene glycol 1000 succinate and alpha-tocopherol succinate in isolated hepatocytes and liver microsomal suspensions. *Biochem Pharmacol* 39 (10): 1597–1601.
10. Prasad, K. N., C. Hernandez, J. Edwards-Prasad, J. Nelson, T. Borus, and W. A. Robinson. 1994. Modification of the effect of tamoxifen, *cis*-platin, DTIC, and interferon-alpha 2b on human melanoma cells in culture by a mixture of vitamins. *Nutr Cancer* 22 (3): 233–245.
11. Vile, G. F., and C. C. Winterbourn. 1988. Inhibition of adriamycin-promoted microsomal lipid peroxidation by beta-carotene, alpha-tocopherol and retinol at high and low oxygen partial pressures. *FEBS Lett* 238 (2): 353–356.
12. Niki, E. 1987. Interaction of ascorbate and alpha-tocopherol. *Ann N Y Acad Sci* 498: 186–199.
13. Sies, H., V. S. Sharov, L. O. Klotz, and K. Briviba. 1997. Glutathione peroxidase protects against peroxynitrite-mediated oxidations. A new function for selenoproteins as peroxynitrite reductase. *J Biol Chem* 272 (44): 27812–27817.
14. Witschi, A., S. Reddy, B. Stofer, and B. H. Lauterburg. 1992. The systemic availability of oral glutathione. *Eur J Clin Pharmacol* 43 (6): 667–669.
15. Niki, E. 1997. Mechanisms and dynamics of antioxidant action of ubiquinol. *Mol Aspects Med* 18 (Suppl): S63–S70.
16. Stoyanovsky, D. A., A. N. Osipov, P. J. Quinn, and V. E. Kagan. 1995. Ubiquinone-dependent recycling of vitamin E radicals by superoxide. *Arch Biochem Biophys* 323 (2): 343–351.
17. Albanes, D., O. P. Heinonen, J. K. Huttunen, P. R. Taylor, J. Virtamo, B. K. Edwards, J. Haapakoski et al. 1995. Effects of alpha-tocopherol and beta-carotene supplements on cancer incidence in the Alpha-Tocopherol Beta-Carotene Cancer Prevention Study. *Am J Clin Nutr* 62 (6 Suppl): 1427S–1430S.
18. Omenn, G. S., G. E. Goodman, M. D. Thornquist, J. Balmes, M. R. Cullen, A. Glass, J. P. Keogh. 1996. Effects of a combination of beta carotene and vitamin A on lung cancer and cardiovascular disease. *N Engl J Med* 334 (18): 1150–1155.
19. Bowen, D. J., M. Thornquist, K. Anderson, M. Barnett, C. Powell, G. Goodman, and G. Omenn. 2003. Stopping the active intervention: CARET. *Control Clin Trials* 24 (1): 39–50.
20. Hennekens, C. H., J. E. Buring, J. E. Manson, M. Stampfer, B. Rosner, N. R. Cook, C. Belanger et al. 1996. Lack of effect of long-term supplementation with beta carotene on the incidence of malignant neoplasms and cardiovascular disease. *N Engl J Med* 334 (18): 1145–1149.
21. Bairati, I., F. Meyer, M. Gelinas, A. Fortin, A. Nabid, F. Brochet, J. P. Mercier et al. 2005. Randomized trial of antioxidant vitamins to prevent acute adverse effects of radiation therapy in head and neck cancer patients. *J Clin Oncol* 23 (24): 5805–5813.
22. Yusuf, S., G. Dagenais, J. Pogue, J. Bosch, and P. Sleight. 2000. Vitamin E supplementation and cardiovascular events in high-risk patients. The Heart Outcomes Prevention Evaluation Study Investigators. *N Engl J Med* 342 (3): 154–160.
23. Lonn, E., S. Yusuf, V. Dzavik, C. Doris, Q. Yi, S. Smith, A. Moore-Cox, J. Bosch, W. Riley, and K. Teo. 2001. Effects of ramipril and vitamin E on atherosclerosis: The study to evaluate carotid ultrasound changes in patients treated with ramipril and vitamin E (SECURE). *Circulation* 103 (7): 919–925.
24. Lonn, E., S. Yusuf, B. Hoogwerf, J. Pogue, Q. Yi, B. Zinman, J. Bosch, G. Dagenais, J. F. Mann, and H. C. Gerstein. 2002. Effects of vitamin E on cardiovascular and microvascular outcomes in high-risk patients with diabetes: Results of the HOPE study and MICRO-HOPE substudy. *Diabetes Care* 25 (11): 1919–1927.

25. Mann, J. F., E. M. Lonn, Q. Yi, H. C. Gerstein, B. J. Hoogwerf, J. Pogue, J. Bosch, G. R. Dagenais, and S. Yusuf. 2004. Effects of vitamin E on cardiovascular outcomes in people with mild-to-moderate renal insufficiency: Results of the HOPE study. *Kidney Int* 65 (4): 1375–1380.
26. Lonn, E., J. Bosch, S. Yusuf, P. Sheridan, J. Pogue, J. M. Arnold, C. Ross, A. Arnold, P. Sleight, J. Probstfield, and G. R. Dagenais. 2005. Effects of long-term vitamin E supplementation on cardiovascular events and cancer: A randomized controlled trial. *JAMA* 293 (11): 1338–1347.
27. Dagenais, G. R., Q. Yi, E. Lonn, P. Sleight, J. Ostergren, and S. Yusuf. 2005. Impact of cigarette smoking in high-risk patients participating in a clinical trial. A substudy from the Heart Outcomes Prevention Evaluation (HOPE) trial. *Eur J Cardiovasc Prev Rehabil* 12 (1): 75–81.
28. Weinberg, R. B., B. S. VanderWerken, R. A. Anderson, J. E. Stegner, and M. J. Thomas. 2001. Pro-oxidant effect of vitamin E in cigarette smokers consuming a high polyunsaturated fat diet. *Arterioscler Thromb Vasc Biol* 21 (6): 1029–1033.
29. Blankenberg, S., M. J. McQueen, M. Smieja, J. Pogue, C. Balion, E. Lonn, H. J. Rupprecht et al. 2006. Comparative impact of multiple biomarkers and N-terminal pro-brain natriuretic peptide in the context of conventional risk factors for the prediction of recurrent cardiovascular events in the Heart Outcomes Prevention Evaluation (HOPE) Study. *Circulation* 114 (3): 201–208.
30. Isaac, M. G., R. Quinn, and N. Tabet. 2008. Vitamin E for Alzheimer's disease and mild cognitive impairment. *Cochrane Database Syst Rev* (3): CD002854.
31. Sano, M., C. Ernesto, R. G. Thomas, M. R. Klauber, K. Schafer, M. Grundman, P. Woodbury, et al. 1997. A controlled trial of selegiline, alpha-tocopherol, or both as treatment for Alzheimer's disease. The Alzheimer's Disease Cooperative Study. *N Engl J Med* 336 (17): 1216–1222.
32. Shoulson, I. 1998. DATATOP: A decade of neuroprotective inquiry. Parkinson Study Group. Deprenyl and Tocopherol Antioxidative Therapy of Parkinsonism. *Ann Neurol* 44 (3 Suppl 1): S160–S166.
33. Group, T. P. S. 1993. Effects of tocopherol and deprenyl on the progression of disability in early Parkinson's disease. *N Engl J Med* 328: 176–183.
34. Prasad, K. N., and R. Kumar. 1996. Effect of individual and multiple antioxidant vitamins on growth and morphology of human nontumorigenic and tumorigenic parotid acinar cells in culture. *Nutr Cancer* 26 (1): 11–19.
35. Lamm, D. L., D. R. Riggs, J. S. Shriver, P. F. vanGilder, J. F. Rach, and J. I. DeHaven. 1994. Megadose vitamins in bladder cancer: A double-blind clinical trial. *J Urol* 151 (1): 21–26.
36. Roncucci, L., P. Di Donato, L. Carati, A. Ferrari, M. Perini, G. Bertoni, G. Bedogni et al. 1993. Antioxidant vitamins or lactulose for the prevention of the recurrence of colorectal adenomas. Colorectal Cancer Study Group of the University of Modena and the Health Care District 16. *Dis Colon Rectum* 36 (3): 227–234.
37. Greenberg, E. R., J. A. Baron, T. D. Tosteson, D. H. Freeman Jr., G. J. Beck, J. H. Bond, T. A. Colacchio et al. 1994. A clinical trial of antioxidant vitamins to prevent colorectal adenoma. Polyp Prevention Study Group. *N Engl J Med* 331 (3): 141–147.
38. DeCosse, J. J., H. H. Miller, and M. L. Lesser. 1989. Effect of wheat fiber and vitamins C and E on rectal polyps in patients with familial adenomatous polyposis. *J Natl Cancer Inst* 81 (17): 1290–1297.
39. Blot, W. J., J. Y. Li, P. R. Taylor, W. Guo, S. Dawsey, G. Q. Wang, C. S. Yang et al. 1993. Nutrition intervention trials in Linxian, China: Supplementation with specific vitamin/mineral combinations, cancer incidence, and disease-specific mortality in the general population. *J Natl Cancer Inst* 85 (18): 1483–1492.
40. Qiao, Y. L., S. M. Dawsey, F. Kamangar, J. H. Fan, C. C. Abnet, X. D. Sun, L. L. Johnson et al. 2009. Total and cancer mortality after supplementation with vitamins and minerals: Follow-up of the Linxian General Population Nutrition Intervention Trial. *J Natl Cancer Inst* 101 (7): 507–518.
41. Biasco, G., and G. M. Paganelli. 1999. European trials on dietary supplementation for cancer prevention. *Ann N Y Acad Sci* 889: 152–156.
42. Hoenjet, K. M., P. C. Dagnelie, K. P. Delaere, N. E. Wijckmans, J. V. Zambon, and G. O. Oosterhof. 2005. Effect of a nutritional supplement containing vitamin E, selenium, vitamin C and coenzyme Q_{10} on serum PSA in patients with hormonally untreated carcinoma of the prostate: A randomised placebo-controlled study. *Eur Urol* 47 (4): 433–439; discussion 439–440.
43. Lippman, S. M., E. A. Klein, P. J. Goodman, M. S. Lucia, I. M. Thompson, L. G. Ford, H. L. Parnes et al. 2009. Effect of selenium and vitamin E on risk of prostate cancer and other cancers: The Selenium and Vitamin E Cancer Prevention Trial (SELECT). *JAMA* 301 (1): 39–51.
44. Beresford, S. A., K. C. Johnson, C. Ritenbaugh, N. L. Lasser, L. G. Snetselaar, H. R. Black, G. L. Anderson et al. 2006. Low-fat dietary pattern and risk of colorectal cancer: The Women's Health Initiative Randomized Controlled Dietary Modification Trial. *JAMA* 295 (6): 643–654.

45. Shike, M., L. Latkany, E. Riedel, M. Fleisher, A. Schatzkin, E. Lanza, D. Corle, and C. B. Begg. 2002. Lack of effect of a low-fat, high-fruit, -vegetable, and -fiber diet on serum prostate-specific antigen of men without prostate cancer: Results from a randomized trial. *J Clin Oncol* 20 (17): 3592–3598.
46. Alberts, D. S., M. E. Martinez, D. J. Roe, J. M. Guillen-Rodriguez, J. R. Marshall, J. B. van Leeuwen et al. 2000. Lack of effect of a high-fiber cereal supplement on the recurrence of colorectal adenomas. Phoenix Colon Cancer Prevention Physicians' Network. *N Engl J Med* 342 (16): 1156–1162.
47. Pierce, J. P., L. Natarajan, B. J. Caan, B. A. Parker, E. R. Greenberg, S. W. Flatt, C. L. Rock et al. 2007. Influence of a diet very high in vegetables, fruit, and fiber and low in fat on prognosis following treatment for breast cancer: The Women's Healthy Eating and Living (WHEL) randomized trial. *JAMA* 298 (3): 289–298.
48. Prasad, K. N. 2003. Antioxidants in cancer care: When and how to use them as an adjunct to standard and experimental therapies. *Expert Rev Anticancer Ther* 3 (6): 903–915.
49. Ishitani, K., J. Lin, J. E. Manson, J. E. Buring, and S. M. Zhang. 2008. Caffeine consumption and the risk of breast cancer in a large prospective cohort of women. *Arch Intern Med* 168 (18): 2022–2031.
50. Carter, C. A., M. Pogribny, A. Davidson, C. D. Jackson, L. J. McGarrity, and S. M. Morris. 1996. Effects of retinoic acid on cell differentiation and reversion toward normal in human endometrial adenocarcinoma (RL95-2) cells. *Anticancer Res* 16 (1): 17–24.
51. Meyskens, F. J. 1995. Role of vitamin A and its derivatives in the treatment of human cancer. In *Nutrients in Cancer Prevention and Treatment*, ed. K. N. Prasad and R. M. Williams. Totawa, NJ: Humana Press. pp. 349–362.
52. Krinsky, N. I. 1989. Antioxidant functions of carotenoids. *Free Radic Biol Med* 7 (6): 617–635.

4 Micronutrients in Healthy Aging

INTRODUCTION

Aging in humans is the result of complex biological processes that are influenced by genetics and environmental, dietary, and lifestyle-related factors. Aging in general terms can be defined as a process in which the function of individual organs gradually declines. Most chronic diseases in humans are a reflection of deterioration of the function of individual organs, each of which loses its function at a different rate, depending on genetics and environmental, dietary, and lifestyle-related stressors. The higher the levels of one or more of these stressors, the greater would be the rate of loss of organ function. Individual organs may exhibit differential sensitivity to these stressors; therefore, loss of function in the individual organs may appear at a different rate. The loss of function of cholinergic neurons in the brain can lead to Alzheimer's disease (AD), just as dopaminergic neurons in the brain can lead to Parkinson's disease. In the case of familial gene defects, the processes of loss of function in these neurons are accelerated; therefore, these neurological diseases appear at an early age.

The loss of function in one organ may seriously affect other organs, eventually causing death. For example, damage to the vascular system such as occlusion of major arteries can cause damage to the heart muscle that can lead to death. Similarly, cancer, in which cells gain function, should not be considered part of the normal aging process. Such causes of death should not be taken into consideration when estimating the life span of a population.

Aging on the cellular level has been defined on the basis of programmed cell death, which presumes that all cells are genetically programmed to die within a specified time and that no intervention with pharmacological or physiological agents can change this destiny. However, the concept of programmed cell death can be applicable to those dividing cells that are eliminated during embryogenesis, and also those adult precursor cells that divide, differentiate cells, and die within a specified time interval. These precursor cells have a finite life span that varies depending on the organ. I suggest that the concept of programmed cell death should not apply to nondividing cells such as liver cells, muscle cells, and neurons. In these cells, it is the accumulation of the level of epigenetic damage, rather than the genetic damage that determines the rate of cell death. The epigenetic damages include mitochondrial dysfunction, reduction of proteasome activity, and oxidation and nitration of proteins that progress gradually and eventually lead to cell death. The extent of epigenetic damage is dependent on the levels of exposure to environmental, dietary, and lifestyle-related stressors.

Aging on the genetic level is difficult to define. This is because of the fact that complex regulatory mechanisms of gene expressions, phosphorylation of certain proteins, and translocation of some proteins from one compartment to another within the same cell are altered during aging.

Healthy aging is defined as a process during which the rate of loss of organ function is markedly reduced; thereby, providing a good quality of life for a long period of time. At present, it is unknown whether the rate of normal aging can be reduced by intervening with pharmacological or physiological agents. Despite decades of laboratory research, it has not been possible to develop a rational guideline for healthy aging (reduced rate of loss of function). Among various biochemical and genetic changes that can influence the rate of aging, oxidative stress and proinflammatory cytokines released during chronic inflammation appear to play a dominant role in determining the rate of aging in humans. If this is the case, supplementation with nontoxic agents that can reduce oxidative stress and chronic inflammation would reduce the rate of aging. The linkage between the increased oxidative stress and aging appears to be also applicable to lower organisms, such as *Drosophila melanogaster*, nematodes, and birds. This chapter discusses the role of oxidative stress and chronic inflammation in affecting the rate of aging, the role of individual antioxidants in reducing oxidative stress and chronic inflammation, and the rationale for recommending multiple micronutrients containing dietary and endogenous antioxidants together with modifications in diet and lifestyle for healthy aging.

OXIDATIVE STRESS DURING AGING

Increased production of free radicals causes oxidative damage to cells. This damage is referred to as oxidative stress. Among various theories of aging, the free radical theory has strong support from data obtained from different organisms including flies, birds, and mammals, including humans. This theory proposes that increased production of free radicals by mitochondria contributes to the cellular damage that occurs with age.[1,2] The mitochondria are the main site where free radicals are generated during generation of ATP. During normal aerobic respiration, the mitochondria of one nerve cell of a rat will process about 10^{12} oxygen molecules and reduce them to water. During this process, superoxide anion ($O_2^{\cdot-}$), hydrogen peroxide (H_2O_2) and hydroxyl ($OH^{\cdot}$) radicals are produced. It has been estimated that about 2% of the partially reduced oxygen leaks out from the mitochondria to generate approximately 20 billion molecules of superoxide anion and hydrogen peroxide per cell.[3,4] The mitochondria are very susceptible to oxidative damage because the mitochondrial DNA (mtDNA) is not protected by histones or DNA-binding proteins. Therefore, it is not surprising that they are easily damaged by free radicals during aging. The damaged mitochondria can produce more free radicals. The role of oxidative stress in aging has been reviewed.[5,6] Based on published studies, I propose that free radical-induced damage to mitochondria is the first damage that initiates the cascade of events such as more production of free radicals, shortening of telomeres, and reduced proteasome activity and immune function that are associated with aging. These cellular abnormalities contribute to age-related decline in organ function and chronic diseases.

Sources of Oxidative Stress

Mitochondria remain the main site where free radicals derived from oxygen and nitrogen are generated.[4,7,8] They include superoxide (O_2^-), hydrogen peroxide (H_2O_2), hydroxyl radical ($HO^{\cdot}$), and nitric oxide ($NO^{\cdot}$). The oxidation of $NO^{\cdot}$ forms another type of free radical called peroxynitrite, which is very damaging to cells, especially nerve cells.

Phagocytes also produce free radicals that include superoxide, hydrogen peroxide, nitric oxide (NO), and hypochlorous (HOCl).[7,9,10] Hypochlorous is a strong inducer of inflammation and also acts as a strong oxidizing and chlorinating agent and can form nitryl chloride (NO_2Cl) and nitrogen dioxide ($NO_2^{\cdot}$), in the presence of nitrite,[11] all of which are toxic to cells. In addition to phagocytes, activated human polymorphonuclear neutrophils convert nitrite into NO_2Cl and $NO_2^{\cdot}$.[12] Thus, increased production of reactive oxygen, reactive nitrogen, and chlorinated species that can increase oxidative stress could increase the rate of aging.

Influence of Environmental, Dietary, Metabolic, and Lifestyle-Related Stressors on Oxidative Stress

Environmental stressors that can increase oxidative stress in humans include extreme heat and cold, high levels of ozone in air, excessive amounts of dust particles in air, intense sound or vibration, and pathogenic bacteria or viruses. Dietary factors include high caloric intake, daily consumption of increased amounts of iron or copper, and ingestion of xenobiotic substances. Free radicals are produced during the normal metabolism of certain compounds. During the degradation of fatty acids and oxidative metabolism of ingested xenobiotic substances, free radicals are produced. Some enzymes during their normal degradation of their substrates generate free radicals. Monoamine oxidase, tyrosine hydroxylase, and L-amino acid oxidases produce hydrogen peroxide as a normal byproduct of their activity.[13] Other enzymes such as xanthine oxidase and aldehyde oxidase also form superoxide anions during metabolism of their substrates. Auto-oxidation of ascorbate and catecholamines generate free radicals.[14] Calcium-dependent activation of phospholipase A_2 releases arachidonic acid, which liberates $O_2^{\cdot-}$ during the synthesis of eicosanoids.[15] Stimulation of glutamate receptor NMDA (N-methyl-D-aspartate) produces excessive amounts of $O_2^{\cdot-}$ and $OH^{\cdot}$.[16] Certain lifestyle-related factors such as cigarette smoking can increase the level of NO[17,18] and the oxidation of NO produces peroxynitrite, a highly reactive species of radicals. Smoking also depletes antioxidants,[19,20] and, thereby, further increases the oxidative stress in smokers. Free iron and copper also can increase oxidative stress by combining with molecules like vitamin C.[21]

In addition to reactive oxygen and nitrogen species, there are other damaging molecules produced by lipid peroxidation. For example, peroxidation of membrane phospholipids acyl chains generates reactive carbonyl species (alpha and beta-unsaturated aldehydes, di-aldehydes, and keto-aldehydes), which are relatively stable. These carbonyl species can diffuse from one subcellular compartment to another within the same cell or they can escape from the cells and damage targets far away from the site of formation. These carbonyl species react with cellular constituents and form advanced lipoxidation end products (ALEs), and they play an important role in accelerating the aging process.[22] This is supported by the fact that the level of ALEs in several tissues and species increases with age, and a dietary restriction that increases the life span decreases the levels of ALEs.

The oxidation and nitration of intracellular proteins play an important role in aging because they can induce loss of function.[23] The oxidized proteins can easily form aggregates that also contribute to the loss of cell function. Normally, damaged proteins are removed by the proteosome pathway; however, if this pathway is impaired, these damaged proteins will accumulate to cause progressive loss in cell function and, eventually, cell death. A progressive increase in oxidative stress in the brain is strongly implicated in the gradual decline of cognitive function with aging.

Heavy metals at high concentrations are toxic to humans and animals. Metal homeostasis is regulated by a metal-responsive transcriptional factor (MTF-1). Mutation in the MTF-1 reduced the life span of *D. melanogaster*, suggesting that the wild-type MTF-1 is an essential component for maintaining the normal life span. The overexpression of MTF-1 in neurons protects against oxidative damage and prolongs the life span of Cu/Zn superoxide-dismutase–deficient flies.[24]

OXIDATIVE STRESS INFLUENCES MITOCHONDRIA, LYSOSOME, AND PROTEASOME FUNCTION DURING AGING

Among various organelles in the cells, mitochondria exhibit unique functions. They are present in all cells, but most abundantly in nondividing cells such as liver cells, neurons, and muscle cells. Their main function is to generate energy. However, they are the major source of free radicals derived from oxygen and nitrogen and, at the same time, they are very vulnerable to free radicals. Damaged mitochondria produce more free radicals, and this creates a vicious cycle of damage by free radicals and production of more free radicals.

Mitochondrial Dysfunction

Various organs may age at a different rate depending on the levels of oxidative damage to the mitochondria in the individual cells of that organ. Several studies suggest that damage to mitochondria may initiate degenerative changes in the cells during the aging of at least nondividing organs such as liver, brain, muscle, and bone. Several animal studies have shown that age-associated increases in the generation of free radicals by mitochondria occur. For example, the levels of $O_2^{\bullet-}$ and H_2O_2 increased with age in mitochondria isolated from aged hearts of gerbils.[25] The generation of H_2O_2 by mitochondria from older hepatocyte of rats increases by 23%.[26] In the house fly, the rate of the production of H_2O_2 progressively increases with age.[27]

The increased production of free radicals by mitochondria with age may cause an increased rate of mutation in mtDNA and oxidative damage to proteins. Indeed, it has been proposed that mutations in mitochondria may contribute to accelerated aging.[28] The mtDNA is especially sensitive to oxidative damage because it is not protected by histones or by DNA-binding proteins. It also has either no repair mechanisms or repair mechanisms that are less efficient in comparison to nuclear DNA.[29] The progressive damage to mitochondria may reduce the production of energy and, therefore, can cause progressive degenerative changes in the cells during aging and, eventually, the loss of function of the organs involved. Mitochondrial dysfunction leads to reduced life span in yeast.[30] In mammals, aged tissue produces reduced amounts of ATP by oxidative phosphorylation.[31] Indeed, aging of the mammalian brain exhibits a gradual but continuous decrease in production of ATP by oxidative phosphorylation in the mitochondria.[32]

Mitochondrial dysfunction also plays a major role in vascular aging.[33,34] Vascular aging is primarily characterized by an impaired endothelium-dependent vasodilation that is regulated by NO. The expression of endothelial nitric oxide synthase (eNOS) is markedly up-regulated in the endothelial cells with increasing age, resulting in production of excessive amounts of NO. Increased levels of super oxide (O_2^-) are also produced. The combination of superoxide and NO can form peroxynitrite ($ONOO^-$). Peroxynitrite causes oxidative modification of proteins that contributes to vascular aging.

The plasma cysteine/acid soluble thiol ratio, an indicator of redox state, is increased in old age and this may account for the loss of body cell mass that is associated with aging in humans. This is further supported by the fact that supplementation with N-acetylcysteine (NAC) caused an increase in body cell mass of healthy subjects with a high plasma cysteine/thiol ratio.[35,36] Increased oxidative stress and mitochondrial dysfunction are also associated with some age-related neurological diseases such as AD and Parkinson disease,[37-39] as well as the genetic basis of these neurological diseases.

Impairment of Proteasome and Lysosomal-Mediated Proteolytic Activities

Progressive loss of muscle mass (sarcopenia) during aging occurs in both humans and rodents. There could be several reasons for this. It has been proposed that reduced degradation of oxidized proteins may be one of the factors that contribute to sarcopenia.[40] The cells can respond successfully to the oxidative damage of proteins only when the ability of proteasome and lysosome to degrade altered proteins remains intact. Increased oxidative stress can impair proteasome activity as well as lysosomal-mediated proteolytic activity. Indeed, during aging, these two biological processes are impaired.[40-43]

OXIDATIVE STRESS INFLUENCES THE LENGTH OF TELOMERE DURING AGING

The data on the role of telomere in human aging come primarily from normal human fibroblasts or other normal cells in culture. These studies suggest that telomere-shortening is associated with aging and that increased oxidative stress accelerates its rate.[44,45] Increased oxidative stress induces translocation of nuclear telomerase reverse transcriptase (TERT) from the nucleus to the cytoplasm.[46] Treatment with NAC reduced the translocation of nuclear TERT from the nucleus to the cytoplasm.[46] The increase in oxidative stress caused premature aging of normal endothelial cells in culture. The role of oxidative stress in telomere-shortening is further supported by the fact that the dietary antioxidants vitamin C[47] and vitamin E[48] reduced the rate of telomere-shortening. These studies suggest that increased oxidative stress causes shortening of telomeres and that it is possible to prevent this shortening by protecting the telomeres from oxidative damage. Daily supplementation with antioxidants is likely to reduce the rate of shortening of the length of telomeres and, thereby, slow down the rate of aging.

CHRONIC INFLAMMATION DURING AGING

During chronic inflammation, proinflammatory cytokines such as tumor necrosis factor-alpha (TNF-alpha), and interleukin-6 (IL-6) are released. Prostaglandins, adhesion molecules, and complement proteins are also released, all of which are toxic to the cells. The increased levels of these products in chronic inflammation can enhance the rate of degenerative changes in the cells and enhance the rate of aging and the risk of chronic diseases. The microglia in the aged brain has increased levels of the proinflammatory cytokine, TNF-alpha.[49] Treatment with TNF-alpha plus beta-amyloid (Ab-42), a fragment of amyloid precursor protein (APP), caused more toxicity in the older neurons than in the younger neurons.[49] It has been suggested[50] that TNF-alpha treatment caused nuclear translocation of nuclear factor kappa-beta (NF-kappa-B) in neurons. This phenomenon, together with the lower level of Bcl-2, promoted cell death in older neurons.[50] It has been reported that treatment of neurons obtained from middle-aged rats with TNF-alpha and Ab-42 increased TNF receptors (TNFR1 and TNFR2); however, similarly treated older neurons do not increase these surface receptors of TNF-alpha.[51] Chronic inflammation also has been linked with several age-related neurological disorders such as AD, cardiovascular disease, and type 2 diabetes.[38,52]

Increased mitochondrial oxidative stress activates NF-kappa-B in the endothelial cells of blood vessels that enhances the expression of inflammatory genes.[53] Age-related increases in oxidative stress may promote vascular inflammation.[54] Thus, aged blood vessels exhibit increased NF-kappaB activity. This was attributed to increased oxidative stress that occurs during aging.[53]

Higher plasma concentrations of IL-6 and TNF-alpha are associated with lower muscle mass and lower muscle strength in well-functioning older men and women.[55] This suggests that proinflammatory cytokines contribute to the loss of muscle mass and muscle strength that are associated with aging. In another study, higher plasma levels of IL-6 and C-reactive proteins increased the risk of loss of muscle strength in older men and women, whereas higher levels of alpha1-antichymotrypsin decreased the risk of muscle strength loss.[56] Higher plasma levels of IL-6 predict onset of disability in older individuals.[57] This may be due to the fact that increased levels of IL-6 contribute to muscle atrophy and may increase the risk of certain chronic diseases.

AGING INFLUENCES IMMUNE FUNCTION

Phagocytes are one of the major sources of free radicals and represent one of the functions of the immune system. Normally, phagocytes attack and eliminate invading pathogenic organisms by generating excessive amounts of oxidants such as superoxide ($O^{\cdot-}$), nitric oxide ($NO^{\cdot}$), H_2O_2, and HOCl, and engulfing through phagocytosis. The engulfed microorganisms are killed and eliminated by a combination of oxidants and lysosomal digestive enzymes.[58]

It has been reported that oxidant production is a function of aging. For example, older macrophages produce reduced levels of oxidants,[59–61] suggesting that the phagocytic activity of macrophages may be reduced in older individuals. Others have reported that production of reactive oxygen species appears to increase in older peritoneal macrophages.[62]

In mice, the antitumor activity of macrophages is reduced in older animals.[63,64] Furthermore, macrophages from old mice were less responsive to the activation signals of lipopolysaccharide (LPS) plus interferon-gamma (INF-gamma) for macrophage-mediated tumoricidal activity.[65] It has been shown that natural killer (NK) activity decreases as a function of age,[66] and that this activity can be suppressed by adherent cells from the spleen and peritoneal cavity. The decline in NK activity found in older mice is due to an increase in the suppressor function of adherent cells.[66] These studies suggest that the immune functions are impaired in older individuals, possibly because of increased oxidative damage caused by free radicals and proinflammatory cytokines.

AGING INFLUENCING ANTIOXIDANT DEFENSE SYSTEMS

ANTIOXIDANT ENZYMES

Antioxidant enzymes, represented by glutathione peroxidase, catalase, and cytosolic Cu/Zn-SOD and mitochondrial Mn-SOD, play an important role in protecting cells against oxidative damage. Glutathione peroxidase is one of the major antioxidant enzymes that neutralize hydrogen peroxide and lipid peroxide and is present in both cytosol and mitochondria. Catalase found in cytosol and mitochondria also metabolized H_2O_2 into water and oxygen. There are two forms of SOD distributed differently within the cell. Cu/Zn-SOD is present in the cytosol, whereas Mn-SOD is present in the mitochondria. Some of these enzymes respond to increased oxidative stress by elevating their activities. This response is referred to as an adaptive response that is an indicator of the presence of high oxidative stress in the cells. However, the activities of some of these antioxidant enzymes may not change or may even decline as a function of aging.

Changes in Antioxidant Enzyme Activities in Animals

Changes in the activities of antioxidant enzymes in animals (primarily rodents) as a function of aging vary, depending on the organs. It has been reported that antioxidant enzymes activities gradually increase as a function of aging in the skeletal muscle of rats.[67] The increase in the activity of catalase in the heart, skeletal muscle, brain, and Cu/Zn-SOD in the skeletal muscle was observed in rats.[67,68] The increase in antioxidant enzyme activities is considered an adaptive response to the increased oxidative stress because markers of oxidative damage and chronic inflammation are elevated in spite of an increase in activities of antioxidant enzymes. These studies suggest that the increased levels of certain antioxidant enzymes are not sufficient to down-regulate the level of oxidative stress and chronic inflammation.

The activity of glutathione peroxidase in the brain and Cu/Zn SOD in the heart showed no significant changes in enzyme activity in rats as a function of aging.[68] However, in other organs such as the liver, brain, and heart, decreases in catalase activity were reported.[68] Prostaglandin E_2 (PGE2) is one of the toxic products released during chronic inflammation. PGA1, which is formed during extraction of PGE2, is stable and is used in experimental systems. We have reported that PGA1-induced degeneration of murine differentiated neurons increased the expression of the catalase gene and decreased the expression of the glutathione peroxidase and Mn-SOD genes without changing the expression of Cu/Zn-SOD as determined by gene array and confirmed by real time PCR.[69] The protein levels of glutathione peroxidase increased, whereas the protein level of Mn-SOD decreased and the levels of catalase and Cu/Zn-SOD did not change as determined by the Western blot.[69]

The activities of antioxidant enzymes as a function of aging vary in different organs. The phenomenon of adaptive response to increased oxidative stress was observed for only certain antioxidant enzymes and in certain organs. The markers of oxidative damage and chronic inflammation were elevated, and immune functions were impaired in older animals irrespective of changes in the activities of antioxidant enzymes. Thus, the increased activities of certain antioxidant enzymes are not sufficient to down-regulate increased oxidative stress and chronic inflammation. Additional studies are needed in which antioxidant enzyme activities and markers of oxidative damage and chronic inflammation are measured at the same time and in the same animals during aging.

Changes in Antioxidant Enzyme Activities in Humans

There is very limited information on changes in antioxidant enzyme activities as a function of aging in humans. However, based on a few studies, it appears that changes in enzyme activities as a function of aging are, in part, different from those observed in rodents. One major difference is that the adaptive response of certain antioxidant enzymes to increased oxidative stress that is found in rodents has not been observed in humans thus far. In older humans, the serum concentrations of SOD, glutathione peroxidase, and albumin were lower than those found in younger individuals, but the activity of catalase did not change.[70] The total antioxidant capacity decreased and the level of lipid peroxides increased in older subjects, as compared to younger ones.[70] In another study, the activities of catalase and SOD in serum did not change as a function of aging; however, the activity of glutathione peroxidase declined in older subjects.[71] Furthermore, age-related increases in lipid peroxidation and protein oxidation were observed.[71] In human skeletal muscle, total SOD decreased as a function of aging, although Mn-SOD increased in older individuals.[72] The activities of catalase and glutathione peroxidase did not change.[72] These observations are opposite those observed in the skeletal muscle of rats.[67] Thus, the results on changes in antioxidant enzyme activities in rodents cannot be extrapolated to humans, in whom no increase in enzyme activity as an adaptive response to increased oxidative stress was observed. This may be due to the fact that the adaptive response of enzymes to increased oxidative stress in humans is very resistant to damage or that the increased levels of oxidative damage in humans overwhelms the adaptive response of antioxidant enzymes.

In an older individual with a disease, the changes in antioxidant enzyme activity were different from those found in older individuals without the disease. It is established that age-related macular degeneration (AMD) is the leading cause of irreversible blindness in developed countries. It appears that an increase in oxidative stress and a decrease in certain antioxidant enzymes play an important role in the pathophysiology of AMD. It has been reported that SOD and glutathione peroxidase were lower in both the plasma and RBC of patients with maculopathy in comparison to those found in age- and sex-matched control subjects; however, the catalase activity in RBC remained unchanged.[73] The activity of alpha-ketoglutarate dehydrogenase complex (KGDHC), a mitochondrial enzyme, is decreased in the brains of AD patients compared to matched control subjects.[74] It is interesting to observe that, in AD patients who carry the ApoE4 allele of the ApoE gene, the Clinical Dementia Rating (CDR) correlated better with KGDHC activity than with the densities of extracellular neuritic plaques and intracellular neurofibrillary tangles. However, in patients with AD who do not carry the ApoE4 allele, the CDR correlated better with the densities of extracellular neuritic plaques and intracellular neurofibrillary tangles. The activity of glutamine synthetase decreased in the autopsied samples of the brain of AD patients,[75] and the levels of glutathione peroxidase in ventricular cerebral spinal fluid also decreased in AD patients compared to age-matched control subjects.[76] Substantia nigra samples from autopsied brains of patients with Parkinson's disease showed reduced levels of antioxidant enzymes.[77,78] These studies suggest that the activities of certain antioxidant enzymes in the brain of patients with neurodegenerative diseases decline more than those found in age-matched control subjects.

DIETARY AND ENDOGENOUS ANTIOXIDANT LEVELS

In addition to antioxidant enzymes, dietary [vitamin A, beta-carotene (BC), vitamin C, vitamin E, and selenium] and endogenous (glutathione, coenzyme Q_{10}, L-carnitine, and alpha-lipoic acid) antioxidants play an important role in reducing oxidative stress and chronic inflammation. The organ, cellular, and subcellular distributions of these antioxidants appear to be highly variable for the same antioxidant. The levels of different dietary and endogenous antioxidants also differ in their distributions. Therefore, measurements of the plasma, whole tissue, or cell levels may not be true reflections of changes in the levels of antioxidants in the subcellular fractions that may be critical in determining the rate of progression of aging or the risk of age-related chronic diseases. The levels of different antioxidants distributed in the subcellular fractions of most mammals (primarily rodents) may be different from those found in humans because most mammals, except guinea pigs, synthesize their own vitamin C, which could affect the level of other antioxidants in the body. Therefore, it is impossible to extrapolate the value of antioxidant levels obtained from the animal studies to humans. Most studies in animals or humans have measured antioxidant levels primarily in plasma.

Vitamin C

Vitamin C is a water-soluble antioxidant that has multiple biological functions. One of them includes regeneration of oxidized glutathione and vitamin E to reduced form in order to maintain their antioxidant function. The plasma level of vitamin C declines as a function of age in various species.[33,79–81] This result cannot be extrapolated to humans because they do not synthesize their own vitamin C; they primarily rely on dietary sources for vitamin C, and consumption of this vitamin is highly variable among the U.S. population. Therefore, changes in the vitamin C levels as a function of aging are meaningless with respect to its role in aging. This is further compounded by the fact that the plasma half-life of vitamin C is rather short (a few hours).

Glutathione

Glutathione is also a water-soluble antioxidant present in cells in millimolar concentrations. It maintains glutathione peroxidase activity and prevents oxidation of vitamin E and vitamin C, along with several other functions. Some studies have shown that glutathione levels increase in the brain of mice as a function of aging,[82,83] but others have reported no significant change in the brains of old rats.[84] Increased glutathione levels have been found in the plasma, heart, and liver.[83,84] Some studies have reported that the level of glutathione in the skeletal muscle increases as a function of aging.[67,83] Other studies have reported no change in the level of glutathione in the liver of rodents.[83,85,86] In contrast, some studies have reported a decline in glutathione levels in the brain[85,86] and eye lens[81] as a function of aging. These studies suggest that the levels of glutathione in most tissues of rodents increase or show no significant change as a function of aging. In contrast to the level of glutathione found in whole tissues of rodents, the levels in the subcellular fractions consistently showed declines as a function of aging. For example, the level of glutathione in the cerebral cortex synaptosomes[87] and mitochondria of the liver, kidney, and brain[88] declined as a function of aging. In a model of prematurely aging mice, the level of glutathione decreased and the level of melondialdehyde (MDA) increased in comparison to normal mice.[89]

Changes in the level of glutathione as a function of aging are not available in humans; however, in age-related diseases such as Parkinson's disease, the autopsied brain tissues consistently show declines in the level of glutathione.[90–92] The serum levels of vitamins A, E, and BC were lower in (well-nourished) patients with AD.[93]

Vitamin E

Like the levels of water-soluble antioxidants, the lipid soluble antioxidant vitamin E level also revealed variable changes in rodents as a function of aging. For example, vitamin E levels increased in certain regions of the brain, lung, and liver,[94] aortic wall of the blood vessel,[33] and serum.[95] There was, however, no change in vitamin E levels in the heart,[96] liver,[79] blood,[97] and membranes.[95] There was a decline in the levels in plasma[79] and in the substantia nigra region of the brain[98] as a function of aging. These studies suggest that the level of vitamin E increased, decreased, and also showed no changes as a function of aging in most studies in rodents.

In elderly humans, the plasma level of vitamin E declined by 70% from that of younger subjects, whereas the plasma level of retinol did not change significantly. However, on the basis of the ratio of lipid-adjusted vitamin E to plasma lipids, only 12% showed declines in vitamin E levels.[99] No data are available on changes in tissue vitamin E levels as a function of aging.

Coenzyme Q_{10}

Coenzyme Q_{10} recycles vitamin C and vitamin E. Tissue levels of coenzyme Q_{10} decrease with age.[98] Many studies with rodents revealed that the activities of antioxidant enzymes and the levels of certain antioxidants (vitamin E and glutathione) increased as a function of aging, although some studies reported no changes or decline in their levels. How can one explain the existence of increased oxidative stress and increased levels of certain markers of proinflammatory cytokines (tumor necrosis factor-alpha and IL-6) in the presence of increased, decreased, or no change in antioxidant enzymes and antioxidants? I propose that the increased physiological activity of antioxidant enzymes or antioxidant level is not sufficient to decrease oxidative stress or chronic inflammation. To reduce these two biological processes that play a crucial role in aging and age-related chronic diseases, pharmacological doses of dietary and endogenous antioxidants are needed. Indeed, supplementation with high doses of one or more dietary or endogenous antioxidants decreased oxidative stress and chronic inflammation in rodents. These studies are described below.

ANTIOXIDANT SUPPLEMENTATION INFLUENCES AGE-RELATED FUNCTIONAL DEFICITS

VITAMIN E

Supplementation with vitamin E restores mitochondrial dysfunction (to produce ATP by oxidative phosphorylation) in aged brains and livers.[31] In healthy elderly humans, supplementation with vitamin E and fish oil was more effective in reducing the levels of proinflammatory cytokines (IL-6 and tumor necrosis factor-alpha) than fish oil alone.[100] Age-dependent loss of T helper 1 (Th1) cytokines, especially INF-gamma that plays an important role in defending against influenza infection, occurs.[101] The production of PGE2 that suppresses Th1 cytokines increases with age in mice. Vitamin E supplementation reduced influenza titer in old mice. This antiviral effect of vitamin E is mediated through reduced production of PGE2 and enhanced production of Th1 cytokines.[101] Other antioxidants such as glutathione, melatonin, or strawberry extract, which reduced oxidative stress, did not affect the level of influenza titer.[102]

Vitamin E supplementation increased the activity of SOD in old trainee rats; however, exercise alone failed to increase SOD activity and reduce oxidative damage in these older animals.[103] It has been shown that vitamin supplementation plus exercise improved age-related deficits in antioxidant enzymes in the cerebral cortex and hippocampus regions of rat brains.[104] Age-related increases in lipid peroxidation and protein oxidation are reduced in the brain of older rats by vitamin E supplementation.[105] Reduced levels of SOD were found in the cerebral cortexes of old rats, where it was highest in the hippocampus region of the brain; however, vitamin E supplementation increased it.[105] Vitamin E, in combination with fish oil, reduced proinflammatory cytokines more than fish oil alone in healthy elderly subjects.[100] In contrast, the immune-enhancing effect of vitamin E alone was reduced in healthy elderly men and women when fish oil was taken concomitantly. This may be due to the fact that plasma levels of vitamin E increased by smaller amounts in the presence of fish oil.[106] From this one study, it appears that supplementation with fish oil interferes with the absorption of vitamin E. Additional studies are needed to substantiate this observation.

COENZYME Q_{10}

Supplementation with coenzyme Q_{10} prolonged the life span of animals fed a polyunsaturated fatty acids-6–enriched diet. It decreased oxidative stress and cardiovascular risk, and regulated inflammation during the aging process.[107,108] Combination of vitamin E and coenzyme Q_{10} improved age-related learning deficits in mice, but the individual agent failed to do so.[109] Administration of coenzyme Q_{10} increased the level of vitamin E in the mitochondria that was related to the regenerating effect of coenzyme Q_{10}.[110] In mice and rats, ingestion of coenzyme Q_{10} elevated coenzyme Q_9, the predominant homologue in mitochondria. It has been reported that the rate of mitochondrial superoxide anion radical generation is directly proportional to mitochondrial coenzyme Q_9 and inversely proportional to coenzyme Q_{10}.[111]

CAROTENOIDS

Intake of dietary lutein and zeaxanthin or zinc reduced the risk of age-related macular degeneration (AMD); however, higher consumption of BC was associated with increased risk of AMD.[112] Another study showed no effect of vitamin E or BC supplementation on the risk of AMD.[113]

MELATONIN

Supplementation with melatonin for 30 days reversed age-related retention deficits in mice.[114] Melatonin regulates circadian rhythms through hypothalamic suprachiasmatic nucleus (SCN). Age-related loss of sensitivity to melatonin occurs in the SCN of mice.[115]

FLAVONOIDS

Quercetin is a bioflavonoid that exhibits strong antioxidant properties. Supplementation with quercetin for 30 days reversed age-related retention deficits in mice.[116] Others have reported that supplementation with flavonoids (apigenin-7-glucoside and quercetin) reversed age-related and LPS-induced retention deficits in mice.[117]

GLUTATHIONE AND N-ACETYLCYSTEINE

In a model of prematurely aging mice, treatment with NAC plus thioproline increased chemotaxis, phagocytosis, and IL-beta release and decreased superoxide levels and TNF-alpha production.[118] This suggests that antioxidant supplementation can protect against early decline in immune function in prematurely aging mice. These antioxidants also reversed age-related behavioral dysfunction in prematurely aging mice.[119]

ALPHA-LIPOIC ACID

A combination of alpha-lipoic acid and acetyl-L-carnitine reduced mitochondrial decay and oxidative damage in rat brains during aging.[120] These results support many other studies discussed previously that show oxidative damage of mitochondria plays a central role in increasing the risk of age-related chronic diseases and functional deficits. Alpha-lipoic acid and acetyl-L-carnitine are substrates for mitochondrial enzyme carnitine acetyltransferase (CAT). In the brains of older rats, the activity of CAT and its binding affinity with substrates declined in comparison to younger rats.[121] Feeding old rats high doses of acetyl-L-carnitine and alpha-lipoic acid can ameliorate oxidative damage, CAT activity and its binding affinity with substrates, and mitochondrial dysfunction.[121]

MULTIPLE DIETARY ANTIOXIDANTS

The effects of supplementation with antioxidants (vitamin C, 500 mg; vitamin E, 400 IU; BC, 15 mg; zinc, 80 mg as zinc oxide; and copper, 2 mg as cupric oxide) or antioxidant plus zinc on AMD were investigated.[122] The results showed that antioxidants or zinc reduced the risk of developing advanced AMD in higher-risk groups; however, the combination was more effective than the individual agents. Diet supplementation with antioxidants protected against early decline in immune function and behavior in prematurely aging mice.[89] It has been shown that the macrophages of prematurely aging mice exhibit depressed chemotaxis and phagocytosis activity. However, supplementation with dietary antioxidants (vitamin C, vitamin E, BC, zinc, and selenium) decreased the levels of proinflammatory cytokines and improved the natural killing cell activity, lymphocyte chemotaxis activity, and proliferation response of lymphocytes to concanavalin A,[123] as well as decreased oxidative stress.[124] Dietary antioxidant supplementation protects immune function against oxidative damage and increases life span.[125] Psychomotor performance is decreased with aging, and this could be related to increased oxidative damage and increased levels of proinflammatory cytokine IL-6. Supplementation with dietary antioxidants improved psychomotor performance in old mice, and decreased the level of oxidative damage and IL-6.[126]

RATIONALE FOR NOT USING A SINGLE DIETARY ANTIOXIDANT TO REDUCE AGE-RELATED FUNCTIONAL DEFICITS

Animal studies with a single antioxidant have produced expected beneficial results in reducing the risk of diseases. However, the experimental paradigm of using a single antioxidant in humans at high risk of developing chronic diseases has produced inconsistent results varying from beneficial effects, to no effect, to harmful effects. Therefore, it should not be used in any future investigations in humans. The most widely quoted studies are those that were performed with BC in heavy tobacco smokers,[127–129] and those using vitamin E in high-risk heart disease.[130–132] The results showed that BC increased the risk of lung cancer,[127–129] and vitamin E increased the risk of heart failure and mortality in patients with heart disease, and secondary cancer in cancer survivors.[130–132] Based on the biology of individual antioxidants and the high internal oxidative environments in the individuals of high-risk populations, these results could have been predicted. It is known that an individual antioxidant, when oxidized, may act as a pro-oxidant. It is also known that heavy tobacco smokers, patients with heart disease, and cancer survivors have a high internal oxidative environment. Therefore, administration of a single antioxidant in these high-risk populations results in oxidation of this antioxidant, and thereby, increases the risk of chronic diseases. Therefore, conclusions drawn from these studies are inaccurate; nevertheless, they have remained major sources on which the recommendations for not taking antioxidant supplements are made by the physicians.

RATIONALE FOR RECOMMENDING MULTIPLE MICRONUTRIENTS TO REDUCE THE RATE OF AGING

The scientific rationale of using multiple micronutrients, including dietary and endogenous antioxidants, to reduce the rate of aging is described below. Several different types of free radicals are produced in the body, and each antioxidant has a different affinity for each of these free radicals, depending on the cellular environment. They exhibit different mechanisms of action. For example, BC was more effective in quenching oxygen radicals than most other antioxidants.[133] BC can perform certain biological functions that cannot be produced by its metabolite, vitamin A, and vice versa.[134,135] BC treatment enhanced the expression of the connexin gene, a gap junction protein gene, whereas vitamin A treatment did not produce such an effect.[135] Vitamin A induced cell differentiation in certain normal and cancer cells, whereas BC did not.[136,137] The gradient of oxygen pressure varies within the cell and tissues. Vitamin E was more effective as a quencher of free radicals in reduced oxygen pressure, whereas BC and vitamin A were more effective at higher atmospheric pressures.[138] Vitamin C is necessary to protect cellular components in aqueous environments, whereas carotenoids, and vitamins A and E protect cellular components in nonaqueous environments. Vitamin C also plays an important role in maintaining cellular levels of vitamin E by recycling the vitamin E radical (oxidized) to the reduced (antioxidant) form.[139] Also, the DNA damage produced by oxidized vitamin C can be ameliorated by vitamin E. The form and type of vitamin E used are also important to improve beneficial effects of vitamin E. It is known that various organs of rats selectively absorb the natural form of vitamin E.[140] It has been established that alpha tocopheryl-succinate (α-TS) is the most effective form of vitamin E.[141,142] We have reported that oral ingestion of α-TS (800 IU/day) for more than 6 months in humans increased plasma levels of not only α-tocopherol, but also of α-TS, suggesting that α-TS can be absorbed from the intestinal tract without hydrolysis to α-tocopherol, provided the pool of alpha-tocopherol in the body has become saturated.[142] Selenium, a cofactor of glutathione peroxidase, acts as an antioxidant. Therefore, selenium supplementation, together with other dietary and endogenous antioxidants, is also essential for healthy aging.

Glutathione, one of the endogenously made compounds, represents a potent intracellular protective agent against oxidative damage. It catabolizes H_2O_2 and anions and is very effective (in the presence of glutathione peroxidase) at quenching peroxynitrite.[143] Therefore, increasing the intracellular levels of glutathione may be important for maintaining healthy aging. Oral supplementation with glutathione failed to significantly increase plasma levels of glutathione in human subjects,[144] suggesting that this tripeptide is completely hydrolyzed in the gastrointestinal tract. NAC and alpha-lipoic acid increase the intracellular levels of glutathione, and therefore, they can also be used in combination with dietary antioxidants. Coenzyme Q_{10} is required for generating ATP by mitochondria. Mitochondrial dysfunction that is associated with aging may not have adequate amounts of coenzyme Q_{10}; therefore, supplementation with coenzyme Q_{10} may be necessary for maintaining healthy aging. It also scavenges peroxy radicals faster than α-tocopherol,[145] and, like vitamin C, can regenerate vitamin E in a redox cycle.[146] The inclusion of all B-vitamins into a multiple micronutrient preparation is needed for healthy aging.

RECOMMENDED MICRONUTRIENTS FOR ADULTS AND CHILDREN

A formulation of multiple micronutrients may include vitamin A (retinyl palmitate), vitamin E (both D-alpha-tocopherol and D-alpha-tocopheryl succinate), natural mixed carotenoids, vitamin C (calcium ascorbate), coenzyme Q_{10}, R-alpha-lipoic acid, NAC, L-carnitine, vitamin D, all B-vitamins, selenium, zinc, and chromium. No iron, copper, or manganese would be included because these trace minerals are known to interact with vitamin C to produce free radicals. These trace minerals are absorbed from the intestinal tract, more in the presence of antioxidants than in their absence, and that could result in increased body stores of the free forms of these minerals. Increased iron stores have been linked to increased risk of several chronic diseases.[114] Omega-3 fatty acids are included because they are known to have anti-inflammation effects. Antioxidants from herbs, fruits, and vegetables were not included because they do not produce any unique biological effects that cannot be produced by antioxidants and omega-3 fatty acids present in the micronutrient preparation.

The micronutrient preparation for children is similar to those for adults, except that the doses of each micronutrient are lower than those found in adult preparations, and that no omega-3 fatty acids are added. The recommended micronutrient supplements should be taken orally and be divided into two doses, half in the morning and the other half in the evening, with a meal. This is because the biological half-lives of micronutrients are highly variable, which can create high levels of fluctuation in the tissue levels of micronutrients. A twofold difference in the levels of certain micronutrients such as alpha-TS can cause a marked difference in the expression of gene profiles (our unpublished data). To maintain relatively consistent levels of micronutrients in the body, the proposed micronutrients should be taken twice a day.

The efficacy of this formulation in humans should be tested by well-designed clinical studies. Meanwhile, the proposed micronutrient recommendations may be adopted by the individuals in consultation with their physicians or health professionals. It is expected that the proposed recommendations would reduce the rate of aging.

CHANGES IN DIET AND LIFESTYLE

Dietary recommendations include consuming a daily low-fat, high-fiber diet with plenty of fresh fruits and vegetables, avoiding excessive amounts of protein, carbohydrates, and calories, and restricting intake of nitrite-rich cured meat, charcoal-broiled or smoked meat or fish, caffeine-containing beverages (cold or hot), and pickled fruits and vegetables.

Lifestyle-related changes include stopping smoking and chewing tobacco; avoiding secondhand smoke and overexposure to sun, UV light for tanning, and hyperbaric therapy for energy; restricting intake of alcohol; reducing stress by vacation, yoga, or meditation; and performing moderate exercise four to five times a week.

CONCLUSIONS

Increased oxidative stress caused by the generation of excessive amounts of free radicals and proinflammatory cytokines produced during chronic inflammation contribute to the age-related decline in organ function and chronic diseases. Mitochondria are not only the first target to be damaged by free radicals but they are also the most sensitive to oxidative stress. Damaged mitochondria produce more free radicals that initiate a cascade of events that reduce proteasome activity, the length of telomeres, and immune function, and improve lysosomal proteolytic activity.

Changes in the antioxidant enzymes during aging have been investigated more in rodents than in humans, and they are highly variable. In rodents, an increase, no change, or a decline in antioxidant enzyme activities in the presence of elevated levels of markers of oxidative damage and inflammation have been observed; however, in humans, the activities of antioxidant enzymes consistently showed either decreases or no changes as a function of aging. An increase in the activities of certain antioxidant enzymes in the presence of elevated levels of markers of oxidative stress and inflammation suggests that they were not sufficient to down-regulate oxidative stress and chronic inflammation. An adaptive response of certain antioxidant enzymes to increased oxidative stress is found in rodents, but is not observed in humans.

Very limited data exist with respect to changes in the levels of dietary and endogenous antioxidants as a function of aging in rodents or in humans. In rodents, plasma vitamin C and tissue coenzyme Q_{10} levels declined, but plasma glutathione and vitamin E levels were elevated as a function of aging. In contrast, the plasma level of vitamin E decreased, and retinol did not change in elderly humans.

Since increased oxidative stress and chronic inflammation occur in the elevated presence of certain antioxidant enzymes and antioxidants,[69] doses of antioxidants higher than those within physiological ranges are needed to reduce oxidative stress and inflammation and age-related decline in organ function. This is supported by the fact that the individual antioxidants at high doses reduce the rate of aging. For example, supplementation with individual antioxidants such as vitamin E, coenzyme Q_{10}, carotenoids, melatonin, flavonoids, glutathione-elevating agents (NAC and alpha-lipoic acid), and L-acetyl-carnitine decreased the rate of age-related decline in organ function by reducing oxidative stress and chronic inflammation in rodents.

Animal studies with antioxidants have produced expected beneficial results in reducing the risk of diseases. However, this experimental paradigm of using single antioxidants in humans with a high risk of developing chronic diseases has produced inconsistent results varying from beneficial effects, to no effect, to harmful effects and, therefore, should not be used in any future investigations in humans. Because of this and other scientific rationale discussed in this chapter, I recommend consumption of multiple micronutrients including high doses of dietary and endogenous antioxidants together with changes in the diet and lifestyle for healthy aging. The efficacy of the proposed recommendations should be tested by well-designed clinical studies. Meanwhile, the proposed recommendations may be adopted by individuals in consultation with their physicians or health professionals. It is expected that the proposed recommendations would reduce the rate of aging.

REFERENCES

1. Harman, D. 1996. Aging and disease: Extending functional life span. *Ann N Y Acad Sci* 786: 321–336.
2. Harman, D. 1998. Aging: Phenomena and theories. *Ann N Y Acad Sci* 854: 1–7.
3. Ames, B. N., M. K. Shigenaga, and T. M. Hagen. 1993. Oxidants, antioxidants, and the degenerative diseases of aging. *Proc Natl Acad Sci U S A* 90 (17): 7915–7922.
4. Boveris, A., and B. Chance. 1973. The mitochondrial generation of hydrogen peroxide. General properties and effect of hyperbaric oxygen. *Biochem J* 134 (3): 707–716.

5. Pollack, M., and C. Leeuwenburgh. 1999. Molecular mechanisms of oxidative stress in aging: Free radicals, aging, antioxidants and disease. In *Handbook of Oxidants and Antioxidants in Exercise*, ed. C. K. Sen, L. Packer, and O. Hanninen, 881–923. New York, NY: Elsevier Science.
6. Droge, W. 2003. Oxidative stress and aging. *Adv Exp Med Biol* 543, 191–200.
7. Chance, B., H. Sies, and A. Boveris. 1979. Hydroperoxide metabolism in mammalian organs. *Physiol Rev* 59 (3): 527–605.
8. Giulivi, C., J. J. Poderoso, and A. Boveris. 1998. Production of nitric oxide by mitochondria. *J Biol Chem* 273 (18): 11038–11043.
9. Hurst, J. K., and W. C. Barrette Jr. 1989. Leukocytic oxygen activation and microbicidal oxidative toxins. *Crit Rev Biochem Mol Biol* 24 (4): 271–328.
10. Klebanoff, S. J. 1980. Oxygen metabolism and the toxic properties of phagocytes. *Ann Intern Med* 93 (3): 480–489.
11. Eiserich, J. P., C. E. Cross, A. D. Jones, B. Halliwell, and A. van der Vliet. 1996. Formation of nitrating and chlorinating species by reaction of nitrite with hypochlorous acid. A novel mechanism for nitric oxide–mediated protein modification. *J Biol Chem* 271 (32): 19199–19208.
12. Eiserich, J. P., M. Hristova, C. E. Cross, A. D. Jones, B. A. Freeman, B. Halliwell, and A. van der Vliet. 1998. Formation of nitric oxide–derived inflammatory oxidants by myeloperoxidase in neutrophils. *Nature* 391 (6665): 393–397.
13. Coyle, J. T., and P. Puttfarcken. 1993. Oxidative stress, glutamate, and neurodegenerative disorders. *Science* 262 (5134): 689–695.
14. Graham, D. G. 1978. Oxidative pathways for catecholamines in the genesis of neuromelanin and cytotoxic quinones. *Mol Pharmacol* 14 (4): 633–643.
15. Chan, P. H., and R. A. Fishman. 1980. Transient formation of superoxide radicals in polyunsaturated fatty acid-induced brain swelling. *J Neurochem* 35 (4): 1004–1007.
16. Lafon-Cazal, M., S. Pietri, M. Culcasi, and J. Bockaert. 1993. NMDA-dependent superoxide production and neurotoxicity. *Nature* 364 (6437): 535–537.
17. Kiyosawa, H., M. Suko, H. Okudaira, K. Murata, T. Miyamoto, M. H. Chung, H. Kasai, and S. Nishimura. 1990. Cigarette smoking induces formation of 8-hydroxydeoxyguanosine, one of the oxidative DNA damages in human peripheral leukocytes. *Free Radic Res Commun* 11 (1–3): 23–27.
18. Reznick, A. Z., C. E. Cross, M. L. Hu, Y. J. Suzuki, S. Khwaja, A. Safadi, P. A. Motchnik, L. Packer, and B. Halliwell. 1992. Modification of plasma proteins by cigarette smoke as measured by protein carbonyl formation. *Biochem J* 286 (Pt 2): 607–611.
19. Duthie, G. G., J. R. Arthur, and W. P. James. 1991. Effects of smoking and vitamin E on blood antioxidant status. *Am J Clin Nutr* 53 (4 Suppl): 1061S–1063S.
20. Schectman, G., J. C. Byrd, and R. Hoffmann. 1991. Ascorbic acid requirements for smokers: Analysis of a population survey. *Am J Clin Nutr* 53 (6): 1466–1470.
21. Winterbourn, C. C. 1995. Toxicity of iron and hydrogen peroxide: The Fenton reaction. *Toxicol Lett* 82–83: 969–974.
22. Pamplona, R. 2008. Membrane phospholipids, lipoxidative damage and molecular integrity: A causal role in aging and longevity. *Biochim Biophys Acta*.
23. Squier, T. C. 2001. Oxidative stress and protein aggregation during biological aging. *Exp Gerontol* 36 (9): 1539–1550.
24. Bahadorani, S., S. Mukai, D. Egli, and A. J. Hilliker. 2008. Overexpression of metal-responsive transcription factor (MTF-1) in *Drosophila melanogaster* ameliorates life-span reductions associated with oxidative stress and metal toxicity. *Neurobiol Aging*.
25. Sohal, R. S., S. Agarwal, and B. H. Sohal. 1995. Oxidative stress and aging in the Mongolian gerbil (*Meriones unguiculatus*). *Mech Ageing Dev* 81 (1): 15–25.
26. Hagen, T. M., D. L. Yowe, J. C. Bartholomew, C. M. Wehr, K. L. Do, J. Y. Park, and B. N. Ames. 1997. Mitochondrial decay in hepatocytes from old rats: Membrane potential declines, heterogeneity and oxidants increase. *Proc Natl Acad Sci U S A* 94 (7): 3064–3069.
27. Sohal, R. S. 1991. Hydrogen peroxide production by mitochondria may be a biomarker of aging. *Mech Ageing Dev* 60 (2): 189–198.
28. Miquel, J. 1998. An update on the oxygen stress-mitochondrial mutation theory of aging: Genetic and evolutionary implications. *Exp Gerontol* 33 (1–2): 113–126.
29. Yakes, F. M., and B. Van Houten. 1997. Mitochondrial DNA damage is more extensive and persists longer than nuclear DNA damage in human cells following oxidative stress. *Proc Natl Acad Sci U S A* 94 (2): 514–519.

30. Aerts, A. M., P. Zabrocki, G. Govaert, J. Mathys, D. Carmona-Gutierrez, F. Madeo, J. Winderickx, B. P. Cammue, and K. Thevissen. 2008. Mitochondrial dysfunction leads to reduced chronological lifespan and increased apoptosis in yeast. *FEBS Lett* 583: 113–117.
31. Navarro, A., and A. Boveris. 2007. The mitochondrial energy transduction system and the aging process. *Am J Physiol Cell Physiol* 292 (2): C670–686.
32. Boveris, A., and A. Navarro. 2008. Brain mitochondrial dysfunction in aging. *IUBMB Life* 60 (5): 308–314.
33. van der Loo, B., R. Koppensteiner, and T. F. Luscher. 2004. How do blood vessels age? Mechanisms and clinical implications. *Vasa* 33 (1): 3–11.
34. van der Loo, B., S. Schildknecht, R. Zee, and M. M. Bachschmid. 2008. Signaling processes in endothelial aging in relation to chronic oxidative stress and their potential therapeutic implications. *Exp Physiol* 94(3): 305–310.
35. Hack, V., R. Breitkreutz, R. Kinscherf, H. Rohrer, P. Bartsch, F. Taut, A. Benner, and W. Droge. 1998. The redox state as a correlate of senescence and wasting and as a target for therapeutic intervention. *Blood* 92 (1): 59–67.
36. Droge, W. 2002. Aging-related changes in the thiol/disulfide redox state: Implications for the use of thiol antioxidants. *Exp Gerontol* 37 (12): 1333–1345.
37. Pope, S., J. M. Land, and S. J. Heales. 2008. Oxidative stress and mitochondrial dysfunction in neurodegeneration; cardiolipin a critical target? *Biochim Biophys Acta* 1777 (7–8): 794–799.
38. Prasad, K. N., W. C. Cole, and K. C. Prasad. 2002. Risk factors for Alzheimer's disease: Role of multiple antioxidants, non-steroidal anti-inflammatory and cholinergic agents alone or in combination in prevention and treatment. *J Am Coll Nutr* 21 (6): 506–522.
39. Prasad, K. N., W. C. Cole, and B. Kumar. 1999. Multiple antioxidants in the prevention and treatment of Parkinson's disease. *J Am Coll Nutr* 18 (5): 413–423.
40. Combaret, L., D. Dardevet, D. Bechet, D. Taillandier, L. Mosoni, and D. Attaix. 2009. Skeletal muscle proteolysis in aging. *Curr Opin Clin Nutr Metab Care* 12 (1): 37–41.
41. Shringarpure, R., and K. J. Davies. 2002. Protein turnover by the proteasome in aging and disease. *Free Radic Biol Med* 32 (11): 1084–1089.
42. Dirks, A. J., T. Hofer, E. Marzetti, M. Pahor, and C. Leeuwenburgh. 2006. Mitochondrial DNA mutations, energy metabolism and apoptosis in aging muscle. *Ageing Res Rev* 5 (2): 179–195.
43. Davies, K. J., and R. Shringarpure. 2006. Preferential degradation of oxidized proteins by the 20S proteasome may be inhibited in aging and in inflammatory neuromuscular diseases. *Neurology* 66 (2 Suppl 1): S93–S96.
44. Kawanishi, S., and S. Oikawa. 2004. Mechanism of telomere shortening by oxidative stress. *Ann N Y Acad Sci* 1019: 278–284.
45. Kurz, D. J., S. Decary, Y. Hong, E. Trivier, A. Akhmedov, and J. D. Erusalimsky. 2004. Chronic oxidative stress compromises telomere integrity and accelerates the onset of senescence in human endothelial cells. *J Cell Sci* 117 (Pt 11): 2417–2426.
46. Haendeler, J., J. Hoffmann, J. F. Diehl, M. Vasa, I. Spyridopoulos, A. M. Zeiher, and S. Dimmeler. 2004. Antioxidants inhibit nuclear export of telomerase reverse transcriptase and delay replicative senescence of endothelial cells. *Circ Res* 94 (6): 768–775.
47. Furumoto, K., E. Inoue, N. Nagao, E. Hiyama, and Miwa. 1998. Age-dependent telomere shortening is slowed down by enrichment of intracellular vitamin C via suppression of oxidative stress. *Life Sci* 63 (11): 935–948.
48. Tanaka, Y., Y. Moritoh, and N. Miwa. 2007. Age-dependent telomere-shortening is repressed by phosphorylated alpha-tocopherol together with cellular longevity and intracellular oxidative-stress reduction in human brain microvascular endotheliocytes. *J Cell Biochem* 102 (3): 689–703.
49. Viel, J. J., D. Q. McManus, S. S. Smith, and G. J. Brewer. 2001. Age- and concentration-dependent neuroprotection and toxicity by TNF in cortical neurons from beta-amyloid. *J Neurosci Res* 64 (5): 454–465.
50. Patel, J. R., and G. J. Brewer. 2008. Age-related differences in NFkappaB translocation and Bcl-2/Bax ratio caused by TNFalpha and Abeta42 promote survival in middle-age neurons and death in old neurons. *Exp Neurol* 213 (1): 93–100.
51. Patel, J. R., and G. J. Brewer. 2008. Age-related changes to tumor necrosis factor receptors affect neuron survival in the presence of beta-amyloid. *J Neurosci Res* 86 (10): 2303–2313.
52. You, T., and B. J. Nicklas. 2006. Chronic inflammation: Role of adipose tissue and modulation by weight loss. *Curr Diabetes Rev* 2 (1): 29–37.
53. Ungvari, Z., Z. Orosz, N. Labinskyy, A. Rivera, Z. Xiangmin, K. Smith, and A. Csiszar. 2007. Increased mitochondrial H_2O_2 production promotes endothelial NF-kappaB activation in aged rat arteries. *Am J Physiol Heart Circ Physiol* 293 (1): H37–H47.

54. Csiszar, A., M. Wang, E. G. Lakatta, and Z. Ungvari. 2008. Inflammation and endothelial dysfunction during aging: Role of NF-kappaB. *J Appl Physiol* 105 (4): 1333–1341.
55. Visser, M., M. Pahor, D. R. Taaffe, B. H. Goodpaster, E. M. Simonsick, A. B. Newman, M. Nevitt, and T. B. Harris. 2002. Relationship of interleukin-6 and tumor necrosis factor-alpha with muscle mass and muscle strength in elderly men and women: The Health ABC Study. *J Gerontol A Biol Sci Med Sci* 57 (5): M326–M332.
56. Schaap, L. A., S. M. Pluijm, D. J. Deeg, and M. Visser. 2006. Inflammatory markers and loss of muscle mass (sarcopenia) and strength, *Am J Med* 119 (6): 526, e9–e17.
57. Ferrucci, L., T. B. Harris, J. M. Guralnik, R. P. Tracy, M. C. Corti, H. J. Cohen, B. Penninx, M. Pahor, R. Wallace, and R. J. Havlik. 1999. Serum IL-6 level and the development of disability in older persons. *J Am Geriatr Soc* 47 (6): 639–646.
58. Pollack, M., and C. Leewenburg. 1999. Molecular mechanisms of oxidative stress in aging: Free radicals, aging, antioxidants and disease. In *Handbook of Oxidants and Antioxidants in Exercise*. Eds. C. K. Sen, L. Packer, and O. Hanninen. New York: Elsevier B.V. pp. 881–923.
59. Alvarez, E., A. Machado, F. Sobrino, and C. Santa Maria. 1996. Nitric oxide and superoxide anion production decrease with age in resident and activated rat peritoneal macrophages. *Cell Immunol* 169 (1): 152–155.
60. Alvarez, E., and C. Santa Maria. 1996. Influence of the age and sex on respiratory burst of human monocytes. *Mech Ageing Dev* 90 (2): 157–161.
61. Santa Maria, C., A. Ayala, and E. Revilla. 1996. Changes in superoxide dismutase activity in liver and lung of old rats. *Free Radic Res* 25 (5): 401–405.
62. Lavie, L., and O. Weinreb. 1996. Age- and strain-related changes in tissue transglutaminase activity in murine macrophages: The effects of inflammation and induction by retinol. *Mech Ageing Dev* 90 (2): 129–143.
63. Khare, V., A. Sodhi, and S. M. Singh. 1999. Age-dependent alterations in the tumoricidal functions of tumor-associated macrophages. *Tumour Biol* 20 (1): 30–43.
64. Wallace, P. K., T. K. Eisenstein, J. J. Meissler Jr., and P. S. Morahan. 1995. Decreases in macrophage mediated antitumor activity with aging. *Mech Ageing Dev* 77 (3): 169–184.
65. Khare, V., A. Sodhi, and S. M. Singh. 1996. Effect of aging on the tumoricidal functions of murine peritoneal macrophages. *Nat Immun* 15 (6): 285–294.
66. Irimajiri, N., E. T. Bloom, and T. Makinodan. 1985. Suppression of murine natural killer cell activity by adherent cells from aging mice. *Mech Ageing Dev* 31 (2): 155–162.
67. Leeuwenburgh, C., R. Fiebig, R. Chandwaney, and L. L. Ji. 1994. Aging and exercise training in skeletal muscle: Responses of glutathione and antioxidant enzyme systems. *Am J Physiol* 267 (2 Pt 2): R439–R445.
68. Yu, B. 1993. *Free Radicals in Aging*, Boca Raton, FL: CRC Press.
69. Yan, X. D., B. Kumar, P. Nahreini, A. J. Hanson, J. E. Prasad, and K. N. Prasad. 2005. Prostaglandin-induced neurodegeneration is associated with increased levels of oxidative markers and reduced by a mixture of antioxidants. *J Neurosci Res* 81 (1): 85–90.
70. Tokunaga, K., K. Kanno, M. Ochi, T. Nishimiya, K. Shishino, M. Murase, H. Makino, and S. Tokui. 1998. Lipid peroxide and antioxidants in the elderly. *Rinsho Byori* 46 (8): 783–789.
71. Kasapoglu, M., and T. Ozben. 2001. Alterations of antioxidant enzymes and oxidative stress markers in aging. *Exp Gerontol* 36 (2): 209–220.
72. Pansarasa, O., L. Bertorelli, J. Vecchiet, G. Felzani, and F. Marzatico. 1999. Age-dependent changes of antioxidant activities and markers of free radical damage in human skeletal muscle. *Free Radic Biol Med* 27 (5–6): 617–622.
73. Evereklioglu, C., H. Er, S. Doganay, M. Cekmen, Y. Turkoz, B. Otlu, and E. Ozerol. 2003. Nitric oxide and lipid peroxidation are increased and associated with decreased antioxidant enzyme activities in patients with age-related macular degeneration. *Doc Ophthalmol* 106 (2): 129–136.
74. Gibson, G. E., V. Haroutunian, H. Zhang, L. C. Park, Q. Shi, M. Lesser, R. C. Mohs, R. K. Sheu, and J. P. Blass. 2000. Mitochondrial damage in Alzheimer's disease varies with apolipoprotein E genotype. *Ann Neurol* 48 (3): 297–303.
75. Koppal, T., J. Drake, S. Yatin, B. Jordan, S. Varadarajan, L. Bettenhausen, and D. A. Butterfield. 1999. Peroxynitrite-induced alterations in synaptosomal membrane proteins: Insight into oxidative stress in Alzheimer's disease. *J Neurochem* 72 (1): 310–317.
76. Lovell, M. A., C. Xie, and W. R. Markesbery. 1998. Decreased glutathione transferase activity in brain and ventricular fluid in Alzheimer's disease. *Neurology* 51 (6): 1562–1566.
77. Ambani, L. M., M. H. Van Woert, and S. Murphy. 1975. Brain peroxidase and catalase in Parkinson disease. *Arch Neurol* 32 (2): 114–118.

78. Kish, S. J., C. Morito, and O. Hornykiewicz. 1985. Glutathione peroxidase activity in Parkinson's disease brain. *Neurosci Lett* 58 (3): 343–346.
79. De, A. K., and R. Darad. 1991. Age-associated changes in antioxidants and antioxidative enzymes in rats. *Mech Ageing Dev* 59 (1–2): 123–128.
80. Panda, A. K., R. P. Ruth, and S. N. Padhi. 1984. Effect of age and sex on the ascorbic acid content of kidney, skeletal muscle and pancreas of common Indian toad, *Bufo melanostictus*. *Exp Gerontol* 19 (2): 95–100.
81. Rikans, L. E., and D. R. Moore. 1988. Effect of aging on aqueous-phase antioxidants in tissues of male Fischer rats. *Biochim Biophys Acta* 966 (3): 269–275.
82. Hussain, S., W. Slikker Jr., and S. F. Ali. 1995. Age-related changes in antioxidant enzymes, superoxide dismutase, catalase, glutathione peroxidase and glutathione in different regions of mouse brain. *Int J Dev Neurosci* 13 (8): 811–817.
83. Ohkuwa, T., Y. Sato, and M. Naoi. 1997. Glutathione status and reactive oxygen generation in tissues of young and old exercised rats. *Acta Physiol Scand* 159 (3): 237–244.
84. Barja de Quiroga, G., R. Perez-Campo, and M. Lopez Torres. 1990. Anti-oxidant defences and peroxidation in liver and brain of aged rats. *Biochem J* 272 (1): 247–250.
85. Farooqui, M. Y., W. W. Day, and D. M. Zamorano. 1987. Glutathione and lipid peroxidation in the aging rat. *Comp Biochem Physiol B* 88 (1): 177–180.
86. Ravindranath, V., B. R. Shivakumar, and H. K. Anandatheerthavarada. 1989. Low glutathione levels in brain regions of aged rats. *Neurosci Lett* 101 (2): 187–190.
87. Favilli, F., T. Iantomasi, P. Marraccini, M. Stio, B. Lunghi, C. Treves, and M. T. Vincenzini. 1994. Relationship between age and GSH metabolism in synaptosomes of rat cerebral cortex. *Neurobiol Aging* 15 (4): 429–433.
88. de la Asuncion, J. G., A. Millan, R. Pla, L. Bruseghini, A. Esteras, F. V. Pallardo, J. Sastre, and J. Vina. 1996. Mitochondrial glutathione oxidation correlates with age-associated oxidative damage to mitochondrial DNA. *FASEB J* 10 (2): 333–338.
89. Viveros, M. P., L. Arranz, A. Hernanz, J. Miquel, and M. De la Fuente. 2007. A model of premature aging in mice based on altered stress-related behavioral response and immunosenescence. *Neuroimmunomodulation* 14 (3–4): 157–162.
90. Perry, T. L., D. V. Godin, and S. Hansen. 1982. Parkinson's disease: A disorder due to nigral glutathione deficiency? *Neurosci Lett* 33 (3): 305–310.
91. Riederer, P., E. Sofic, W. D. Rausch, B. Schmidt, G. P. Reynolds, K. Jellinger, and M. B. Youdim. 1989. Transition metals, ferritin, glutathione, and ascorbic acid in parkinsonian brains. *J Neurochem* 52 (2): 515–520.
92. Sofic, E., K. W. Lange, K. Jellinger, and P. Riederer. 1992. Reduced and oxidized glutathione in the substantia nigra of patients with Parkinson's disease. *Neurosci Lett* 142 (2): 128–130.
93. Zaman, Z., S. Roche, P. Fielden, P. G. Frost, D. C. Niriella, and A. C. Cayley. 1992. Plasma concentrations of vitamins A and E and carotenoids in Alzheimer's disease. *Age Ageing* 21 (2): 91–94.
94. Matsuo, M., F. Gomi, and M. M. Dooley. 1992. Age-related alterations in antioxidant capacity and lipid peroxidation in brain, liver, and lung homogenates of normal and vitamin E–deficient rats. *Mech Ageing Dev* 64 (3): 273–292.
95. Laganiere, S., and B. P. Yu. 1989. Effect of chronic food restriction in aging rats. I. Liver subcellular membranes. *Mech Ageing Dev* 48 (3): 207–219.
96. Vatassery, G. T., C. K. Angerhofer, and C. A. Knox. 1984. Effect of age on vitamin E concentrations in various regions of the brain and a few selected peripheral tissues of the rat, and on the uptake of radioactive vitamin E by various regions of rat brain. *J Neurochem* 43 (2): 409–412.
97. Sawada, M., and J. C. Carlson. 1987. Changes in superoxide radical and lipid peroxide formation in the brain, heart and liver during the lifetime of the rat. *Mech Ageing Dev* 41 (1–2): 125–137.
98. Albano, C. B., D. Muralikrishnan, and M. Ebadi. 2002. Distribution of coenzyme Q homologues in brain. *Neurochem Res* 27 (5): 359–368.
99. Panemangalore, M., and C. J. Lee. 1992. Evaluation of the indices of retinol and alpha-tocopherol status in free-living elderly. *J Gerontol* 47 (3): B98–B104.
100. Wu, D., S. N. Han, M. Meydani, and S. N. Meydani. 2004. Effect of concomitant consumption of fish oil and vitamin E on production of inflammatory cytokines in healthy elderly humans. *Ann N Y Acad Sci* 1031, 422–424.
101. Han, S. N., D. Wu, W. K. Ha, A. Beharka, D. E. Smith, B. S. Bender, and S. N. Meydani. 2000. Vitamin E supplementation increases T helper 1 cytokine production in old mice infected with influenza virus. *Immunology* 100 (4): 487–493.

102. Han, S. N., M. Meydani, D. Wu, B. S. Bender, D. E. Smith, J. Vina, G. Cao, R. L. Prior, and S. N. Meydani. 2000. Effect of long-term dietary antioxidant supplementation on influenza virus infection. *J Gerontol A Biol Sci Med Sci* 55 (10), B496–B503.
103. Asha Devi, S., S. Prathima, and M. V. Subramanyam. 2003. Dietary vitamin E and physical exercise: II. Antioxidant status and lipofuscin-like substances in aging rat heart. *Exp Gerontol* 38 (3): 291–297.
104. Devi, S. A., and T. R. Kiran. 2004. Regional responses in antioxidant system to exercise training and dietary vitamin E in aging rat brain. *Neurobiol Aging* 25 (4): 501–508.
105. Jolitha, A. B., M. V. Subramanyam, and S. Asha Devi. 2006. Modification by vitamin E and exercise of oxidative stress in regions of aging rat brain: Studies on superoxide dismutase isoenzymes and protein oxidation status. *Exp Gerontol* 41 (8): 753–763.
106. Wu, D., S. N. Han, M. Meydani, and S. N. Meydani. 2006. Effect of concomitant consumption of fish oil and vitamin E on T cell mediated function in the elderly: A randomized double-blind trial. *J Am Coll Nutr* 25 (4): 300–306.
107. Santos-Gonzalez, M., C. Gomez Diaz, P. Navas, and J. M. Villalba. 2007. Modifications of plasma proteome in long-lived rats fed on a coenzyme Q_{10}–supplemented diet. *Exp Gerontol* 42 (8): 798–806.
108. Quiles, J. L., J. J. Ochoa, J. R. Huertas, and J. Mataix. 2004. Coenzyme Q supplementation protects from age-related DNA double-strand breaks and increases lifespan in rats fed on a PUFA-rich diet. *Exp Gerontol* 39 (2): 189–194.
109. McDonald, S. R., R. S. Sohal, and M. J. Forster. 2005. Concurrent administration of coenzyme Q_{10} and alpha-tocopherol improves learning in aged mice. *Free Radic Biol Med* 38 (6): 729–736.
110. Lass, A., and R. S. Sohal. 2000. Effect of coenzyme Q(10) and alpha-tocopherol content of mitochondria on the production of superoxide anion radicals. *FASEB J* 14 (1): 87–94.
111. Sohal, R. S., and M. J. Forster. 2007. Coenzyme Q, oxidative stress and aging. *Mitochondrion* 7 (Suppl): S103–S111.
112. Tan, J. S., J. J. Wang, V. Flood, E. Rochtchina, W. Smith, and P. Mitchell. 2008. Dietary antioxidants and the long-term incidence of age-related macular degeneration: The Blue Mountains Eye Study. *Ophthalmology* 115 (2): 334–341.
113. Evans, J. R., and K. Henshaw. 2008. Antioxidant vitamin and mineral supplements for preventing age-related macular degeneration. *Cochrane Database Syst Rev* (1): CD000253.
114. Raghavendra, V., and S. K. Kulkarni. 2001. Possible antioxidant mechanism in melatonin reversal of aging and chronic ethanol-induced amnesia in plus-maze and passive avoidance memory tasks. *Free Radic Biol Med* 30 (6): 595–602.
115. von Gall, C., and D. R. Weaver. 2008. Loss of responsiveness to melatonin in the aging mouse suprachiasmatic nucleus. *Neurobiol Aging* 29 (3): 464–470.
116. Singh, A., P. S. Naidu, and S. K. Kulkarni. 2003. Reversal of aging and chronic ethanol-induced cognitive dysfunction by quercetin a bioflavonoid. *Free Radic Res* 37 (11): 1245–1252.
117. Patil, C. S., V. P. Singh, P. S. Satyanarayan, N. K. Jain, A. Singh, and S. K. Kulkarni. 2003. Protective effect of flavonoids against aging- and lipopolysaccharide-induced cognitive impairment in mice. *Pharmacology* 69 (2), 59–67.
118. Guayerbas, N., M. Puerto, P. Alvarez, and M. de la Fuente. 2004. Improvement of the macrophage functions in prematurely ageing mice by a diet supplemented with thiolic antioxidants. *Cell Mol Biol (Noisy-le-grand)* 50: Online Pub, OL677-81.
119. Guayerbas, N., M. Puerto, A. Hernanz, J. Miquel, and M. De la Fuente. 2005. Thiolic antioxidant supplementation of the diet reverses age-related behavioural dysfunction in prematurely ageing mice. *Pharmacol Biochem Behav* 80 (1): 45–51.
120. Long, J., F. Gao, L. Tong, C. W. Cotman, B. N. Ames, and J. Liu. 2009. Mitochondrial decay in the brains of old rats: Ameliorating effect of alpha-lipoic acid and acetyl-L-carnitine, *Neurochem Res* 34: 755–763.
121. Liu, J., D. W. Killilea, and B. N. Ames. 2002. Age-associated mitochondrial oxidative decay: Improvement of carnitine acetyltransferase substrate-binding affinity and activity in brain by feeding old rats acetyl-L-carnitine and/or *R*-alpha-lipoic acid. *Proc Natl Acad Sci U S A* 99 (4): 1876–1881.
122. Group, A.-R. E. D. S. 2001. A randomized, placebo-controlled, clinical trial of high-dose supplementation with vitamins C and E, beta-carotene, and zinc for age-related macular degeneration and vision loss: AREDS report no. 8. *Arch Ophthalmol* 119: 1417–1436.
123. Alvarado, C., P. Alvarez, L. Jimenez, and M. De la Fuente. 2005. Improvement of leukocyte functions in young prematurely aging mice after a 5-week ingestion of a diet supplemented with biscuits enriched in antioxidants. *Antioxid Redox Signal* 7 (9–10): 1203–1210.

124. Alvarado, C., P. Alvarez, M. Puerto, N. Gausseres, L. Jimenez, and M. De la Fuente. 2006. Dietary supplementation with antioxidants improves functions and decreases oxidative stress of leukocytes from prematurely aging mice. *Nutrition* 22 (7–8): 767–777.
125. De la Fuente, M. 2002. Effects of antioxidants on immune system ageing. *Eur J Clin Nutr* 56 (Suppl 3): S5–S8.
126. Richwine, A. F., J. P. Godbout, B. M. Berg, J. Chen, J. Escobar, D. K. Millard, and R. W. Johnson. 2005. Improved psychomotor performance in aged mice fed diet high in antioxidants is associated with reduced ex vivo brain interleukin-6 production. *Brain Behav Immun* 19 (6): 512–520.
127. Albanes, D., O. P. Heinonen, J. K. Huttunen, P. R. Taylor, J. Virtamo, B. K. Edwards, J. Haapakoski, et al. 1995. Effects of alpha-tocopherol and beta-carotene supplements on cancer incidence in the Alpha-Tocopherol Beta-Carotene Cancer Prevention Study. *Am J Clin Nutr* 62 (6 Suppl): 1427S–1430S.
128. Alpha-Tocopherol, BCCPSG. 1994. The effect of vitamin E and beta-carotene on the incidence of lung cancer and other cancers in male smokers. *N Eng J Med* 330: 1029–1035.
129. Omenn, G. S., G. E. Goodman, M. D. Thornquist, J. Balmes, M. R. Cullen, A. Glass, J. P. Keogh, et al. 1996. Effects of a combination of beta carotene and vitamin A on lung cancer and cardiovascular disease. *N Engl J Med* 334 (18): 1150–1155.
130. Bairati, I., F. Meyer, M. Gelinas, A. Fortin, A. Nabid, F. Brochet, J. P. Mercier, et al. 2005. Randomized trial of antioxidant vitamins to prevent acute adverse effects of radiation therapy in head and neck cancer patients. *J Clin Oncol* 23 (24): 5805–5813.
131. Lonn, E., J. Bosch, S. Yusuf, P. Sheridan, J. Pogue, J. M. Arnold, C. Ross, et al. 2005. Effects of long-term vitamin E supplementation on cardiovascular events and cancer: A randomized controlled trial. *JAMA* 293 (11): 1338–1347.
132. Weinberg, R. B., B. S. VanderWerken, R. A. Anderson, J. E. Stegner, and M. J. Thomas. 2001. Pro-oxidant effect of vitamin E in cigarette smokers consuming a high polyunsaturated fat diet. *Arterioscler Thromb Vasc Biol* 21 (6): 1029–1033.
133. Krinsky, N. I. 1989. Antioxidant functions of carotenoids. *Free Radic Biol Med* 7 (6): 617–635.
134. Hazuka, M. B., J. Edwards-Prasad, F. Newman, J. J. Kinzie, and K. N. Prasad. 1990. Beta-carotene induces morphological differentiation and decreases adenylate cyclase activity in melanoma cells in culture. *J Am Coll Nutr* 9 (2): 143–149.
135. Zhang, L. X., R. V. Cooney, and J. S. Bertram. 1992. Carotenoids up-regulate connexin43 gene expression independent of their provitamin A or antioxidant properties. *Cancer Res* 52 (20): 5707–5712.
136. Carter, C. A., M. Pogribny, A. Davidson, C. D. Jackson, L. J. McGarrity, and S. M. Morris. 1996. Effects of retinoic acid on cell differentiation and reversion toward normal in human endometrial adenocarcinoma (RL95-2) cells. *Anticancer Res* 16 (1): 17–24.
137. Meyskens, Jr., F. 1995. Role of vitamin A and its derivatives in the human cancer. In *Nutrients in Cancer Prevention and Treatment*. Eds. K. N. Prasad, and R. M. Williams, Totowa, NJ: Humana Press. pp. 349–362.
138. Vile, G. F., and C. C. Winterbourn. 1988. Inhibition of adriamycin-promoted microsomal lipid peroxidation by beta-carotene, alpha-tocopherol and retinol at high and low oxygen partial pressures. *FEBS Lett* 238 (2): 353–356.
139. Niki, E. 1987. Interaction of ascorbate and alpha-tocopherol. *Ann N Y Acad Sci* 498: 186–199.
140. Ingold, K. U., G. W. Burton, D. O. Foster, L. Hughes, D. A. Lindsay, and A. Webb. 1987. Biokinetics of and discrimination between dietary *RRR*- and *SRR*-alpha-tocopherols in the male rat. *Lipids* 22 (3): 163–172.
141. Carini, R., G. Poli, M. U. Dianzani, S. P. Maddix, T. F. Slater, and K. H. Cheeseman. 1990. Comparative evaluation of the antioxidant activity of alpha-tocopherol, alpha-tocopherol polyethylene glycol 1000 succinate and alpha-tocopherol succinate in isolated hepatocytes and liver microsomal suspensions. *Biochem Pharmacol* 39 (10): 1597–1601.
142. Prasad, K. N., B. Kumar, X. D. Yan, A. J. Hanson, and W. C. Cole. 2003. alpha-Tocopheryl succinate, the most effective form of vitamin E for adjuvant cancer treatment: A review. *J Am Coll Nutr* 22 (2): 108–117.
143. Sies, H., V. S. Sharov, L. O. Klotz, and K. Briviba. 1997. Glutathione peroxidase protects against peroxynitrite-mediated oxidations. A new function for selenoproteins as peroxynitrite reductase. *J Biol Chem* 272 (44): 27812–27817.
144. Witschi, A., S. Reddy, B. Stofer, and B. H. Lauterburg. 1992. The systemic availability of oral glutathione. *Eur J Clin Pharmacol* 43 (6): 667–669.
145. Niki, E. 1997. Mechanisms and dynamics of antioxidant action of ubiquinol. *Mol Aspects Med* 18 (Suppl): S63–S70.
146. Stoyanovsky, D. A., A. N. Osipov, P. J. Quinn, and V. E. Kagan. 1995. Ubiquinone-dependent recycling of vitamin E radicals by superoxide. *Arch Biochem Biophys* 323 (2): 343–351.

5 Role of Micronutrients in the Prevention of Coronary Artery Disease and Improvement of the Standard Therapy

INTRODUCTION

Despite current prevention recommendations and improved treatment outcomes due to advances in surgical techniques, early detection equipment, and the discovery of cholesterol-lowering drugs, coronary artery disease (CAD) remains the number one cause of death in the United States. The exact reasons for the failure of the current approaches to affect the incidence of and mortality from heart disease are unknown. However, it is possible that the major risk factors that initiate and promote damage have not been addressed at the same time, either in prevention or treatment of CAD. These risk factors include increased oxidative stress,[1,2] oxidized LDL-cholesterol,[3-6] and high levels of C-reactive proteins, a marker of chronic inflammation,[7] and homocysteine.[8] Currently, cholesterol-lowering drugs, with or without niacin, and low-dose aspirin are recommended for reducing the risk and progression of CAD. These recommendations do not affect all risk factors simultaneously. For example, they do not affect oxidative stress and inflammation in an optimal manner. In addition, they do not affect either the homocysteine level or its mechanism of action that is mediated via free radicals. Therefore, the use of antioxidants that neutralize free radicals and reduce inflammation and B-vitamins that reduce homocysteine levels may affect major risk factors that initiate CAD and, thereby, may reduce the incidence of this disease. A similar approach may improve the efficacy of standard therapy in the treatment of CAD. Modifications in diet and lifestyle may improve the efficacy of micronutrient supplements in both prevention and treatment of this disease. Currently, cardiologists recommend modifications in diet and lifestyle, but they do not recommend micronutrients, including dietary and endogenous antioxidants for prevention or improving the treatment outcomes of CAD. Previous clinical studies primarily with vitamin E alone in high-risk populations have produced inconsistent results.

This chapter briefly describes the incidence and cost, major risk factors, role of increased oxidative stress, chronic inflammation, and laboratory, epidemiologic, and intervention studies utilizing antioxidants and B-vitamins in CAD. This chapter also proposes a scientific rationale and evidence for using multiple micronutrients, including dietary and endogenous antioxidants, low-dose aspirin, and diet and lifestyle modifications for the prevention of CAD. A similar approach, in combination with cholesterol-lowering drugs for the treatment of CAD, is proposed.

INCIDENCE AND COST

About 1.5 million new cases are detected annually, and approximately 1 million people die of this disease every year. The current estimate is that about 62 million Americans have one or more types of cardiovascular disease,[9] and about 14 million per year suffer heart attacks or angina. The direct and indirect financial cost in the United States of this disease is estimated to be about $329 billion annually.[9]

PRIMARY RISK FACTORS AND INVOLVEMENT OF OXIDATIVE STRESS AND INFLAMMATION IN CAD

The primary diet-, lifestyle-, and disease-related risk factors for CAD include cigarette smoking, obesity, diabetes mellitus, and aging. These risk factors are associated with increased oxidative stress and chronic inflammation that initiate and promote damage to the vascular system leading to CAD. A high homocysteine level, a risk factor for CAD, also causes damage to the endothelial cells of arterial walls via increased oxidative stress.[10] Increased levels of free iron and copper and impaired mitochondria can also increase the production of free radicals.

CONSEQUENCES OF INCREASED OXIDATIVE STRESS AND CHRONIC INFLAMMATION

LDL cholesterol is commonly referred to as "bad cholesterol" because it is easily oxidized by free radicals. Oxidized LDL cholesterol may be one of the early events that initiate plaque formation by increasing the formation of foam cells, enhancing platelet adhesion and aggregation, triggering thrombosis, and impairing elasticity of the coronary arteries.[4,6] Oxidized LDL cholesterol can also increase vascular smooth muscle cell proliferation by activating c-*myc* oncogene and its binding partner MAX, the carboxyl-terminal domain-binding factors activator protein-2 (AP-2), and elongation 2 factor (E2F) in human coronary artery smooth muscle cells.[3] The importance of c-*myc* in the progression of atherosclerotic lesions was demonstrated by the fact that gene therapy by decoy oligodeoxynucleotide, which inactivates E2F, delivered to human bypass vein grafts intraoperatively, caused fewer graft occlusions and critical stenosis after 12 months.[5] Oxidized LDL cholesterol is engulfed by the macrophages to form foam cells, and C-reactive protein increases the uptake of oxidized LDL cholesterol by the macrophages and, thereby, increases the number of foam cells.[7] Both foam cells and increased proliferation of vascular smooth muscle cells contribute to the formation of plaque in the coronary arteries. Once the plaque is formed, it serves as a continuous stimulus for increased inflammatory reactions that release reactive oxygen species (ROS) and proinflammatory cytokines. Using cultured monocyte and mononuclear cells obtained from CAD patients and normal persons, it was demonstrated that long-term exposure to oxidized LDL cholesterol enhanced cytoplasmic IkappaB phosphorylation and NF-kappaB translocation, and increased endothelial adhesiveness of monocyte/mononuclear. Oxidized LDL cholesterol also significantly enhanced TNF-alpha–stimulated ROS production and endothelial adhesiveness of monocyte/mononuclear cells. This increase in oxidative stress contributes to atherogenesis.[11] Thus, lowering the level of LDL cholesterol and preventing its oxidation should reduce the risk of developing plaques.

Endothelial cells of the vascular wall are damaged by free radicals, secretary products of inflammatory reactions (ROS, proinflammatory cytokines, adhesion molecules, compliment proteins, and prostaglandin E_2), and homocysteine. It is now recognized that endothelial cell dysfunction may also be one of the early events in the development of CAD.[12,13] Damage to endothelial cells may impair the nitric oxide synthase (NOS) pathway, which in turn may reduce endothelium-dependent coronary artery dilation. Thus, a deficiency in the production of NO may interfere with the function of the vessel wall. The levels of inducible NOS (iNOS) mRNA in vascular smooth muscle cells of a healthy arterial wall is low, but the levels of iNOS, mRNA, and protein in macrophages, and smooth muscle cells are high in CAD.[14] This suggests that high levels of iNOS may release excessive amounts of NO that could be oxidized to form peroxynitrite, which can induce arterial dysfunction. Thus, the role of NO in maintaining normal vascular function depends upon maintaining the proper levels of NO. Both deficiency and excess production of NO can impair vasomotion and enhance endothelial dysfunction. Therefore, protecting the endothelial cells from damage produced by free radicals should be considered useful in reducing the risk and progression of CAD.

LOW-DOSE ASPIRIN IN CAD

Low-dose aspirin (acetylsalicylic acid) is commonly recommended for reducing the risk and progression of CAD. Aspirin has been shown to reduce major cardiac or cerebral events by 25%.[15] It does so by irreversibly inhibiting cyclooxygenase-1 enzyme activity, and thus preventing the production of thromboxane-A2, which is responsible for aggregation of platelets.[16] However, it has been reported that about 5–12% of patients with CAD develop resistance to aspirin,[17,18] and about 24% of patients taking aspirin become semiresponders.[19] Another study estimated that 8–45% of patients taking aspirin develop aspirin resistance.[16] This has required physicians to increase aspirin doses. However, the aspirin resistance continued to be present in some cases, in spite of increased aspirin doses. Aspirin resistance may increase the risk of major cardiac events. The exact mechanisms of aspirin resistance remain to be elucidated. The proposed mechanisms include genetic polymorphism, alternate pathways of platelet activation, insensitivity of the cyclooxygenase-1 enzyme, and drug interactions.[20] It has also been reported that endothelial dysfunction is one of the mechanisms of aspirin resistance, and increased oxidative stress plays no significant role in this process.[20] It has been reported that the risk of major cardiac events may increase by about threefold in aspirin-resistant patients.[18] Therefore, resolving the issue of aspirin resistance has become a new challenge for researchers in cardiology.

ROLE OF ANTIOXIDANTS IN CAD

Since increased oxidative stress and chronic inflammation are early events that initiate and promote damage leading to CAD, and since antioxidants can neutralize free radicals and reduce inflammation, they should be considered one of the rational strategies for the prevention of CAD. Indeed, the U.S. Prevention Service Task Force recommends multiple vitamin supplements to reduce the risk of cancer and CAD.[21,22] However, these recommendations do not provide guidelines with respect to the type of micronutrients that should be included or excluded. The doses and dose schedule were also not described in the above recommendation.

ANIMAL STUDIES AFTER TREATMENT WITH ANTIOXIDANTS

Animal studies consistently show that individual antioxidants, such as vitamin E alone reduced the incidence and/or rate of progression of CAD.[23–26] In rats, supplementation with vitamin C and vitamin E reduced hyperhomocysteinemia-induced increases in myocardial oxidative stress and myocardial fibrosis.[27] The beneficial effects of one or two dietary antioxidants on cardiac events in animals have not been consistently observed in patients with CAD. This suggests that the data obtained from animal models should not be extrapolated to humans, because the absorption, distribution, and metabolism of antioxidants are different in each. Furthermore, rodents, except guinea pigs, make their own vitamin C, while humans do not.

EPIDEMIOLOGIC STUDIES WITH ANTIOXIDANTS

Despite numerous confounding factors associated with epidemiologic investigations, six out of eight studies on vitamin E alone showed an inverse relationship between vitamin E intake and the risk of CAD. The remaining two studies showed no beneficial effects. In a WHO/Multinational MONItoring of Trends and Determinants in Cardiovascular Disease (MONICA) study, there was a high inverse association between age-specific mortality from ischemic heart disease and lipid-standardized vitamin E levels.[28] In a Polish study, plasma levels of vitamin E were significantly lower in patients with stable and unstable angina compared to healthy control persons.[29] In a UK study, an inverse association between plasma vitamin E levels and the risk of angina was reported.[30]

In a Harvard study of 39,910 male health professionals, a 36% lower relative risk of CAD was demonstrated among those who consumed 60 IU of vitamin E per day, compared to those who consumed less than 7.5 IU of vitamin E per day.[31] Men who took at least 100 IU of vitamin E per day for at least 2 years had a 37% lower risk of CAD than those who did not take vitamin E. Another Harvard study of 87,245 healthy nurses with a follow-up period of 8 years revealed that women in the top fifth of vitamin E intake had a 34% lower relative risk of major cardiac events compared to those in the lowest fifth.[32] The relative risk of CAD was 48% lower in women taking vitamin E supplements of more than 100 mg/day for at least 2 years. Vitamin E obtained only from the diet provided no such protection.

In another U.S. study of 11,000 people aged 67 and over with a follow-up period of 6 years found that vitamin E supplementation was associated with a 47% reduction in mortality from CAD.[33] Further reduction was observed in people who were taking vitamin E supplements together with vitamin C.

In contrast to the above six investigations, two studies failed to observe any association between serum selenium, vitamin A, or vitamin E and the risk of death from CAD.[34,35] None of the epidemiologic studies have examined the role of endogenous antioxidants such as glutathione, alpha-lipoic acid, L-carnitine, or coenzyme Q_{10} in reducing the risk of CAD.

It has been reported that the serum levels of neopterin, a marker of inflammation, were elevated in patients with CAD compared to controls.[36] The average serum levels of vitamin C, gamma-tocopherol, lycopene, lutein, zeanthin, alpha-carotene, and beta-carotene (BC) were lower in patients with CAD compared to controls. These results suggest that the serum level of neopterin was inversely related to the serum levels of antioxidants in patients with CAD, and that increased inflammation plays an important role in the etiology of CAD.

INTERVENTION HUMAN STUDIES AFTER TREATMENT WITH ONE OR MORE DIETARY ANTIOXIDANTS

Based on the consistency of data on the beneficial effects of vitamin E alone, vitamin C alone, or both in combination on CAD obtained from animal and epidemiologic studies, it was tempting to think that similar beneficial effects of these dietary antioxidants could be observed when used individually or in combination in human populations at high risk for developing CAD. However, in view of the fact that the high-risk populations, such as heavy tobacco smokers and patients with type 2 diabetes, have a high internal oxidative environment, and that administration of vitamin E or vitamin C alone can result in oxidation of these antioxidants, such a temptation should have been resisted. Nevertheless, a few clinical studies with vitamin E alone were initiated in patients with CAD, and as expected, they all produced inconsistent results varying from no effect, to beneficial effects, to harmful effects. Other reasons were that the form, type, number, dose, and dose schedule of antioxidants, study end points, observation periods, and patient populations differ from one study to another (Tables 5.1–5.3). When endogenous antioxidants were used individually, similar inconsistent results were obtained. When dietary antioxidants were used in combination with cholesterol-lowering drugs, similar inconsistent results were also noted (Tables 5.4–5.5). The published intervention trials utilizing antioxidants with or without cholesterol-lowering drugs can be divided into five groups:

- Dietary antioxidants producing beneficial effects
- Dietary antioxidants producing no effects or adverse effects
- Endogenous antioxidants producing no effects or beneficial effects
- Dietary antioxidants in combination with cholesterol-lowering drugs producing beneficial effects
- Dietary antioxidants in combination with cholesterol-lowering drugs producing no effects or adverse effects

TABLE 5.1
Summary of Intervention Trials with Vitamin E Alone in High-Risk CAD Patients Showing Beneficial Effects

Name of Study	No. of Patients	Type of Antioxidant	Criteria of Study	Follow-Up Period	Results
CHAOS	2002[a]	Vitamin E (d-α), 400 or 800 IU	Death, nonfatal MI	510 days	Reduced[41]
–	42[b]	Vitamin E (α-TA), 544 IU	FMD	4 months	Improved[39]
–	100[c]	Vitamin E, 1200 IU	Stenosis	4 months	Reduced[37]
–	75[d]	Vitamin E, 1200 IU	C-reactive protein	5 months	Reduced[38]
–	33[e]	Vitamin E (d-αT), 800 IU	LDL oxidation	12 weeks	Reduced[40]

Note: CHAOS, Cambridge Heart Antioxidant Study; MI, myocardial infarction; FMD, endothelial-dependent, flow-mediated dilation.

All vitamins were given once a day unless specified otherwise. The number in parentheses indicates reference number.

[a] Proven atherosclerosis disease.
[b] Hypercholesterolemia, smokers, and smokers with hypercholesterolemia.
[c] Angioplasty.
[d] Type 2 diabetes.
[e] Patients undergoing peritoneal dialysis ($N = 17$) or hemodialysis ($N = 16$).

VITAMIN E ALONE PRODUCING BENEFICIAL EFFECTS

Table 5.1 summarizes the effect of vitamin E alone on various cardiac risk factors.[37–41] It can be noted that the dose of vitamin E varied from 400 to 1200 IU and that the number and type of patients, criteria of study, and follow-up period also varied. It is well established that when vitamin E is oxidized, it acts as a pro-oxidant. Since the observation period was short, the adverse effects of oxidized vitamin E were not apparent. Table 5.2 primarily shows the effect of vitamin E in combination with vitamin C on the risk factors for CAD.[42–45] The variables described in Table 5.1 are

TABLE 5.2
Summary of Intervention Trials with Vitamin E in Combination with Vitamin C in High-Risk CAD Patients Showing Beneficial Effects

No. of Patients	Type of Antioxidant	Criteria of Study	Follow-Up Period	Results
19[a]	Vitamin E, 400 IU Vitamin C, 500 mg	Coronary atherosclerosis	1 year	Reduced[43]
520[b]	Vitamin E, slow-release vitamin C	Atherosclerosis	6 years	Reduced[45]
20[c]	Vitamin E, 800 IU Vitamin C, 1 g	FMD	6 hours	Increased[44]
182[b]	Multivitamins	Homocysteine	6 months	Reduced[42]

Note: FMD, endothelial-dependent, flow-mediated dilation; LDL-C, LDL cholesterol.

All vitamins were given once a day unless specified otherwise. The number in parentheses indicates reference number.

[a] Cardiac transplant.
[b] Hypercholesterolemia.
[c] Normal individuals consuming high-fat meals.

also shown in Table 5.2. These studies showed that the beneficial effects of two dietary antioxidants on CAD risk factors can be observed. Even though these studies produced some short-term beneficial effects, I do not recommend the use of one or two dietary antioxidants for the prevention or improved treatment of CAD because they do not take into account other cardiac risk factors and do not utilize other antioxidants.

VITAMIN C ALONE PRODUCING BENEFICIAL EFFECTS

During a 10-year follow-up, 4647 major cardiac events occurred in 293,172 subjects who were free of CAD at baseline. The results showed that supplemental vitamin C at high doses reduced major cardiac events.[46]

DIETARY ANTIOXIDANTS PRODUCING NO EFFECTS OR ADVERSE EFFECTS

A prospective cohort study of 29,092 Finnish male smokers aged 50 to 69 years who participated in the Alpha-Tocopherol, Beta-Carotene Cancer Prevention (ATBC) study was carried out to determine the risk of cardiac events. The fasting baseline of serum alpha-tocopherol concentration was determined. Only about 10% of participants reported the use of a vitamin E supplement. The analysis of data presented in four separate publications has produced inconsistent results (Table 5.3). The results showed that higher serum concentrations of alpha-tocopherol were associated with lower total and cause-specific (cancer and cardiovascular disease) mortality in male heavy smokers.[47] In the ATBC study, the effect of daily oral supplementation with a once-a-day dose of synthetic

TABLE 5.3
Dietary Antioxidants Producing No Effects or Adverse Effects in High-Risk CAD Patients

Name of Study	Treatment	End Points	Results
ATBC Trial	High serum alpha-T	Mortality	Decreased[47]
	DL-alpha-T (50 mg/day)	CAD risk	No effect[48]
	DL-alpha-T (50 mg/day)	Cerebral infarction	Decreased[49]
	DL-alpha-T (50 mg/day)		Increased[50]
ATBC Trial	Synthetic beta-carotene (50 mg/day)	CAD risk	Increased[48]
	Synthetic beta-carotene (50 mg/day)	Intracerebral hemorrhage	Increased[49]
	Synthetic beta-carotene (50 mg/day)	Cerebral infarction	No effect[50]
HOPE Trial	Natural alpha-T (400 IU/day)	Major cardiac events (myocardial infarction, stroke, and death)	No effect[51-55]
		Secondary cardiac events (unstable angina, renal insufficiency, nephropathy)	No effect[51-54]
		Risk for heart failure	Increased[55]
WAVE Trial	Vitamin E (400 IU) + vitamin C (500 mg)	MLD	No effect[59]
			Decreased[59a]
	Vitamin E (400 IU) + vitamin C (500 mg)	FMD	No effect[60]
	Vitamin E (400 IU) + vitamin C (500 mg)	MDL	Increased[61b]

Note: ATBC, Alpha-Tocopherol, Beta-Carotene cancer Prevention; HOPE, Heart Outcomes Prevention Evaluation; WAVE, Women's Angiographic Vitamin and Estrogen; Alpha-T, alpha-tocopherol; CAD, coronary artery disease; MLD, median luminal diameter; FMD, flow-mediated dilation.

All vitamins were given once a day unless specified otherwise. The number in parentheses indicates reference number.

[a] Potential harm (decrease in MLD) was suggested only when patients who died or had myocardial infarction during the trial period was included in the analysis.

[b] Patients with haptoglobin allele showing beneficial effect.

(DL)-alpha-tocopherol (50 mg) or synthetic BC (20 mg) on CAD was investigated 6 years after the completion of the trial period of 5 to 8 years. At the beginning of the post-trial follow-up, 23,144 men were at risk for a first major cardiac event, and 1255 men with a pretrial history of myocardial infarction (MI) were at risk for major cardiac events. The results showed that alpha-tocopherol supplementation did not significantly affect the outcomes in either patient populations compared to placebo control subjects. However, BC supplementation increased the risk of major cardiac events by about 14%, nonfatal MI by about 16%, and fatal coronary heart disease by about 11%. However, no such effects were observed in the population that had a history of pretrial MI.[48] In the same study population, vitamin E prevented cerebral infarction, but increased the risk of fatal hemorrhagic strokes; BC increased the risk of intracerebral hemorrhage.[49] In the same study population, another investigation showed that alpha-tocopherol increased the risk of cerebral infarction, while BC had no effect.[50] The reasons for this discrepancy in the analysis of the same population are unknown. During a 10-year follow-up, 4647 major cardiac events occur in 293,172 subjects who were free of CAD at the baseline. The results showed that supplementation with vitamin E alone did not reduce major cardiac events.[46]

A randomized, double-blind, placebo-controlled international trial, Heart Outcomes Prevention Evaluation (HOPE) was conducted from December 21, 1993 to April 15, 1999. One of the objectives of this trial was to evaluate the efficacy of natural vitamin E (400 IU/day) in reducing the risk of CAD for patients at least 55 years of age with vascular disease or diabetes, many of whom were heavy cigarette smokers. The analysis of data from this study presented in five separate publications has produced inconsistent results (Table 5.3).

In the analysis published in 2000, the primary end points were major cardiac events (MI, stroke, and death due to coronary heart disease), and the secondary end points were unstable angina, heart failure, revascularization, amputation, death due to coronary heart disease, and complications of diabetes. No significant effect of vitamin E supplementation on the primary or the secondary end points was observed.[51]

In the analysis published in 2001, the effect of vitamin E on carotid intimal medial thickness as measured by ultrasound was evaluated in a subset of the study population. The results showed that vitamin E supplementation had no effect on the progression of atherosclerosis.[52] In the analysis published in 2002, the primary end points were the same as those in the analysis of 2000, but the secondary end points included an additional criterion, nephropathy. The results showed that vitamin E had no effect on either the primary or the secondary end points.[53]

In the analysis published in 2004, the primary end points were the same as those in the analysis of 2000, but the secondary end points included an additional criterion, clinical proteinuria (renal insufficiency). The results showed that in people with mild to moderate renal insufficiency, vitamin E had no effect on the primary or the secondary end points.[54]

In the analysis published in 2005, the primary and secondary end points were the same as those in the analysis of 2000. The results showed that vitamin E supplementation had no effect on the primary or most secondary end points; however, it increased the risk of two secondary end points: heart failure by about 13%, and hospitalization for heart failure by about 21%.[55] The analysis of the subpopulation of heavy tobacco smokers revealed that smoking increased the risk of morbidity and mortality among the high-risk patients, despite the treatment with gold standard medications known to reduce cardiovascular disease.[56] This is consistent with an independent study outside of the HOPE study in which daily consumption of 800 IU of vitamin E increased the levels of oxidative stress markers in heavy smokers.[57] These studies suggest that smoking plays a dominant role in increasing morbidity and mortality. If these major cardiac events increased despite the gold standard medications that were given to reduce the risk of cardiovascular disease in this population, it is not surprising that administration of vitamin E alone either had no significant effect on any primary end points or most secondary end points, or increased the risk of two of the secondary end points (heart failure and hospitalization for heart failure) in one study. Individual antioxidants in high-risk populations, such as tobacco smokers and patients with type 2 diabetes, may be oxidized because of high internal oxidative environment and, thereby, act as pro-oxidants rather than as antioxidants.

A recent analysis of the HOPE study population showed that the levels of markers of inflammation were significantly related to future cardiovascular risk; however, the combination of traditional risk factors and the levels of N-terminal pro-brain natriuretic peptide (NT proBNP) were the best clinical predictive for future cardiac events.[58]

The Women's Angiographic Vitamin and Estrogen (WAVE) trial was conducted on postmenopausal women suffering from progressive CAD with at least one 15% to 75% coronary stenosis at baseline coronary angiography. The trial was conducted from July 1997 to January 2002. Antioxidants (400 IU vitamin E + 500 mg vitamin C, twice daily) were administered orally. The primary end point was annualized mean changes in minimum luminal diameter (MLD). The results showed that in postmenopausal women with progressive coronary disease, antioxidant supplements provided no cardiovascular benefits in these patients (Table 5.3). The potential for harm was suggested only when patients who died or had MIs during the trial period were included in the data analysis.[59] In the analysis published in 2005, antioxidant treatment did not improve flow-mediated dilation (FMD).[60] The analysis of the subgroup of patients with haptoglobin (hp) alleles showed a significant benefit of changes in MLD with antioxidant therapy compared with placebo in patients with Hp 1-allele homozygote (Hp-1-1). This effect was more pronounced in women with diabetes.[61] Again, because of inconsistencies of the results with one or two dietary antioxidants, I do not recommend the use of such antioxidants in the prevention or improved treatment of CAD.

Administration of vitamin E (400 IU) plus vitamin C (1000 mg) for 8 weeks improved arterial stiffness and endothelial-dependent vasodilation in patients with essential hypertension.[62] The combination of vitamin E and vitamin C reduced 30-day cardiac mortality in diabetic patients with acute myocardial infarction (AMI) by about 14%, but this beneficial effect was not observed in patients with AMI who did not have diabetes.[63] Another study revealed that dietary intake of vitamins C and E, and supplemental intake of vitamin E had an inverse association with CAD risk.[64] In contrast, administration of vitamin E (800 IU) plus vitamin C (1000 mg) for 6 months did not improve coronary and brachial endothelial vasomotor function.[65] A combination of 400 IU vitamin E, 500 mg vitamin C, and 12 mg BC, or 800 IU vitamin E, 1000 mg vitamin C, and 24 mg BC did not significantly affect brachial reactivity.[66] These studies suggest that supplementation with dietary antioxidants alone may not be sufficient to reduce the risk of CAD. Addition of endogenous antioxidants and other micronutrients may be necessary.

In a recent analysis of published data on the use of diet, and dietary or supplemental dietary antioxidants,[67] it has been suggested that a strong inverse relationship between intake of vegetables, nuts, and Mediterranean diet patterns with CAD exists. A moderate inverse relationship exists between the intake of fish, marine omega-3 fatty acids, folate, whole grain, dietary vitamins E, C, and BC, alcohol, fruits, and fiber with CAD. However, insufficient evidence exists regarding the value of supplemental vitamin E, vitamin C, saturated and polyunsaturated fatty acids, total fats, alpha-linolenic acid (ALA), meat, eggs, and milk in reducing the risk of CAD when used individually. These studies revealed that diet modifications together with other micronutrients may also be important in reducing the risk of CAD.

ENDOGENOUS ANTIOXIDANTS PRODUCING NO EFFECT OR BENEFICIAL EFFECTS

Like dietary antioxidants, endogenous antioxidants, such as glutathione-elevating agent *N*-acetylcysteine (NAC) and alpha-lipoic acid, produced inconsistent results when used individually. In a study with 100 patients, prophylactic use of NAC in patients undergoing coronary artery bypass grafting (100 patients study) did not improve clinical outcomes or biochemical markers.[68] However, in another study involving 40 patients, prophylactic administration of NAC attenuated myocardial oxidative stress in the heart of patients undergoing cardiopulmonary bypass.[69] In a short-term (8 weeks) study involving 36 patients, oral administration of NAC and alpha-lipoic acid increased

TABLE 5.4
Beneficial or No Effects of Antioxidants in Combination with Cholesterol-Lowering Drugs in High-Risk CAD Patients

Name of Study	No. of Patients	Type of Antioxidant + Cholesterol-Lowering Drug	Criteria of Study	Follow-Up Period	Results
–	7[a]	Simvastatin + Vitamin E, 300 IU	FMD NMD	8 weeks	Improved[71]
–	126[b]	Standard therapy + Coenzyme Q_{10}, 33 mg (three/day)	Cardiac muscle function	6 years	Improved[72–73]
CLAS	156[c]	Colestipol + Niacin Vitamin E, 100 IU or more	Progressive atherosclerosis	2 years	Reduced[74]
HPS	20,500[a]	Simvastatin + Vitamin E, 650 mg Vitamin C, 250 mg Beta-carotene, 20 mg	Cardiac events	5.5 years	No better than drug alone

Note: HPS, Heart Protection Study; CLAS, Cholesterol-Lowering Atherosclerosis Study; NMD, endothelium-independent nitroglycerine-mediated dilation.

All vitamins were given once a day unless specified otherwise. The number in parentheses indicates reference number.

[a] Hypercholesterolemia.
[b] Idiopathic dilated cardiomyopathy.
[c] Coronary bypass surgery.

brachial artery diameter and reduced arterial tone as well as decreased systolic blood pressure in patients with CAD.[70] Based on these results, I do not recommend the use of one or two endogenous antioxidants in any prevention or treatment strategy for CAD.

DIETARY AND ENDOGENOUS ANTIOXIDANTS WITH CHOLESTEROL-LOWERING DRUGS

A summary of three interventional trials in high-risk patients with vitamin E or coenzyme Q_{10}, alone or in combination with cholesterol-lowering drugs, is described in Table 5.4. The number, type, dose, and dose schedules of antioxidants, patient population, observation period and criteria of study were different. It has been reported[71] that vitamin E supplementation (300 IU/day) together with simvastatin for an 8-week period improved endothelial-dependent FMD as well as endothelial-dependent, nitroglycerine-mediated dilation (NMD) in the brachial artery of patients with hypercholesterolemia more that that produced by simvastatin alone. Similarly, coenzyme Q_{10}, in combination with standard therapy, improved the function of damaged cardiac muscle associated with congestive heart failure[72] and idiopathic dilated cardiomyopathy.[73] One study using 156 men with previous coronary bypass surgery who were receiving a cholesterol-lowering drug combination (colestipol–niacin) alone or in combination with vitamin E, 100 IU/day, showed that the vitamin E–treated group revealed less progression of the narrowing of their coronary arteries in comparison to cholesterol-lowering drugs alone during a 4-year trial period.[74] In the Heart Protection Study[75] involving 20,500 patients at high risk, supplementation with antioxidants (vitamin E, 650 mg; vitamin C, 250 mg; and β-carotene, 20 mg) together with simvastatin for a period of 5.5 years did not interfere with the efficacy of cholesterol-lowering drugs.

MULTIPLE DIETARY ANTIOXIDANTS WITH CHOLESTEROL-LOWERING DRUGS

In the HDL Atherosclerosis Treatment Study (HATS), the effects of the dietary antioxidants in combination with cholesterol-lowering drugs on stenosis and HDL cholesterol were evaluated in

CAD patients with low HDL.[76,77] Dietary antioxidants included vitamin C (1000 mg/day), vitamin E as D-α-tocopherol (800 IU/day), natural BC (25 mg/day), and selenium (100 μg/day), were given together with simvastatin–niacin in a subset of patients with a low level of HDL cholesterol (Table 5.5). The results revealed that niacin-induced elevation of HDL cholesterol was reduced by antioxidant supplements. The same group of investigators using the same formulation reported that a mixture of dietary antioxidants reduced the degree of proximal artery stenosis in comparison to placebo controls; however, in combination with simvastatin–niacin antioxidant supplementation was less effective than the simvastatin–niacin treatment alone in reducing the degree of stenosis. Because of the small sample size (40 patients per group) and unusually large variations in the results (200–700% variation around the mean value),[76] no conclusion regarding the value of antioxidants in combination with standard therapy in the management of stenosis can be drawn. This was further confirmed by the analysis of plasma levels of markers of cholesterol synthesis and absorption in the same study population. In this study, simvastatin–niacin treatment reduced plasma levels of desmosterol and lathosterol (markers of cholesterol synthesis) by 46% and 36%, respectively; whereas, simvastatin–niacin plus antioxidant reduced each of them by 37% and 31%, respectively, suggesting no significant difference between the two groups. Similarly, simvastatin–niacin treatment increased plasma levels of campesterol and beta-sitosterol (markers of cholesterol absorption) by 70% and 59%, respectively; whereas, simvastatin–niacin plus antioxidant increased each of them by 54% and 46%, respectively, suggesting a small difference between the two groups.[78] Nevertheless, the authors concluded that mean changes in percent stenosis was positively associated with a percent change in the lathosterol level and negatively associated with a percent change in the β-sitosterol level. This conclusion does not appear to be consistent with their data on the markers of cholesterol synthesis and absorption. Thus, the conclusion that antioxidant supplementation can increase the level of stenosis in the group of CAD patients with low HDL receiving simvastatin–niacin therapy may not be valid. These intervention studies, with one or multiple dietary antioxidants in combination with cholesterol-lowering drugs, produced inconsistent results because other cardiac risk factors were not addressed, and multiple endogenous antioxidants were not used in these studies.

TABLE 5.5
Summary of Intervention Trials with One or More Dietary Antioxidants in Combination with Cholesterol-Lowering Drugs in High-Risk Patients Showing No Effects or Adverse Effects

Name of Study	No. of Patients	Type of Antioxidant and Cholesterol-Lowering Drug	Criteria of Study	Follow-Up Period	Results
HATS	160[b]	Simvastatin + Niacin + vitamin E, 800 IU Vitamin C, 1 g Beta-carotene, 25 mg Selenium, 100 μg ($N = 46$)	Stenosis	3 years	Reduced drug effectiveness,[76,77] more effective than control
HATS	153[b]	Same	HDL	1 year	Reduced drug effectiveness[76]
HATS		Same	Markers of cholesterol synthesis and absorption		No effect[78]

Note: HATS, HDL Atherosclerosis Treatment Study; HDL, high-density lipoprotein cholesterol; N, sample size for the group.

All vitamins were given once a day unless specified otherwise. The number in parentheses indicates the reference number.

[a] Women with diabetes.
[b] Coronary disease with low HDL cholesterol.

RESVERATROL AND OMEGA-3 FATTY ACIDS

Resveratrol

Several epidemiological and experimental studies have shown that mild to moderate drinking of wine, particularly red wine, reduced the risks for cardiovascular, cerebrovascular, and peripheral vascular diseases.[79–82] The cardioprotective effects of wine were primarily due to the presence of antioxidants, primarily resveratrol (*trans*-3,5,4'-trihydroxystilbene), found in grape skin, and proanthocyanidins, found in grape seed. The white wine also appears to provide cardioprotection in animal models due primarily to the presence of antioxidants, especially tyrosol and hydroxytyrosol.[83] These antioxidants increased the activities of mitochondrial complex (I–IV). Resveratrol reduced infarct size and prevented cardiac mitochondrial swelling in rats during reperfusion injury.[84] It also protected against H_2O_2-induced apoptosis in cardiomyocytes.[85] This effect of resveratrol on apoptosis is mediated through activation of AMP-activated kinase in cardiomyocytes.[86] Administration of resveratrol significantly reduced the MI-induced ventricular tachycardia and ventricular fibrillation. The infarct size and mortality were reduced in resveratrol-treated rats.[87] It has been demonstrated that lower doses of resveratrol provided cardioprotection on the criteria of improved postischemic ventricular recovery, reduction of myocardial infarct size, and cardiomyocyte apoptosis by up-regulating antiapoptotic and redox proteins Akt and Bcl-2 in ischemic and reperfusion rats. However, higher doses of resveratrol produced adverse effects on the heart by down-regulating redox proteins and up-regulating proapoptotic proteins.[88] The biphasic effects of resveratrol, depending upon the dose, should be carefully considered while considering the doses to be used in any clinical studies.

The identified mechanisms of cardioprotection by components of red or white wine include antioxidant, anti-inflammatory and antifibrotic. Oxidized LDL reduced antiplatelet activity of endothelial cells, and NOS protein in endothelial cells, but pretreatment of these cells with resveratrol attenuated the above effects of oxidized HDL.[89] Resveratrol and quercetin inhibited the expression of C-reactive proteins induced by IL-1 beta + IL-6) by activating phosphorylation of p38 and p44/42 MAP kinases.[90] Resveratrol inhibited ICAM-1 gene expression induced by cytokines [tumor necrosis factor-alpha (TNF-alpha) and IL-6] by reducing STAT3 phosphorylation.[91]

Treatment with resveratrol inhibited collagen- and epinephrine-induced aggregation of platelets obtained from patients who exhibited aspirin resistance.[92] In ischemic and reperfusion rats with hypercholesterolemia, it was observed that treatment with resveratrol, statin, or resveratrol plus statin improved left ventricular function recovery and reduced infarct size compared to control animals. The lipid levels were decreased in all treatment groups compared to controls, but more so in the statin- and resveratrol-plus-statin–treated groups than in the resveratrol-treated group. The reduction in apoptosis was more in the group treated with statin plus resveratrol than in other treated groups.[93] In a rat MI model, it was demonstrated that resveratrol treatment up-regulated the protein expression profiles of vascular endothelial growth factor and its tyrosine kinase receptor, FIK-1, after inducing MI. Pretreatment with resveratrol also increased iNOS and eNOS, together with increased antiapoptotic and proangiogenic factors NF-kappaB and specificity (SP)-1. Resveratrol treatment also improved left ventricular function and increased capillary density 3 weeks after MI.[94]

Omega-3 Fatty Acids

Omega-3 fatty acids are essential fatty acids consisting of ALA, eicosapentaenoic acid (EPA), and docosahexaenoic acid (DHA). These fatty acids are not synthesized in the body but are obtained from the diet. EPA and DHA are formed from ALA in the body. Several reviews on the efficacy of omega-3 fatty acids have revealed that supplementation with omega-3 from fish or capsules reduced the risk of cardiac events in patients with CAD.[95–100] It has been reported that certain CAD patients with angina and some individuals with a history of ventricular arrhythmia may not derive any benefit from omega-3 fatty acid supplementation.[101] Atrial fibrillation is a common complication after a coronary artery bypass grafting operation. A review of studies suggests that omega-3 fatty acids supplementation is associated with a lower incidence of atrial fibrillation in patients who underwent cardiac surgery. It also reduced the incidence of sudden death in survivors of myocardial infarction.[102] Oral administration of omega-3 fatty acids significantly reduced the rate of postoperative atrial fibrillation. Preoperative intravenous infusion of omega-3 fatty acids also reduced the incidence of atrial fibrillation after cardiac surgery, and shortened stays in intensive care units and in hospitals.[103,104] An analysis of published studies on the effects of omega-3 fatty acids on the incidence of recurrent ventricular arrhythmia in patients with implantable cardioverter defibrillator (ICD) showed that these fatty acids did not provide any protection in these patients.[105] Prescription omega-3 fatty acids, in combination with statin, improved lipid profiles better than statin alone.[106] An analog of omega-3 fatty acids and omega-3 ethyl esters in combination with simvastatin improved lipid profiles better than simvastatin alone.[107] Administration of omega-3 fatty acids without statin (rosuvastatin) significantly reduced death and admission to hospital for cardiovascular reasons.[108] Chronic kidney disease is associated with increased risk of CAD. In a randomized, double-blind, placebo-controlled trial involving 85 nondiabetic patients with chronic kidney disease, it was observed that omega-3 fatty acid supplementation reduced blood pressure, heart rate, and triglycerides.[109] A review of literatures has confirmed that supplementation with omega-3 fatty acids significantly improved arterial hypertension.[110] Omega-3 fatty acids exhibit a wide range of biological activity, including regulation of both vasomotor tone and renal sodium excretion. They also reduce angiotensin-converting enzyme (ACE) activity, angiotensin II formation, tumor growth factor-beta (TGF-beta) expression, as well as enhance production of endothelial nitric oxide and activate the parasympathetic nervous system.

Based on cellular and animal models, the mechanisms of action of omega-3 fatty acids involve reduction of inflammation and platelet aggregation and improvement of endothelial dysfunction.[111] The western diet contains a high ratio of omega-6 fatty acids to omega-3 fatty acids that has been suggested to associate with increased incidence of chronic diseases including CAD. Omega-3 fatty acids reduced the levels of interleukin-1beta (IL-1beta), TNF-alpha, and interleukin-6 (IL-6).[112] The studies discussed here convincingly suggest that supplementation with omega-3 fatty acids, together with micronutrients, diet, and lifestyle modifications, may be necessary for an optimal effect in prevention or improved treatment of CAD.

INTERVENTION STUDIES WITH B-VITAMINS TO LOWER HOMOCYSTEINE LEVELS

All patients included in four studies (Table 5.6) were at high risk for MI, stroke, and death from coronary heart disease. It is interesting to note that a high dose of folic acid plus vitamins B_6 and B_{12} increased the risk of recurrence of MI, stroke, and death from CAD in one study,[113] but had no significant effect in the other three studies.[114–116] The exact reasons for this discrepancy are unknown; however, the patient population and criteria of end points in these studies were different. In the first study,[113] the patients who had MIs within 1 week were randomized, whereas, in the other studies,[114–116] patients with vascular disease and diabetes were randomized for the study. The latter patient population was considered at the lower risk for CAD compared to those in the first study. These studies concluded that high doses of B-vitamins should not be recommended to these patients in order to reduce the risk of cardiac events. These well-designed studies were performed in order to reduce the risk of major cardiac events; however, they did not take into account the oxidative stress through which homocysteine mediated its action on endothelial cells of the vessel walls. Therefore, a modest reduction in homocysteine levels is not expected to have any significant effect on any of the major cardiac events. Other risk factors, such as increased oxidative stress generated by mechanisms other than homocysteine, chronic inflammation, and oxidation of LDL cholesterol were not affected by supplementation with B-vitamins alone. Therefore, consumption of B-vitamins alone is not expected to produce any beneficial effects on cardiac events in high-risk populations.

TABLE 5.6
Effects of B-Vitamins on Cardiac Events Showing No Effects or Adverse Effects

Patient Type	Vitamin Treatment	End Points	Results
3749 patients with MI	Folic acid (0.8 mg) Vitamin B_6 (40 mg) Vitamin B_{12} (0.4 mg)	MI, stroke, death	Increase[113]
5522 patients with vascular disease or diabetes	Folic acid (2.5 mg) Vitamin B_6 (50 mg) Vitamin B_{12} (1 mg)	MI, stroke, death	No effect[114]
Same patients	Same B-vitamins	Thrombosis	No effect[115]
3680 patients with nondisabling cerebral infarction	Multiple vitamins with high-dose or low-dose B-vitamins	MI, stroke, death	No effect[116]

Note: MI, myocardial infarction.

SCIENTIFIC RATIONALE FOR USING MULTIPLE MICRONUTRIENTS INCLUDING DIETARY AND ENDOGENOUS ANTIOXIDANTS IN PREVENTION AND IMPROVED TREATMENT OF CAD

Since increased production of free radicals and chronic inflammation may be involved in the initiation and progression of damage leading to CAD, and since antioxidants can neutralize free radicals and reduce chronic inflammation, the use of antioxidants appears to be one of the rational choices for prevention and improved treatment of CAD. Multiple dietary and endogenous antioxidants should be added to a multiple micronutrient preparation, because many different types of free radicals are produced, and each antioxidant has a different affinity for each of these free radicals, depending upon the cellular environment. They also exhibit different mechanisms of action. For example, BC was more effective in quenching oxygen radicals than most other antioxidants.[117] BC can perform certain biological functions that cannot be produced by its metabolite, vitamin A, and vice versa.[118,119] BC treatment enhanced the expression of the connexin gene, a gap junction protein gene, whereas vitamin A treatment did not produce such an effect.[119] Vitamin A induced cell differentiation in certain normal and cancer cells, whereas BC did not.[120,121] The gradient of oxygen pressure varies within the cell and tissues. Vitamin E was more effective as a quencher of free radicals in reduced oxygen pressure, whereas BC and vitamin A were more effective in higher atmospheric pressure.[122] Vitamin C is necessary to protect cellular components in aqueous environments, whereas carotenoids, and vitamins A and E protect cellular components in nonaqueous (lipid) environments. Vitamin C also plays an important role in maintaining cellular levels of vitamin E by recycling the vitamin E radical (oxidized) to the reduced (antioxidant) form.[123] Also, the DNA damage produced by oxidized vitamin C can be ameliorated by vitamin E. The form and type of vitamin E used in the micronutrient preparation are also important to improving the beneficial effects of vitamin E. It is known that various organs of rats selectively absorb the natural form of vitamin E.[124] Therefore, the natural form of vitamin E should be used. It has been established that alpha tocopheryl-succinate (α-TS) is the most effective form of vitamin E.[125,126] We have reported that oral ingestion of α-TS (800 IU/day) for more than 6 months in humans increased plasma levels of not only α-tocopherol, but also of α-TS, suggesting that α-TS can be absorbed from the intestinal tract without hydrolysis to α-tocopherol, provided the pool of alpha-tocopherol in the body has become saturated.[126] Therefore, alpha-TS should be utilized in addition to alpha-tocopherol or alpha-tocopheryl acetate to increase the efficacy of vitamin E in the micronutrient preparation.

Seleno-L-methionine instead of selenium oxide should be utilized in the micronutrient preparation, because it is absorbed better than selenium oxide. Selenium, a cofactor of glutathione peroxidase, acts as an antioxidant.

Glutathione, one of the endogenously made compounds, represents a potent intracellular protective agent against oxidative damage. It catabolizes H_2O_2 and anions and is very effective in quenching peroxynitrite.[127] Therefore, increasing the intracellular levels of glutathione in vascular endothelial cells, vascular smooth muscle cells, and cardiac muscles may be very useful in the prevention or improved treatment of CAD. Oral supplementation with glutathione failed to significantly increase plasma levels of glutathione in human subjects,[128] suggesting that this tripeptide is completely hydrolyzed in the gastrointestinal tract. NAC and alpha-lipoic acid increase the intracellular levels of glutathione by different mechanisms; and therefore, they can also be used in the preparation of multiple micronutrients. Damaged vascular endothelial cells and cardiac muscle cells may not produce sufficient amounts of ATP due to a reduction in the level of coenzyme Q_{10}. It also scavenges peroxy radicals faster than α-tocopherol,[129] and, like vitamin C, can regenerate vitamin E in a redox cycle.[130] Therefore, supplementation with coenzyme Q_{10} may be necessary to improve the efficacy of preparation of multiple micronutrients. L-Carnitine, which facilitates oxidation of fatty acids, should be added to the micronutrient preparation. The inclusion of B-vitamins into a multiple micronutrient preparation is also essential, because vitamins B_6, B_{12}, and folic acid are needed to reduce the levels of homocysteine.[113,116,131]

PROPOSED MULTIPLE MICRONUTRIENT PREPARATION

I propose a multiple micronutrient preparation containing multiple dietary and endogenous antioxidants, B-vitamins, vitamin D, mercury-free omega-3 fatty acids, and certain minerals, including selenium, but no iron, copper, manganese, heavy metals (vanadium, zirconium, and molybdenum), herbs, or herbal antioxidants. Iron and copper are not added because they are known to interact with vitamin C and generate excessive amounts of free radicals. In addition, prolonged consumption of these trace minerals in the presence of antioxidants may increase the levels of free iron or copper stores in the body, because there are no significant mechanisms of excretion of iron among men of all ages and women after menopause. Increased stores of free iron may increase the risk of some human chronic diseases including CAD. Heavy metals are not added, because prolonged consumption of these metals may increase their levels in the body, because there is no significant mechanism of excretion. High levels of these metals are considered neurotoxic. Herbs are not added because some herbs are known to interact adversely with prescription and nonprescription drugs. Herbal antioxidants and resveratrol are not added because they do not produce any unique biological effects that cannot be produced by the dietary and endogenous antioxidants.

IMPORTANCE OF DOSE SCHEDULE

Almost all clinical studies have utilized a once-a-day dose schedule. Most consumers of multiple vitamins take a once-a-day dose. This dose-schedule may not be sufficient for an optimal beneficial effect on CAD, because the biological half-lives of the ingredients present in the micronutrient preparation in the plasma vary markedly, depending upon their solubility and turnover. Taking a micronutrient preparation once a day may create large fluctuations in their levels in the cells and tissues. A twofold change in the treatment dose of alpha-TS caused marked alterations in the expression of gene profiles of neuroblastoma cells in culture. This suggests that large fluctuations in the levels of antioxidants may force cells to constantly adjust genetic activity that can cause cellular stress over a long period. Therefore, the dose schedule of once a day may cause genetic stress over a long period. Taking a micronutrient preparation twice a day may reduce the levels of fluctuation of micronutrients and, thus, avoid potential problems in the future.

ANTIOXIDANTS AND ASPIRIN RESISTANCE

Aspirin resistance is associated with an increased risk of adverse clinical outcomes in stable patients with CAD.[132] The patients exhibiting aspirin resistance to a low dose receive a gradual increase in aspirin doses, until the toxic limit is reached. The mechanisms of aspirin-resistance are not known. I suggest that the addition of antioxidants such as vitamin E may enhance the efficacy of low-dose aspirin in reducing platelet aggregation, at least for certain periods of time. This is because vitamin E in combination with aspirin is more effective in inhibiting cyclooxygenase-1-enzyme activity than the individual agent.[133] Thus, supplementation with multiple dietary and endogenous antioxidants can prolong the efficacy of aspirin among semiresponders, as well as in patients who developed total resistance to aspirin in reducing platelet aggregation. This should be tested in a well-designed clinical study.

SCIENTIFIC RATIONALE FOR USING MULTIPLE MICRONUTRIENT PREPARATIONS IN COMBINATION WITH CHOLESTEROL-LOWERING DRUGS AND ASPIRIN FOR REDUCING THE PROGRESSION OF CAD

Increased oxidative stress and chronic inflammation continue to occur during treatment with cholesterol lowering drugs in high-risk populations. This is evidenced by the fact that tobacco smoking increased the risk of morbidity and mortality among heavy tobacco smokers despite the treatment with gold standard medications known to reduce cardiovascular disease.[56] Therefore, the addition of multiple micronutrients such as those described in Proposed Multiple Micronutrient Preparation to the regimen of cholesterol-lowering drugs and low-dose aspirin appears to be one of the rational choices for reducing the progression of CAD.

MODIFICATIONS IN DIET AND LIFESTYLE

Dietary recommendations include daily consumption of a low-fat, high-fiber diet with plenty of fresh fruits and vegetables, avoiding excessive amounts of protein, carbohydrates, or calories, restricting intake of nitrite-rich cured meat, charcoal-broiled, or smoked meat or fish, caffeine-containing beverages (cold or hot), and pickled fruits and vegetables.

Lifestyle-related changes include stopping smoking and chewing tobacco, avoiding secondhand smoke, restricting intake of alcohol, reducing stress by vacation, yoga, or meditation, and performing moderate exercise four to five times a week.

CONCLUSIONS

Despite current prevention recommendations and improved treatment outcomes due to advances in surgical technique, early detection equipment, and the discovery of cholesterol-lowering drugs, CAD remains the number one cause of death in the United States. The risk factors for CAD include increased oxidative stress, oxidized LDL cholesterol, and high levels of C-reactive proteins, a marker of chronic inflammation, and homocysteine. Therefore, the use of multiple micronutrients including dietary and endogenous antioxidants that neutralize free radicals and reduce inflammation and B-vitamins that reduce homocysteine levels appears to be a rational choice for reducing the risk and progression of CAD. However, previous clinical studies have utilized primarily dietary antioxidants such as vitamin E alone or vitamin C alone in populations at high risk of developing CAD or in patients at various stages of the disease. Sometimes, these antioxidants have been used in combination in these high-risk populations. These studies have produced inconsistent results ranging from beneficial effects, to no effects, to harmful effects. This may be partly because none of the clinical studies have utilized agents that can reduce the major risk factors of CAD, including increased oxidative stress, oxidized LDL cholesterol, and high levels of C-reactive proteins and homocysteine at the same time. Most studies have utilized only one or more dietary antioxidants that may not be sufficient. None of the clinical studies have attempted to elevate the level of glutathione, one of the most abundant intracellular antioxidants, by NAC and alpha-lipoic acid. Coenzyme Q_{10} is in the same pathway as cholesterol. Statins are well known to decrease the levels of cholesterol and, therefore, are expected to decrease the level of coenzyme Q_{10} as well. However, coenzyme Q_{10} has never been used in combination with other antioxidants in any clinical studies that include statins. I have proposed that a multiple micronutrient preparation, together with modification in diet and lifestyle, be tested in a normal population with no risk factor for CAD for reducing the incidence of this disease. The same strategy can also be used in high-risk populations who are on cholesterol-lowering drugs and low-dose aspirin. The proposed strategy is expected to reduce all major risk factors at the same time and, thereby, reduce the rate of progression of CAD and improve the efficacy of standard therapy. The efficacy of proposed recommendations can be tested by well-designed clinical trials. Meanwhile, individuals interested in reducing the risk of, or improving the treatment of CAD may like to adopt the proposed recommendations in consultation with their doctors.

REFERENCES

1. Jessup, W. 1996. Oxidized lipoproteins and nitric oxide. *Curr Opin Lipidol* 7 (5): 274–280.
2. Witztum, J. L. 1994. The oxidation hypothesis of atherosclerosis. *Lancet* 344 (8925): 793–795.
3. de Nigris, F., T. Youssef, S. Ciafre, F. Franconi, V. Anania, G. Condorelli, W. Palinski, and C. Napoli. 2000. Evidence for oxidative activation of c-Myc–dependent nuclear signaling in human coronary smooth muscle cells and in early lesions of Watanabe heritable hyperlipidemic rabbits: Protective effects of vitamin E. *Circulation* 102 (17): 2111–2117.
4. Holvoet, P., and D. Collen. 1994. Oxidized lipoproteins in atherosclerosis and thrombosis. *FASEB J* 8 (15): 1279–1284.
5. Mann, M. J., A. D. Whittemore, M. C. Donaldson, M. Belkin, M. S. Conte, J. F. Polak, E. Orav, et al. 1999. Ex-vivo gene therapy of human vascular bypass grafts with E2F decoy: The PREVENT single-centre, randomised, controlled trial. *Lancet* 354 (9189): 1493–1498.
6. Reaven, P. D., A. Khouw, W. F. Beltz, S. Parthasarathy, and J. L. Witztum. 1993. Effect of dietary antioxidant combinations in humans. Protection of LDL by vitamin E but not by beta-carotene. *Arterioscler Thromb* 13 (4): 590–600.
7. Becker, A. E., O. J. de Boer, and A. C. van Der Wal. 2001. The role of inflammation and infection in coronary artery disease. *Annu Rev Med* 52: 289–297.
8. Verhoef, P., F. J. Kok, D. A. Kruyssen, E. G. Schouten, J. C. Witteman, D. E. Grobbee, P. M. Ueland, and H. Refsum. 1997. Plasma total homocysteine, B vitamins, and risk of coronary atherosclerosis. *Arterioscler Thromb Vasc Biol* 17 (5): 989–995.
9. American Heart Association. 2001. *Heart and Stroke Statistical Update.* Dallas, TX: American Heart Association.
10. Perez-de-Arce, K., R. Foncea, and F. Leighton. 2005. Reactive oxygen species mediates homocysteine-induced mitochondrial biogenesis in human endothelial cells: Modulation by antioxidants. *Biochem Biophys Res Commun* 338 (2): 1103–1109.
11. Chen, J. W., Y. H. Chen, and S. J. Lin. 2006. Long-term exposure to oxidized low-density lipoprotein enhances tumor necrosis factor-alpha–stimulated endothelial adhesiveness of monocytes by activating superoxide generation and redox-sensitive pathways. *Free Radic Biol Med* 40 (5): 817–826.
12. Anderson, T. J., M. D. Gerhard, I. T. Meredith, F. Charbonneau, D. Delagrange, M. A. Creager, A. P. Selwyn, and P. Ganz. 1995. Systemic nature of endothelial dysfunction in atherosclerosis. *Am J Cardiol* 75 (6): 71B–74B.
13. Drexler, H. 1999. Nitric oxide and coronary endothelial dysfunction in humans. *Cardiovasc Res* 43 (3): 572–579.
14. Luoma, J. S., and S. Yla-Herttuala. 1999. Expression of inducible nitric oxide synthase in macrophages and smooth muscle cells in various types of human atherosclerotic lesions. *Virchows Arch* 434 (6): 561–568.
15. Macchi, L., N. Sorel, and L. Christiaens. 2006. Aspirin resistance: Definitions, mechanisms, prevalence, and clinical significance. *Curr Pharm Des* 12 (2): 251–258.

16. Patel, D., and M. Moonis. 2007. Clinical implications of aspirin resistance. *Expert Rev Cardiovasc Ther* 5 (5): 969–975.
17. Cotter, G., E. Shemesh, M. Zehavi, I. Dinur, A. Rudnick, O. Milo, Z. Vered, R. Krakover, E. Kaluski, and A. Kornberg. 2004. Lack of aspirin effect: Aspirin resistance or resistance to taking aspirin? *Am Heart J* 147 (2): 293–300.
18. Gum, P. A., K. Kottke-Marchant, P. A. Welsh, J. White, and E. J. Topol. 2003. A prospective, blinded determination of the natural history of aspirin resistance among stable patients with cardiovascular disease. *J Am Coll Cardiol* 41 (6): 961–965.
19. Gum, P. A., M. Thamilarasan, J. Watanabe, E. H. Blackstone, and M. S. Lauer. 2001. Aspirin use and all-cause mortality among patients being evaluated for known or suspected coronary artery disease: A propensity analysis. *JAMA* 286 (10): 1187–1194.
20. Sztriha, L. K., K. Sas, and L. Vecsei. 2005. Aspirin resistance in stroke: 2004. *J Neurol Sci* 229–230: 163–169.
21. U.S. Preventive Services Task Force. 2003. Routine vitamin supplementation to prevent cancer and cardiovascular disease: Recommendation and rationale. *Ann Intern Med* 139: 51–55.
22. Riley, S. J., and G. A. Stouffer. 2002. Cardiology Grand Rounds from the University of North Carolina at Chapel Hill. The antioxidant vitamins and coronary heart disease: Part 1. Basic science background and clinical observational studies. *Am J Med Sci* 324 (6): 314–320.
23. Lynch, S., and B. Frei. 1994. *Antioxidants as Antiatherogens: Animal Studies*. New York, NY: Academic Press.
24. Smith, T. L., and F. A. Kummerow. 1989. Effect of dietary vitamin E on plasma lipids and atherogenesis in restricted ovulator chickens. *Atherosclerosis* 75 (2–3): 105–109.
25. Verlangieri, A. J., and M. J. Bush. 1992. Effects of D-alpha-tocopherol supplementation on experimentally induced primate atherosclerosis. *J Am Coll Nutr* 11 (2): 131–138.
26. Wojcicki, J., L. Rozewicka, B. Barcew-Wiszniewska, L. Samochowiec, S. Juzwiak, D. Kadlubowska, S. Tustanowski, and Z. Juzyszyn. 1991. Effect of selenium and vitamin E on the development of experimental atherosclerosis in rabbits. *Atherosclerosis* 87 (1): 9–16.
27. Joseph, J., L. Joseph, S. Devi, and R. H. Kennedy. 2008. Effect of anti-oxidant treatment on hyperhomocysteinemia-induced myocardial fibrosis and diastolic dysfunction. *J Heart Lung Transplant* 27 (11): 1237–1241.
28. Gey, K. F., and P. Puska. 1989. Plasma vitamins E and A inversely correlated to mortality from ischemic heart disease in cross-cultural epidemiology. *Ann N Y Acad Sci* 570: 268–282.
29. Sklodowska, R. W., W. Gromadzinska, J. Miroslaw, and W. Malczyk. 1991. Selenium and vitamin E concentrations in plasma and erythrocytes of angina pectoris patients. *Trace Elem Med* 8: 113–117.
30. Riemersma, R. A., D. A. Wood, C. C. Macintyre, R. A. Elton, K. F. Gey, and M. F. Oliver. 1991. Risk of angina pectoris and plasma concentrations of vitamins A, C, and E and carotene. *Lancet* 337 (8732): 1–5.
31. Rimm, E. B., M. J. Stampfer, A. Ascherio, E. Giovannucci, G. A. Colditz, and W. C. Willett. 1993. Vitamin E consumption and the risk of coronary heart disease in men. *N Engl J Med* 328 (20): 1450–1456.
32. Stampfer, M. J., C. H. Hennekens, J. E. Manson, G. A. Colditz, B. Rosner, and W. C. Willett. 1993. Vitamin E consumption and the risk of coronary disease in women. *N Engl J Med* 328 (20): 1444–1449.
33. Losonczy, K. G., T. B. Harris, and R. J. Havlik. 1996. Vitamin E and vitamin C supplement use and risk of all-cause and coronary heart disease mortality in older persons: The Established Populations for Epidemiologic Studies of the Elderly. *Am J Clin Nutr* 64 (2): 190–196.
34. Kok, F. J., A. M. de Bruijn, R. Vermeeren, A. Hofman, A. van Laar, M. de Bruin, R. J. Hermus, and H. A. Valkenburg. 1987. Serum selenium, vitamin antioxidants, and cardiovascular mortality: A 9-year follow-up study in the Netherlands. *Am J Clin Nutr* 45 (2): 462–468.
35. Salonen, J. T., R. Salonen, I. Penttila, J. Herranen, M. Jauhiainen, M. Kantola, R. Lappetelainen, P. H. Maenpaa, G. Alfthan, and P. Puska. 1985. Serum fatty acids, apolipoproteins, selenium and vitamin antioxidants and the risk of death from coronary artery disease. *Am J Cardiol* 56 (4): 226–231.
36. Murr, C., B. M. Winklhofer-Roob, K. Schroecksnadel, M. Maritschnegg, H. Mangge, B. O. Bohm, B. R. Winkelmann, W. Marz, and D. Fuchs. 2009. Inverse association between serum concentrations of neopterin and antioxidants in patients with and without angiographic coronary artery disease. *Atherosclerosis* 202 (2): 543–549.
37. DeMaio, S. J., S. B. King, 3rd, N. J. Lembo, G. S. Roubin, J. A. Hearn, H. N. Bhagavan, and D. S. Sgoutas. 1992. Vitamin E supplementation, plasma lipids and incidence of restenosis after percutaneous transluminal coronary angioplasty (PTCA). *J Am Coll Nutr* 11 (1): 68–73.

38. Devaraj, S., and I. Jialal. 2000. Alpha tocopherol supplementation decreases serum C-reactive protein and monocyte interleukin-6 levels in normal volunteers and type 2 diabetic patients. *Free Radic Biol Med* 29 (8), 790–792.
39. Heitzer, T., S. Yla Herttuala, E. Wild, J. Luoma, and H. Drexler. 1999. Effect of vitamin E on endothelial vasodilator function in patients with hypercholesterolemia, chronic smoking or both. *J Am Coll Cardiol* 33 (2): 499–505.
40. Islam, K. N., D. O'Byrne, S. Devaraj, B. Palmer, S. M. Grundy, and I. Jialal. 2000. Alpha-tocopherol supplementation decreases the oxidative susceptibility of LDL in renal failure patients on dialysis therapy. *Atherosclerosis* 150 (1): 217–224.
41. Stephens, N. G., A. Parsons, P. M. Schofield, F. Kelly, K. Cheeseman, and M. J. Mitchinson. 1996. Randomised controlled trial of vitamin E in patients with coronary disease: Cambridge Heart Antioxidant Study (CHAOS). *Lancet* 347 (9004): 781–786.
42. Earnest, C. P., K. A. Wood, and T. S. Church. 2003. Complex multivitamin supplementation improves homocysteine and resistance to LDL-C oxidation. *J Am Coll Nutr* 22 (5): 400–407.
43. Fang, J. C., S. Kinlay, J. Beltrame, H. Hikiti, M. Wainstein, D. Behrendt, J. Suh, et al. 2002. Effect of vitamins C and E on progression of transplant-associated arteriosclerosis: A randomised trial. *Lancet* 359 (9312): 1108–1113.
44. Plotnick, G. D., M. C. Corretti, and R. A. Vogel. 1997. Effect of antioxidant vitamins on the transient impairment of endothelium-dependent brachial artery vasoactivity following a single high-fat meal. *JAMA* 278 (20): 1682–1686.
45. Salonen, J. T. 2002. Clinical trials testing cardiovascular benefits of antioxidant supplementation. *Free Radic Res* 36 (12): 1299–1306.
46. Knekt, P., J. Ritz, M. A. Pereira, E. J. O'Reilly, K. Augustsson, G. E. Fraser, et al. 2004. Antioxidant vitamins and coronary heart disease risk: A pooled analysis of 9 cohorts. *Am J Clin Nutr* 80 (6): 1508–1520.
47. Wright, M. E., K. A. Lawson, S. J. Weinstein, P. Pietinen, P. R. Taylor, J. Virtamo, and D. Albanes. 2006. Higher baseline serum concentrations of vitamin E are associated with lower total and cause-specific mortality in the Alpha-Tocopherol, Beta-Carotene Cancer Prevention Study. *Am J Clin Nutr* 84 (5): 1200–1207.
48. Tornwall, M. E., J. Virtamo, P. A. Korhonen, M. J. Virtanen, P. R. Taylor, D. Albanes, and J. K. Huttunen. 2004. Effect of alpha-tocopherol and beta-carotene supplementation on coronary heart disease during the 6-year post-trial follow-up in the ATBC study. *Eur Heart J* 25 (13): 1171–1178.
49. Leppala, J. M., J. Virtamo, R. Fogelholm, J. K. Huttunen, D. Albanes, P. R. Taylor, and O. P. Heinonen. 2000. Controlled trial of alpha-tocopherol and beta-carotene supplements on stroke incidence and mortality in male smokers. *Arterioscler Thromb Vasc Biol* 20 (1): 230–235.
50. Tornwall, M. E., J. Virtamo, P. A. Korhonen, M. J. Virtanen, D. Albanes, and J. K. Huttunen. 2004. Postintervention effect of alpha tocopherol and beta carotene on different strokes: A 6-year follow-up of the Alpha Tocopherol, Beta Carotene Cancer Prevention Study. *Stroke* 35 (8): 1908–1913.
51. Yusuf, S., G. Dagenais, J. Pogue, J. Bosch, and P. Sleight. 2000. Vitamin E supplementation and cardiovascular events in high-risk patients. The Heart Outcomes Prevention Evaluation Study Investigators. *N Engl J Med* 342 (3): 154–160.
52. Lonn, E., S. Yusuf, V. Dzavik, C. Doris, Q. Yi, S. Smith, A. Moore-Cox, J. Bosch, W. Riley, and K. Teo. 2001. Effects of ramipril and vitamin E on atherosclerosis: The study to evaluate carotid ultrasound changes in patients treated with ramipril and vitamin E (SECURE). *Circulation* 103 (7): 919–925.
53. Lonn, E., S. Yusuf, B. Hoogwerf, J. Pogue, Q. Yi, B. Zinman, J. Bosch, G. Dagenais, J. F. Mann, and H. C. Gerstein. 2002. Effects of vitamin E on cardiovascular and microvascular outcomes in high-risk patients with diabetes: Results of the HOPE study and MICRO-HOPE substudy. *Diabetes Care* 25 (11): 1919–1927.
54. Mann, J. F., E. M. Lonn, Q. Yi, H. C. Gerstein, B. J. Hoogwerf, J. Pogue, J. Bosch, G. R. Dagenais, and S. Yusuf. 2004. Effects of vitamin E on cardiovascular outcomes in people with mild-to-moderate renal insufficiency: Results of the HOPE study. *Kidney Int* 65 (4): 1375–1380.
55. Lonn, E., J. Bosch, S. Yusuf, P. Sheridan, J. Pogue, J. M. Arnold, C. Ross, A. Arnold, P. Sleight, J. Probstfield, and G. R. Dagenais. 2005. Effects of long-term vitamin E supplementation on cardiovascular events and cancer: A randomized controlled trial. *JAMA* 293 (11): 1338–1347.
56. Dagenais, G. R., Q. Yi, E. Lonn, P. Sleight, J. Ostergren, and S. Yusuf. 2005. Impact of cigarette smoking in high-risk patients participating in a clinical trial. A substudy from the Heart Outcomes Prevention Evaluation (HOPE) trial. *Eur J Cardiovasc Prev Rehabil* 12 (1): 75–81.

57. Weinberg, R. B., B. S. VanderWerken, R. A. Anderson, J. E. Stegner, and M. J. Thomas. 2001. Pro-oxidant effect of vitamin E in cigarette smokers consuming a high polyunsaturated fat diet. *Arterioscler Thromb Vasc Biol* 21 (6): 1029–1033.
58. Blankenberg, S., M. J. McQueen, M. Smieja, J. Pogue, C. Balion, E. Lonn, H. J. Rupprecht, et al. 2006. Comparative impact of multiple biomarkers and N-Terminal pro-brain natriuretic peptide in the context of conventional risk factors for the prediction of recurrent cardiovascular events in the Heart Outcomes Prevention Evaluation (HOPE) Study. *Circulation* 114 (3): 201–208.
59. Waters, D. D., E. L. Alderman, J. Hsia, B. V. Howard, F. R. Cobb, W. J. Rogers, P. Ouyang, et al. 2002. Effects of hormone replacement therapy and antioxidant vitamin supplements on coronary atherosclerosis in postmenopausal women: A randomized controlled trial. *JAMA* 288 (19): 2432–2440.
60. Kelemen, M., D. Vaidya, D. D. Waters, B. V. Howard, F. Cobb, N. Younes, M. Tripputi, and P. Ouyang. 2005. Hormone therapy and antioxidant vitamins do not improve endothelial vasodilator function in postmenopausal women with established coronary artery disease: A substudy of the Women's Angiographic Vitamin and Estrogen (WAVE) trial. *Atherosclerosis* 179 (1): 193–200
61. Levy, A. P., P. Friedenberg, R. Lotan, P. Ouyang, M. Tripputi, L. Higginson, F. R. Cobb, J. C. Tardif, V. Bittner, and B. V. Howard. 2004. The effect of vitamin therapy on the progression of coronary artery atherosclerosis varies by haptoglobin type in postmenopausal women. *Diabetes Care* 27 (4): 925–930.
62. Plantinga, Y., L. Ghiadoni, A. Magagna, C. Giannarelli, F. Franzoni, S. Taddei, and A. Salvetti. 2007. Supplementation with vitamins C and E improves arterial stiffness and endothelial function in essential hypertensive patients. *Am J Hypertens* 20 (4): 392–397.
63. Jaxa-Chamiec, T., B. Bednarz, K. Herbaczynska-Cedro, P. Maciejewski, and L. Ceremuzynski. 2009. Effects of vitamins C and E on the outcome after acute myocardial infarction in diabetics: A retrospective, hypothesis-generating analysis from the MIVIT study. *Cardiology* 112 (3): 219–223.
64. Ye, Z., and H. Song. 2008. Antioxidant vitamins intake and the risk of coronary heart disease: Meta-analysis of cohort studies. *Eur J Cardiovasc Prev Rehabil* 15 (1): 26–34.
65. Kinlay, S., D. Behrendt, J. C. Fang, D. Delagrange, J. Morrow, J. L. Witztum, N. Rifai, A. P. Selwyn, M. A. Creager, and P. Ganz. 2004. Long-term effect of combined vitamins E and C on coronary and peripheral endothelial function. *J Am Coll Cardiol* 43 (4):629–634.
66. McKechnie, R., M. Rubenfire, and L. Mosca. 2002. Antioxidant nutrient supplementation and brachial reactivity in patients with coronary artery disease. *J Lab Clin Med* 139 (3): 133–139.
67. Mente, A., L. de Koning, H. S. Shannon, and S. S. Anand. 2009. A systematic review of the evidence supporting a causal link between dietary factors and coronary heart disease. *Arch Intern Med* 169 (7): 659–669.
68. El-Hamamsy, I., L. M. Stevens, M. Carrier, M. Pellerin, D. Bouchard, P. Demers, R. Cartier, P. Page, and L. P. Perrault. 2007. Effect of intravenous *N*-acetylcysteine on outcomes after coronary artery bypass surgery: A randomized, double-blind, placebo-controlled clinical trial. *J Thorac Cardiovasc Surg* 133 (1): 7–12.
69. Tossios, P., W. Bloch, A. Huebner, M. R. Raji, F. Dodos, O. Klass, M. Suedkamp, S. M. Kasper, M. Hellmich, and U. Mehlhorn. 2003. *N*-Acetylcysteine prevents reactive oxygen species-mediated myocardial stress in patients undergoing cardiac surgery: Results of a randomized, double-blind, placebo-controlled clinical trial. *J Thorac Cardiovasc Surg* 126 (5): 1513–1520,
70. McMackin, C. J., M. E. Widlansky, N. M. Hamburg, A. L. Huang, S. Weller, M. Holbrook, N. Gokce, T. M. Hagen, J. F. Keaney, Jr., and J. A. Vita. 2007. Effect of combined treatment with alpha-lipoic acid and acetyl-L-carnitine on vascular function and blood pressure in patients with coronary artery disease. *J Clin Hypertens (Greenwich)* 9 (4): 249–255.
71. Neunteufl, T., K. Kostner, R. Katzenschlager, M. Zehetgruber, G. Maurer, and F. Weidinger. 1998. Additional benefit of vitamin E supplementation to simvastatin therapy on vasoreactivity of the brachial artery of hypercholesterolemic men. *J Am Coll Cardiol* 32 (3): 711–716.
72. Judy, W. V., K. Folkers, and J. H. Hall. 1991. Improved long-term survival in coenzyme Q_{10} treated congestive heart failure patients compared to conventionally treated patients. In *Biomedical and Clincial Aspects of Coenzyme Q*, ed. K. Folkers, G. P. Littarro, and T. Yamagami, 291–298. Amsterdam: Elsevier.
73. Langsjoen, P. H., P. H. Langsjoen, and K. Folkers. 1990. Long-term efficacy and safety of coenzyme Q_{10} therapy for idiopathic dilated cardiomyopathy. *Am J Cardiol* 65 (7): 521–523.
74. Hodis, H. N., W. J. Mack, L. LaBree, L. Cashin-Hemphill, A. Sevanian, R. Johnson, and S. P. Azen. 1995. Serial coronary angiographic evidence that antioxidant vitamin intake reduces progression of coronary artery atherosclerosis. *JAMA* 273 (23): 1849–1854.

75. Collins, R., R. Peto, and J. Armitage. 2002. The MRC/BHF Heart Protection Study: Preliminary results. *Int J Clin Pract* 56 (1): 53–56.
76. Brown, B. G., X. Q. Zhao, A. Chait, L. D. Fisher, M. C. Cheung, J. S. Morse, A. A. Dowdy, et al. 2001. Simvastatin and niacin, antioxidant vitamins, or the combination for the prevention of coronary disease. *N Engl J Med* 345 (22): 1583–1592.
77. Cheung, M. C., X. Q. Zhao, A. Chait, J. J. Albers, and B. G. Brown. 2001. Antioxidant supplements block the response of HDL to simvastatin–niacin therapy in patients with coronary artery disease and low HDL. *Arterioscler Thromb Vasc Biol* 21 (8): 1320–1326.
78. Matthan, N. R., A. Giovanni, E. J. Schaefer, B. G. Brown, and A. H. Lichtenstein. 2003. Impact of simvastatin, niacin, and/or antioxidants on cholesterol metabolism in CAD patients with low HDL. *J Lipid Res* 44 (4): 800–806.
79. Bertelli, A. A., and D. K. Das. 2009. Grapes, wines, resveratrol and heart health. *J Cardiovasc Pharmacol* 54: 468–476.
80. Penumathsa, S. V., and N. Maulik. 2009. Resveratrol: A promising agent in promoting cardioprotection against coronary heart disease. *Can J Physiol Pharmacol* 87 (4), 275–286.
81. Das, S., and D. K. Das. 2007. Resveratrol: A therapeutic promise for cardiovascular diseases. *Recent Pat Cardiovasc Drug Discov* 2 (2): 133–138.
82. Baur, J. A., and D. A. Sinclair. 2006. Therapeutic potential of resveratrol: The in vivo evidence. *Nat Rev Drug Discov* 5 (6): 493–506.
83. Dudley, J. I., I. Lekli, S. Mukherjee, M. Das, A. A. Bertelli, and D. K. Das. 2008. Does white wine qualify for French paradox? Comparison of the cardioprotective effects of red and white wines and their constituents: Resveratrol, tyrosol, and hydroxytyrosol. *J Agric Food Chem* 56 (20): 9362–9373.
84. Xi, J., H. Wang, R. A. Mueller, E. A. Norfleet, and Z. Xu. 2009. Mechanism for resveratrol-induced cardioprotection against reperfusion injury involves glycogen synthase kinase 3beta and mitochondrial permeability transition pore. *Eur J Pharmacol* 604 (1–3): 111–116.
85. Yu, W., Y. C. Fu, X. H. Zhou, C. J. Chen, X. Wang, R. B. Lin, and W. Wang. 2009. Effects of resveratrol on H(2)O(2)-induced apoptosis and expression of SIRTs in H9c2 cells. *J Cell Biochem* 107 (4): 741–747.
86. Hwang, J. T., D. Y. Kwon, O. J. Park, and M. S. Kim. 2008. Resveratrol protects ROS-induced cell death by activating AMPK in H9c2 cardiac muscle cells. *Genes Nutr* 2 (4): 323–326.
87. Chen, Y. R., F. F. Yi, X. Y. Li, C. Y. Wang, L. Chen, X. C. Yang, P. X. Su, and J. Cai. 2008. Resveratrol attenuates ventricular arrhythmias and improves the long-term survival in rats with myocardial infarction. *Cardiovasc Drugs Ther* 22 (6): 479–485.
88. Dudley, J., S. Das, S. Mukherjee, and D. K. Das. 2009. Resveratrol, a unique phytoalexin present in red wine, delivers either survival signal or death signal to the ischemic myocardium depending on dose. *J Nutr Biochem* 20 (6): 443–452.
89. Chen, Y. J., J. S. Wang, and S. E. Chow. 2007. Resveratrol protects vascular endothelial cell from ox-LDL-induced reduction in antithrombogenic activity. *Chin J Physiol* 50 (1): 22–28
90. Kaur, G., L. V. Rao, A. Agrawal, and U. R. Pendurthi. 2007. Effect of wine phenolics on cytokine-induced C-reactive protein expression. *J Thromb Haemost* 5 (6): 1309–1317.
91. Wung, B. S., M. C. Hsu, C. C. Wu, and C. W. Hsieh. 2005. Resveratrol suppresses IL-6–induced ICAM-1 gene expression in endothelial cells: Effects on the inhibition of STAT3 phosphorylation. *Life Sci* 78 (4): 389–397.
92. Stef, G., A. Csiszar, K. Lerea, Z. Ungvari, and G. Veress. 2006. Resveratrol inhibits aggregation of platelets from high-risk cardiac patients with aspirin resistance. *J Cardiovasc Pharmacol* 48 (2): 1–5.
93. Penumathsa, S. V., M. Thirunavukkarasu, S. Koneru, B. Juhasz, L. Zhan, R. Pant, V. P. Menon, H. Otani, and N. Maulik. 2007. Statin and resveratrol in combination induces cardioprotection against myocardial infarction in hypercholesterolemic rat. *J Mol Cell Cardiol* 42 (3): 508–516.
94. Fukuda, S., S. Kaga, L. Zhan, D. Bagchi, D. K. Das, A. Bertelli, and N. Maulik. 2006. Resveratrol ameliorates myocardial damage by inducing vascular endothelial growth factor-angiogenesis and tyrosine kinase receptor Flk-1. *Cell Biochem Biophys* 44 (1): 43–49.
95. Lee, J. H., J. H. O'Keefe, C. J. Lavie, and W. S. Harris. 2009. Omega-3 fatty acids: Cardiovascular benefits, sources and sustainability. *Nat Rev Cardiol* 6: 753–758.
96. He, K. 2009. Fish, long-chain omega-3 polyunsaturated fatty acids and prevention of cardiovascular disease—eat fish or take fish oil supplement? *Prog Cardiovasc Dis* 52 (2): 95–114.
97. Marchioli, R., M. G. Silletta, G. Levantesi, and R. Pioggiarella. 2009. Omega-3 Fatty acids and heart failure. *Curr Atheroscler Rep* 11 (6): 440–447.
98. Lavie, C. J., R. V. Milani, M. R. Mehra, and H. O. Ventura. 2009. Omega-3 polyunsaturated fatty acids and cardiovascular diseases. *J Am Coll Cardiol* 54 (7): 585–594.

99. Marik, P. E., and J. Varon. 2009. Omega-3 dietary supplements and the risk of cardiovascular events: A systematic review. *Clin Cardiol* 32 (7): 365–372.
100. Holub, B. J. 2009. Docosahexaenoic acid (DHA) and cardiovascular disease risk factors. *Prostaglandins Leukot Essent Fatty Acids* 81 (2–3): 199–204.
101. Jenkins, D. J., A. R. Josse, P. Dorian, M. L. Burr, R. LaBelle Trangmar, C. W. Kendall, and S. C. Cunnane. 2008. Heterogeneity in randomized controlled trials of long chain (fish) omega-3 fatty acids in restenosis, secondary prevention and ventricular arrhythmias. *J Am Coll Nutr* 27 (3): 367–378.
102. Lombardi, F., and P. Terranova. 2007. Anti-arrhythmic properties of N-3 poly-unsaturated fatty acids (n-3 PUFA). *Curr Med Chem* 14 (19): 2070–2080.
103. Heidt, M. C., M. Vician, S. K. Stracke, T. Stadlbauer, M. T. Grebe, A. Boening, P. R. Vogt, and A. Erdogan. 2009. Beneficial effects of intravenously administered N-3 fatty acids for the prevention of atrial fibrillation after coronary artery bypass surgery: A prospective randomized study. *Thorac Cardiovasc Surg* 57 (5): 276–280.
104. Calo, L., L. Bianconi, F. Colivicchi, F. Lamberti, M. L. Loricchio, A. de Ruvo, A. Meo, C. Pandozi, M. Staibano, and M. Santini. 2005. N-3 Fatty acids for the prevention of atrial fibrillation after coronary artery bypass surgery: A randomized, controlled trial. *J Am Coll Cardiol* 45 (10): 1723–1728.
105. Brouwer, I. A., M. H. Raitt, C. Dullemeijer, D. F. Kraemer, P. L. Zock, C. Morris, M. B. Katan, et al. 2009. Effect of fish oil on ventricular tachyarrhythmia in three studies in patients with implantable cardioverter defibrillators. *Eur Heart J* 30 (7): 820–826.
106. Dall, T. L., and H. Bays. 2009. Addressing lipid treatment targets beyond cholesterol: A role for prescription omega-3 fatty acid therapy. *South Med J* 102 (4): 390–396.
107. Davidson, M. H., E. A. Stein, H. E. Bays, K. C. Maki, R. T. Doyle, R. A. Shalwitz, C. M. Ballantyne, and H. N. Ginsberg. 2007. Efficacy and tolerability of adding prescription omega-3 fatty acids 4 g/d to simvastatin 40 mg/d in hypertriglyceridemic patients: An 8-week, randomized, double-blind, placebo-controlled study. *Clin Ther* 29 (7): 1354–1367.
108. Marchioli, R., G. Levantesi, M. G. Silletta, S. Barlera, M. Bernardinangeli, E. Carbonieri, F. Cosmi et al. 2009. Effect of n-3 polyunsaturated fatty acids and rosuvastatin in patients with heart failure: Results of the GISSI-HF trial. *Expert Rev Cardiovasc Ther* 7 (7): 735–748.
109. Mori, T. A., V. Burke, I. Puddey, A. Irish, C. A. Cowpland, L. Beilin, G. Dogra, and G. F. Watts. 2009. The effects of [omega]3 fatty acids and coenzyme Q_{10} on blood pressure and heart rate in chronic kidney disease: A randomized controlled trial. *J Hypertens* 27 (9): 1863–1872.
110. Cicero, A. F., S. Ertek, and C. Borghi. 2009. Omega-3 polyunsaturated fatty acids: Their potential role in blood pressure prevention and management. *Curr Vasc Pharmacol* 7 (3): 330–337.
111. Dimitrow, P. P., and M. Jawien. 2009. Pleiotropic, cardioprotective effects of omega-3 polyunsaturated fatty acids. *Mini Rev Med Chem* 9 (9): 1030–1039.
112. Simopoulos, A. P. 2008. The omega-6/omega-3 fatty acid ratio, genetic variation, and cardiovascular disease. *Asia Pac J Clin Nutr* 17 (Suppl 1): 131–134.
113. Bonaa, K. H., I. Njolstad, P. M. Ueland, H. Schirmer, A. Tverdal, T. Steigen, H. Wang, J. E. Nordrehaug, E. Arnesen, and K. Rasmussen. 2006. Homocysteine lowering and cardiovascular events after acute myocardial infarction. *N Engl J Med* 354 (15): 1578–1588.
114. Lonn, E., S. Yusuf, M. J. Arnold, P. Sheridan, J. Pogue, M. Micks, M. J. McQueen. et al. 2006. Homocysteine lowering with folic acid and B vitamins in vascular disease. *N Engl J Med* 354 (15): 1567–1577.
115. Ray, J. G., C. Kearon, Q. Yi, P. Sheridan, and E. Lonn. 2007. Homocysteine-lowering therapy and risk for venous thromboembolism: A randomized trial. *Ann Intern Med* 146 (11): 761–767.
116. Toole, J. F., M. R. Malinow, L. E. Chambless, J. D. Spence, L. C. Pettigrew, V. J. Howard, E. G. Sides, C. H. Wang, and M. Stampfer. 2004. Lowering homocysteine in patients with ischemic stroke to prevent recurrent stroke, myocardial infarction, and death: The Vitamin Intervention for Stroke Prevention (VISP) randomized controlled trial. *JAMA* 291 (5): 565–575.
117. Krinsky, N. I. 1989. Antioxidant functions of carotenoids. *Free Radic Biol Med* 7 (6): 617–635.
118. Hazuka, M. B., J. Edwards-Prasad, F. Newman, J. J. Kinzie, and K. N. Prasad. 1990. Beta-carotene induces morphological differentiation and decreases adenylate cyclase activity in melanoma cells in culture. *J Am Coll Nutr* 9 (2): 143–149.
119. Zhang, L. X., R. V. Cooney, and J. S. Bertram. 1992. Carotenoids up-regulate connexin43 gene expression independent of their provitamin A or antioxidant properties. *Cancer Res* 52 (20): 5707–5712.
120. Carter, C. A., M. Pogribny, A. Davidson, C. D. Jackson, L. J. McGarrity, and S. M. Morris. 1996. Effects of retinoic acid on cell differentiation and reversion toward normal in human endometrial adenocarcinoma (RL95-2) cells. *Anticancer Res* 16 (1): 17–24.

121. Meyskens, Jr., F. 1995. Role of vitamin A and its derivatives in the treatment of human cancer. In *Nutrients in Cancer Prevention and Treatment*. Eds. K. N. Prasad and R. M. Williams. Totowa, NJ: Humana Press. pp. 349–362.
122. Vile, G. F., and C. C. Winterbourn. 1988. Inhibition of adriamycin-promoted microsomal lipid peroxidation by beta-carotene, alpha-tocopherol and retinol at high and low oxygen partial pressures. *FEBS Lett* 238 (2): 353–356.
123. Niki, E. 1987. Interaction of ascorbate and alpha-tocopherol. *Ann N Y Acad Sci* 498: 186–199.
124. Ingold, K. U., G. W. Burton, D. O. Foster, L. Hughes, D. A. Lindsay, and A. Webb. 1987. Biokinetics of and discrimination between dietary *RRR*- and *SRR*-alpha-tocopherols in the male rat. *Lipids* 22 (3): 163–172.
125. Carini, R., G. Poli, M. U. Dianzani, S. P. Maddix, T. F. Slater, and K. H. Cheeseman. 1990. Comparative evaluation of the antioxidant activity of alpha-tocopherol, alpha-tocopherol polyethylene glycol 1000 succinate and alpha-tocopherol succinate in isolated hepatocytes and liver microsomal suspensions. *Biochem Pharmacol* 39 (10): 1597–1601.
126. Prasad, K. N., B. Kumar, X. D. Yan, A. J. Hanson, and W. C. Cole. 2003. Alpha-tocopheryl succinate, the most effective form of vitamin E for adjuvant cancer treatment: A review. *J Am Coll Nutr* 22 (2): 108–117.
127. Sies, H., V. S. Sharov, L. O. Klotz, and K. Briviba. 1997. Glutathione peroxidase protects against peroxynitrite-mediated oxidations. A new function for selenoproteins as peroxynitrite reductase. *J Biol Chem* 272 (44): 27812–27817.
128. Witschi, A., S. Reddy, B. Stofer, and B. H. Lauterburg. 1992. The systemic availability of oral glutathione. *Eur J Clin Pharmacol* 43 (6): 667–669.
129. Niki, E. 1997. Mechanisms and dynamics of antioxidant action of ubiquinol. *Mol Aspects Med* 18 (Suppl): S63–S70.
130. Stoyanovsky, D. A., A. N. Osipov, P. J. Quinn, and V. E. Kagan. 1995. Ubiquinone-dependent recycling of vitamin E radicals by superoxide. *Arch Biochem Biophys* 323 (2): 343–351.
131. Schnyder, G., M. Roffi, Y. Flammer, R. Pin, and O. M. Hess. 2002. Effect of homocysteine-lowering therapy with folic acid, vitamin B_{12}, and vitamin B_6 on clinical outcome after percutaneous coronary intervention: The Swiss Heart study: A randomized controlled trial. *JAMA* 288 (8): 973–979.
132. Chen, W. H., X. Cheng, P. Y. Lee, W. Ng, J. Y. Kwok, H. F. Tse, and C. P. Lau. 2007. Aspirin resistance and adverse clinical events in patients with coronary artery disease. *Am J Med* 120 (7): 631–635.
133. Abate, A., G. Yang, P. A. Dennery, S. Oberle, and H. Schroder. 2000. Synergistic inhibition of cyclooxygenase-2 expression by vitamin E and aspirin. *Free Radic Biol Med* 29 (11): 1135–1142.

6 Micronutrients for the Prevention of Diabetes and Improvement of the Standard Therapy

INTRODUCTION

Diabetes mellitus is a chronic disease characterized by high levels of blood glucose that can result from defects in insulin production, insulin transport and/or utilization, or both. Diabetes can lead to serious complications and premature death if untreated. Diabetes has become a serious health problem throughout the world, including in the United States, and has reached epidemic proportions. Despite development of new medications to control glucose and recommendations for losing weight, daily moderate exercise, and a balanced diet, the incidence of diabetes continues to increase in the United States. Severe diabetic-related complications eventually develop in spite of medications. Although the compliance for medications is very good, compliance is not consistent for diet and lifestyle modifications. The analysis of published data suggests that increased oxidative stress and chronic inflammation are associated with the development of all diabetes-related complications. They may also be associated with the initiation of diabetes. Antioxidants are known to reduce oxidative stress and inflammation; therefore, they should be useful in reducing the incidence of diabetes as well as diabetes-related complications. However, several laboratory and human studies utilizing a single dietary, endogenous antioxidant, certain B-vitamins, omega-3 fatty acids, the mineral chromium, or aspirin alone have been performed to evaluate their efficacy in prevention and improved treatment. The results of these studies showed that different individual agents improved different risk factors and reduced different markers of oxidative stress and inflammation, producing inconsistent results. Antioxidants in combination with the standard therapy appear to be more effective than the individual agents.

This chapter describes the incidence, cost, types of diabetes, and the involvement of oxidative stress and chronic inflammation in the initiation and progression of diabetes and diabetes-related complications. The laboratory and clinical studies on the effects of antioxidants, omega-3 fatty acids, aspirin, and chromium in reducing risks and improving the efficacy of standard therapy are discussed. This chapter also presents a scientific rationale and evidence in support of the hypothesis that daily supplementation with multiple micronutrients, including dietary and endogenous antioxidants, may reduce the incidence of diabetes and improve the efficacy of standard therapy.

INCIDENCE AND COST

A total of 1.6 million new cases of diabetes were diagnosed in the U.S. population aged 20 years or older in 2007. It has been estimated that the total number of diabetic cases (diagnosed and undiagnosed) in the United States was 23.6 million, out of which 17.9 million were diagnosed and 5.7 million were undiagnosed.[1] Of the total number of diabetic cases, about 12 million were men and about 11.5 million were women. About 14.9 million were non-Hispanic whites and 3.7 million were non-Hispanic blacks, suggesting that the incidence of disease (percentage of population of each race) is higher in the black population compared to the white population.

Based on data collected from 2003 to 2006 in the U.S. population aged 20 years or older, the incidence of impaired fasting glucose after adjusting for population age and sex differences was 25.1% in non-Hispanic whites, 21.1% in non-Hispanic blacks, and 26.1% in Mexican-Americans.

The estimated direct and indirect cost (disability, work loss, and premature death) of diabetes in the United States in 2007 was $174 billion, and the direct medical cost alone was $116 billion.

TYPES OF DIABETES

There are four types of diabetes in humans. They include type 1 diabetes, type 2 diabetes, gestational diabetes, and other types of diabetes. Prediabetic condition and metabolic syndrome are considered high risk for developing type 2 diabetes.

TYPE 1 DIABETES

Type 1 diabetes was previously called insulin-dependent diabetes mellitus, or juvenile-onset diabetes. This form of diabetes develops when the body's immune system destroys pancreatic beta cells that are responsible for synthesizing and releasing insulin, which regulates blood levels of glucose. Type 1 diabetes primarily affects children and young adults, although onset of the disease can occur at any age. In adults, type 1 diabetes accounts for 5–10% of all diagnosed cases of diabetes.[1] Risk factors for type 1 diabetes include autoimmune disease, genetics, or environmental factors.

TYPE 2 DIABETES

The type 2 diabetes was previously called noninsulin-dependent diabetes mellitus, or adult-onset diabetes. This form of diabetes develops when cells become resistant to insulin, possibly due to defects in the glucose transport protein or in insulin receptors (IRs). This forces the beta cells of the pancreas to produce more insulin. Pancreatic beta cells are gradually damaged, leading to a progressive decrease in insulin production. Type 2 diabetes primarily affects older individuals; however, this form of diabetes is being diagnosed more frequently in children of American Indians, African-Americans, Hispanic/Latino Americans, and Asians/Pacific Islanders.[1] The primary risk factors include older age, obesity, a family history of diabetes, a history of gestational diabetes, impaired glucose metabolism, physical inactivity, and race/ethnicity.

GESTATIONAL DIABETES

Gestational diabetes is characterized by glucose intolerance that usually develops during pregnancy. This form of diabetes is commonly observed in African-Americans, American Indians, and Hispanic/Latino Americans. It is also more common among obese women and women with a family history of diabetes. About 5–10% of women with gestational diabetes develop type 2 diabetes 5 to 10 years later.[1]

OTHER TYPES OF DIABETES

These forms of diabetes result from genetic defects, surgery, medications, pancreatic disease, and infections that damage the pancreas. Such types of diabetes account for 1–5% of all diagnosed cases.[1]

PREDIABETES AND METABOLIC SYNDROME

Prediabetes is a condition in which individuals have blood glucose levels higher than normal, but not high enough to be classified as diabetes. Prediabetic individuals with fasting blood glucose levels of 100 to 125 mg/dl may be due to an impaired fasting glucose (IFG), or with glucose levels of 140 to 199 mg/dl, due to an impaired glucose tolerance (IGT). Individuals with prediabetic conditions have an increased risk of developing type 2 diabetes, heart disease, and stroke. The metabolic syndrome is a common and complex health issue combining obesity, abnormal lipid profiles, hypertension, and insulin resistance.

COMPLICATIONS OF DIABETES

There are severe complications associated with diabetes. They include heart disease, stroke, high blood pressure, blindness, kidney disease, impaired function of nerves including peripheral neuropathy, numbness of extremities, erectile dysfunction, amputation, periodontal disease, and birth defects in pregnant women. Adults with diabetes have death rates about two to four times higher from heart disease compared to those without diabetes.[1] The risk of stroke in diabetic individuals is about two to four times higher than in individuals without diabetes. Diabetes is the leading cause of new cases of blindness among the U.S. population aged 20 to 74 years. The annual incidence of diabetic retinopathy is about 12,000 to 24,000 cases. About 60% to 70% of diabetic patients have mild to severe forms of damage to the nervous system. Severe forms of diabetic nerve disease are major contributing factors to lower-extremity amputations. Diabetes is the leading cause of kidney failure, accounting for about 44% of new cases in 2005.[1]

EVIDENCE FOR INCREASED OXIDATIVE STRESS IN DIABETES

TYPE 1 DIABETES

Several human and animal studies have suggested that the markers of oxidative stress are elevated in children with type 1 diabetes.[2] The frequency of sister chromatid exchange was evaluated in blood-cell cultures from 35 type 1 diabetic patients and 5 healthy age- and sex-matched individuals as the controls. The results showed that the frequency of sister chromatid exchange was higher in patients with type 1 diabetes compared to the controls. It was concluded that hyperglycemia-induced oxidative stress may be primarily responsible for this genetic instability.[3] The levels of protein glycation and oxidative stress parameters in blood and serum from 81 patients with type 1 diabetes (61 patients with long-term poor glycemic control and 20 patients with long-term good glycemic control) and 31 healthy children were evaluated. The results showed that the levels of glycation end-products and advanced oxidation protein products in diabetics were higher compared to the controls; the highest levels were found in patients with poor glycemic control.[4]

The patients with type 1 diabetes eventually developed insulin resistance and other characteristics of type 2 diabetes. The exact mechanisms are unknown. However, it was demonstrated that prolonged exposure of cultured mouse hepatocytes to insulin increased oxidative stress that accounts for the development of insulin resistance. The insulin resistance was associated with impaired mitochondrial function, and overexpression of mitochondrial MnSOD prevented insulin-induced insulin resistance.[5] The levels of oxidant/antioxidant defense systems in 20 children with type 1 diabetes, 22 obese children, and 16 age- and sex-matched controls were evaluated. The results showed that the levels of lipoperoxides and malondialdehyde (MDA) and protein oxidation were significantly higher in both patients with diabetes and obese children compared to control, although the levels of MDA were highest in children with diabetes. The serum levels of alpha-tocopherol and beta-carotene, red cell glutathione peroxidase activity, and reduced glutathione levels in patients with diabetes were lower compared to obese children. It was concluded that oxidative stress is elevated in both children with type 1 diabetes and obesity.[6] Although increased oxidative stress is associated with type 1 diabetes, it is not certain whether increased oxidative stress precedes or merely reflects consequences of the disease. Therefore, the levels of markers of oxidative stress were evaluated in 30 patients with type 1 diabetes (10 without diabetic complications, 10 with retinopathy, and 10 with nephropathy), 36 nondiabetic siblings, 37 nondiabetic parents of type 1 diabetic patients, and 3 control subjects without a familial history of diabetes were evaluated. The results revealed that the levels of MDA in plasma and red blood cells (RBC) were elevated in diabetic patients and their relatives, compared to the control subjects. However, the levels of reduced glutathione in RBC were lower in diabetic patients. It was concluded that increased oxidative stress occurs in nondiabetic relatives of diabetic patients; therefore, increased oxidative stress may precede type 1 diabetes.[7] In a clinical study involving 59 patients with type 1 diabetes, it was observed that lower plasma vitamin C levels were associated with adverse changes in the microcirculation, peripheral arteries, and ventricular repolarization.[8]

Type 2 Diabetes

There are substantial experimental and clinical studies that suggest that increased oxidative stress plays a major role in the pathogenesis of both types of diabetes mellitus.[9–13] In another clinical study, the levels of markers of oxidative stress and DNA damage in 92 subjects with normal glucose tolerance (NGT), 78 patients with IGT, and 113 patients with newly diagnosed diabetes were evaluated. The results showed that patients with IGT had reduced erythrocyte SOD activity compared to subjects with NGT; however, the patients with diabetes had higher levels of plasma MDA, but lower levels of total antioxidative capacity and erythrocyte SOD activity than the subjects with NGT. The damage to DNA was slight in IGT subjects, but the level increased in patients with diabetes.[14] Oxidative stress induces beta-cell dysfunction by activating the JNK pathway.[11] Diabetic-related complications such as microalbuminuria, periodontitis, nephropathy, retinopathy, and cardiovascular disease are due to increased oxidative stress induced by hyperglycemia.[15–20]

NAD(P)H oxidases are major sources of reactive oxygen species (ROS), and Nox4, one of these ubiquitous oxidases, is localized in the mitochondria of many cells and in the kidneys of diabetic rats. The expression of mitochondrial Nox4 expression was elevated in the kidney cortex of diabetic rats, suggesting that Nox4 is a major source of ROS in the kidneys during early stages of diabetes.[21,22] Thus, Nox4-derived ROS contributes to renal hypertrophy and increased fibronectin expression in the cell.[22] It has been reported that the exercise capacity and mitochondrial function in the skeletal muscle of mice were impaired in type 2 diabetes, which was related to increased oxidative stress.[23]

Metabolic Syndrome

Increased oxidative stress also occurs in individuals with metabolic syndrome. Increased levels of insulin and impaired glycemic control were associated with higher levels of oxidized low density lipids (LDL).[24] This suggests that increased oxidative stress occurs in individuals with metabolic syndrome.

EVIDENCE FOR INCREASED CHRONIC INFLAMMATION IN DIABETES

Inflammatory molecules and their transcriptional factor, NF-kappa B, appear to play an important role in diabetes-induced cardiac dysfunction. In diabetic mice, increased NF-kappa B activity was associated with enhanced oxidative stress. Administration of pyrrolidine dithiocarbamates (PDTC), a NF-kappaB inhibitor, reduced oxidative stress and improved mitochondrial dysfunction in diabetic mice.[25] In rat models of diabetes, elevated levels of IL-1 beta in islet cells promotes cytokines and chemokine expression, leading to the recruitment of innate immune cells. Therefore, IL-1 beta may not produce direct toxic effects on islet beta cells, but may induce tissue inflammation that causes beta cell death and insulin resistance in type 2 diabetes.[26] In mice models of type 2 diabetes, the interaction between NF-kappa B and tumor necrosis factor (TNF)-alpha signaling induced the activation of IKK-beta and amplified oxidative stress, leading to endothelial dysfunction.[27]

The histology of islet cells from patients with type 2 diabetes exhibited the presence of inflammatory products such as cytokines, immune cell infiltration, amyloid deposits associated with apoptotic cells, and fibrosis.[28] Inflammatory molecules such as IL-beta, interferon-gamma (IFN-gamma), and TNF-alpha contribute to pancreatic beta cell death by activating NF-kappaB activity. This was confirmed by the fact that blocking NF-kappaB activation protected beta cells in culture against IL-beta + IFN-gamma, or TNF-alpha + IFN-gamma–induced apoptosis.[29] Thus, activation of NF-kappaB activity appears to be a primary event in the progressive loss of beta cells from the pancreas.

In obesity, white adipose tissue is infiltrated by macrophages that release excessive amounts of inflammatory molecules, including TNF-alpha and IL-6, which contribute to insulin resistance in type 2 diabetes.[30,31] It has been reported that increased expression of p53 in mice adipose tissue contributes to insulin resistance caused by enhanced inflammatory responses.[32] In a clinical study involving 10 normal-weight and 8 obese subjects, the effects of a high-fat and high-carbohydrate meal on markers of oxidative stress and inflammation after an overnight fast were evaluated. The results showed that high-fat, high-carbohydrate meals induced a significantly more prolonged and greater oxidative stress and inflammation compared to normal-weight subjects.[33] This may increase the risk of cardiac disease and insulin resistance.

BENEFICIAL EFFECTS OF ANTIOXIDANTS AND OTHER NUTRIENTS IN DIABETES

Most animal and human studies have utilized one antioxidant, certain B-vitamins, aspirin, chromium, and omega-3 fatty acids in prevention and improved treatment of diabetes. The results of these studies have produced inconsistent results with respect to prevention, markers of oxidative stress and inflammation, insulin sensitivity, glycemic index, and diabetic-related complications. The results on the effects of individual agents in diabetes are described below.

Vitamin A

It has been suggested that decreased production of nerve growth factor (NGF) may contribute to diabetic neuropathy; however, administration of exogenous NGF produced only a modest benefit. Retinoic acid (RA), a metabolite of retinol (vitamin A), induced expression of NGF and its receptor. Therefore, it was thought that administration of retinoic acid may be useful in improving some of the symptoms of diabetic retinopathy. Treatment of diabetic rats with RA increased the levels of NGF in serum and nerve, and induced nerve regeneration;[34,35] however, the levels of plasma glucose did not change, and there was no difference in pain threshold between treated and untreated groups of diabetic animals.[35] Type 1 diabetes is characterized by inflammation as evidenced by the infiltration of activated T lymphocytes and monocytes into the islet cells of the pancreas resulting into loss of beta cells. Supplementation with vitamin A (retinyl acetate) through diet caused a marked reduction in inflammatory reaction and loss of beta cells in diabetic mice.[36] Similar effects of polyphenols present in the freeze-dried grape powder were observed in the above study.

Vitamin C

In a randomized clinical study involving 36 elderly patients with type 2 diabetes, a dose-dependent increase in the cellular levels of reduced glutathione and vitamin E was observed after treatment with vitamin C; however, these changes were not sufficient to reduce LDL susceptibility to peroxidation.[37] Endothelial dysfunction is associated with hyperglycemia-induced type 2 diabetes, and this may become aggravated in patients with insulin resistance. Both intra-arterial and oral administration of high-dose vitamin C improved plasma vitamin C levels and endothelial dysfunction and insulin resistance in diabetic patients.[38,39]

Treatment of streptozotocin-induced diabetic rats with vitamin C suppressed leukocyte adhesion and endothelial dysfunction and, thus, improved blood flow in the iris microvessels.[40] This suggests that administration of vitamin C could be useful in preventing diabetic retinopathy. Vitamin C treatment of diabetic rats also prevented diabetic-induced endothelial dysfunction in mesenteric microcirculation.[41] Oxidative stress appears to play an important role in diabetic nephropathy. Supplementation with vitamin C in a diabetic rat model reduced the number of apoptotic kidney cells, albuminuria, and proteinuria, glomerular and tubulointerstitial sclerosis, and renal MDA without changing the level of plasma glucose.[42] This suggests that vitamin C reduces oxidative stress, but that it has no role in regulating plasma glucose levels.

Vitamin D

In a rat model of diabetes, administration of 1alpha-, 25 dihydroxyvitamin D3 [1alpha, 25(OH) 2 VD3] increased plasma insulin levels, normalized the hepatic glycogen concentration, and maintained the normal plasma glucose level. In addition, treatment with 1alpha, 25(OH) 2VD3 enhanced SOD, catalase and glutathione peroxidase activities, compared to control diabetic rats. It also reduced lipid peroxidation and reduced toxicity in the liver and kidneys.[43] Vitamin D deficiency may be associated with both type 1 and type 2 diabetes and it impairs biosynthesis and release of insulin in animals and humans with type 2 diabetes. Epidemiologic studies have supported the role of vitamin D deficiency in the etiology of diabetes. In nonobese diabetic mice, supplementation with 1alpha, 25(OH) vD3 or its structural analogs delay the onset of diabetes.[44,45] Therefore, supplementation with vitamin D3 may be one of the necessary ingredients of any multiple micronutrient preparation for the prevention or improved treatment of diabetes.

Vitamin E

It has been reported that an oral administration of vitamin E reduced kidney MDA in both diabetic and control rats.[46] Haptoglobin (Hp) is an antioxidant protein that protects against oxidative damage caused by extracorpuscular hemoglobin. There are two alleles at the Hp locus, 1 and 2. Hp-1 is a superior antioxidant compared to Hp-2. The haptoglobin (Hp) 2-2 genotype is associated with increased risk of cardiovascular disease in diabetes. This genotype is also associated with increased risk of diabetic neuropathy and appears to be associated with a more rapid progression to end-stage renal disease. Using transgenic mice it was demonstrated that vitamin E supplementation provided significant protection against the development of functional and histological features of diabetic neuropathy in Hp 2-2 mice but not in Hp 1-1 mice.[47] It has been reported that administration of tocotrienol was more effective in protecting against diabetic neuropathy in streptozotocin-induced diabetic rats than alpha-tocopherol.[48] In a rat model of type 1 diabetes, supplementation with vitamin E reduced the incidence of cardiac failure and myocardial markers of oxidative stress.[49]

Diabetes is associated with increased risk of complications following coronary bypass graft, in which increased oxidative stress and proinflammatory markers and adhesion molecules play an important role. The efficacy of vitamin E as an adjunctive therapy on markers of oxidative damage, proinflammatory cytokines, and adhesion molecules in diabetic patients with coronary bypass graft were evaluated. The results showed that supplementation with vitamin E reduced oxidative stress, inflammation markers, and adhesion molecules.[50] Memory impairment is observed in patients with type 2 diabetes and this becomes aggravated after a high-fat meal possibly due to generation of excessive amounts of free radicals.

In the Women's Antioxidant Cardiovascular Study involving 8171 female health professionals with either a history of cardiovascular disease, or more cardiovascular risk factors, the efficacy of vitamin C (ascorbic acid, 500 mg/day), vitamin E (*RRR*-alpha-tocopheryl acetate, 600 IU every other day), beta-carotene (50 mg every other day), or their respective placebos on the risk of developing type 2 diabetes was evaluated. The results showed that none of these antioxidants, when used individually, was effective in reducing the risk of type 2 diabetes.[51] Although the selection of the high-risk population for type 2 diabetes was rational, the use of only one dietary antioxidant was not. Inconsistent results with a single antioxidant have been obtained with other chronic diseases including cancer, heart disease, and neurological diseases. Therefore, the above results were not unexpected. However, these results should not be extrapolated to the potential efficacy of multiple dietary and endogenous antioxidants in reducing the risk of diabetes or improving the treatment of diabetes.

ALPHA-LIPOIC ACID

A recent review on the role of alpha-lipoic acid in the management of type 2 diabetes showed that alpha-lipoic acid produced beneficial effects in diabetic patients by improving uptake and utilization of glucose.[52–54] Alpha-lipoic acid also reduced oxidative stress and the formation of advanced glycation end-products (AEGs) and improved insulin sensitivity to glucose in skeletal muscle and the liver. The inhibitor of AEG, pyridoxamine (PM), prevented irreversible protein glycation. In a randomized, double-blind, placebo-controlled trial involving over 1500 patients with type 1 and type 2 diabetes, the efficacy of supplementation with alpha lipoic acid on neuropathic symptoms and neuropathic deficits was evaluated. The results showed that supplementation with alpha-lipoic acid (600 mg/day, IV) over a 3-week period significantly improved neuropathic symptoms and neuropathic deficits in diabetic patients with polyneuropathy,[55–57] and autonomic neuropathy in patients with type 1 diabetes.[58] An oral administration of alpha-lipoic acid (600 mg, twice a day, or 600, 1200, or 1800 mg once a day) increased peripheral insulin sensitivity in patients with type 2 diabetes and improved neuropathic symptoms and deficits in patients with diabetic polyneuropathy.[59–61] Several studies have demonstrated that the combination of enduring exercise and alpha-lipoic acid produced better improvement in insulin sensitivity to glucose in skeletal muscle than either agent alone.[62]

It has been reported that the combination of alpha-lipoic acid and pyridoxamine produced better results in insulin-mediated glucose transport in the soleus muscle of obese Zucker rats with insulin resistance disease.[63] In a diabetic rat model, supplementation with alpha-lipoic acid reduced proteinuria by attenuating expressions of transforming growth factor-beta1 (TGF-beta1) and fibronectin proteins that contribute to diabetic nephropathy.[64] It has been reported that supplementation with alpha-lipoic acid reduced neural tube defects, cardiovascular malformations, and skeletal muscle malformations in the offspring of diabetic mice at term delivery.[65] Lipoic acid synthase is involved in the biosynthesis of alpha-lipoic acid. In the animal model of diabetes type 2, the expression of lipoic acid synthase expression in tissues is significantly reduced. TNF-alpha and hyperglycemia decreased the alpha-lipoic acid synthase expression in the endothelial cells in culture. Down-regulation of alpha-lipoic acid synthase aggravated the inflammatory responses, whereas overexpression of this gene ameliorated the inflammatory responses in the diabetic animals.[66] Supplementation with alpha-lipoic acid delayed development and progression of diabetic cataracts in streptozotocin-induced diabetic rats.[67]

N-ACETYLCYSTEINE

In a clinical study involving 10 patients with type 2 diabetes and 10 normal subjects, the effect of *N*-acetylcysteine (NAC) on the markers of oxidative stress and chronic inflammation after a high-glucose meal was evaluated. The results showed that the levels of 4-hydroxynonenal (HNE) and MDA increased after high-glucose meal consumption in patients with diabetes who did not receive NAC, while the glycemic index, markers of inflammation, and insulinemia remained unchanged. However, in diabetic patients consuming a high-glucose meal after NAC administration, the levels of HNE, MDA, and vascular adhesion molecule-1 (VCAM-1) decreased. The control subjects consuming a high-glucose meal before or after NAC administration did not show any significant changes in any parameters of oxidative or inflammation markers.[68]

In a rat model of type 1 diabetes, administration of NAC reduced the levels of hyperglycemia-induced oxidative stress.[69] Increased markers of oxidative stress and inflammation appear to be associated with diabetic retinopathy. Supplementation with NAC reduced the levels of these markers in streptozotocin-induced diabetic rats[70] and, therefore, may reduce the risk of retinopathy. Oxidative stress–mediated activation of membrane-bound protein kinase C-beta 2 (PKC-beta 2) in the myocardium is involved in the development of cardiomyopathy associated with diabetes. Supplementation with NAC reduced markers of oxidative stress and prevented hyperglycemia-induced cardiomyocyte hypertrophy in cultured neonatal cardiomyocites.[71] Diabetic encephalopathy caused by hyperglycemia-induced oxidative stress is associated with impaired cognitive function. Supplementation with NAC through drinking water significantly reduced cognitive deficits and oxidative stress in streptozotocin-induced diabetic rats.[72] Diabetes during pregnancy increases the risk for congenital heart disease in the offspring. Administration of NAC together with a high concentration of glucose directly into the chick embryos decreased the frequency of heart malformations from 82% to 27%.[73] NAC treatment reduced diabetic myocardial dysfunction by restoring myocardial MnSOD activity.[74] It has been reported that the blood levels of glutathione were significantly reduced in patients with type 1 diabetes; however, supplementation with low levels of cysteine, a precursor of glutathione, failed to restore glutathione levels in patients with poorly controlled type 1 diabetes.[75] This is in contrast to animal studies in which supplementation with high doses of L-cysteine can lower the glycemic index and markers of vascular inflammation by preventing the activation of NF-kappaB.[76]

L-Carnitine

L-Carnitine, the L-beta-hydroxy-gamma-N-trimethylaminobutyric acid, is synthesized from lysine and methionine primarily in the liver and kidneys. It plays an important role in lipid metabolism. It acts as an obligatory cofactor for beta oxidation of fatty acids by transporting the long-chain fatty acids to the mitochondrial membrane as acyl-carnitine esters. Since L-carnitine shuttles acetyl groups from inside to outside the mitochondrial membrane, it plays a key role in glucose metabolism. Any reduction in the transport of fatty acids inside the mitochondria can lead to the cytosolic accumulation of triglycerides, which contribute to insulin resistance. Indeed, it has been reported that L-carnitine and acetyl-L-carnitine improved insulin-mediated glucose metabolism in normal healthy subjects, as well as in patients with type 2 diabetes.[77] It has been reported that the accumulation of fatty acyl CoA derivatives and metabolites in muscle inhibited insulin signaling and glucose oxidation. Supplementation with L-carnitine improved insulin-stimulated glucose utilization by reversing abnormalities in lipid metabolism.[78] Diabetes is associated with peripheral neuropathy. A review of two clinical trials involving 1679 patients with diabetes revealed that a dose of 2 g daily was well tolerated and caused a reduction in pain scores. One study shows improvements in nerve conduction velocities, while the other did not. Evidence of nerve regeneration was found in some trials.[79,80] The results of these investigations suggest that supplementation with high-dose L-carnitine may reduce some of the symptoms of diabetic peripheral neuropathy. Type 2 diabetes is associated with increased levels of oxidized LDL. In a randomized, placebo-controlled trial involving 81 patients with type 2 diabetes, supplementation with L-carnitine reduced the levels of oxidized LDL.[81] In a randomized clinical trial involving 52 patients with type 2 diabetes, supplementation with L-carnitine and simvastatin lowered serum lipoproteins levels more than that produced by simvastatin treatment alone.[82] Obese subjects with insulin resistance have elevated levels of free fatty acid that contribute to the endothelial dysfunction. In a clinical study involving 7 normal lean subjects, supplementation with L-carnitine improved free fatty acids associated with endothelial dysfunction.[83] The role of L-carnitine in diabetes is further supported by the fact that the mean serum-free L-carnitine levels in diabetic patients with complications were almost 25% lower than in diabetic patients without complications.[84]

Obesity can contribute to glucose intolerance. It has been reported that supplementation with L-carnitine improved insulin-stimulated glucose disposal in genetically induced diabetic mice and wild-type mice fed a high-fat diet. It increased circulating levels of acetyl-L-carnitine and several medium- and long-chain acyl-carnitine species in both plasma and tissue.[85] Diabetes is known to cause defects in nerve conduction. Using streptozotocin-induced diabetic rats, it has been demonstrated that supplementation with high-dose acetyl-L-carnitine improved nerve conduction velocity of the sural nerve; however, a lower dose of acetyl-L-carnitine was less effective.[86] Increased levels of AGEs are observed in patients with diabetes. High-fructose diets induced hyperglycemia and glycation of hemoglobin; however, supplementation with L-carnitine significantly reduced glycation of hemoglobin. The efficacy of L-carnitine in reducing glycation was compared with a well-known antiglycation agent, aminoguanidine, using bovine serum albumin in vitro. The results showed that L-carnitine was more effective than aminoguanidine in inhibiting glycation in vitro.[87] Streptozotocin-induced diabetes in rats is associated with L-carnitine deficiency, bradycardia, and left ventricular enlargement. An oral supplementation of L-carnitine normalized serum L-carnitine, heart rate regulation, and left ventricular size.[88] Excessive administration of insulin can cause hypoglycemia, which can induce mitochondrial swelling followed by neuronal death in the brain. Administration of L-carnitine in insulin-induced hypoglycemic rats prevented neuronal damage in the hippocampus by improving mitochondrial function.[89]

Coenzyme Q_{10}

In a clinical study involving 28 patients with type 2 diabetes (10 men and 18 women) and 10 healthy individuals (age- and sex-matched), the effect of coenzyme Q_{10} on markers of oxidative stress (MDA in platelets and serum) was evaluated. The levels of MDA in platelets and serum were higher, and the plasma coenzyme Q_{10} levels were lower in patients with diabetes than in control subjects. There was a negative correlation between plasma coenzyme Q_{10} concentrations and glycosylated hemoglobin. This suggests that patients with type 2 diabetes have a high internal oxidative environment that may cause impaired glycemic control in diabetic patients.[90]

Maternally inherited diabetes mellitus and deafness (MIDD) is due to a mutation in mitochondrial DNA (mtDNA) 3243 (A-G), and is characterized by a progressive insulin secretory defect and neurosensory deafness. In a clinical study involving 28 MIDD patients, 7 mutant subjects with IGT and 15 mutant subjects with NGT, the efficacy of coenzyme Q_{10} (150 mg/day for a period of 3 years) on insulin secretory response, hearing disorders, and clinical symptoms of MIDD were evaluated. The results showed that the insulin secretory response in MIDD patients was significantly higher than in the control MIDD patients.[91] Coenzyme Q_{10} treatment also improved hearing loss; however, it did not affect the diabetic complications or other clinical symptoms of MIDD. Furthermore, coenzyme Q_{10} treatment did not affect insulin secretory responses in the Mutant IGT or NGT subjects. There were no side effects of coenzyme Q_{10} during the therapy period of 3 years. In a randomized, double-blind, placebo-controlled 2 × 2 factorial clinical study involving 74 patients with uncomplicated type 2 diabetes and dyslipidemia, an oral supplementation with coenzyme Q_{10} (100 mg twice a day), 200 mg fenofibrate once a day, or both for 12 weeks showed that coenzyme Q_{10} improved blood pressure (systolic and diastolic) and long-term glycemic control, whereas fenofibrate, a cholesterol-lowering drug that improves lipid profiles, did not alter blood pressure or glycemic control.[92]

Diabetes and obesity can be induced by the consumption of excessive dietary fat that increases the levels of markers of oxidative stress and inflammation. It has been reported that supplementation with coenzyme Q_{10} reduced global hepatic mRNA expressions of inflammatory and metabolic stressor genes without changing the levels of lipid peroxides in mice fed high-fat diets, compared to control mice receiving a high-fat diet alone.[93] This suggests that the action of coenzyme Q_{10} does not involve a reduction in oxidative stress. Treatment of human umbilical vein epithelial cells in culture with coenzyme Q_{10} prevented hyperglycemia-induced increased oxidative stress and markers of adhesion molecules.[94] This suggests that coenzyme Q_{10} can protect against hyperglycemia-induced endothelial dysfunction that increases the progression of cardiovascular disease. Neuropathy, a disorder of nerve conduction, is associated with type 2 diabetes. Supplementation with coenzyme Q_{10} improved nerve conduction by the sciatic nerve in diabetic rats.[95]

ANTIOXIDANT MIXTURES

A mixture of vitamin C, vitamin E, and selenium protected the lens of the eye of streptozotocin-induced diabetic rats against oxidative damage by reducing markers of oxidative damage and improving the antioxidant defense system.[96] In a single-blind, controlled clinical study involving 46 patients with type 2 diabetes, 46 subjects with IGT and 46 control subjects, the efficacy of a mixture of antioxidants (vitamin E, vitamin C, and NAC) on the markers of oxidative stress and inflammation was evaluated. The results showed that the plasma levels of markers of oxidative stress (MDA, 4-hydroxynonenal, and oxidized LDL), markers of endothelial function (NO, endothelin-1, and von Willebrand factor) and a marker of inflammation, VCAM-1, were increased in all groups before supplementation with antioxidants. However, after supplementation, the levels of these markers of oxidative stress and inflammation were reduced.[97] In a clinical study involving 16 patients with type 2 diabetes, it was observed that supplementation with tablets containing vitamin C (1000 mg) and vitamin E (800 IU) reduced high-fat–induced memory impairment and markers of oxidative stress.[98]

In the Myocardial Infarction and Vitamins Study involving 800 patients with acute myocardial infarction (AMI), of which 122 (15%) patients had confirmed diabetes, the efficacy of vitamin E and vitamin C on the mortality was evaluated. The results revealed that supplementation with vitamin E and vitamin C reduced cardiac mortality in patients with AMI and diabetes.[99] In a randomized, double-blind, placebo-controlled trial involving 30 patients with type 2 diabetes, it was observed that supplementation with chromium (1000 μg), alone or in combination with vitamin C (1000 mg) and vitamin E (800 IU), reduced oxidative stress and improved glucose metabolism.[100] Treatment of diabetic rats with beta-carotene, pycnogenol, and alpha-lipoic acid, alone or in combination, normalized lipid peroxidation in the liver, kidneys, and heart, and elevated hepatic-reduced glutathione levels and cardiac glutathione peroxidase activity, or had no effect on hepatic catalase and SOD activities in all tissues.[101] In streptozotocin-induced diabetic rats, supplementation with curcumin and vitamin C was more effective in reducing blood glucose, glycosylated hemoglobin (HbA1c), dyslipidemia, leukocyte adhesion, and MDA than the individual agents.[102] It has been reported that the combination of vitamin E and magnesium was more effective in improving plasma lipid parameters and blood viscosity in diabetic rats than the individual agents.[103]

The overexpression of CuZn SOD or Mn SOD, together with catalase, reduced H_2O_2-induced oxidative stress in islet beta cells in culture.[104] Dexamethasone-induced impairment of beta cell function may be mediated via increased oxidative stress. This is confirmed by the fact that overexpression of catalase prevented dexamethasone-induced toxicity in beta cells in culture.[105]

VITAMIN A AND INSULIN

In a rat model of diabetes, insulin treatment was not as effective in reducing oxidative stress as vitamin A; however, a combination of the two was more effective in reducing oxidative stress in the heart than the individual agents.[106]

FOLIC ACID AND THIAMINE

Patients with type 1 diabetes have reduced levels of endothelial progenitor cells with impaired function. Reduced NO and increased oxidative stress contribute to the endothelial progenitor cells dysfunction. The analysis of gene expression profiles of endothelial progenitor cells from patients with type 1 diabetes revealed marked alterations in the expressions of 1591 genes involved in processes regulating development, cell communication, cell adhesion, and localization compared to healthy control subjects. Supplementation with folic acid normalized gene expression profiles in diabetic patients.[107] This is a remarkable observation that treatment of patients with type 1 diabetes with a single micronutrient can restore alterations in gene expression profiles to a normal level.

In the Women's Antioxidants and Folic Acid Cardiovascular Study involving 5442 female health professionals with a history of cardiovascular disease or more cardiovascular disease risk factors, the efficacy of a mixture of 2.5 mg folic acid, 50 mg vitamin B_6, and 1 mg vitamin B_{12} on the risk of type 2 diabetes was evaluated. The results showed that lowering homocysteine levels by B-vitamins in women at high risk for cardiovascular disease did not reduce the risk of type 2 diabetes.[108]

Diabetes can lead to thiamine deficiency. Treatment of streptozotocin-induced diabetic mice with benfotiamine, a lipophilic derivative of thiamine, reduced cerebral oxidative stress without affecting the levels of AGE, protein carbonyl, tissue factor, and TNF-alpha.[109] These results suggest that the primary action of benfotiamine is mediated via antioxidation. In a clinical study involving nine patients with type 1 diabetes, the effect of benfotiamine together with slow-release alpha-lipoic acid on glycemic status was evaluated by measuring hyperglycemia, intracellular AGE formation, hexosamine pathway activity, and prostacyclin. The results showed that the levels of AGE and monocyte hexosamine–modified proteins were increased, whereas the activity of prostacyclin synthase was decreased in diabetic patients. Treatment with benfotiamine together with slow-release alpha-lipoic acid did not affect hyperglycemia, but it normalized the AGE level and the activity of prostacyclin synthase and reduced monocyte hexosamine–modified proteins.[110] Zycose is a new drug released in 2006 for the treatment of diabetes. It contains benfotiamine (150 mg), benzamine (850 mg), a proprietary blend of *para*-aminobenzoic acid (PABA), vitamin E, and alpha-lipoic acid. Zycose has been shown to improve vascular dysfunction, neuropathy, nephropathy, and nerve function.[111]

CHROMIUM

A review of 15 published studies, including 11 randomized, controlled studies, on the efficacy of chromium picolinate (Crpic) in improving some of the markers of type 2 diabetes revealed that supplementation with Crpic reduced hyperglycemia, hyperinsulinemia, and requirements for hyperglycemic medication.[112] In a randomized, double-blind, placebo-controlled trial involving patients with metabolic syndrome (obese and nondiabetic), the efficacy of Crpic on insulin sensitivity to glucose was evaluated. The results showed that after 16 weeks of treatment, there was no significant change in the insulin sensitivity index, body weight, serum lipids, or markers of oxidative stress and inflammation between the control and treated groups. However, Crpic treatment increased acute insulin response to glucose.[113] This study has no conflict with the above studies, because all the above studies were performed in patients with type 2 diabetes. It is possible that the mechanisms of action of Crpic in diabetic patients and obese nondiabetic subjects are, in part, different.

ANTIOXIDANTS IN COMBINATION WITH DIABETIC/CARDIOVASCULAR DRUGS AND/OR INSULIN

In a rat model of insulin resistance induced by feeding 10% glucose for 20 weeks, the increased levels of insulin resistance associated with a higher production of markers of oxidative stress and systolic blood pressure were observed. Treatment with NAC prevented these alterations, except for systolic blood pressure; however, treatment with ramipril, an inhibitor of an angiotensin I-converting enzyme, did not effectively reduce insulin resistance or oxidative stress.[114] In a randomized clinical study with 80 patients with type 2 diabetes associated with dyslipidemia, the efficacy of combination treatment with fenofibrate and coenzyme Q_{10} on endothelial-dependent and endothelial-independent vasodilator function of the forearm microcirculation was tested. The results showed that the combination of two agents were more effective in improving vasodilator function of the forearm microcirculation than the individual agents.[115]

OMEGA-3 FATTY ACIDS

ANIMAL STUDIES

High dietary intake of omega-3 fatty acids reduced diabetic-related renal disease in diabetic models of rodents.[116] Supplementation with omega-3 fatty acids reduced the levels of MDA and the activities of SOD and catalase, and decreased the number of cerebral apoptotic neurons that were elevated in diabetic animals.[117] Long-term consumption of a diet rich in omega-3 fatty acids improved blood lipids and vascular function in an animal model of insulin resistance and type 2 diabetes; however, only dietary monosaturated fatty acids and alpha linolenic acid enhanced insulin sensitivity and glycemic responses.[118] Increased inflammation in white adipose tissue appears to be associated with obesity and type 2 diabetes. In obese mice with diabetes, treatment with omega-3 fatty acids prevented inflammation in white adipose tissue induced by a high-fat diet.[119] Dietary intake of low-dose omega-3 fatty acids attenuated leukocyte adhesion and infiltration into the tissues of diabetic mice complicated with sepsis.[120] Supplementation with omega-3 fatty acids in pregnant female diabetic rats improved lipid profiles and antioxidant enzyme activities and the levels of antioxidants (vitamins A, C, and E) in mothers as well as in their offspring.

HUMAN EPIDEMIOLOGIC STUDIES WITH OMEGA-3 FATTY ACIDS

Epidemiologic studies have suggested that populations consuming large amounts of omega-3 fatty acids (n-3 long-chain polyunsaturated fatty acids) found mainly in fish reduced the incidence of IGT, type 2 diabetes, and cardiovascular disease. This was not confirmed by a recent epidemiologic study. A large epidemiologic study involving 195,000 U.S. adults (152,700 women and 42,504 men) without preexisting chronic disease at baseline with a follow-up period of 14 to 18 years was conducted. The results showed that higher consumption of omega-3 fatty acids and fish was not associated with reduced risk of type 2 diabetes. Instead, it was modestly associated with increased incidence of the disease.[121] This study suggests that supplementation with omega-3 fatty acids will have no impact on the incidence of type 2 diabetes. However, this suggestion needs to be confirmed by intervention studies before it is accepted. Epidemiologic studies have suggested that supplementation with high amounts of omega-3 fatty acids protects against the development of depression; and a review of intervention studies with omega-3 fatty acids in nondiabetic subjects showed some benefit in reducing the level of depression.[122]

HUMAN INTERVENTION STUDIES WITH OMEGA-3 FATTY ACIDS ALONE

In a randomized intervention study involving 162 healthy individuals, it was found that moderate supplementation with fish oil did not affect insulin sensitivity, insulin secretion, beta-cell function, or glucose tolerance.[123] A review of published data showed that supplementation with omega-3 fatty acids in type 2 diabetes has no significant effect on glycemic control or fasting insulin; however, it lowered triglycerides and very low density lipoprotein (VLDL)-cholesterol levels, but it may raise LDL cholesterol.[124] Several intervention studies to evaluate the efficacy of various doses of omega-3 fatty acids on prevention and diabetic-related complications have produced inconsistent results. In a cross-sectional study involving 454 Alaskan Eskimos, the efficacy of omega-3 on the incidence of cardiovascular disease was evaluated. The American population consumes omega-3 fatty acids about 0.2 g/day and Eskimos about 3–4 g/day. The intervention dose of omega-3 fatty acids was 1–2 g/day. The results showed that there was no association between omega-3 fatty acids consumption and the presence of cardiovascular disease.[125] In a systematic review and meta-analysis of several randomized, placebo-controlled trials involving 1075 patients with type 2 diabetes, the effects of dietary and nondietary intake of omega-3 fatty acids on lipid profiles were evaluated. The results revealed that supplementation with omega-3 fatty acids decreased the levels of triglycerides, VLDL cholesterol, and VLDL triglycerides, but slightly enhanced the level of LDL cholesterol. It also showed improvement in thrombogenesis, but had no beneficial effects on cardiovascular disease risk factors such as HDL cholesterol, LDL particle size, glycemia, insulinemia, inflammatory biomarkers, and blood pressure.[126,127] In a clinical study involving 30 patients with type 2 diabetes and hypertriglyceridemia (16 men and 14 women), it was found that after supplementation with omega-3 fatty acids, the levels of triglycerides, non-HDL cholesterol, C-reactive protein, and TNF-alpha were decreased, whereas the levels of HDL cholesterol increased, and there was no change in the levels of IL-6.[128] In a randomized, double-blind, placebo-controlled trial involving 81 patients with type 2 diabetes, the efficacy of omega-3 fatty acids on the levels of homocysteine and MDA was determined. The results revealed that supplementation with omega-3 fatty acids (3 g/day) for a period of 2 months decreased the levels of homocysteine without changing the levels of MDA, fasting blood sugar, and CRP. This study showed that supplementation with omega-3 fatty acids does not reduce the glycemic index and some other risk factors associated with cardiovascular disease.[129] Supplementation with omega-3 fatty acids (3 g/day) for a period of 2 months failed to alter insulin sensitivity in 27 women with type 2 diabetes.[130,131]

HUMAN STUDIES WITH OMEGA-3 FATTY ACIDS, ANTIDIABETIC DRUGS AND HEART MEDICATIONS

In a clinical study involving 34 patients with type 2 diabetes who were treated with antidiabetic drugs for a month and then were administered omega-3 fatty acids in combination with antidiabetic drugs for a period of 2 months, the effects of omega-3 fatty acids on lipid peroxidation and antioxidant enzyme were evaluated. The results showed that supplementation with omega-3 fatty acids reduced the levels of serum triglycerides, MDA, and increased HDL cholesterol levels and erythrocytes glutathione peroxidase activity; however, it did not produce significant change in erythrocyte catalase and SOD activities.[132] The addition of 4 g of omega-3 fatty acids to treatment with a statin improved the lipid profiles better than statin treatment alone.[133,134] In a randomized, placebo-controlled trial involving 24 patients with type 2 diabetes, supplementation with omega-3 fatty acids in combination with a statin and fibrate decreased the risk of cardiovascular disease, and delayed the onset and progression of nephropathy in these patients.[135,136] These studies show that supplementation with omega-3 fatty acids in combination with antidiabetic drugs or heart medications yields better clinical outcomes than supplementation with omega-3 fatty acids alone.

In a clinical trial involving 1770 children at increased risk of developing type 1 diabetes, the efficacy of omega-3 fatty acids on the risk of developing islet autoimmunity was evaluated. The results showed that dietary intake of omega-3 fatty acids decreased the risk of developing islet autoimmunity in children at increased risk for type 1 diabetes.[137]

TREATMENTS OF DIABETES

STANDARD TREATMENTS

At present, treatments of diabetes are based primarily on control of glycemia. The main classes of oral antidiabetic medications include stimulators of insulin secretion (rapid-acting secretagogues and sulphanylureas), inhibitors of hepatic glucose production (biguanides), drugs dealing with digestion and absorption of intestinal carbohydrates (alpha-glucosidase inhibitors), or stimulators of insulin action (thiazolidinediones). It also involves a combination of diet modification and other antidiabetic oral medications including metformin, glynides, acarbose, troglitazone, and insulin or its analogs. Other adjunctive therapy may include antihypertensive drugs and cholesterol-lowering medications.[138,139] These standard therapies do not address the issues of increased oxidative stress and increased chronic inflammation that are the primary events in the initiation and progression of diabetes. This is one of the reasons why diabetic complications develop in spite of these multiple medications, although gradually. Therefore, additional approaches must be developed to address these issues. Such approaches would prevent the incidence of diabetes in high-risk populations, improve the efficacy of standard therapy in diabetic patients, and reduce diabetic-related complications.

Aspirin

Cardiovascular disease is associated with diabetes. Low-dose aspirin is widely recommended to reduce the risk of cardiac events in patients with cardiovascular disease. Supplementation with aspirin failed to reduce the risk of cardiovascular disease in patients with type 2 diabetes in some major clinical trials.[140–142] Although some studies have suggested minor beneficial effects on cardiac events,[143] its continued use has been suggested by many current diabetic guidelines.[144–146] The role of aspirin in the prevention of diabetes has also become controversial. An epidemiologic study involving 22,071 healthy men taking aspirin for a period of 22 years revealed that the incidence of type 2 diabetes decreased by about 14%.[147] Although the decrease in the incidence of type 2 diabetes after aspirin intake is small, the results are very impressive because aspirin, which does not affect oxidative stress, one of the primary events that contribute to the risk of type 2 diabetes, can decrease the incidence of this disease. In a randomized, double-blind, placebo-controlled trial involving 38,716 women free of clinical diabetes (19,326 received aspirin and 19,390 received placebo) and a follow-up period of 10 years, the efficacy of aspirin treatment on the incidence of type 2 diabetes was evaluated. The results showed that long-term consumption of low-dose aspirin failed to prevent the development of diabetes type 2 in initially healthy women.[148] A combination of aspirin and statin increased the weight loss in patients with type 2 diabetes.[149] A review of several studies has revealed that aspirin treatment did not lower the risk of diabetic retinopathy.[150] In a rat model of diabetes, treatment with aspirin prevented diabetes-induced tear secretion from the lacrimal gland and reduced diabetes-induced degenerative changes in the lacrimal glands.[151]

Aspirin Resistance

Although aspirin has become an essential component of the treatment of cardiovascular disease associated with or without type 2 diabetes because of its antiplatelet aggregation activity, the phenomenon of aspirin resistance has become of great interest because of its implication in increasing cardiac events. A review of studies on aspirin has revealed that about 20–30% of aspirin-treated patients exhibit platelet hyperactivity, despite adequate inhibition of cyclooxygenase-1 (COX-1) activity, and several meta-analyses suggest that residual platelet hyperactivity could be a risk factor for the recurrence of ischemic events in aspirin-treated patients.[152–154] The exact reasons for aspirin resistance are unknown. The suggested mechanisms include genetic polymorphism of COX-1, nonenzymatic formation of prostaglandins responsible for platelet aggregation, and inadequate doses.

Animal Studies with Aspirin

Although clinical studies failed to show any beneficial effect of aspirin in the prevention of type 2 diabetes, supplementation with aspirin prevented the development of type 2 diabetes by reducing insulin resistance, and elevating the level of fasting insulin and insulin sensitivity in streptozotocin-treated rats. It also protected the pancreas against streptozotocin-induced damage and maintained near-normal levels of glucose in diabetic rats.[155] Aspirin treatment protected the lacrimal gland against damage produced by increased oxidative stress and inflammation in streptozotocin-induced diabetic rats.[151] Pretreatment with aspirin attenuated cerebral ischemia in diabetic rats, and decreased neurological deficits. It also reduced platelet aggregation. However, aspirin treatment did not alter the levels of glucose and insulin in diabetic rats.[156] In diet-induced obese rats, the levels of iNOS and S-nitrosylation of IR-beta, IRS-1, and protein kinase B (Akt) were increased. Aspirin treatment not only reduced the levels of the above biomarkers of oxidative damage and inflammation, but also improved insulin resistance and insulin sensitivity.[157] Thus, in contrast to the results from human intervention studies, aspirin treatment consistently produced beneficial effects in the prevention and progression of diabetes in animals. Hence, the information gained from diabetic animal models cannot readily be extrapolated to human with respect to the efficacy of aspirin in prevention or treatment of diabetes.

PROBLEMS ASSOCIATED WITH USING A SINGLE AGENT IN DIABETIC PATIENTS

Laboratory studies of animal models with diabetes consistently showed that supplementation with a single micronutrient such as an antioxidant may reduce the risk of diabetes and improve insulin sensitivity and the glycemic index. In contrast, epidemiologic studies with a single agent produced inconsistent results with respect to the incidence of type 2 diabetes, insulin resistance, the glycemic index, or cardiovascular disease. Similarly, intervention studies with a single micronutrient or varying doses of omega-3 fatty acids also failed to produce consistent results on all diabetic and cardiac risk factors (lipid profiles, homocysteine levels, and markers of oxidative stress and inflammation). The reasons for these inconsistent results with a single agent in patients with type 2 diabetes are unknown. It is possible that doses of a single agent used in the studies were not sufficient to produce a full benefit on the incidence or progression of the disease. Since diabetes is a complex disease involving several risk factors that play an important role in the initiation and progression of diabetes, a single agent cannot attenuate the effects of all these risk factors. Therefore, I recommend the use of multiple micronutrients including dietary and endogenous antioxidants, B-vitamins, and certain minerals for reducing the incidence of diabetes in high-risk populations, and improving the risk of diabetic-related complications when combined with the standard therapy. Additional rationales for using multiple micronutrients are described below.

RATIONALE FOR USING MULTIPLE MICRONUTRIENTS IN DIABETIC PATIENTS

Because of the potential for increased levels of oxidative stress and chronic inflammation in high-risk populations (obese individuals, individuals with metabolic syndrome, older individuals, and individuals with a familial history of diabetes), an oral supplementation with appropriate multiple micronutrients appears to be one of the rational choices for the prevention of diabetes in these populations. Experimental designs of most clinical studies in patients with type 2 diabetes have utilized primarily only one antioxidant for reducing the complications associated with diabetes. These designs are not suitable for determining the efficacy of multiple micronutrients in reducing the incidence of diabetes or improved treatment of the disease when combined with the standard therapy. This is because their mechanisms of action and distribution at the cellular and organ levels differ, their cellular and organ environments (oxygenation, aqueous, and lipid components) differ, and their affinity for various types of free radicals differs. For example, beta-carotene (BC) is more effective in quenching oxygen radicals than most other antioxidants.[158] BC can perform certain biological functions that cannot be produced by its metabolite vitamin A, and vice versa.[159,160] It has been reported that BC treatment enhances the expression of the connexin gene, which codes for a gap junction protein in mammalian fibroblasts in culture, whereas, vitamin A treatment does not produce such an effect.[160] Vitamin A can induce differentiation in certain normal and cancer cells, whereas BC and other carotenoids do not.[161,162] Thus, BC and vitamin A have, in part, different biological functions.

The gradient of oxygen pressure varies within cells. Some antioxidants, such as vitamin E, are more effective as quenchers of free radicals in reduced oxygen pressure, whereas BC and vitamin A are more effective at higher atmospheric pressures.[163] Vitamin C is necessary to protect cellular components in aqueous environments, whereas carotenoids and vitamins A and E protect cellular components in lipid environments. In addition, vitamin C is necessary for the activity of tyrosine hydroxylase, which is the rate-limiting enzyme in the synthesis of catecholamines. Vitamin C also plays an important role in maintaining cellular levels of vitamin E by recycling vitamin E radical (oxidized) to the reduced (antioxidant) form.[164] Also, oxidative DNA damage produced by high levels of vitamin C could be protected by vitamin E. The oxidized form of vitamin C or vitamin E can also act as a radical; therefore, excessive amounts of any one of these forms of antioxidants could be harmful over a long period.

The form of vitamin E used in any clinical trial is also important. It has been established that D-alpha-tocopheryl succinate (alpha-TS) is the most effective form of vitamin E both in vitro and in vivo.[165,166] This form of vitamin E is more soluble than alpha-tocopherol and enters cells more readily. We have reported that an oral ingestion of alpha-TS (800 IU/day) in humans increased plasma levels of not only alpha-tocopherol, but also alpha-TS, suggesting that a portion of alpha-TS can be absorbed from the intestinal tract before hydrolysis.[167] This observation is important because the conventional assumption based on the rodent studies has been that esterified forms of vitamin E such as alpha-TS, alpha-tocopheryl nicotinate, or alpha-tocopheryl acetate, can be absorbed from the intestinal tract only after they are hydrolyzed to alpha-tocopherol. Our preliminary data shows that this assumption may not be true for the absorption of alpha-TS in humans.

Glutathione is effective in catabolizing H_2O_2 and anions. However, an oral supplementation with glutathione failed to significantly increase plasma levels of glutathione in human subjects,[168] suggesting that this tripeptide is completely hydrolyzed in the gastrointestinal tract. Therefore, I propose to utilize NAC and alpha-lipoic acid that increase the cellular levels of glutathione by different mechanisms in a multiple micronutrient preparation. In addition, R-alpha-lipoic acid and acetyl-L-carnitine together promoted mitochondrial biogenesis in murine adipocytes in culture; however, no effect was observed when these antioxidants were used individually.[169] These types of studies further emphasized the value of using more than one antioxidants in any clinical or laboratory studies involving type 1 or type 2 diabetes.

Other endogenous antioxidants, such as coenzyme Q_{10}, may also have some potential value in the prevention and improved treatment of diabetes. Since mitochondrial dysfunction occurs in patients with diabetes and coenzyme Q_{10} is needed for the generation of ATP by mitochondria, it is essential to add this antioxidant in multiple micronutrient preparation to improve the function of mitochondria. A study has shown that Ubiquinol (coenzyme Q_{10}) scavenges peroxy radicals faster than alpha-tocopherol,[170] and, like vitamin C, can regenerate vitamin E in a redox cycle.[171] However, it is a weaker antioxidant than alpha-tocopherol. Coenzyme Q_{10} administration has been shown to improve clinical symptoms in patients with mitochondrial encephalomyopathies[172] and has shown some benefits in diabetic patients. Selenium is a cofactor of glutathione peroxidase, and Se-glutathione peroxidase increases the intracellular level of glutathione, which is a powerful antioxidant. There may be some other mechanisms of action of selenium. Therefore, selenium and coenzyme Q_{10} should be added to a multiple micronutrient preparation for the prevention and improved treatment of diabetes.

Certain B-vitamins have produced some beneficial effects in patients with diabetes. Therefore, in addition to dietary and endogenous antioxidants, all B-vitamins that are necessary for general health should be added to a multiple micronutrient preparation for reducing the incidence or improved treatment of diabetes in combination with the standard therapy.

RECOMMENDED MICRONUTRIENT SUPPLEMENT FOR THE PREVENTION OF DIABETES IN HIGH-RISK POPULATIONS

High-risk populations include those with a family history of diabetes, prediabetic individuals, overweight individuals, and individuals with metabolic syndrome. They provide an excellent opportunity to study the efficacy of multiple micronutrients on reducing the incidence of diabetes. A formulation of multiple micronutrients may include vitamin A (retinyl palmitate), vitamin E (both D-alpha-tocopherol and D-TS), natural mixed carotenoids, vitamin C (calcium ascorbate), coenzyme Q_{10}, R-alpha-lipoic acid, NAC, L-carnitine, vitamin D, all B-vitamins, selenium, zinc, and chromium. The levels of alpha-lipoic acid, L-carnitine and chromium in a multiple micronutrient preparation would be higher than those for other chronic diseases. No iron, copper, or manganese would be included because these trace minerals are known to interact with vitamin C to produce free radicals. These trace minerals are absorbed from the intestinal tract more in the presence of antioxidants than in their absence, which could result in increased body stores of free forms of these minerals. Increased iron stores have been linked to increased risk of several chronic diseases.[173] Aspirin and omega-3 fatty acids were not included because they were not effective in reducing the incidence of type 2 diabetes. Antioxidants from herbs, fruits, and vegetables were also not included because they do not produce any unique biological effects that can not be produced by antioxidants present in the micronutrient preparation.

The recommended micronutrient supplements should be taken orally and divided into two doses, half in the morning and the other half in the evening with meal. This is because the biological half-lives of micronutrients are highly variable, which can create high levels of fluctuations in the tissue levels of micronutrients. A twofold difference in the levels of certain micronutrients such as alpha-TS can cause a marked difference in the expression of gene profiles (our unpublished data). To maintain relatively consistent levels of micronutrients in the body, the proposed micronutrients should be taken twice a day.

The efficacy of this formulation in high-risk populations should be tested by well-designed clinical studies. Meanwhile, the proposed micronutrient recommendations may be adopted by individuals who are at high risk for developing diabetes in consultation with their physicians or health professionals. It is expected that the proposed recommendations would reduce the incidence of diabetes in these populations.

RECOMMENDED MICRONUTRIENT SUPPLEMENT IN COMBINATION WITH STANDARD THERAPY IN DIABETIC PATIENTS

Increased oxidative stress and chronic inflammation have been linked to diabetic-related complications. The current antidiabetic medications, including insulin, do not affect these processes. Therefore, diabetic-related complications develop in spite of antidiabetic medications. The addition of a formulation of multiple micronutrients such as described in Recommended Micronutrient Supplement for the Prevention of Diabetes in High-Risk Populations on diabetic prevention may improve the efficacy of standard therapy. The efficacy of this formulation in combination with standard therapy should be tested in well-designed clinical studies in patients with type 1 and type 2 diabetes. Meanwhile, the proposed micronutrient recommendations may be adopted by diabetic patients receiving standard therapy in consultation with their physicians or health professionals. It is expected that the proposed recommendations would enhance the efficacy of standard therapy and reduce diabetic-related complications.

DIET AND LIFESTYLE RECOMMENDATIONS FOR PREDIABETIC INDIVIDUALS AND DIABETIC PATIENTS

A balanced diet is very necessary, in addition to supplementation with multiple micronutrients, for the prevention and improved treatment of diabetes. I recommend a balanced low-fat diet containing plenty of fruits and vegetables. Lifestyle recommendations include daily moderate exercise, reduced stress, no tobacco smoking, and maintaining a normal weight.

CONCLUSIONS

Diabetes mellitus is a chronic disease characterized by high levels of blood glucose that can result from defects in insulin production, insulin transport and/or utilization, or both. Diabetes leads to serious complications such as retinopathy, neuropathy, and nephropathy and can cause premature death if untreated. Diabetes has become a serious health problem throughout the world, including in the United States, and it has reached epidemic proportions. Despite the development of new medications to control glucose and recommendations of weight loss, daily moderate exercise, and a balanced diet, the incidence of diabetes continues to increase in the U.S. Severe diabetic-related complications eventually develop in spite of multiple diabetic medications. The analysis of published data suggests that increased oxidative stress and chronic inflammation are major factors in the initiation and progression of diabetes, as well as in the development of all diabetes-related complications. Antioxidants are known to reduce oxidative stress and inflammation; therefore, they should be useful in reducing the incidence of diabetes as well as diabetic-related complications. The results of several laboratory and human studies on the prevention and improved treatment of diabetes in which a single dietary antioxidant, endogenous antioxidant, certain B-vitamins, omega-3 fatty acids, mineral chromium, or aspirin alone was used showed inconsistent results. Therefore, I propose a preparation of multiple micronutrients including dietary and endogenous antioxidants, vitamin D, all B-vitamins, selenium, chromium, and certain other minerals, but not iron, copper, or manganese. This micronutrient preparation can be used for the prevention of, as well as in combination with standard therapy for the treatment of, type 1 and type 2 diabetes. It is expected that the use of multiple micronutrients alone may reduce the incidence of diabetes in high-risk populations and, in combination with standard therapy, may improve the clinical outcomes produced by standard therapy alone.

REFERENCES

1. National Diabetes Statistics. 2007. Fact Sheet. Bethesda, MD: U.S. Department of Health and Human Services, National Institutes of Health, 2008.
2. Martin-Gallan, P., A. Carrascosa, M. Gussinye, and C. Dominguez. 2003. Biomarkers of diabetes-associated oxidative stress and antioxidant status in young diabetic patients with or without subclinical complications. *Free Radic Biol Med* 34 (12): 1563–1574.
3. Cinkilic, N., S. Kiyici, S. Celikler, O. Vatan, O. Oz Gul, E. Tuncel, and R. Bilaloglu. 2009. Evaluation of chromosome aberrations, sister chromatid exchange and micronuclei in patients with type-1 diabetes mellitus. *Mutat Res* 676 (1–2): 1–4.
4. Kostolanska, J., V. Jakus, and L. Barak. 2009. HbA1c and serum levels of advanced glycation and oxidation protein products in poorly and well controlled children and adolescents with type 1 diabetes mellitus. *J Pediatr Endocrinol Metab* 22 (5): 433–442.
5. Liu, H. Y., S. Y. Cao, T. Hong, J. Han, Z. Liu, and W. Cao. 2009. Insulin is a stronger inducer of insulin resistance than hyperglycemia in mice with type 1 diabetes mellitus (T1DM). *J Biol Chem* 284: 27090–27100.
6. Codoner-Franch, P., S. Pons-Morales, L. Boix-Garcia, and V. Valls-Belles. 2009. Oxidant/antioxidant status in obese children compared to pediatric patients with type 1 diabetes mellitus. *Pediatr Diabetes* in press.
7. Matteucci, E., and O. Giampietro. 2000. Oxidative stress in families of type 1 diabetic patients. *Diabetes Care* 23 (8): 1182–1186.
8. Odermarsky, M., J. Lykkesfeldt, and P. Liuba. 2009. Poor vitamin C status is associated with increased carotid intima-media thickness, decreased microvascular function, and delayed myocardial repolarization in young patients with type 1 diabetes. *Am J Clin Nutr* 90 (2): 447–452.
9. Maritim, A. C., R. A. Sanders, and J. B. Watkins, 3rd. 2003. Diabetes, oxidative stress, and antioxidants: A review. *J Biochem Mol Toxicol* 17 (1): 24–38.
10. Kahler, W. K., B. Kuklinski, C. Ruhlmann, and C. Plotz. 1993. Diabetes mellitus—a free radical-associated disease. Effects of adjuvant supplementation with antioxidants. In *The Role of Antioxidants in Diabetes Mellitus: Oxygen Radicals and Antioxidants in Diabetes*, ed. F. A. Gries and K. Wessel, 33–53. Frankfurt, Germany: pmi Verlag Gruppe.
11. Kajimoto, Y., and H. Kaneto. 2004. Role of oxidative stress in pancreatic beta-cell dysfunction. *Ann N Y Acad Sci* 1011: 168–176.

12. Osorio, J. M., C. Ferreyra, A. Perez, J. M. Moreno, and A. Osuna. 2009. Prediabetic States, subclinical atheromatosis, and oxidative stress in renal transplant patients. *Transplant Proc* 41 (6): 2148–2150.
13. Lodovici, M., E. Bigagli, G. Bardini, and C. Rotella. 2009. Lipoperoxidation and antioxidant capacity in patients with poorly controlled type 2 diabetes. *Toxicol Ind Health* 25 (4–5): 337–341.
14. Song, F., W. Jia, Y. Yao, Y. Hu, L. Lei, J. Lin, X. Sun, and L. Liu. 2007. Oxidative stress, antioxidant status and DNA damage in patients with impaired glucose regulation and newly diagnosed type 2 diabetes. *Clin Sci (Lond)* 112 (12): 599–606.
15. de Lauzon-Guillain, B., A. Fournier, A. Fabre, N. Simon, S. Mesrine, M. C. Boutron-Ruault, B. Balkau, and F. Clavel-Chapelon. 2009. Menopausal hormone therapy and new-onset diabetes in the French Etude Epidemiologique de Femmes de la Mutuelle Generale de l'Education Nationale (E3N) cohort. *Diabetologia* 52 (10): 2092–2100.
16. Costford, S. R., S. A. Crawford, R. Dent, R. McPherson, and M. E. Harper. 2009. Increased susceptibility to oxidative damage in post-diabetic human myotubes. *Diabetologia* 52: 2405–2415.
17. El-Mesallamy, H., N. Hamdy, S. Suwailem, and S. Mostafa. 2009. Oxidative stress and platelet activation: Markers of myocardial infarction in type 2 diabetes mellitus. *Angiology* 61: 14–18.
18. Mellor, K. M., R. H. Ritchie, and L. M. Delbridge. 2010. Reactive oxygen species and insulin resistant cardiomyopathy. *Clin Exp Pharmacol Physiol* 37: 222–228.
19. Morales-Indiano, C., R. Lauzurica, M. C. Pastor, B. Bayes, A. Sancho, M. Troya, and R. Romero. 2009. Greater posttransplant inflammation and oxidation are associated with worsening kidney function in patients with pretransplant diabetes mellitus. *Transplant Proc* 41 (6): 2126–2128.
20. Allen, E. M., J. B. Matthews, R. O'Connor, D. O'Halloran, and I. L. Chapple. 2009. Periodontitis and type 2 diabetes: Is oxidative stress the mechanistic link? *Scott Med J* 54 (2): 41–47.
21. Block, K., Y. Gorin, and H. E. Abboud. 2009. Subcellular localization of Nox4 and regulation in diabetes. *Proc Natl Acad Sci U S A* 106 (34): 14385–14390.
22. Gorin, Y., K. Block, J. Hernandez, B. Bhandari, B. Wagner, J. L. Barnes, and H. E. Abboud. 2005. Nox4 NAD(P)H oxidase mediates hypertrophy and fibronectin expression in the diabetic kidney. *J Biol Chem* 280 (47): 39616–39626.
23. Yokota, T., S. Kinugawa, K. Hirabayashi, S. Matsushima, N. Inoue, Y. Ohta, S. Hamaguchi, et al. 2009. Oxidative stress in skeletal muscle impairs mitochondrial respiration and limits exercise capacity in type 2 diabetic mice. *Am J Physiol Heart Circ Physiol* 297 (3): H1069–H1077.
24. Holvoet, P. 2008. Relations between metabolic syndrome, oxidative stress and inflammation and cardiovascular disease. *Verh K Acad Geneeskd Belg* 70 (3): 193–219.
25. Mariappan, N., C. M. Elks, S. Sriramula, A. Guggilam, Z. Liu, O. Borkhsenious, and J. Francis. 2010. NF-{kappa}B-induced oxidative stress contributes to mitochondrial and cardiac dysfunction in type II diabetes. *Cardiovasc Res* 85: 473–483.
26. Ehses, J. A., G. Lacraz, M. H. Giroix, F. Schmidlin, J. Coulaud, N. Kassis, J. C. Irminger, et al. 2009. IL-1 antagonism reduces hyperglycemia and tissue inflammation in the type 2 diabetic GK rat. *Proc Natl Acad Sci U S A* 106 (33): 13998–14003.
27. Yang, J., Y. Park, H. Zhang, X. Xu, G. A. Laine, K. C. Dellsperger, and C. Zhang. 2009. Feed-forward signaling of TNF-alpha and NF-kappaB via IKK-beta pathway contributes to insulin resistance and coronary arteriolar dysfunction in type 2 diabetic mice. *Am J Physiol Heart Circ Physiol* 296 (6): H1850–H1858.
28. Donath, M. Y., D. M. Schumann, M. Faulenbach, H. Ellingsgaard, A. Perren, and J. A. Ehses. 2008. Islet inflammation in type 2 diabetes: From metabolic stress to therapy. *Diabetes Care* 31 (Suppl 2): S161–S164.
29. Ortis, F., P. Pirot, N. Naamane, A. Y. Kreins, J. Rasschaert, F. Moore, E. Theatre, et al. 2008. Induction of nuclear factor-kappaB and its downstream genes by TNF-alpha and IL-1beta has a pro-apoptotic role in pancreatic beta cells. *Diabetologia* 51 (7): 1213–1225.
30. Bastard, J. P., M. Maachi, C. Lagathu, M. J. Kim, M. Caron, H. Vidal, J. Capeau, and B. Feve. 2006. Recent advances in the relationship between obesity, inflammation, and insulin resistance. *Eur Cytokine Netw* 17 (1): 4–12.
31. Heilbronn, L. K., and L. V. Campbell. 2008. Adipose tissue macrophages, low grade inflammation and insulin resistance in human obesity. *Curr Pharm Des* 14 (12): 1225–1230.
32. Minamino, T., M. Orimo, I. Shimizu, T. Kunieda, M. Yokoyama, T. Ito, A. Nojima, et al. 2009. A crucial role for adipose tissue p53 in the regulation of insulin resistance. *Nat Med* 15 (9): 1082–1087.
33. Patel, C., H. Ghanim, S. Ravishankar, C. L. Sia, P. Viswanathan, P. Mohanty, and P. Dandona. 2007. Prolonged reactive oxygen species generation and nuclear factor-kappaB activation after a high-fat, high-carbohydrate meal in the obese. *J Clin Endocrinol Metab* 92 (11): 4476–4479.

34. Arrieta, O., R. Garcia-Navarrete, S. Zuniga, G. Ordonez, A. Ortiz, G. Palencia, D. Morales-Espinosa, N. Hernandez-Pedro, and J. Sotelo. 2005. Retinoic acid increases tissue and plasma contents of nerve growth factor and prevents neuropathy in diabetic mice. *Eur J Clin Invest* 35 (3): 201–207.
35. Hernandez-Pedro, N., G. Ordonez, A. Ortiz-Plata, G. Palencia-Hernandez, A. C. Garcia-Ulloa, D. Flores-Estrada, J. Sotelo, and O. Arrieta. 2008. All-*trans* retinoic acid induces nerve regeneration and increases serum and nerve contents of neural growth factor in experimental diabetic neuropathy. *Transl Res* 152 (1): 31–37.
36. Zunino, S. J., D. H. Storms, and C. B. Stephensen. 2007. Diets rich in polyphenols and vitamin A inhibit the development of type I autoimmune diabetes in nonobese diabetic mice. *J Nutr* 137 (5): 1216–1221.
37. Tessier, D. M., A. Khalil, L. Trottier, and T. Fulop. 2009. Effects of vitamin C supplementation on antioxidants and lipid peroxidation markers in elderly subjects with type 2 diabetes. *Arch Gerontol Geriatr* 48 (1): 67–72.
38. Chen, H., R. J. Karne, G. Hall, U. Campia, J. A. Panza, R. O. Cannon, 3rd, Y. Wang, A. Katz, M. Levine, and M. J. Quon. 2006. High-dose oral vitamin C partially replenishes vitamin C levels in patients with type 2 diabetes and low vitamin C levels but does not improve endothelial dysfunction or insulin resistance. *Am J Physiol Heart Circ Physiol* 290 (1): H137–H145.
39. Anderson, R. A., L. M. Evans, G. R. Ellis, N. Khan, K. Morris, S. K. Jackson, A. Rees, M. J. Lewis, and M. P. Frenneaux. 2006. Prolonged deterioration of endothelial dysfunction in response to postprandial lipaemia is attenuated by vitamin C in Type 2 diabetes. *Diabet Med* 23 (3): 258–264.
40. Jariyapongskul, A., T. Rungjaroen, N. Kasetsuwan, S. Patumraj, J. Seki, and H. Niimi. 2007. Long-term effects of oral vitamin C supplementation on the endothelial dysfunction in the iris microvessels of diabetic rats. *Microvasc Res* 74 (1): 32–38.
41. Sridulyakul, P., D. Chakraphan, and S. Patumraj. 2006. Vitamin C supplementation could reverse diabetes-induced endothelial cell dysfunction in mesenteric microcirculation in STZ-rats. *Clin Hemorheol Microcirc* 34 (1–2): 315–321.
42. Lee, E. Y., M. Y. Lee, S. W. Hong, C. H. Chung, and S. Y. Hong. 2007. Blockade of oxidative stress by vitamin C ameliorates albuminuria and renal sclerosis in experimental diabetic rats. *Yonsei Med J* 48 (5): 847–855.
43. Hamden, K., S. Carreau, K. Jamoussi, S. Miladi, S. Lajmi, D. Aloulou, F. Ayadi, and A. Elfeki. 2009. 1Alpha, 25 dihydroxyvitamin D3: Therapeutic and preventive effects against oxidative stress, hepatic, pancreatic and renal injury in alloxan-induced diabetes in rats. *J Nutr Sci Vitaminol (Tokyo)* 55 (3): 215–222.
44. Mathieu, C., C. Gysemans, A. Giulietti, and R. Bouillon. 2005. Vitamin D and diabetes. *Diabetologia* 48 (7): 1247–1257.
45. Palomer, X., J. M. Gonzalez-Clemente, F. Blanco-Vaca, and D. Mauricio. 2008. Role of vitamin D in the pathogenesis of type 2 diabetes mellitus. *Diabetes Obes Metab* 10 (3): 185–197.
46. Ulusu, N. N., M. Sahilli, A. Avci, O. Canbolat, G. Ozansoy, N. Ari, M. Bali, M. Stefek, S. Stolc, A. Gajdosik, and C. Karasu. 2003. Pentose phosphate pathway, glutathione-dependent enzymes and antioxidant defense during oxidative stress in diabetic rodent brain and peripheral organs: Effects of stobadine and vitamin E. *Neurochem Res* 28 (6): 815–823.
47. Nakhoul, F. M., R. Miller-Lotan, H. Awad, R. Asleh, K. Jad, N. Nakhoul, R. Asaf, N. Abu-Saleh, and A. P. Levy. 2009. Pharmacogenomic effect of vitamin E on kidney structure and function in transgenic mice with the haptoglobin 2-2 genotype and diabetes mellitus. *Am J Physiol Renal Physiol* 296 (4): F830–F838.
48. Kuhad, A., and K. Chopra. 2009. Attenuation of diabetic nephropathy by tocotrienol: Involvement of NFkB signaling pathway. *Life Sci* 84 (9–10): 296–301.
49. Hamblin, M., H. M. Smith, and M. F. Hill. 2007. Dietary supplementation with vitamin E ameliorates cardiac failure in type I diabetic cardiomyopathy by suppressing myocardial generation of 8-isoprostaglandin F2alpha and oxidized glutathione. *J Card Fail* 13 (10): 884–892.
50. Hamdy, N. M., S. M. Suwailem, and H. O. El-Mesallamy. 2009. Influence of vitamin E supplementation on endothelial complications in type 2 diabetes mellitus patients who underwent coronary artery bypass graft. *J Diabetes Complications* 23 (3): 167–173.
51. Song, Y., N. R. Cook, C. M. Albert, M. Van Denburgh, and J. E. Manson. 2009. Effects of vitamins C and E and beta-carotene on the risk of type 2 diabetes in women at high risk of cardiovascular disease: A randomized controlled trial. *Am J Clin Nutr* 90 (2): 429–437.
52. Poh, Z. 2009. A current update on the use of alpha lipoic acid in the management of type 2 diabetes mellitus. *Endocr Metab Immune Disord Drug Targets*.

53. Packer, L., K. Kraemer, and G. Rimbach. 2001. Molecular aspects of lipoic acid in the prevention of diabetes complications. *Nutrition* 17 (10): 888–895.
54. Singh, U., and I. Jialal. 2008. Alpha-lipoic acid supplementation and diabetes. *Nutr Rev* 66 (11): 646–657.
55. Ziegler, D., H. Nowak, P. Kempler, P. Vargha, and P. A. Low. 2004. Treatment of symptomatic diabetic polyneuropathy with the antioxidant alpha-lipoic acid: A meta-analysis. *Diabet Med* 21 (2): 114–121.
56. Burekovic, A., M. Terzic, S. Alajbegovic, Z. Vukojevic, and N. Hadzic. 2008. The role of alpha-lipoic acid in diabetic polyneuropathy treatment. *Bosn J Basic Med Sci* 8 (4): 341–345.
57. Liu, F., Y. Zhang, M. Yang, B. Liu, Y. D. Shen, W. P. Jia, and K. S. Xiang. 2007. Curative effect of alpha-lipoic acid on peripheral neuropathy in type 2 diabetes: A clinical study. *Zhonghua Yi Xue Za Zhi* 87 (38): 2706–2709.
58. Tankova, T., D. Koev, and L. Dakovska. 2004. Alpha-lipoic acid in the treatment of autonomic diabetic neuropathy (controlled, randomized, open-label study). *Rom J Intern Med* 42 (2): 457–464.
59. Kamenova, P. 2006. Improvement of insulin sensitivity in patients with type 2 diabetes mellitus after oral administration of alpha-lipoic acid. *Hormones* (Athens) 5 (4): 251–258.
60. Jacob, S., P. Ruus, R. Hermann, H. J. Tritschler, E. Maerker, W. Renn, H. J. Augustin, G. J. Dietze, and K. Rett. 1999. Oral administration of RAC-alpha-lipoic acid modulates insulin sensitivity in patients with type-2 diabetes mellitus: A placebo-controlled pilot trial. *Free Radic Biol Med* 27 (3–4): 309–314.
61. Ziegler, D., A. Ametov, A. Barinov, P. J. Dyck, I. Gurieva, P. A. Low, U. Munzel, et al. 2006. Oral treatment with alpha-lipoic acid improves symptomatic diabetic polyneuropathy: The SYDNEY 2 trial. *Diabetes Care* 29 (11): 2365–2370.
62. Henriksen, E. J. 2006. Exercise training and the antioxidant alpha-lipoic acid in the treatment of insulin resistance and type 2 diabetes. *Free Radic Biol Med* 40 (1): 3–12.
63. Muellenbach, E. A., C. J. Diehl, M. K. Teachey, K. A. Lindborg, T. L. Archuleta, N. B. Harrell, G. Andersen, V. Somoza, O. Hasselwander, M. Matuschek, and E. J. Henriksen. 2008. Interactions of the advanced glycation end product inhibitor pyridoxamine and the antioxidant alpha-lipoic acid on insulin resistance in the obese Zucker rat. *Metabolism* 57 (10): 1465–1472.
64. Lee, S. J., J. G. Kang, O. H. Ryu, C. S. Kim, S. H. Ihm, M. G. Choi, H. J. Yoo, D. S. Kim, and T. W. Kim. 2009. Effects of alpha-lipoic acid on transforming growth factor beta1–p38 mitogen-activated protein kinase-fibronectin pathway in diabetic nephropathy. *Metabolism* 58 (5): 616–623.
65. Sugimura, Y., T. Murase, K. Kobayashi, K. Oyama, S. Hayasaka, Y. Kanou, Y. Oiso, and Y. Murata. 2009. Alpha-lipoic acid reduces congenital malformations in the offspring of diabetic mice. *Diabetes Metab Res Rev* 25 (3): 287–294.
66. Padmalayam, I., S. Hasham, U. Saxena, and S. Pillarisetti. 2009. Lipoic acid synthase (LASY): A novel role in inflammation, mitochondrial function, and insulin resistance. *Diabetes* 58 (3): 600–608.
67. Kojima, M., L. Sun, I. Hata, Y. Sakamoto, H. Sasaki, and K. Sasaki. 2007. Efficacy of alpha-lipoic acid against diabetic cataract in rat. *Jpn J Ophthalmol* 51 (1): 10–13.
68. Masha, A., L. Brocato, S. Dinatale, C. Mascia, F. Biasi, and V. Martina. 2009. N-Acetylcysteine is able to reduce the oxidation status and the endothelial activation after a high-glucose content meal in patients with type 2 diabetes mellitus. *J Endocrinol Invest* 32 (4): 352–356.
69. Kamboj, S. S., K. Chopra, and R. Sandhir. 2009. Hyperglycemia-induced alterations in synaptosomal membrane fluidity and activity of membrane bound enzymes: Beneficial effect of N-acetylcysteine supplementation. *Neuroscience* 162 (2): 349–358.
70. Tsai, G. Y., J. Z. Cui, H. Syed, Z. Xia, U. Ozerdem, J. H. McNeill, and J. A. Matsubara. 2009. Effect of N-acetylcysteine on the early expression of inflammatory markers in the retina and plasma of diabetic rats. *Clin Experiment Ophthalmol* 37 (2): 223–231.
71. Xia, Z., K. H. Kuo, P. R. Nagareddy, F. Wang, Z. Guo, T. Guo, J. Jiang, and J. H. McNeill. 2007. N-Acetylcysteine attenuates PKCbeta2 overexpression and myocardial hypertrophy in streptozotocin-induced diabetic rats. *Cardiovasc Res* 73 (4): 770–782.
72. Kamboj, S. S., K. Chopra, and R. Sandhir. 2008. Neuroprotective effect of N-acetylcysteine in the development of diabetic encephalopathy in streptozotocin-induced diabetes. *Metab Brain Dis* 23 (4): 427–443.
73. Roest, P. A., L. van Iperen, S. Vis, L. J. Wisse, R. E. Poelmann, R. P. Steegers-Theunissen, D. G. Molin, U. J. Eriksson, and A. C. Gittenberger-De Groot. 2007. Exposure of neural crest cells to elevated glucose leads to congenital heart defects, an effect that can be prevented by N-acetylcysteine. *Birth Defects Res A Clin Mol Teratol* 79 (3): 231–235.

74. Xia, Z., Z. Guo, P. R. Nagareddy, V. Yuen, E. Yeung, and J. H. McNeill. 2006. Antioxidant *N*-acetylcysteine restores myocardial Mn-SOD activity and attenuates myocardial dysfunction in diabetic rats. *Eur J Pharmacol* 544 (1–3): 118–125.
75. Darmaun, D., S. D. Smith, S. Sweeten, B. K. Hartman, S. Welch, and N. Mauras. 2008. Poorly controlled type 1 diabetes is associated with altered glutathione homeostasis in adolescents: Apparent resistance to *N*-acetylcysteine supplementation. *Pediatr Diabetes* 9 (6): 577–582.
76. Jain, S. K., T. Velusamy, J. L. Croad, J. L. Rains, and R. Bull. 2009. L-Cysteine supplementation lowers blood glucose, glycated hemoglobin, CRP, MCP-1, and oxidative stress and inhibits NF-kappaB activation in the livers of Zucker diabetic rats. *Free Radic Biol Med* 46 (12): 1633–1638.
77. Mingrone, G. 2004. Carnitine in type 2 diabetes. *Ann N Y Acad Sci* 1033: 99–107.
78. Mynatt, R. L. 2009. Carnitine and type 2 diabetes. *Diabetes Metab Res Rev* 25 (Suppl 1): S45–S49.
79. Evans, J. D., T. F. Jacobs, and E. W. Evans. 2008. Role of acetyl-L-carnitine in the treatment of diabetic peripheral neuropathy. *Ann Pharmacother* 42 (11): 1686–1691.
80. Sima, A. A. 2007. Acetyl-L-carnitine in diabetic polyneuropathy: Experimental and clinical data. *CNS Drugs* 21 (Suppl 1): 13–23; discussion 45–46.
81. Malaguarnera, M., M. Vacante, T. Avitabile, L. Cammalleri, and M. Motta. 2009. L-Carnitine supplementation reduces oxidized LDL cholesterol in patients with diabetes. *Am J Clin Nutr* 89 (1): 71–76.
82. Solfrizzi, V., C. Capurso, A. M. Colacicco, A. D'Introno, C. Fontana, S. A. Capurso, F. Torres, et al. 2006. Efficacy and tolerability of combined treatment with L-carnitine and simvastatin in lowering lipoprotein(a) serum levels in patients with type 2 diabetes mellitus. *Atherosclerosis* 188 (2): 455–461.
83. Shankar, S. S., B. Mirzamohammadi, J. P. Walsh, and H. O. Steinberg. 2004. L-Carnitine may attenuate free fatty acid-induced endothelial dysfunction. *Ann N Y Acad Sci* 1033: 189–197.
84. Poorabbas, A., F. Fallah, J. Bagdadchi, R. Mahdavi, A. Aliasgarzadeh, Y. Asadi, H. Koushavar, and M. Vahed Jabbari. 2007. Determination of free L-carnitine levels in type II diabetic women with and without complications. *Eur J Clin Nutr* 61 (7): 892–895.
85. Power, R. A., M. W. Hulver, J. Y. Zhang, J. Dubois, R. M. Marchand, O. Ilkayeva, D. M. Muoio, and R. L. Mynatt. 2007. Carnitine revisited: Potential use as adjunctive treatment in diabetes. *Diabetologia* 50 (4): 824–832.
86. Soneru, I. L., T. Khan, Z. Orfalian, and C. Abraira. 1997. Acetyl-L-carnitine effects on nerve conduction and glycemic regulation in experimental diabetes. *Endocr Res* 23 (1–2): 27–36.
87. Rajasekar, P., and C. V. Anuradha. 2007. L-Carnitine inhibits protein glycation in vitro and in vivo: Evidence for a role in diabetic management. *Acta Diabetol* 44 (2): 83–90.
88. Malone, J. I., D. D. Cuthbertson, M. A. Malone, and D. D. Schocken. 2006. Cardio-protective effects of carnitine in streptozotocin-induced diabetic rats. *Cardiovasc Diabetol* 5: 2.
89. Hino, K., M. Nishikawa, E. Sato, and M. Inoue. 2005. L-Carnitine inhibits hypoglycemia-induced brain damage in the rat. *Brain Res* 1053 (1–2): 77–87.
90. El-ghoroury, E. A., H. M. Raslan, E. A. Badawy, G. S. El-Saaid, M. H. Agybi, I. Siam, and S. I. Salem. 2009. Malondialdehyde and coenzyme Q10 in platelets and serum in type 2 diabetes mellitus: Correlation with glycemic control. *Blood Coagul Fibrinolysis* 20 (4): 248–251.
91. Suzuki, S., Y. Hinokio, M. Ohtomo, M. Hirai, A. Hirai, M. Chiba, S. Kasuga, Y. Satoh, H. Akai, and T. Toyota. 1998. The effects of coenzyme Q10 treatment on maternally inherited diabetes mellitus and deafness, and mitochondrial DNA 3243 (A to G) mutation. *Diabetologia* 41 (5): 584–588.
92. Hodgson, J. M., G. F. Watts, D. A. Playford, V. Burke, and K. D. Croft. 2002. Coenzyme Q10 improves blood pressure and glycaemic control: A controlled trial in subjects with type 2 diabetes. *Eur J Clin Nutr* 56 (11): 1137–1142.
93. Sohet, F. M., A. M. Neyrinck, B. D. Pachikian, F. C. de Backer, L. B. Bindels, P. Niklowitz, T. Menke, P. D. Cani, and N. M. Delzenne. 2009. Coenzyme Q10 supplementation lowers hepatic oxidative stress and inflammation associated with diet-induced obesity in mice. *Biochem Pharmacol* 78: 1391–1400.
94. Tsuneki, H., N. Sekizaki, T. Suzuki, S. Kobayashi, T. Wada, T. Okamoto, I. Kimura, and T. Sasaoka. 2007. Coenzyme Q10 prevents high glucose-induced oxidative stress in human umbilical vein endothelial cells. *Eur J Pharmacol* 566 (1–3): 1–10.
95. Ayaz, M., S. Tuncer, N. Okudan, and H. Gokbel. 2008. Coenzyme Q(10) and alpha-lipoic acid supplementation in diabetic rats: Conduction velocity distributions. *Methods Find Exp Clin Pharmacol* 30 (5): 367–374.
96. Naziroglu, M., N. Dilsiz, and M. Cay. 1999. Protective role of intraperitoneally administered vitamins C and E and selenium on the levels of lipid peroxidation in the lens of rats made diabetic with streptozotocin. *Biol Trace Elem Res* 70 (3): 223–232.

97. Neri, S., S. S. Signorelli, B. Torrisi, D. Pulvirenti, B. Mauceri, G. Abate, L. Ignaccolo, et al. 2005. Effects of antioxidant supplementation on postprandial oxidative stress and endothelial dysfunction: A single-blind, 15-day clinical trial in patients with untreated type 2 diabetes, subjects with impaired glucose tolerance, and healthy controls. *Clin Ther* 27 (11): 1764–1773.
98. Chui, M. H., and C. E. Greenwood. 2008. Antioxidant vitamins reduce acute meal-induced memory deficits in adults with type 2 diabetes. *Nutr Res* 28 (7): 423–439.
99. Jaxa-Chamiec, T., B. Bednarz, K. Herbaczynska-Cedro, P. Maciejewski, and L. Ceremuzynski. 2009. Effects of vitamins C and E on the outcome after acute myocardial infarction in diabetics: A retrospective, hypothesis-generating analysis from the MIVIT study. *Cardiology* 112 (3), 219–223.
100. Lai, M. H. 2008. Antioxidant effects and insulin resistance improvement of chromium combined with vitamin C and E supplementation for type 2 diabetes mellitus. *J Clin Biochem Nutr* 43 (3): 191–198.
101. Berryman, A. M., A. C. Maritim, R. A. Sanders, and J. B Watkins, 3rd. 2004. Influence of treatment of diabetic rats with combinations of pycnogenol, beta-carotene, and alpha-lipoic acid on parameters of oxidative stress. *J Biochem Mol Toxicol* 18 (6): 345–352.
102. Patumraj, S., N. Wongeakin, P. Sridulyakul, A. Jariyapongskul, N. Futrakul, and S. Bunnag. 2006. Combined effects of curcumin and vitamin C to protect endothelial dysfunction in the iris tissue of STZ-induced diabetic rats. *Clin Hemorheol Microcirc* 35 (4): 481–489.
103. Dou, M., A. G. Ma, Q. Z. Wang, H. Liang, Y. Li, X. M. Yi, and S. C. Zhang. 2009. Supplementation with magnesium and vitamin E were more effective than magnesium alone to decrease plasma lipids and blood viscosity in diabetic rats. *Nutr Res* 29 (7): 519–524.
104. Lortz, S., and M. Tiedge. 2003. Sequential inactivation of reactive oxygen species by combined overexpression of SOD isoforms and catalase in insulin-producing cells. *Free Radic Biol Med* 34 (6): 683–688.
105. Roma, L. P., J. R. Bosqueiro, D. A. Cunha, E. M. Carneiro, E. Gurgul-Convey, S. Lenzen, A. C. Boschero, and K. L. Souza. 2009. Protection of insulin-producing cells against toxicity of dexamethasone by catalase overexpression. *Free Radic Biol Med*.
106. Zobali, F., A. Avci, O. Canbolat, and C. Karasu. 2002. Effects of vitamin A and insulin on the antioxidative state of diabetic rat heart: A comparison study with combination treatment. *Cell Biochem Funct* 20 (2): 75–80.
107. van Oostrom, O., D. P. de Kleijn, J. O. Fledderus, M. Pescatori, A. Stubbs, A. Tuinenburg, S. K. Lim, and M. C. Verhaar. 2009. Folic acid supplementation normalizes the endothelial progenitor cell transcriptome of patients with type 1 diabetes: A case-control pilot study. *Cardiovasc Diabetol* 8: 47.
108. Song, Y., N. R. Cook, C. M. Albert, M. Van Denburgh, and J. E. Manson. 2009. Effect of homocysteine-lowering treatment with folic Acid and B vitamins on risk of type 2 diabetes in women: A randomized, controlled trial. *Diabetes* 58 (8): 1921–1928.
109. Wu, S., and J. Ren. 2006. Benfotiamine alleviates diabetes-induced cerebral oxidative damage independent of advanced glycation end-product, tissue factor and TNF-alpha. *Neurosci Lett* 394 (2): 158–162.
110. Du, X., D. Edelstein, and M. Brownlee. 2008. Oral benfotiamine plus alpha-lipoic acid normalises complication-causing pathways in type 1 diabetes. *Diabetologia* 51 (10): 1930–1932.
111. Stirban, A. 2008. Drugs for the treatment of diabetes complications. Zycose: A new player in the field? *Drugs Today (Barc)* 44 (10): 783–796.
112. Broadhurst, C. L., and P. Domenico. 2006. Clinical studies on chromium picolinate supplementation in diabetes mellitus—a review. *Diabetes Technol Ther* 8 (6): 677–687.
113. Iqbal, N., S. Cardillo, S. Volger, L. T. Bloedon, R. A. Anderson, R. Boston, and P. O. Szapary. 2009. Chromium picolinate does not improve key features of metabolic syndrome in obese nondiabetic adults. *Metab Syndr Relat Disord* 7 (2): 143–150.
114. El Midaoui, A., M. A. Ismael, H. Lu, I. G. Fantus, J. de Champlain, and R. Couture. 2008. Comparative effects of N-acetyl-L-cysteine and ramipril on arterial hypertension, insulin resistance, and oxidative stress in chronically glucose-fed rats. *Can J Physiol Pharmacol* 86 (11): 752–760.
115. Playford, D. A., G. F. Watts, K. D. Croft, and V. Burke. 2003. Combined effect of coenzyme Q10 and fenofibrate on forearm microcirculatory function in type 2 diabetes. *Atherosclerosis* 168 (1): 169–179.
116. Garman, J. H., S. Mulroney, M. Manigrasso, E. Flynn, and C. Maric. 2009. Omega-3 fatty acid rich diet prevents diabetic renal disease. *Am J Physiol Renal Physiol* 296 (2): F306–F316.
117. Cosar, M., A. Songur, O. Sahin, E. Uz, R. Yilmaz, M. Yagmurca, and O. A. Ozen. 2008. The neuroprotective effect of fish n-3 fatty acids in the hippocampus of diabetic rats. *Nutr Neurosci* 11 (4): 161–166.
118. Mustad, V. A., S. Demichele, Y. S. Huang, A. Mika, N. Lubbers, N. Berthiaume, J. Polakowski, and B. Zinker. 2006. Differential effects of n-3 polyunsaturated fatty acids on metabolic control and vascular reactivity in the type 2 diabetic ob/ob mouse. *Metabolism* 55 (10): 1365–1374.

119. Todoric, J., M. Loffler, J. Huber, M. Bilban, M. Reimers, A. Kadl, M. Zeyda, W. Waldhausl, and T. M. Stulnig. 2006. Adipose tissue inflammation induced by high-fat diet in obese diabetic mice is prevented by n-3 polyunsaturated fatty acids. *Diabetologia* 49 (9): 2109–2119.
120. Chiu, W. C., Y. C. Hou, C. L. Yeh, Y. M. Hu, and S. L. Yeh. 2007. Effect of dietary fish oil supplementation on cellular adhesion molecule expression and tissue myeloperoxidase activity in diabetic mice with sepsis. *Br J Nutr* 97 (4): 685–691.
121. Kaushik, M., D. Mozaffarian, D. Spiegelman, J. E. Manson, W. C. Willett, and F. B. Hu. 2009. Long-chain omega-3 fatty acids, fish intake, and the risk of type 2 diabetes mellitus. *Am J Clin Nutr* 90 (3): 613–620.
122. Pouwer, F., G. Nijpels, A. T. Beekman, J. M. Dekker, R. M. van Dam, R. J. Heine, and F. J. Snoek. 2005. Fat food for a bad mood. Could we treat and prevent depression in Type 2 diabetes by means of omega-3 polyunsaturated fatty acids? A review of the evidence. *Diabet Med* 22 (11): 1465–1475.
123. Giacco, R., V. Cuomo, B. Vessby, M. Uusitupa, K. Hermansen, B. J. Meyer, G. Riccardi, and A. A. Rivellese. 2007. Fish oil, insulin sensitivity, insulin secretion and glucose tolerance in healthy people: Is there any effect of fish oil supplementation in relation to the type of background diet and habitual dietary intake of n-6 and n-3 fatty acids? *Nutr Metab Cardiovasc Dis* 17 (8): 572–580.
124. Hartweg, J., R. Perera, V. Montori, S. Dinneen, H. A. Neil, and A. Farmer. 2008. Omega-3 polyunsaturated fatty acids (PUFA) for type 2 diabetes mellitus. *Cochrane Database Syst Rev* (1): CD003205.
125. Ebbesson, S. O., P. M. Risica, L. O. Ebbesson, and J. M. Kennish. 2005. Eskimos have CHD despite high consumption of omega-3 fatty acids: The Alaska Siberia project. *Int J Circumpolar Health* 64 (4): 387–395.
126. Hartweg, J., A. J. Farmer, R. Perera, R. R. Holman, and H. A. Neil. 2007. Meta-analysis of the effects of n-3 polyunsaturated fatty acids on lipoproteins and other emerging lipid cardiovascular risk markers in patients with type 2 diabetes. *Diabetologia* 50 (8): 1593–1602.
127. Hartweg, J., A. J. Farmer, R. R. Holman, and A. Neil. 2009. Potential impact of omega-3 treatment on cardiovascular disease in type 2 diabetes. *Curr Opin Lipidol* 20 (1): 30–38.
128. De Luis, D. A., R. Conde, R. Aller, O. Izaola, M. Gonzalez Sagrado, J. L. Perez Castrillon, A. Duenas, and E. Romero. 2009. Effect of omega-3 fatty acids on cardiovascular risk factors in patients with type 2 diabetes mellitus and hypertriglyceridemia: An open study. *Eur Rev Med Pharmacol Sci* 13 (1): 51–55.
129. Pooya, S., M. D. Jalali, A. D. Jazayery, A. Saedisomeolia, M. R. Eshraghian, and F. Toorang. 2010. The efficacy of omega-3 fatty acid supplementation on plasma homocysteine and malondialdehyde levels of type 2 diabetic patients. *Nutr Metab Cardiovasc Dis* 20 (5): 326–331.
130. Kabir, M., G. Skurnik, N. Naour, V. Pechtner, E. Meugnier, S. Rome, A. Quignard-Boulange, et al. 2007. Treatment for 2 mo with n 3 polyunsaturated fatty acids reduces adiposity and some atherogenic factors but does not improve insulin sensitivity in women with type 2 diabetes: A randomized controlled study. *Am J Clin Nutr* 86 (6): 1670–1679.
131. Mostad, I. L., K. S. Bjerve, S. Lydersen, and V. Grill. 2008. Effects of marine n-3 fatty acid supplementation on lipoprotein subclasses measured by nuclear magnetic resonance in subjects with type II diabetes. *Eur J Clin Nutr* 62 (3): 419–429.
132. Kesavulu, M. M., B. Kameswararao, C. Apparao, E. G. Kumar, and C. V. Harinarayan. 2002. Effect of omega-3 fatty acids on lipid peroxidation and antioxidant enzyme status in type 2 diabetic patients. *Diabetes Metab* 28 (1): 20–26.
133. Valdivielso, P., J. Rioja, C. Garcia-Arias, M. A. Sanchez-Chaparro, and P. Gonzalez-Santos. 2009. Omega 3 fatty acids induce a marked reduction of apolipoprotein B48 when added to fluvastatin in patients with type 2 diabetes and mixed hyperlipidemia: A preliminary report. *Cardiovasc Diabetol* 8: 1.
134. Davidson, M. H., E. A. Stein, H. E. Bays, K. C. Maki, R. T. Doyle, R. A. Shalwitz, C. M. Ballantyne, and H. N. Ginsberg. 2007. Efficacy and tolerability of adding prescription omega-3 fatty acids 4 g/d to simvastatin 40 mg/d in hypertriglyceridemic patients: An 8-week, randomized, double-blind, placebo-controlled study. *Clin Ther* 29 (7): 1354–1367.
135. Zeman, M., A. Zak, M. Vecka, E. Tvrzicka, A. Pisarikova, and B. Stankova. 2006. N-3 fatty acid supplementation decreases plasma homocysteine in diabetic dyslipidemia treated with statin–fibrate combination. *J Nutr Biochem* 17 (6): 379–384.
136. Zeman, M., A. Zak, M. Vecka, E. Tvrzicka, A. Pisarikova, and B. Stankova. 2005. Effect of n-3 polyunsaturated fatty acids on plasma lipid, LDL lipoperoxidation, homocysteine and inflammation indicators in diabetic dyslipidemia treated with statin + fibrate combination. *Cas Lek Cesk* 144 (11): 737–741.
137. Norris, J. M., X. Yin, M. M. Lamb, K. Barriga, J. Seifert, M. Hoffman, and H. D. Orton. 2007. Omega-3 polyunsaturated fatty acid intake and islet autoimmunity in children at increased risk for type 1 diabetes. *JAMA* 298 (12): 1420–1428.

138. Triggiani, V., F. Resta, E. Guastamacchia, C. Sabba, B. Licchelli, S. Ghiyasaldin, and E. Tafaro. 2006. Role of antioxidants, essential fatty acids, carnitine, vitamins, phytochemicals and trace elements in the treatment of diabetes mellitus and its chronic complications. *Endocr Metab Immune Disord Drug Targets* 6 (1): 77–93.
139. Krentz, A. J., and C. J. Bailey. 2005. Oral antidiabetic agents: Current role in type 2 diabetes mellitus. *Drugs* 65 (3): 385–411.
140. Price, H. C., and R. R. Holman. 2009. Primary prevention of cardiovascular events in diabetes: Is there a role for aspirin? *Nat Clin Pract Cardiovasc Med* 6 (3): 168–169.
141. Ogawa, H., M. Nakayama, T. Morimoto, S. Uemura, M. Kanauchi, N. Doi, H. Jinnouchi, S. Sugiyama, and Y. Saito. 2008. Low-dose aspirin for primary prevention of atherosclerotic events in patients with type 2 diabetes: A randomized controlled trial. *JAMA* 300 (18): 2134–2141.
142. Belch, J., A. MacCuish, I. Campbell, S. Cobbe, R. Taylor, R. Prescott, R. Lee, et al. 2008. The prevention of progression of arterial disease and diabetes (POPADAD) trial: Factorial randomised placebo controlled trial of aspirin and antioxidants in patients with diabetes and asymptomatic peripheral arterial disease. *Br Med J* 337: a1840.
143. Sacco, M., F. Pellegrini, M. C. Roncaglioni, F. Avanzini, G. Tognoni, and A. Nicolucci. 2003. Primary prevention of cardiovascular events with low-dose aspirin and vitamin E in type 2 diabetic patients: Results of the Primary Prevention Project (PPP) trial. *Diabetes Care* 26 (12): 3264–3272.
144. Younis, N., S. Williams, and H. Soran. 2009. Aspirin therapy and primary prevention of cardiovascular disease in diabetes mellitus. *Diabetes Obes Metab*.
145. Colwell, J. A. 2004. Antiplatelet agents for the prevention of cardiovascular disease in diabetes mellitus. *Am J Cardiovasc Drugs* 4 (2): 87–106.
146. Nobles-James, C., E. A. James, and J. R. Sowers. 2004. Prevention of cardiovascular complications of diabetes mellitus by aspirin. *Cardiovasc Drug Rev* 22 (3): 215–226.
147. Hayashino, Y., C. H. Hennekens, and T. Kurth. 2009. Aspirin use and risk of type 2 diabetes in apparently healthy men. *Am J Med* 122 (4): 374–379.
148. Pradhan, A. D., N. R. Cook, J. E. Manson, P. M. Ridker, and J. E. Buring. 2009. A randomized trial of low-dose aspirin in the prevention of clinical type 2 diabetes in women. *Diabetes Care* 32 (1): 3–8.
149. Boaz, M., L. Lisy, G. Zandman-Goddard, and J. Wainstein. 2009. The effect of anti-inflammatory (aspirin and/or statin) therapy on body weight in type 2 diabetic individuals: EAT, a retrospective study. *Diabet Med* 26 (7): 708–713.
150. Bergerhoff, K., C. Clar, and B. Richter. 2002. Aspirin in diabetic retinopathy. A systematic review. *Endocrinol Metab Clin North Am* 31 (3): 779–793.
151. Jorge, A. G., C. M. Modulo, A. C. Dias, A. M. Braz, R. B. Filho, A. A. Jordao Jr., J. S. de Paula, and E. M. Rocha. 2009. Aspirin prevents diabetic oxidative changes in rat lacrimal gland structure and function. *Endocrine* 35 (2): 189–197.
152. Reny, J. L., R. F. Bonvini, I. Barazer, P. Berdague, P. de Moerloose, J. F. Schved, J. C. Gris, and P. Fontana. 2009. The concept of aspirin "resistance": Mechanisms and clinical relevance. *Rev Med Intern* in press.
153. Miyata, S., T. Miyata, A. Kada, and K. Nagatsuka. 2008. Aspirin resistance. *Brain Nerve* 60 (11): 1357–1364.
154. Patel, D., and M. Moonis. 2007. Clinical implications of aspirin resistance. *Expert Rev Cardiovasc Ther* 5 (5): 969–975.
155. Martha, S., K. R. Devarakonda, R. N. Anreddy, and N. Pantam. 2009. Effect of aspirin treatment in streptozotocin-induced type 2 diabetic rats. *Methods Find Exp Clin Pharmacol* 31 (5): 331–335.
156. Wang, T., F. H. Fu, B. Han, M. Zhu, X. Yu, and L. M. Zhang. 2009. Aspirin attenuates cerebral ischemic injury in diabetic rats. *Exp Clin Endocrinol Diabetes* 117 (4): 181–185.
157. Carvalho-Filho, M. A., E. R. Ropelle, R. J. Pauli, D. E. Cintra, D. M. Tsukumo, L. R. Silveira, R. Curi, J. B. Carvalheira, L. A. Velloso, and M. J. Saad. 2009. Aspirin attenuates insulin resistance in muscle of diet-induced obese rats by inhibiting inducible nitric oxide synthase production and S-nitrosylation of IRbeta/IRS-1 and Akt. *Diabetologia* 52: 2425–2435.
158. Krinsky, N. I. 1989. Antioxidant functions of carotenoids. *Free Radic Biol Med* 7 (6): 617–635.
159. Hazuka, M. B., J. Edwards-Prasad, F. Newman, J. J. Kinzie, and K. N. Prasad. 1990. Beta-carotene induces morphological differentiation and decreases adenylate cyclase activity in melanoma cells in culture. *J Am Coll Nutr* 9 (2): 143–149.
160. Zhang, L. X., R. V. Cooney, and J. S. Bertram. 1992. Carotenoids up-regulate connexin43 gene expression independent of their provitamin A or antioxidant properties. *Cancer Res* 52 (20): 5707–5712.

161. Carter, C. A., M. Pogribny, A. Davidson, C. D. Jackson, L. J. McGarrity, and S. M. Morris. 1996. Effects of retinoic acid on cell differentiation and reversion toward normal in human endometrial adenocarcinoma (RL95-2) cells. *Anticancer Res* 16 (1): 17–24.
162. Meyskens Jr, F. L. 1995. Role of vitamin A and its derivatives in the treatment of human cancer. In *Nutrients in Cancer Prevention and Treatment*, ed. K. N. Prasad, L. Santamaria, and R. M. Williams, 349–362. Totowa, NJ: Humana Press.
163. Vile, G. F., and C. C. Winterbourn. 1988. Inhibition of adriamycin-promoted microsomal lipid peroxidation by beta-carotene, alpha-tocopherol and retinol at high and low oxygen partial pressures. *FEBS Lett* 238 (2): 353–356.
164. McCay, P. B. 1985. Vitamin E: Interactions with free radicals and ascorbate. *Annu Rev Nutr* 5: 323–340.
165. Prasad, K. N., B. Kumar, X. D. Yan, A. J. Hanson, and W. C. Cole. 2003. Alpha-Tocopheryl succinate, the most effective form of vitamin E for adjuvant cancer treatment: A review. *J Am Coll Nutr* 22 (2): 108–117.
166. Schwartz, J. L. 1995. Molecular and biochemical control of tumor growth following treatment with carotenoids or tocopherols. In *Nutrients in Cancer Prevention and Treatment*, ed. K. N. Prasad, L. Santamaria, and R. M. Williams, 287–316. Totowa, NJ: Humana Press.
167. Prasad, K. N., and J. Edwards-Prasad. 1992. Vitamin E and cancer prevention: Recent advances and future potentials. *J Am Coll Nutr* 11 (5): 487–500.
168. Witschi, A., S. Reddy, B. Stofer, and B. H. Lauterburg. 1992. The systemic availability of oral glutathione. *Eur J Clin Pharmacol* 43 (6): 667–669.
169. Shen, W., K. Liu, C. Tian, L. Yang, X. Li, J. Ren, L. Packer, C. W. Cotman, and J. Liu. 2008. *R*-alpha-Lipoic acid and acetyl-L-carnitine complementarily promote mitochondrial biogenesis in murine 3T3-L1 adipocytes. *Diabetologia* 51 (1): 165–174.
170. Niki, E. 1997. Mechanisms and dynamics of antioxidant action of ubiquinol. *Mol Aspects Med* 18 (Suppl): S63–S70.
171. Hiramatsu, M., R. D. Velasco, D. S. Wilson, and L. Packer. 1991. Ubiquinone protects against loss of tocopherol in rat liver microsomes and mitochondrial membranes. *Res Commun Chem Pathol Pharmacol* 72 (2), 231–241.
172. Chen, R. S., C. C. Huang, and N. S. Chu. 1997. Coenzyme Q10 treatment in mitochondrial encephalomyopathies. Short-term double-blind, crossover study. *Eur Neurol* 37 (4), 212–218.
173. Olanow, C. W., and G. W. Arendash. 1994. Metals and free radicals in neurodegeneration. *Curr Opin Neurol* 7 (6): 548–558.

7 Micronutrients in Cancer Prevention

INTRODUCTION

In spite of extensive research on cancer prevention during the past several decades, the incidence of cancer appears to be on the rise. A little more than a decade ago, the number of new cases of cancer was about 1.2 million per year; in 2009, it was estimated to be 1.5 million. The current recommendations of consuming a diet rich in antioxidants, low in fat, and high in fiber, although very rational, has not had any significant impact in reducing the incidence of cancer. This may be partly because modifications in diet and lifestyle are difficult to implement in humans. Another possibility is that the recommendations themselves may not be sufficient to reduce the incidence of cancer and additional, mechanistic-based, novel approaches are needed to reduce the incidence of cancer. Despite the new advances in early diagnosis and drug treatment, the death rate from cancer has not changed significantly compared to data in 1950. Hence, an effective cancer prevention strategy remains one of the best approaches to reduce cancer-related mortality.

In an effort to reduce the incidence of cancer, numerous laboratory (cell culture and animal models) and human studies were performed, and several cancer-causing and cancer-protective substances associated with diet, lifestyle, and environment were identified. The cancer-protective agents included multiple dietary and endogenous antioxidants; the cancer-causing agents included several tumor initiators and tumor promoters. Some mechanisms of action for these agents were also clarified from these studies. Most epidemiologic studies in humans confirmed the inverse association between a diet rich in antioxidants, low in fat, and high in fiber and the risk of cancer. Several intervention studies—primarily with one dietary antioxidant, sometimes with two, and occasionally with multiple dietary antioxidants—were performed in populations at high risk for developing cancer. The results of these studies varied, ranging from beneficial effect, to no effect, or to a harmful effect on cancer incidence. Intervention studies with a high-fiber or low-fat diet alone, or in combination, were also performed in high-risk populations, and they yielded inconsistent results varying from beneficial effects to no effect.

This chapter discusses cancer incidence and mortality, proposed stages of human carcinogenesis, and laboratory, epidemiologic, and intervention studies with micronutrients in cancer prevention. This chapter also discusses possible reasons for the conflicting results of intervention studies with individual antioxidants in high-risk populations, and proposes a comprehensive micronutrient strategy, together with changes in diet and lifestyle, that can be tested in clinical trials for reducing the risk of cancer in high-risk populations.

CANCER INCIDENCE, MORTALITY, AND COST

The American Cancer Society estimated that in 2009, the number of new cases of cancer could be 766,130 in men and 713,220 in women, for a total of 1,479,350 cases. In 2008, a total of 1,437 million new cases (745,000 in men and 692,000 in women) were detected (U.S. Mortality Data, 2005, National Center for Health Statistics, Center for Disease Control and Prevention, 2008). This is an increase in cancer incidence from 1.2 million to about 1.5 million new cases in more than a decade.

The incidence of prostate cancer represents about 25% of all cancers, breast cancer about 27%, lung and bronchus cancer about 15% in men and 14% in women, and colon/rectal cancer about 10%

TABLE 7.1
Cancer Mortality in the U.S. Population

Year	Death Rate per 100,000 Persons
1950	194
1991	251.1
2005	184
2006	180.7

Source: U.S. Mortality Data, 2005, National Center for Health and Statistics, Center for Disease Control and Prevention, 2008.

in men and women. During 2003–2005, the American Cancer Society has estimated that the lifetime probability of developing cancer for all sites is 1 in 2 in men and 1 in 3 in women. For prostate cancer, the rate is 1 in 6, and for breast cancer, 1 in 8. For lung and bronchus cancer, the rate is 1 in 13 in men and 1 in 16 in women. For colon/rectal cancer, the rate is 1 in 18 in men and 1 in 20 in women. It appears that the incidence of new cancer is increasing, while there is no significant change in the death rate from cancer since 1950. Therefore, the development and implementation of a cancer prevention strategy that is based on a scientific rationale and evidence should be developed.

The U.S. mortality rate from cancer has not changed significantly during the past several decades in spite of extensive research and the development of new treatment modalities. In 1950, the death rate was about 194 per 100,000 persons; in 2005, this value was about 184 and, in 2006, it was 180.7. However, in 1991, it was estimated to be about 251.1 (see Table 7.1). The cancer death rate data of 1991 may be abnormally high because there is no data for subsequent or previous years. Thus, it appears that cancer deaths were reduced compared to 1991 data, but remained the same compared to 1950 data. It is more likely that the cancer death rate, which was increasing, has been prevented due to advancement of current treatments. In 2006, the total deaths from cancer were 559,888; however, in 2009, the estimated total cancer deaths were 562,340 (292,540 in men and 269,800 in women). Deaths from lung and bronchus cancer were highest in men (30%) and in women (26%). The deaths from other cancers include 9% from prostate cancer, 15% from breast cancer, and 9% from colon/rectal cancer for both men and women. About 26% and 23% of all deaths in men and women, respectively, are due to cancer. An effective cancer preventive strategy remains one of the best approaches to reducing the rate of cancer deaths in humans.

In 2009, the National Institutes of Health estimated that the overall annual direct and indirect cost of cancer in 2008 was $228.1 billion. This cost included $93.2 billion for medical, $18.8 billion for lost productivity due to illness, and $116.1 billion for lost productivity due to premature death.

PROPOSED STAGES OF HUMAN CARCINOGENESIS

Human carcinogenesis is a very complex process with a long latent period (3–30 years) between exposures to carcinogens and clinically detectable cancer. This implies that a preventive strategy can be implemented at any time before cancer detection. The identification of biochemical events that can alter the activities of genes responsible for cancer formation during the latent period can help to select agents that can attenuate cancer-causing events. Spontaneous tumors or familial tumors cannot be distinguished histologically. Despite profound advances in molecular carcinogenesis, the primary genes that initiate development of human cancer remain elusive in most cases.

The various proposed hypotheses of human carcinogenesis include (1) chromosomal aberrations, (2) activation of oncogenes, (3) loss of antioncogenes, (4) infection with certain viruses, and (5) overexpression of proto-oncogenes due to recombinational substitution of strong promoters. These proposed concepts of human carcinogenesis have been critically reviewed.[1–3] Although these concepts are intriguing, none of them alone is sufficient to explain the initial events in human carcinogenesis.

For example, chromosomal aberrations that can occur spontaneously or are induced by carcinogens can be observed in dividing cells. These cells may or may not transform to cancer cells depending upon the subsequent specific genetic changes. Similarly, overexpression and/or mutation of cellular oncogenes are not sufficient to convert normal cells to cancer cells, nor are the induced expression of antioncogenes sufficient to reverse cancer cells to a normal phenotype. Recently, polymorphism of certain genes appears to be associated with increased risk of cancer.[4-6]

To develop a novel biological strategy to reduce the risk of cancer, it is essential to know the potential stages that normal cells go through before they become cancer cells, and what risk factors contribute to the development of cancer at each stage. In an effort to develop a model to study carcinogenesis process, carcinogens were applied topically to the skin of animals, and the development of cancer was followed as function of time after treatment. These studies allowed postulating a two-stage model of carcinogenesis (initiation stage and promotion stage).[7] This model has been useful in identifying carcinogenic and anticarcinogenic substances and characterizing biochemical and genetic changes at each stage.

Normal cells undergo at least through two identifiable stages of carcinogenesis, immortalization and cancerous. Immortalized cells continue to divide without undergoing differentiation, leading to the formation of benign tumors, whereas cancerous cells continue to divide and metastasize to distant organs. Certain oncogenic viruses can induce immortalization when inserted into normal cells in culture. For example, rat and human brain cells can be immortalized by inserting a large T-antigen gene from SV40 and polyoma virus, respectively.[3,8] Viral oncogenes E6 and E7 of human papilloma virus (HPV) increase the risk of several cancers, including benign and malignant cervical cancer.[9-11] HPV can also act as a cocarcinogen in combination with tobacco smoking in increasing the risk of oral squamous cell carcinoma.[12] In the case of HPV-induced cervical cancer, the herpes virus may act as a cofactor in the development of cancer.[13]

When immortalized hepatocytes are transfected with the oncogenic c-Has in culture, they gain the capacity to form tumors in appropriate hosts.[14] This suggests that activation of cellular oncogenes can constitute a cancer risk factor, secondary to a critical step leading to immortalization.

A generic model of carcinogenesis suggests that cancer cells are the result of multiple mutations (gene defects) due to exposure to environmental, dietary, and lifestyle-related carcinogenic agents. Based on the histological progression of cancer formation, we have proposed a three-stage model of human carcinogenesis.[2] A diagrammatic representation of this model is shown below. This model shows that intervention can be made at any time during the first and second stages of carcinogenesis to reduce the risk of cancer. The latent period for each of these stages in humans could vary from a few to several years.

DIAGRAMMATIC REPRESENTATION OF THE PROPOSED STAGES OF HUMAN CARCINOGENESIS

First Stage

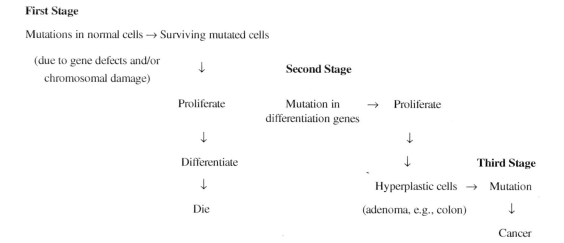

The first stage involves the induction of random mutations caused by gene defects or chromosomal damage in normal dividing cells due to an exposure to cancer-causing substances associated with the environment, diet, or lifestyle, a deficiency in the natural repair system, or a deficiency in protective substances, such as antioxidants. These mutations can also occur spontaneously due to random errors during replication and increased endogenous oxidative stress and chronic inflammation. The mutated cells may die or survive, depending upon the severity of the chromosomal damage. The surviving mutated cells continue to divide, differentiate, and die similar to the patterns observed in normal cells that do not have mutations. The mutated cells continue to accumulate additional mutations at a higher rate, but continue to divide and differentiate like unmutated, normal dividing cells for a long period.

The second stage of carcinogenesis involves the induction of random mutations in specific genes that are responsible for inducing differentiation in normal cells. As a result, the mutated cells continue to divide without achieving differentiation and subsequent cell death. Such cells become immortal and form precancerous or benign growths such as polyps in the colon or cysts in the female breast or ovary. They continue to proliferate while accumulating additional mutations for a long period.

The third stage of carcinogenesis involves the induction of random mutations in the immortal cells. Most such mutations play no role in converting immortal cells to cancer cells; however, when mutations occur in specific cellular genes, oncogenes, or antioncogenes, immortal cells become cancerous. This is well demonstrated in colon polyps and female breast and ovarian cysts, which remain noncancerous for a long time, but if not removed, become cancerous. Because mutation occurs randomly, the colon polyp may carry defects in more than one oncogene. The multiple, heterogeneous foci of cancer cells found in colon polyps are not necessarily clonal with respect to a given oncogene. This heterogeneity may be the reason why, in spite of extensive research in molecular carcinogenesis, it has not been possible to establish any direct relationship between the presence of one defective oncogene or other cellular genes and the tumor type or tumor behavior, although some associations between oncogene or antioncogene and tumor behavior have been documented.

The induction of random mutations in cancer cells may lead to aggressive behavior of cancer cells. Again, most mutations may not have any significant impact on tumor behavior; however, when mutations occur in certain specified genes, the cancer cells become very aggressive and invasive and, as a consequence, cause distant metastasis. Although several studies have tried to establish a relationship between defects in a particular gene and aggressive behavior of tumors, the results have not been consistent for the same tumor type.

Irrespective of the types of mutagenic or carcinogenic agents, increased oxidative stress and chronic inflammation[15–19] are associated with human carcinogenesis and they play a central role in inducing gene mutations and/or chromosomal changes that initiate carcinogenic changes. Therefore, agents that can attenuate oxidative stress and chronic inflammation may reduce the incidence of cancer.

SOME EXAMPLES OF TUMOR INITIATORS AND TUMOR PROMOTERS

Human are exposed to several tumor initiators and promoters daily from environmental, dietary, and lifestyle-related factors. Tumor initiators at any doses can cause cancer, whereas tumor promoters by themselves do not cause cancer, but, in combination with tumor initiators, increase the risk of cancer, and may reduce the latent period. There are two types of tumor initiators (carcinogens): direct-acting carcinogens, such as ionizing radiation, and indirect-acting carcinogens, such as benzo(*a*)pyrene that require conversion to an active form in the liver. Examples of tumor promoters are phorbol ester, excessive fat consumption, and high estrogen levels in women.

CONTRIBUTION OF ENVIRONMENTAL, DIETARY, AND LIFESTYLE-RELATED FACTORS

It has been estimated that the U.S. diet contributes to about 40% of human cancers, tobacco smoking contributes to about 30%, environmental factors contributes to about 29%, and familial gene defects contribute to about 1%. From these data, it appears that cancer can be considered a preventable disease. This issue has been reviewed.[2]

SOME EXAMPLES OF LIFESTYLE-RELATED CARCINOGENS

Alcohol. Several epidemiologic studies have revealed that the daily consumption of high amounts of alcohol is associated with an increased risk of colorectal cancer, pancreatic cancer, and oral cancer.[20–24] Alcohol intake and excessive weight were associated with an increased risk of breast cancer.[25] Although no intervention studies have been performed to establish a causal relationship between the consumption of excessive amounts of alcohol and an increased risk of certain cancers, epidemiologic data have been consistent. Therefore, excessive consumption of alcohol should be avoided in the proposed cancer prevention strategy.

Cell phones. Cell or mobile phone technology and its use have exploded during the past decade throughout the world. It is estimated that between 4 and 5 billion people use cell phones at this time. The fact that radiofrequency electromagnetic radiation from the cell phones can be absorbed into the brain has prompted concerns that the regular use of cell phones for a long period may increase the risk of acoustic neuroma and other brain tumors. The effects of cell phone use on cancer risks have been investigated using primarily epidemiologic methodologies. The results of these studies on cancer incidence have been inconsistent, varying from no effect to an adverse effect.[26–28] Reviews of several studies on the effect of cell phone use on the risk of brain tumors revealed that regular use of cell phones for a period of 10 years or more was associated with an increased risk of acoustic neuroma and glioma.[29,30] Other epidemiologic studies reported no such association between cell phone use and the risk of brain tumor.[31,32] In another epidemiologic study, regular use of cell phones was associated with an increased risk of benign parotid gland tumors.[33] An epidemiologic study on the Egyptian population living near cell phone base stations revealed that they were at increased risk of developing neuropsychiatric problems such as headache, memory changes, dizziness, tremors, depressive symptoms, and sleep disturbance compared to a control population.[34] This observation has not been confirmed in another population.

The laboratory studies with animal and cell culture models are very few. The radiofrequency radiation emitted from a cell phone produced no effect on cancer incidence in mice.[35] Exposure of mammalian cells in culture to 835-MHz radiofrequency radiation electromagnetic field slightly enhanced the levels of chromosomal aberrations induced by a chemical (ethylmethanesulfonate).[36]

It is known that epidemiologic studies reveal an association rather than a causal relationship between cell phone use and cancer risk. A causal relationship can only be established by intervention studies. Unfortunately, the results of epidemiologic studies are often propagated by the media and some professionals as a causal relationship between cell phone use and adverse health effects. Both epidemiologic studies and laboratory data are not sufficient to make any definitive conclusion about the health risk of cell phone use and additional studies should be performed. Because of the long latent period between continuous exposures from radiofrequency electromagnetic radiation from a cell phone and the development of adverse effects, and because of potential interaction with other agents during this period, conclusive data from epidemiologic studies are difficult to obtain.

The current controversies regarding the effects of cell phone use on cancer risk are analogous to those encountered in the early 1960s on the carcinogenic potential of low doses of ionizing radiation. The denial that low-dose ionizing radiation is carcinogenic persisted for decades until recently when it was accepted as a human carcinogen by the federal agencies. The author hopes that the controversy regarding the effects of cell phone use on human health will be settled sooner because of its potential health implications around the world involving billions of people. At this time, it is not necessary or prudent to recommend any limitation on use of the cell phone in any cancer prevention strategy, but caution should be maintained regarding overuse of this communication technology in the proposed cancer prevention strategy.

Smoking. Numerous epidemiologic and laboratory studies have confirmed that cigarette smoking is a major human carcinogen. It increases the risk of not only lung cancer but other cancers as well, and contributes to about 30% of all cancers. Passive smoking also increased the risk of cancer. However, some epidemiologic studies with specific cancers have produced inconsistent results. Lifetime exposure to active or passive tobacco smoking was not associated with alterations in breast cancer[37] or esophageal cancer and gastric adenocarcinoma.[38] Other epidemiologic studies revealed that both active and passive tobacco smoking were associated with an increased risk of breast cancer,[39-41] renal carcinoma,[42] and bladder cancer.[43] Despite some conflicting results, cessation of active and passive tobacco smoking must be included in the proposed cancer prevention strategy.

Coffee and caffeine. Epidemiologic studies on the association between coffee or caffeine consumption and the risk of cancer have produced inconsistent results. For example, some studies showed no association between coffee or caffeine consumption and the risk of renal carcinoma.[44] There was no significant association between caffeinated and decaffeinated coffee and tea consumption and the risk of breast cancer; however, a weak inverse association between caffeine-containing beverages and the risk of breast cancer in postmenopausal women was observed.[45] In another study, no association between caffeine consumption and the risk of breast cancer was found;[46] however, in women carrying a mutated BRCA1 gene, which increases the risk of breast cancer, an inverse association between coffee consumption and the risk of breast cancer was observed. There was no association between coffee consumption and the risk of ovarian cancer;[47,48] however, an increased risk of ovarian cancer was associated with heavy consumption (5 cups or more per day) in postmenopausal women.[49] On the other hand, another study reported an inverse association between caffeine consumption and ovarian cancer risk in women on hormone supplements.[50] An association between coffee and caffeine consumption and an increased risk of bladder cancer was observed,[51] but an inverse association was observed for liver cancer.[52] A meta-analysis of data on coffee consumption and the risk of lung cancer revealed that increased consumption of coffee was associated with an enhanced risk of lung cancer.[53] From these studies, it is difficult to draw any specific conclusions with respect to the impact of coffee, decaffeinated coffee, or caffeine consumption on the risk of overall cancer. In my view, 1 or 2 cups of coffee or an equivalent amount of caffeine-containing beverages may have no effect on the incidence of any type of cancer; however, excessive consumption of coffee or caffeine should be avoided in the proposed cancer prevention strategy until definitive data from intervention studies become available.

SOME EXAMPLES OF ENVIRONMENT-RELATED CARCINOGENS

There are numerous carcinogens and mutagens in atmospheric and work-related environments. They include ozone, ionizing radiation and ultraviolet radiation from the sun, burning wood in the forest, or buildings that release high levels of polycyclic hydrocarbons such as benzo(*a*)pyrene, asbestos, benzene, and vinyl chloride.

SOME EXAMPLES OF DIET-RELATED CARCINOGENS

Human diets contain both cancer-protective and cancer-causing substances.[54] Most of the mutagenic and carcinogenic substances that are present in the diet are naturally occurring; however, small amounts of mutagens have been introduced into the diet by the use of pesticides in agriculture production.[54] The relative ratio of protective and mutagenic substances in the human diet can vary markedly from one individual to another and from one day to another in the same individual. Varying levels of mutagens and carcinogens are formed during the storage of food at room temperature (browning of fruits and vegetables), and during the cooking process (browning of vegetables and meat). Flamed-broiled fatty meat may contain much higher levels of carcinogens like benzo(*a*)pyrene than those found in grilled meat. Consumption of a nitrite-rich diet (bacon, sausage, cured meat) can form nitrosamine in the stomach at an acid pH by the combination of nitrites and secondary amines. Diets rich in meat increase the levels of mutagens in the feces compared to vegetarian diets. Excessively high caloric diets and the consumption of diets rich in fat can increase the risk of cancer. Epidemiologic studies have reported that acrylamide, which is formed during the heating of several foods at very high temperatures, is associated with the increased risk of endometrial, ovarian, estrogen-positive breast cancer, and renal cell cancer, but not with lung cancer in men; however, it was inversely associated with lung cancer in women.[55] Aflatoxin alone or in combination with the hepatitis B virus can increase the risk of liver cancer.[56]

SOME EXAMPLES OF DIET-RELATED CANCER PROTECTIVE AGENTS

Protective substances in the diets are antioxidants—the levels and types of which can vary markedly, depending upon the type of food. Generally, fruits and green, red, or yellow vegetables are rich in antioxidants. Consumption of meat or fish provides endogenous antioxidants (made in the body) that may decrease as a function of aging. A lower intake of nutrients, especially antioxidants from the diet, can increase the risk of cancer.

In addition to standard dietary antioxidants such vitamins A, C, and E, carotenoids, and the mineral selenium, there are several other antioxidants including several polyphenolic compounds present in fruits, vegetables, and herbs that exhibit properties relevant to cancer prevention. However, these antioxidants do not exhibit any unique functional relevance to cancer prevention that cannot be produced by standard dietary antioxidants. Therefore, their inclusion in the proposed cancer preventive strategy that contains standard dietary antioxidants and endogenous antioxidants may not be necessary.

In contrast to human diets in the United States, the diet of laboratory rodents is vegetarian and relatively uniform in contents. Therefore, the relative ratio of protective and carcinogenic substances in these animals' diet may not vary significantly during the study period. The human diet, with respect to cancer-protective and cancer-causing substances, varies markedly from day to day and from one individual to another on the same day. In addition, most rodents, except guinea pigs, make their own vitamin C; humans do not. These differences in rodent and human diets are often ignored while extrapolating the results of micronutrient experiments on rodents to design of cancer prevention studies in humans. The analysis of animal and human studies with antioxidants has convinced me that the results of investigation on the effects of micronutrients on cancer prevention in animal models should not be extrapolated to the design of human studies with respect to the number, type, dose, and dose schedule of antioxidants.

FUNCTIONS OF ANTIOXIDANTS RELEVANT TO CANCER PREVENTION

Extensive studies have been published on the functions of antioxidants that explain their protective role in reducing the risk of cancer. This issue has been discussed extensively in a review.[2] Antioxidants can neutralize excessive levels of free radicals that increase the risk of cancer. They can prevent the formation of potential carcinogenic substances. For example, vitamins C and E, alone or in combination, prevent the formation of nitrosamine in the stomach from nitrites (present in a nitrite-rich diet) and secondary amines.[57] These dietary antioxidants also reduce the levels of fecal mutagens that are formed during the digestion of food.[58] The combination of vitamins C and E is more effective than the individual antioxidants in reducing the levels of fecal mutagens. High levels of antioxidants can prevent conversion of indirect carcinogens to an active form in the liver that is needed to increase the risk of cancer. Mutations due to gene mutation and/or chromosomal damage can increase the risk of cancer. Antioxidants can reduce spontaneous and induced mutations in animal as well as human cells and, thus, could play an important role in cancer prevention. For example, vitamins C and E and beta-carotene reduce chromosomal damage produced by ionizing radiation and chemical carcinogens.[59-61]

They can also inhibit overexpression of oncogenes and the expression and levels of mutated oncogenes. A high-fat diet increases the levels of prostaglandins (PGs) in the animal model[62] and may increase the risk of some cancers.[63] Vitamin E and a nonsteroidal anti-inflammatory drug (NSAID), aspirin, inhibit the production of PGs more than that produced by the individual agent.

Although a host's immune system may not play a direct role in human carcinogenesis, it could play an important role in allowing or rejecting newly formed cancer cells. The optimally functioning immune cells (natural killer cells) can recognize newly formed cancer cells and kill them. A weak immune system may allow newly formed cancer cells to establish themselves in the host; these cells will then grow and metastasize to distant organs. Antioxidants stimulate humoral and cellular immunity[7,64,65] and, thus, can reduce the risk of developing cancer.

ANALYSIS OF CELL CULTURES AFTER TREATMENT WITH ANTIOXIDANTS

Tissue culture systems provide a unique opportunity to evaluate the anticancer properties of antioxidants in a cost- and time-effective manner. In addition, detailed studies on the mechanisms of action of antioxidants at the cellular and genetic levels could not be carried out in animal models owing to the inherent complexity of in vivo systems. The availability of a normal-like murine cell line (CH310T1/2) and other mammalian cell cultures of normal cells and immortalized cells provide a new opportunity to investigate the mechanisms of action of antioxidants and their derivatives on cancer prevention. All forms of vitamin E do not exhibit the same efficacy in cancer prevention studies. In 1982, we identified alpha-tocopheryl succinate (alpha-TS) as the most effective form of vitamin E exhibiting anti-cancer properties.[66] It has been reported that alpha-TS, but not alpha-tocopherol or alpha-tocopheryl acetate, reduces the incidence of chemical and ionizing radiation-induced transformation of normal-like murine fibroblasts in culture.[67,68] Beta-carotene also reduced the incidence of chemical and ionizing radiation-induced transformation of normal-like murine fibroblasts in culture.[69,70] Natural beta-carotene was more effective than synthetic beta-carotene in reducing the incidence of radiation-induced transformation in vitro. *N*-Acetylcysteine (NAC) markedly reduced estrogen-induced transformation of E6 cells (a normal mouse epithelial cell line) in culture.[71] A number of studies have revealed that breast cancer formation is related to abnormal estrogen oxidation forming an excess of estrogen-3,4-quinones, which react with DNA to form depurinating adducts and induce mutations. This metabolite of estrogen can induce transformation in normal cells in culture. Thus, NAC can prevent the oxidation of estrogen and thereby reduce the risk of breast cancer. From the cell culture studies, it can be suggested that the addition of natural beta-carotene, NAC, and alpha-TS to the multiple micronutrient preparation would be necessary for the proposed cancer prevention strategy.

The exact mechanisms of protection of induced carcinogenesis in vitro by these antioxidants are unknown; however, I suggest that antioxidants probably prevent those mutagenic changes that initiate immortalization (preneoplastic state) by reducing oxidative damage caused by carcinogens. The results of in vitro studies cannot readily be extrapolated to animals or humans with respect to antioxidant type, dose, or dose schedule. The cell culture models are excellent for investigating the molecular mechanisms of action of antioxidants in chemical- or radiation-induced cancer. Therefore, the use of a single antioxidant to investigate cancer prevention mechanisms is perfectly valid and essential in cell culture models. The use of a single antioxidant may not be useful for prevention of human cancer in high-risk populations, because of the presence of a high internal oxidative environment in which a single antioxidant may act as a pro-oxidant.

ANALYSIS OF CANCER PREVENTION STUDIES IN ANIMALS AFTER TREATMENT WITH ANTIOXIDANTS

The role of antioxidants in cancer prevention was demonstrated in animal models long before any human or in vitro study was initiated. A two-stage model of carcinogenesis was developed and utilized primarily to investigate the mechanisms of carcinogenesis and to determine the efficacy of antioxidants in cancer prevention. The overwhelming majority of studies performed on this model suggest that supplementation with high doses of individual antioxidants such as vitamins C[72] and E,[73] retinoids,[74] and carotenoids[75,76] reduced the risk of chemical-induced tumors. Among various forms of vitamin E, alpha-TS was most effective as an anticancer agent.[73] In the Lady transgenic animal model, the combination of vitamin E, selenium, and lycopene was effective in reducing the risk of prostate cancer, whereas the combination of vitamin E and selenium was ineffective.[77] The result of the combined effect of vitamin E and selenium is consistent with the results of Selenium and Vitamin E Cancer Prevention Trial (SELECT) in which the combination of vitamin E and selenium was found to be ineffective in reducing the risk of prostate cancer.[78] The data from the above animal study also suggest that the addition of other antioxidants may be necessary to reduce the risk of cancer in general and prostate cancer in particular. In p53 knockout pregnant mice, prenatal supplementation with vitamin E (all-rac-alpha-tocopheryl acetate) reduced postnatal malignancies by reducing the levels of DNA oxidation.[79]

Dihydrolipoic acid, a reduced form of alpha-lipoic acid, significantly reduced tumor incidence and tumor multiplicity in dimethylbenzanthracene (DMBA)/tetrachlorohydroquinone (TCHQ)-induced skin tumor formation.[80] TCHQ is a tumor promoter, and DMBA is a tumor initiator. Dihydrolipoic acid also markedly inhibited expression of inducible nitric oxide synthase protein and cyclooxygenase-2 activity, and reduced the tumor incidence and tumor multiplicity of DMBA/12-O-tetradecanoylphorbol-13-acetate (TPA)-induced skin tumors.[81] In mice overexpressing Her2/neu, as an animal model for breast cancer, and APCmin mice for intestinal cancer, supplementation with alpha-lipoic acid did not affect the incidence of breast or colon cancer.[82] The reasons for these contradictory results between transgenic models of cancer and chemical-induced cancer models in animals remain unknown. However, it is possible that susceptibility of the animals with inserted oncogenes to cancer may not involve increased oxidative stress in the formation of cancer. It is equally possible that other antioxidants rather than alpha-lipoic acid alone may be needed to reduce the incidence of cancer in the genetic models of mice.

The hereditary human disorder ataxia telangiectasia (AT) is characterized by an extremely high incidence of lymphoid malignancy. Using AT-deficient mice, it was demonstrated that supplementation with NAC increased lifespan and reduced the incidence and tumor multiplicity of lymphoma.[83] However, supplementation with NAC did not change the incidence of liver tumors, but caused a significant decrease in tumor multiplicity in rats treated with N-diethyl nitrosamine/diethyldithiocarbamate (DEN/DEDTC).[84] On the other hand, using the p53 haploinsufficient Tg.AC (v-H-*ras*) mouse, which contains activated ras oncogenes and an inactivated p53 tumor suppressor gene—frequently found in human cancers—it was demonstrated that supplementation with NAC does not affect the incidence of benzo(*a*)pyrene-induced skin tumors; however, it did reduce tumor multiplicity.[85] Supplementation with NAC did not affect DMBA-induced mammary tumor in the rodent model.[86] In contrast to DMBA-induced mammary tumors, NAC supplementation reduced the incidence of urethane-induced lung cancer.[87] Vitamin E, in combination with NAC, was more effective in reducing the incidence of esophageal cancer in the esophagogastroduodenal anastomosis (EGDA) rat model than the individual agents.[88] The effects of NAC in reducing induced cancers in rodent models are variable, depending upon the type of tumor and tumor-inducing agents. It is interesting to note that both NAC and alpha-lipoic acid, when used individually, produced inconsistent results.

Supplementation with coenzyme Q_{10} reduced azoxymethane-induced, aberrant crypt foci and mucin-depleted foci in the colon of a male rat.[89]

A few studies found that certain antioxidants at very high doses, when used individually, may increase the risk of cancer. For example, vitamin E at very high doses (the equivalent of 40 g per person per day) increased the risk of chemical-induced cancer in the small intestine of mice.[90] Vitamin C, in the form of sodium ascorbate, increased the risk of chemical-induced bladder cancer in rats.[91] It was found that the increased osmolarity of urine caused chronic irritations in the bladder, which may account for the increased risk of chemical-induced cancer following treatments with a high concentration of sodium ascorbate. The use of such high doses of single antioxidants in cancer prevention studies is not relevant to humans except that they can produce harmful effects in animals, and possibly in humans.

Most studies published on animal models have utilized a single dietary or endogenous antioxidant and have yielded sometime inconsistent protective effects against chemical-induced cancers. The efficacy of a mixture of dietary and endogenous antioxidants in reducing the incidence of chemical-induced cancer in animal models has never been tested.

It should be noted that most animal studies in the past used Purina Chow (Ralston Purina, St. Louis, MO), a standard rodent diet, but no information regarding the basal levels of antioxidants was available to the investigators. The antioxidant levels in Purina Chow are known to vary significantly from one batch to another; and this could have an impact in determining the efficacy of supplemented antioxidants in cancer prevention. In my opinion, a well-defined diet that contains multiple dietary and endogenous antioxidants at the levels that are higher than the RDA levels for rodents must be used for any cancer prevention study with antioxidants in animals. The published studies that have failed to use such well-defined diets may not provide accurate results on the efficacy of single or multiple antioxidants in reducing the risk of chemical- or radiation-induced cancer. From animal studies, it can be concluded that antioxidants have the potential to reduce the risk of cancer in humans.

Although animal models are useful for determining the efficacy of antioxidants in cancer prevention, the results obtained from these models cannot be extrapolated to humans with respect to dose, dose schedule, and type of antioxidants because the absorption, tissue distribution, biological turnover, and metabolism of these antioxidants in animals are totally different from those found in humans. Unlike humans, most rodents except guinea pigs make their own vitamin C, which could have an impact on the dose and efficacy of antioxidants in reducing the risk of chemical-induced cancer.

ANALYSIS OF EPIDEMIOLOGIC STUDIES ON ANTIOXIDANTS AND CANCER PREVENTION

Epidemiologic studies utilize two different experimental designs: retrospective case-control studies and prospective case-control studies. The design of a retrospective case-control study involves analysis of the history of dietary intake through questionnaires and personal interviews of cancer patients and compared to age- and sex-matched normal subjects. From this comparison, the association between dietary agents and cancer incidence is determined. A prospective case-control study involves analysis of the intake from dietary records of participating normal subjects and then correlates the relationship of dietary agents with cancer incidence in subsequent years. From the dietary data obtained through questionnaires or records, the levels of intake of antioxidants such as vitamins A, C, and E, and beta-carotene, as well as fat and fiber, are estimated using appropriate nutritional computer software. Occasionally, the plasma or serum levels of antioxidants in participating individuals are measured. Using these epidemiologic experimental designs, several studies[73,92,93] concluded that diets rich in antioxidants but low in fat and high in fiber were associated with a reduced risk of cancer.[94] Consumption of fruits and vegetables and food items rich in carotene and lycopene may reduce the risk of ovarian cancer. A diet low in fat and high in fiber from fruits and vegetables and regular modest consumption of alcohol are associated with reduced risk of benign prostatic hyperplasia.[95] It has been estimated that eating fruits and vegetables can reduce the risk of cancer by about 30%.[96] Another epidemiologic study showed that eating one or more apples a day was associated with a reduced risk of colorectal cancer. This effect was not observed with other fruits.[97] When the risk of cancer was correlated with the level of individual antioxidants in the diet or blood, the inverse association between diet and cancer incidence became weak, nonexistent, or reversed. In a prospective study involving 295 cases and 295 control menopausal women, the plasma levels of retinol, retinyl palmitate, alpha-carotene, beta-carotene, beta-cryptoxanthin, lutein, lycopene, total carotenoids, alpha-tocopherol, and gamma-tocopherol were measured. The results showed that beta-carotene, lycopene, and total carotene were lower in cases compared to controls. The risk of developing breast cancer was inversely proportional to the level of beta-carotene in plasma.[98] In another similar prospective study, the level of alpha-carotene, but not other carotenoids, was inversely related to the risk of breast cancer.[99,100] In a review of six randomized clinical trials and 25 prospective studies, it was concluded that beta-carotene supplementation was not associated with a decreased risk of lung cancer.[101] In the VITamins And Lifestyle (VITAL) cohort study, it was found that long-term intake of beta-carotene, retinol, and lutein was associated with an increased risk of lung cancer.[102] In Brazilian women, dietary intake of folate, vitamin B_6, or vitamin B_{12} had no overall association with breast cancer risk; however, dietary intake of high levels of folate was associated with an increased risk of breast cancer in premenopausal women and MTR2756GG genotype.[103]

Increased intake of dietary flavonoids was associated with reduced risk of lung cancer;[104] however, another study reported no association between individual or multiple flavonoids intake and the risk of breast, ovarian, colorectal, lung, and endometrial cancer.[105] A recent study has reported that the intake of lycopene and lycopene products through diet were associated with a decreased risk of prostate cancer.[106] The Women's Health Initiative (WHI), involving 133,614 postmenopausal women, found that the dietary intake of antioxidants, carotenoids, and vitamin A were not associated with a reduction in ovarian cancer risk.[107] During 8 years of follow-up involving 56,007 French women, it was found that breast cancer risk was inversely associated with alpha-linolenic acid (ALA) intake from fruits, vegetables, and vegetable oils, but it was positively related to ALA intake from nut mixes and processed foods.[108] This suggests that other protective substances in the foods such as antioxidants may be necessary to observe the protective effect of ALA. It was also observed that the risk of breast cancer was inversely associated with intake of omega-3 in women having the highest levels of omega-6. Thus, epidemiologic studies with dietary intake of antioxidants, fat, fiber, and B-vitamins alone have produced conflicting results. This may be because each of these nutrient groups may contribute to a reduction in cancer incidence in different amounts; therefore, they cannot be analyzed separately to obtain consistent results. Also, the human diet contains agents that can produce opposite effects on cancer risk. For example, antioxidants and high fiber are considered cancer-protective substances in the diet, whereas diets rich in fat, meat, calories, and nitrites may increase the risk of cancer. Dietary antioxidants can also influence the metabolism of ingested or inhaled mutagens and carcinogens.[109,110] This may be the reason for the fact that diets rich in fruits and vegetables containing high levels of antioxidants, low in fat, and high in fiber consistently produced cancer-protective effects.

Experimental designs of any epidemiologic study have several inherent technical problems that make it difficult to arrive at any definitive conclusion. These limitations include the following:

- The collection of retrospective dietary history data by questionnaires is unreliable because it is based on the memory of the participants in the study and because quantitative and qualitative information on past daily dietary intake is impossible to recall with any degree of accuracy.
- Dietary records are difficult to express in a quantitative manner because the information on antioxidant intake is based on estimations rather than actual measurements. Thus, the determination of dietary intake of antioxidants, fat, and fiber on the basis of a diet history or a dietary record must be considered unreliable until validated by blood or tissue levels of these nutrients.

There are several other confounding factors associated with lifestyle and environment that could impact cancer incidence, in addition to the diet. It is very difficult to account for all of them in the data analysis. It should be emphasized that epidemiologic studies, despite the best experimental design and correct data interpretation, can only infer a direct or inverse relationship between single or multiple nutrients and the risk of cancer. The cause–effect relationship between micronutrient intake and cancer risk can only be established by a well-designed intervention trial in high-risk populations.

ANALYSIS OF INTERVENTION STUDIES ON ANTIOXIDANTS AND CANCER PREVENTION

High-risk populations such as heavy tobacco smokers, individuals with precancerous lesions, cancer patients in remission, and persons with a family history of cancer are very appropriate models that can be used to evaluate the efficacy of antioxidant supplements on the risk of cancer. However, the experimental design for a clinical trial must consider not only the statistical, bias, end point, and period of observation issues, but also the selection of appropriate types and numbers of micronutrients, as well as the dose, dose schedule, and internal oxidative environment of the participating subjects.

The clinical studies published thus far were sound with respect to selection of high-risk populations, number of patients, and statistical power analysis, but they did not take into consideration the above scientific rationale with respect to antioxidants. The intervention study rarely utilized endogenous antioxidants, which resulted in inconsistent results varying from no effect, to beneficial effects, to harmful effects. For example, some studies used only one antioxidant (mostly synthetic form), while others used more than one antioxidant (only the dietary form). The dose range of antioxidants and the criteria of end points varied markedly from one study to another. All studies utilized a once-a-day dose schedule. The inconsistent results obtained from the intervention studies have created much misinformation and confusion in the minds of health providers and the public alike; as a consequence, antioxidants are being misused by the public and not recommended by most physicians for cancer prevention.

The extrapolation of existing clinical trial models to determine the efficacy of novel drugs that affect specific molecular targets involved in the etiology of a particular disease should not be applied to the clinical trials in which the efficacy of micronutrients to reduce the risk of cancer is determined. Any efforts to do so may produce inconsistent results. Unfortunately, most clinical trials have utilized the experimental design of drugs that is based on the concept of the single drug–single target effect.

CANCER RISK IN HEAVY TOBACCO SMOKERS AFTER TREATMENT WITH A SINGLE DIETARY ANTIOXIDANT

Heavy tobacco smokers represent an excellent model of a high-risk population in which the efficacy of micronutrients to reduce the risk of cancer can be tested by a well-designed clinical trial. In a large randomized, double-blind, placebo-controlled clinical trial, supplementation with synthetic beta-carotene at a dose of 20 mg/day increased the incidence of lung cancer, prostate cancer, and stomach cancer among male heavy tobacco smokers.[111–113] Heavy tobacco smokers are known to have high internal oxidative environments; therefore, this increase in lung cancer incidence could have been predicted because beta-carotene in the high internal oxidative environments of heavy smokers would be oxidized and then act as a pro-oxidant rather than as an antioxidant. This was further confirmed by the fact that the same dose of beta-carotene did not affect the incidence of cancer in normal populations who have lower internal oxidative environments than the heavy tobacco smokers.[114]

Supplementation with NAC reduced certain biomarkers associated with lung cancer in smokers,[115] but it remains uncertain whether NAC supplementation alone can affect the incidence of lung cancer. In a clinical study involving 2592 patients (60% head and neck cancer and 40% lung cancer), a

2-year supplementation with vitamin A (retinyl palmitate, 300,000 IU daily for 1 year, and 150,000 IU daily for the following year) and NAC (600 mg daily for 2 years) alone or in combination produced no benefit with respect to secondary primary tumors.[116] This suggested that using one or two antioxidants was not sufficient to reduce the risk of cancer. This study utilized an unusually high dose of vitamin A that could be toxic after long-term consumption. Even the dose of NAC in this study is high. These clinical studies have failed to consider the biology of antioxidants and the internal oxidative environment of the high-risk populations.

OTHER CANCER RISKS AFTER TREATMENT WITH A SINGLE DIETARY ANTIOXIDANT

Beta-carotene supplementation in patients with a low dietary intake of beta-carotene reduced prostate cancer.[117] High doses of beta-carotene caused regression of leukoplakia (precancerous lesions in the mouth).[118,119]

Supplementation with alpha-tocopherol (50 mg/day) reduced prostate cancer and colorectal cancer, but increased the incidence of stomach cancer.[111] Supplementation with vitamin E (400 IU/day) produced no effect on the prostate-specific antigen (PSA) levels;[120] however, high serum levels of vitamin E were associated with a reduced prostate cancer incidence.[121–123] In another study, supplementation with vitamin E 400 IU/day was associated with a reduced risk of prostate cancer in tobacco smokers, whereas beta-carotene supplementation was associated with a reduced risk of this cancer only in those smokers who have low levels of beta-carotene.[117] Consumption of vitamin E alone increased the incidence of secondary primary cancer or recurrence of the initial tumor after cancer therapy.[124] The causal relationship between vitamin E supplementation and increased mortality as suggested earlier[125] has been contradicted by another statistical analysis.[126] Elevated levels of benzo(a)pyrene (B(a)P)–DNA adducts have been associated with a threefold increase in the risk of lung cancer in heavy tobacco smokers,[127] but supplementation with DL-alpha tocopherol (400 IU/day) and vitamin C (500 mg/day) did not reduce the level of B(a)P–DNA adducts in men, although it did reduce them in women.[127] In a recent double-blind, placebo-controlled $2 \times 2 \times 2$ factorial trial of vitamin C (500 mg/day of ascorbic acid), a natural source of vitamin E (600 IU of alpha-tocopherol, every other day), and beta-carotene (50 mg, every other day), involving 7627 women free of cancer, it was found that supplementation with individual vitamin C, vitamin E, or beta-carotene had no impact on cancer incidence or cancer mortality during a follow-up period of 9.4 years.[128] Using the population of the Alpha-Tocopherol, Beta-Carotene Cancer Prevention Study on male Finnish smokers, it was revealed that higher serum alpha-tocopherol concentrations was associated with a reduced risk of pancreatic cancer.[129]

Supplementation with vitamin A at a dose of 300,000 IU/day for 12 months produces an 11% reduction in recurrence of primary non-small-cell lung carcinoma,[130] but this high dose cannot be given for a prolonged period because of toxicity. Retinoids also caused regression of oral leukoplakia and other cancers.[131]

The results obtained from supplementation with single antioxidants should not be extrapolated to the effect of the same antioxidant present in multiple antioxidant preparations. Nevertheless, many scientists, researchers, and physicians and some press publications are promoting the idea that supplementation with antioxidants can be deleterious to your health, and should not be taken for cancer prevention. Such misleading promotions have no scientific merit.

The use of a single antioxidant in high-risk populations such as heavy tobacco smokers to reduce the risk of cancer has no scientific basis for the following reasons: (1) an individual antioxidant in a high oxidative environment acts as a pro-oxidant because antioxidants are easily oxidized; and (2) heavy tobacco smokers have a very high internal oxidative environment due to inhalation of smoke and depletion of antioxidant levels. Therefore, the use of a single antioxidant in a high-risk population is expected to increase the risk of cancer. The natural forms of vitamin E and beta-carotene are more effective than their synthetic counterparts. For example, natural beta-carotene reduced radiation-induced transformation, but the synthetic beta-carotene did not.[70] Cells accumulated more of the natural form of vitamin E than the synthetic form,[132] and alpha-TS is now considered the most effective form of vitamin E.[133] The use of one or more dietary antioxidants alone may not be sufficient for developing an effective cancer prevention strategy. Endogenous antioxidants such as glutathione, alpha-lipoic acid, N-acetyl cysteine (a glutathione-elevating agent), L-carnitine, and coenzyme Q_{10} represent important natural intracellular antioxidants that have diverse biological actions. Their levels could be reduced due to an increased oxidative environment in the cells. Therefore, the addition of these antioxidants in addition to dietary antioxidants is essential for an optimal effect on the proposed cancer prevention strategy.

The dose schedule is also very important to enhance the efficacy of multiple micronutrients in reducing the risk of cancer. Taking antioxidants once a day may create huge fluctuations in the levels of antioxidants in the body. This is because the biological half-lives (time needed to remove antioxidants from the body by 50%) of antioxidants markedly vary, depending upon their lipid or water solubility, creating a high degree of fluctuation in tissue antioxidant levels. A marked alteration in the expression of gene profiles occurs by different levels of vitamin E succinate;[134] therefore, taking antioxidants once a day can create genetic stress in the cells that may compromise the efficacy of the antioxidant supplementation after long-term consumption. These factors were not taken into consideration while designing antioxidant trials in high-risk populations, resulting in inconsistent results.

CANCER RISK AFTER TREATMENT WITH MULTIPLE DIETARY ANTIOXIDANTS

Supplementation with multiple dietary antioxidants without endogenous antioxidants (alpha-lipoic acid, NAC, a glutathione-elevating agent, coenzyme Q_{10}, and L-carnitine) may produce inconsistent results in high-risk populations. These studies are described below. The administration of multiple dietary antioxidants vitamin A (40,000 IU/day), vitamin C (2000 mg/day), vitamin E (400 IU/day), zinc (90 mg/day), and vitamin B_6 (100 mg/day), in combination with the BCG (Bacilli bilie de Calmette–Guerin) vaccine, caused a 50% reduction in the incidence of recurrence of bladder cancer in 5 years, compared to control patients who received multiple vitamins containing RDA levels of nutrients and BCG.[135]

Supplementation with antioxidants (vitamin A, 30,000 IU/day; vitamin C, 1000 mg/day; vitamin E, 70 mg/day) reduced the incidence of recurrence of colon polyps from 36% to 6%;[136] however, daily consumption of synthetic beta-carotene (25 mg), vitamin C (1000 mg), and vitamin E (400 mg) failed to show any beneficial effects on the recurrence of colon polyps.[137] Daily administration of vitamin C (400 mg) and DL-alpha tocopherol also failed to reduce the incidence of recurrence of colon polyps,[138] In another study, daily supplementation with vitamin C (4000 mg) and vitamin E (400 mg) failed to reduce the risk of colon polyps, but when they were combined with a high-fiber diet (more than 12 g/day) there was a significant reduction in the incidence of recurrence of polyps.[139] This study indicated the importance of a high-fiber diet in combination with antioxidants in cancer prevention.

In Linxian General Population Nutrition Interventional Trial, a preparation of multiple dietary antioxidants (beta-carotene, vitamin E, and selenium at doses two to three times that of the U.S. RDA) reduced mortality by 10% and cancer incidence by 13%.[140] The beneficial effects of this supplementation on mortality were still evident up to 10 years after the cessation of supplementation, and were consistently greater in younger participants.[141]

The combination of vitamins A, C, and E, omega-3 fatty acids, and folic acid significantly reduced recurrence of adenoma in patients after polypectomy.[142] In a randomized placebo-controlled trial involving 80 untreated patients with prostate cancer, daily supplementation with vitamin E, selenium, vitamin C, and coenzyme Q_{10} did not affect serum levels of PSA.[143] In a randomized, placebo-controlled trial referred to as SELECT involving 35,553 healthy men from 427 participating sites in the United States, Canada, and Puerto Rico with a follow-up period of a minimum of 7 years and a maximum of 12 years, it was observed that selenium (200 µg/day) or vitamin E (400 IU/day), alone or in combination, did not reduce the risk of prostate cancer.[78]

From the intervention studies discussed above, it appears that supplementation with dietary antioxidants alone may not be sufficient to produce an optimal and consistent effect on reducing the risk of cancer. Inclusion of endogenous antioxidants may be necessary in any experimental design to test the efficacy of antioxidants in cancer prevention. In recent years, there have been trends to perform meta-analysis of published data in which far-reaching conclusions have been made. Since the total number of participating subjects in such analyses becomes huge, numbering in the hundreds of thousands, the conclusions appear impressive and definitive. However, if the meta-analysis is performed on publications that have flawed experimental design, the conclusions will be the same as were made in the initial publications. The publications of such meta-analyses are of no scientific value except that they add to the existing misinformation about the value of micronutrients in cancer prevention.

CANCER RISK AFTER TREATMENT WITH VITAMIN D AND CALCIUM

In recent years, the role of vitamin D alone or in combination with calcium has been evaluated, often yielding inconsistent results. The results show that vitamin D at a dose of 1000 IU/day reduced colorectal cancer.[144,145] In another study, vitamin D at a dose of 400 IU/day and calcium at a dose of 1000 mg/day produced no effect on colorectal cancer.[146] Administration of vitamin D at a dose of 400 IU/day and calcium at a dose of 1000 mg/day reduced colorectal cancer but, in combination with estrogen, increased the risk of this cancer.[147] In view of the fact that estrogen is known to have tumor-promoting effects, and that vitamin D has no effect on the activity of estrogen, the above increase in cancer incidence is expected. This could have been avoided by the addition of antioxidants that are known to reduce the effect of tumor promoters. In a recent review of several clinical studies, it was concluded that supplementation with elemental calcium may have a modest effect in reducing the risk of colorectal cancer; however, this approach was not recommended for reducing the risk of colorectal cancer in the general population.[148] Supplementation with elemental calcium at 1000 mg/day and vitamin D at 400 IU/day did not reduce the risk of breast cancer.[149] However, in another study, dietary intake of calcium was modestly associated with a reduced risk of breast cancer in postmenopausal women.[94,150] In the Wheat Bran Fiber Trial, a higher intake of calcium (1068 vs. 690 mg/day) decreased the risk of recurrence of colorectal adenoma by about 45%.[151] A possible effect of this treatment was also noted in women with the BRCA mutation. It has been reported that calcium and vitamin D supplementation together reduce the recurrence of colorectal adenoma.[152] The reason for these inconsistencies may be that the contribution of calcium alone, or with vitamin D, to cancer formation may be small, and therefore, additional micronutrients such as antioxidants and B-vitamins may be necessary to produce consistent results. I propose adding vitamin D and calcium into multiple micronutrient preparations to be used in the proposed cancer prevention strategy in high-risk populations.

CANCER RISK AFTER TREATMENT WITH FOLATE AND B-VITAMINS

A diet rich in folate and vitamins B_6 and B_{12} was associated with a reduced risk of breast cancer and colorectal cancer,[153–157] but had no association with pancreatic cancer. However, supplementation with folic acid alone did not reduce the incidence of colorectal adenoma, and may possibly increase the risk.[158] In other studies,[158,159] consumption of folate did not reduce the incidence of colorectal cancer. In a randomized double-blind, placebo-controlled, clinical trial involving 137 patients with polypectomy, supplementation with 5 mg folate daily reduced the recurrence of colonic adenomas.[160] Dietary intake of high amounts of folate and vitamin B_{12} were independently associated with a decreased risk of breast cancer, particularly in postmenopausal women. There was no association between intake of vitamin B_6 and breast cancer.[156] In a recent epidemiologic study, it was found that there may be a nonlinear relationship between folate status and the risk of all cancer mortality, and thus persons with low serum levels of folate may be at risk of cancer.[161] This inconsistency between diet and supplement may be because the diet may also be rich in antioxidants in addition to B-vitamins and folate; therefore, clinical studies with folate and B-vitamins alone are expected to yield different results. I propose combining B-vitamins and folate with multiple micronutrients for the proposed cancer prevention strategy.

Cancer Risk after Treatment with Fat and Fiber

The average American diet contains about 34.1% of calories from fat. Animal experiments and human epidemiologic studies have revealed that this level of fat consumption may increase the risk of cancer. The mechanisms of action of a high-fat diet on carcinogenesis are not well understood, except that high levels of fat can act as a tumor promoter. A high-fat diet may also increase the blood levels of PGs that have been implicated in increasing the risk of cancer. In females, a high-fat, low-fiber, Western-style diet appears to be associated with increased levels of plasma and urinary estrogen, which is significant as this hormone is known to act as a tumor promoter. An intervention study (the WHI Dietary Modification Trial), in which post menopausal women received a low-fat (40% calories from fat) or high-fat (60% calories from fat) diet, showed that a low-fat diet did not reduce the risk of colorectal cancer during the 8.1-year follow-up period.[162] I am not sure if a diet in which the fat content represents 40% should be considered a low-fat diet. Also, the protective effect of a low-fat diet alone may be minor; therefore, the cancer protective effect of low-fat diet alone cannot be assessed in any cancer prevention trial.

The detailed references for this section have been provided in a review.[2] Average American diets are also low in fiber. Human epidemiologic studies revealed a strong inverse relationship between fiber intake and cancer incidence. High fiber would bind increased amounts of intestinal cholesterol, bile acids, mutagens, and carcinogens that are formed during digestion and eliminate them with the feces. This would then reduce the intestinal absorption and exposure time of the intestinal cells to these potentially carcinogenic substances. It was assumed that only cancer of the intestinal tract would be reduced by this mechanism of action of a high-fiber diet. However, the consumption of a high-fiber diet reduced the recurrence of breast cancer. Therefore, additional mechanisms of cancer protection by a high-fiber diet may exist. Indeed, it has been reported that high fiber intake can generate millimolar levels of butyric acid, a 4-carbon fatty acid, with the help of endogenous bacteria that are present in the colon. Butyric acid, being a small fatty acid, is absorbed rapidly. Several studies have reported that butyrate and its analog (phenyl butyrate) have exhibited strong anticancer properties against a variety of tumors in vitro and in vivo. Thus, a high-fiber diet may provide protection not only against colon cancer but also against other tumors. Therefore, the inclusion of a low-fat, high-fiber diet is essential for the proposed cancer prevention strategy.

In the polyp prevention trial, dietary intervention and supplementation, along with reduced fat intake and increased consumption of fruits, vegetables, and fiber, produced no effect on PSA or on the incidence of prostate cancer in normal men.[163] Similarly, adopting a diet low in fat (20% of total calories) and high in fiber (18 g per 1000 kcal) and fruits and vegetables (3.5 serving per 1000 kcal) did not influence the risk of recurrence of colorectal adenomas.[164] In contrast to the above observation, another study reported that vitamin A from food, with or without supplementation, and alpha-carotene from food may protect against recurrence of tumors in nonsmokers and nondrinkers.[165] The current dietary guidelines (fruits, vegetables, whole grains, low-fat dairy, and lean meat) are associated with decreased risk of mortality from all causes.[166] A dietary supplement (13.5 vs. 2 g/day) with wheat-bran fiber did not protect against recurrence of colorectal adenomas.[167] Testing the effect of a high fiber diet alone in which the difference between the control and experimental groups is small may not yield any significant reduction in cancer incidence because the effect of an additional 10 g of fiber alone on the risk of cancer may be too small to be detected. Such an interventional trial does not appear to have any scientific rationale.

In a multi-institutional, randomized, controlled trial involving 3088 women previously treated for early-stage breast cancer, supplementation with a diet high in vegetables, fruits, and fiber and low in fat did not reduce additional breast cancer events or mortality during a 7.3-year follow-up period.[168] The lack of additional micronutrients such as dietary and endogenous antioxidants, B-vitamins, and calcium with vitamin D may have contributed to the failure of detecting protective effects of the high-fiber, low-fat diet in the above study.

CANCER RISK AFTER TREATMENT WITH NSAIDS

Aspirin and indomethacin reduce the risk of cancer in animal models.[169] The use of an NSAID was associated with a small decrease in lung cancer incidence,[170] and other cancers in humans.[171] In a recent study, it was demonstrated that the use of NSAIDs for a shorter period may be more effective in reducing the risk of nonmelanoma skin cancer (squamous-cell carcinoma and basal-cell carcinoma).[172] Since chronic or recurrent prostate inflammation and oxidative stress may be involved in the development of prostate cancer, it has been suggested that a combination of aspirin and antioxidants may be useful in reducing the risk of prostate cancer.[173] These studies have revealed that addition of NSAIDs could be useful in reducing the risk of cancer. Therefore, the addition of low-dose aspirin to multiple micronutrients may be necessary for the proposed cancer prevention strategy in high-risk populations.

PROPOSED CANCER PREVENTION STRATEGIES

To develop a rational cancer prevention strategy, it is essential to know about agents that can increase the risk of cancer and those that can reduce the risk of cancer. Cancer research of the last several decades has identified agents in the environment, diet, and lifestyle that can increase the risk of cancer and agents in the diet that can reduce the risk of cancer. These issues have been reviewed in several publications and books.[2] Cancer-causing agents (carcinogens) can be divided into two categories: tumor initiators and tumor promoters. Tumor initiators are agents that by themselves are sufficient to cause cancer; whereas, tumor promoters by themselves may not cause cancer, but they help tumor initiators to induce cancer at low doses that may not be sufficient normally to cause cancer. Tumor promoters may enhance the incidence of tumor initiator–induced cancer. Some examples of tumor initiators include x-rays, gamma-rays, ultraviolet radiation, nitrosamines and benzo(*a*)pyrene, dioxin, asbestos, pesticides, ozone, tobacco smoking, HPV, and familial gene defects. Some examples of tumor promoters include high levels of estrogen, phorbol esters, and excessive consumption of alcohol, caffeine, and a high-fat diet. Dietary factors that can reduce the risk of cancer include antioxidants, some B-vitamins, selenium, and a low-fat, high-fiber diet.

Cancer prevention strategies can be developed separately for three different populations, cancer-free normal individuals of all ages and gender, cancer-free persons at high risk of developing cancer such as heavy smokers, and cancer survivors with no sign of detectable cancer. The latter population has an increased risk of recurrence of initial tumors or development of new primary tumors induced by cancer treatment agents. The recommendations for reducing the exposure to potential carcinogens and tumor promoters, increasing the intake of a diet rich in fruits and vegetables, and adopting a healthy lifestyle are the same for all three populations; however, the recommendations of micronutrient supplements are different with respect to doses and types of antioxidants, depending upon the population type.

RECOMMENDATIONS FOR CANCER-FREE NORMAL INDIVIDUALS

Reducing exposure to potential carcinogens from diet, environment, and lifestyle appear to be the most effective strategy for reducing the risk of cancer in humans; however, it is the most difficult strategy to implement. In some cases, it is counterproductive, if totally eliminated, and in others, it may be difficult to achieve. For example, diagnostic x-rays are commonly used to detect and diagnose disease earlier; therefore, they should not be avoided. Avoiding ultraviolet radiation from sun exposure appears to be the easiest thing to do to reduce the risk of skin cancer, but the beaches in summer are full of sun bathers in spite of repeated warnings. Because of the addictive nature of tobacco smoking, there has been no significant change in the number of smokers in the United States, in spite of massive education programs and state and federal laws prohibiting smoking in public places. It is difficult to implement the environmental, lifestyle-related, and genetic factors that contribute to cancer risk. Nevertheless, avoiding exposure to potential carcinogens as much as possible must be a part of the proposed cancer prevention strategy.

Dietary habits are difficult to alter in humans. Human diets contain both cancer-protective substances and cancer-causing agents (mutagens and carcinogens).[54] Most of the mutagenic and carcinogenic substances that are present in the diet are naturally occurring; however, small amounts of them have been introduced into the diet by the use of pesticides in agriculture production. These issues are usually beyond our control (the exception being exclusive consumption of certified organic produce). Mutagens (compounds that alter genetic activity) are formed during cooking. Browning of vegetables or meat during cooking is an indication of the formation of mutagens. All mutations do not increase the risk of cancer, but all cancers require mutations. Flame-broiled fatty meat, generally preferred by consumers, contains much higher levels of carcinogens such as benzo(*a*)pyrene than found in oven-cooked meat. The dietary recommendations of eating fresh fruits and vegetables and a low-fat, high-fiber diet are difficult to implement consistently over a long period because human behaviors are not easily changed. Nevertheless, the dietary recommendations must be part of a proposed cancer preventive strategy for this population.

Supplementation with multiple micronutrients must be included in a proposed cancer preventive strategy, in addition to recommendations of avoiding exposure to potential carcinogens and modifications in the diet and lifestyle. Micronutrient formulations for cancer prevention must include dietary (vitamins A, C, and E, natural mixed carotenoids, and selenium) and endogenous antioxidants (alpha-lipoic acid, NAC, a glutathione-elevating agent, L-carnitine, and coenzyme Q_{10}), vitamin D and elemental calcium, B-vitamins, and zinc at appropriate doses. The proposed micronutrient preparation should not contain iron, copper, manganese, or heavy metals. However, the doses of micronutrients for a normal population will be different, depending upon age and gender. For example, a supplement for young persons between the ages of 5 and 17 years would not contain endogenous antioxidants, because they maintain optimal capacity of making them. Endogenous antioxidants will be included for persons of age 18 years and older. Calcium and vitamin D supplementation at high doses would be included for women after the age of 35 years.

RECOMMENDATIONS FOR CANCER-FREE HIGH-RISK INDIVIDUALS

High-risk individuals include heavy tobacco smokers and persons with a family history of cancer. Supplementations for these individuals will have a micronutrient preparation similar to that for persons 18 years or older, except that higher doses of dietary and endogenous antioxidants will be included. Smokers can start the supplementation at any time; however, individuals with a family history of cancer may follow the time schedule beginning at the age of 5 years. It has been presumed that the genetic basis of cancer cannot be delayed or prevented; therefore, such individuals wait until the tumor appears. A recent study on the effect of a mixture of dietary and endogenous antioxidants on proton radiation-induced cancer in *Drosophila melanogaster* suggests that antioxidants can reduce the incidence of the genetic basis of cancer. For example, female flies carrying mutant HOP (TUM-1) become very sensitive to developing a leukemia-like cancer. Exposure to proton radiation markedly enhanced the incidence of this cancer. Supplementation with the antioxidant mixture before and after irradiation completely blocked radiation-induced cancer (in collaboration with Dr. Sharmila Bhattacharya of NASA at Moffat Field, CA). This result obtained from fruit flies cannot be extrapolated to humans, but this study at least suggests that antioxidants have the potential to reduce the risk or delay the appearance of tumors in individuals with a family history of cancer.

Recommendations for Cancer Survivors

An increased number of cancer patients are surviving because of the advancements in cancer therapy (surgery, chemotherapy, and radiation therapy). However, they exhibit short-term and long-term adverse health effects induced by the cancer treatment agents. Short-term effects include dementia, referred to as *chemo brain*, fatigue, peripheral neuropathy, and increased susceptibility to infection because of impaired immune function. Some of these symptoms can last for a long time. Long-term adverse health effects include recurrence of initial primary tumors and development of secondary new tumors induced by the cancer treatment agents. The proposed micronutrient formulation for this high-risk population would be the same as that for other high-risk populations. This formulation can be started a week after completion of standard therapy.

Diet and Lifestyle Recommendations for Individuals of High-Risk Populations

In addition to supplementation with multiple micronutrients, changes in diet and lifestyle are very important for an optimal effect on cancer prevention. Dietary recommendations include daily consumption of a low-fat, high-fiber diet with plenty of fresh fruits and vegetables, avoiding excessive amounts of protein, carbohydrates, or calories, restricting intake of nitrite-rich cured meat, charcoal-broiled or smoked meat or fish, caffeine-containing beverages (cold or hot), and pickled fruits and vegetables.

Lifestyle-related recommendations include stopping smoking and chewing tobacco, avoiding secondhand smoke, and overexposure to sun and UV light for tanning, avoiding hyperbaric therapy for energy, restricting intake of alcohol, reducing stress by vacation, yoga, or meditation, and performing moderate exercise three to five times a week.

RATIONALE FOR USING MULTIPLE MICRONUTRIENTS IN PROPOSED CANCER PREVENTIVE STRATEGY

Multiple micronutrients including dietary and endogenous antioxidants are recommended because many different types of free radicals are produced and each antioxidant has a different affinity for each of these free radicals, depending upon the cellular environment. They are distributed differently in organs and within the same cells. The gradient of oxygen pressure varies within the cell and tissues. Vitamin E was more effective as a quencher of free radicals in reduced oxygen pressure, whereas vitamins C and A were more effective in higher oxygen pressures.[174] Vitamin C is necessary to protect cellular components in aqueous environments, whereas carotenoids, and vitamins A and E protect cellular components in nonaqueous environments. Vitamin C also plays an important role in maintaining cellular levels of vitamin E by recycling the vitamin E radical (oxidized) to the reduced (antioxidant) form.[175] Also, the DNA damage produced by oxidized vitamin C can be ameliorated by vitamin E. The form and type of vitamin E used in micronutrient preparations are also important to improve beneficial effects. It is known that various organs of rats selectively accumulate the natural form of vitamin E.[132] It has been established that alpha-TS is the most effective form of the vitamin E.[133,176] We have reported that oral ingestion of alpha-TS (800 IU/day) for more than 6 months in humans increased plasma levels of not only alpha-tocopherol, but also of alpha-TS, suggesting that alpha alpha-TS can be absorbed from the intestinal tract without hydrolysis to alpha-tocopherol, provided that the pool of alpha-tocopherol in the body has become saturated.[133,176] Selenium, a cofactor of glutathione peroxidase, acts as an antioxidant. Therefore, selenium supplementation, together with other dietary and endogenous antioxidants, is also essential.

Glutathione, one of the endogenously made compounds, represents a potent intracellular protective agent against oxidative damage. It catabolizes H_2O_2 and anions and is very effective (in the presence of glutathione peroxidase) in quenching peroxynitrite.[177] Therefore, increasing the intracellular levels of glutathione is essential for the protection of various organelles within the cells. An oral supplementation with glutathione failed to significantly increase plasma levels of glutathione in human subjects,[178] suggesting that this tripeptide is completely hydrolyzed in the gastrointestinal tract. NAC and alpha-lipoic acid increase the intracellular levels of glutathione and, therefore, they can be used in combination with dietary antioxidants. Coenzyme Q_{10} is needed by the mitochondria to generate energy. It also scavenges peroxy radicals faster than alpha-tocopherol,[179] and, like vitamin C, can regenerate vitamin E in a redox cycle.[180]

In addition to those scientific rationales, clinical trials primarily with one dietary antioxidant, B-vitamins, or elemental calcium, with or without vitamin D, have produced inconsistent results. It has been shown that a single antioxidant such as vitamin C can stimulate the growth of some cancer cells in culture,[2] and when it is oxidized, it can act as a free radical.

UNIQUE FEATURES OF PROPOSED MICRONUTRIENT FORMULATION

The proposed micronutrient formulations do not contain iron, copper, or manganese, because they are known to combine with vitamin C and produce free radicals that could reduce optimal effects of the micronutrient preparation. These trace minerals in the presence of antioxidants are absorbed more efficiently and that could increase the body stores of free forms of these minerals. The increased body stores of free iron or copper have been associated with the enhanced risk of most chronic human diseases including cancer.

All proposed micronutrient preparations should contain both vitamin A and natural mixed carotenoids (90% represent beta-carotene). This is because beta-carotene, in addition to acting as a precursor of vitamin A, performs unique functions that cannot be produced by vitamin A, and vice versa. For example, beta-carotene increases the expression of the connexin gene, which codes for a gap junction protein that holds two normal cells together,[181] whereas vitamin A does not produce such an effect. Vitamin A produces differentiation in normal and cancer cells, but beta-carotene does not.[131,182] Beta-carotene was more effective in quenching oxygen radicals than most other antioxidants.[75] Thus, the addition of both vitamin A and beta-carotene may enhance the efficacy of micronutrient supplementation in cancer prevention. All micronutrient formulations should contain two forms of vitamin E, D-alpha tocopheryl acetate and D-alpha-TS. Alpha-TS is now considered the most effective form of vitamin E.[133] Alpha-TS is more soluble than alpha tocopherol and enters the cells easily where it is converted to alpha-tocopherol and thus, provides intracellular protection against oxidative damage. Alpha-TS can also produce some unique biological effects that cannot be produced by alpha-tocopherol. Therefore, to increase the efficacy of vitamin E, the addition of both forms of vitamin E is essential. The proposed micronutrient preparation does not contain herbs or herbal antioxidants. This is because certain herbs may interact with the prescription and over-the-counter drugs in an adverse manner, and that herbal antioxidants do not produce any unique biological effects that cannot be produced by antioxidants present in the proposed multiple micronutrients preparation.

The recommended micronutrient supplements should be taken orally and divided into two doses, half in the morning and the other half in the evening with a meal. This is because the biological half-lives of micronutrients are highly variable, which can create high levels of fluctuation in the tissue levels of micronutrients. A twofold difference in the levels of certain micronutrients such as alpha-TS can cause a marked difference in the expression of gene profiles (our unpublished data). To maintain relatively consistent levels of micronutrients in the body, the proposed micronutrients should be taken twice a day.

A well-designed clinical trial using the proposed preventive strategy should be initiated in a high-risk, cancer-free population, as well as in cancer survivors. Meanwhile, individuals of high-risk populations may like to adopt the proposed cancer prevention strategy in consultation with their physicians.

TOXICITY OF MICRONUTRIENTS

References listed in this section have been described in a review.[183] Antioxidants at doses higher than those that are recommended for the proposed micronutrient preparations have been consumed by the U.S. population for decades without reported toxicity. However, they could be harmful for some individuals at certain high doses when consumed daily for a long period. For example, vitamin A at doses of 10,000 IU or more can cause birth defects in pregnant women, and beta-carotene can produce bronzing of the skin at doses of 50 mg or more. The discoloration is reversible on discontinuation. Vitamin C as ascorbic acid at high doses, 10 g or more, can cause diarrhea in some individuals Vitamin E at doses of 2000 IU or more can induce clotting defects after long-term consumption and vitamin B_6 at high doses may produce peripheral neuropathy. Selenium at doses of 400 µg or more can cause skin and liver toxicity after long-term consumption. Coenzyme Q_{10} has no known toxicity, and recommended daily doses are from 30 to 400 mg. NAC doses of 250–1500 mg and alpha-lipoic acid doses of 600 mg are used in humans without toxicity. All ingredients present in the proposed micronutrient preparations are safe and come under the category of "Food Supplement," therefore, they do not require FDA approval for their use.

CONCLUSIONS

Cancer incidence in the U.S. population appears to be on the rise. There is no effective cancer preventive strategy that can easily be implemented. The recommendations of modifications in the diet and lifestyle may not be sufficient. Supplementation with a multiple micronutrient preparation, including dietary and endogenous antioxidants, together with diet and lifestyle modifications may be necessary for reducing the risk of cancer in high-risk populations. The clinical studies published thus far have utilized primarily one dietary antioxidants, sometimes two, and occasionally three to four dietary antioxidants alone, folate, with or without vitamin B_6, and vitamin B_{12} alone, elemental calcium with or without vitamin D alone, and fat and fiber, individually or in combination. The results of these studies have been inconsistent, and varied from beneficial effects, to no effect, or to harmful effects. Therefore, there should be a change in the paradigm of clinical trials while using micronutrients for cancer prevention studies. I have proposed a new paradigm in which appropriately prepared multiple micronutrient preparations containing dietary and endogenous antioxidants, B-vitamins, elemental calcium with vitamin D, but no iron, copper, manganese, or heavy metals, together with modifications in diet and lifestyle are utilized. The twice-a-day dose schedule is recommended to maintain relatively steady levels of tissue micronutrient levels.

The proposed micronutrient cancer preventive strategy has a sound mechanistic basis for reducing the risk of cancer. This strategy can be initiated at any time and at any age in the cancer-free normal population and in populations at high risk for developing new cancers (heavy tobacco smokers and individuals with a family history of cancer). However, this proposed micronutrient prevention strategy in cancer survivors can be started only after completion of standard cancer therapy. The efficacy of the proposed cancer prevention strategy should be tested in high-risk populations by a well-designed clinical trial. Meanwhile, individuals belonging to the high-risk populations may like to adopt the proposed cancer prevention strategy in consultation with their physicians.

REFERENCES

1. Duesberg, P. H., and J. R. Schwartz. 1992. Latent viruses and mutated oncogenes: No evidence for pathogenicity. *Prog Nucleic Acid Res Mol Biol* 43: 135–204.
2. Prasad, K. N., W. Cole, and P. Hovland. 1998. Cancer prevention studies: Past, present, and future directions. *Nutrition* 14 (2): 197–210; discussion 237–238.
3. Prasad, K. N., E. Carvalho, J. Edwards-Prasad, F. G. La Rosa, R. Kumar, and S. Kumar. 1994. Establishment and characterization of immortalized cell lines from rat parotid glands. *In Vitro Cell Dev Biol Anim* 30A (5): 321–328.

4. Zhai, R., G. Liu, K. Asomaning, L. Su, M. H. Kulke, R. S. Heist, N. S. Nishioka, T. J. Lynch, J. C. Wain, X. Lin, and D. C. Christiani. 2008. Genetic polymorphisms of VEGF, interactions with cigarette smoking exposure and esophageal adenocarcinoma risk. *Carcinogenesis* 29 (12): 2330–2334.
5. Xu, T., Y. Zhu, Q. K. Wei, Y. Yuan, F. Zhou, Y. Y. Ge, J. R. Yang, H. Su, and S. M. Zhuang. 2008. A functional polymorphism in the *miR-146a* gene is associated with the risk for hepatocellular carcinoma. *Carcinogenesis* 29 (11): 2126–2131.
6. Zhang, Z., S. Wang, M. Wang, N. Tong, and G. Fu. 2008. Genetic variants in RUNX3 and risk of bladder cancer: A haplotype-based analysis. *Carcinogenesis* 29 (10): 1973–1978.
7. Boutwell, R. 1983. Biology and biochemistry of two-steps carcinogenesis. In *Modulation and Mediation of Cancer by Vitamins*, ed. F. J. Meyskens and K. N. Prasad, 2. Basel: Karger.
8. La Rosa, F. G., F. S. Adams, G. E. Krause, A. D. Meyers, J. Edwards-Prasad, R. Kumar, C. R. Freed, and K. N. Prasad. 1997. Inhibition of proliferation and expression of T-antigen in SV40 large T-antigen gene–induced immortalized cells following transplantations. *Cancer Lett* 113 (1–2): 55–60.
9. Cullmann, C., K. Hoppe-Seyler, S. Dymalla, C. Lohrey, M. Scheffner, M. Durst, and F. Hoppe-Seyler. 2009. Oncogenic human papillomaviruses block expression of the B-cell translocation gene-2 (BTG2) tumor suppressor gene. *Int J Cancer*.
10. DiPaolo, J. A., N. C. Popescu, L. Alvarez, and C. D. Woodworth. 1993. Cellular and molecular alterations in human epithelial cells transformed by recombinant human papillomavirus DNA. *Crit Rev Oncog* 4 (4): 337–360.
11. Franceschi, S., N. Munoz, X. F. Bosch, P. J. Snijders, and J. M. Walboomers. 1996. Human papillomavirus and cancers of the upper aerodigestive tract: A review of epidemiological and experimental evidence. *Cancer Epidemiol Biomarkers Prev* 5 (7): 567–575.
12. Chocolatewala, N. M., and P. Chaturvedi. 2009. Role of human papilloma virus in the oral carcinogenesis: An Indian perspective. *J Cancer Res Ther* 5 (2): 71–77.
13. Szostek, S., B. Zawilinska, J. Kopec, and M. Kosz-Vnenchak. 2009. Herpesviruses as possible cofactors in HPV-16–related oncogenesis, *Acta Biochim Pol* 56: 337–342.
14. Jacob, J. R., and B. C. Tennant. 1996. Transformation of immortalized woodchuck hepatic cell lines with the c-Ha-*ras* proto-oncogene. *Carcinogenesis* 17 (4): 631–636.
15. Li, Y., C. B. Ambrosone, M. J. McCullough, J. Ahn, V. L. Stevens, M. J. Thun, and C. C. Hong. 2009. Oxidative stress-related genotypes, fruit and vegetable consumption and breast cancer risk. *Carcinogenesis* 30 (5): 777–784.
16. Matsui, H., and K. Rai. 2008. Oxidative stress in gastric carcinogenesis. *Gan To Kagaku Ryoho* 35 (9): 1451–1456.
17. Nelson, W. G., A. M. De Marzo, T. L. DeWeese, and W. B. Isaacs. 2004. The role of inflammation in the pathogenesis of prostate cancer. *J Urol* 172 (5 Pt 2): S6–S11; discussion S11–S12.
18. Sugar, L. M. 2006. Inflammation and prostate cancer. *Can J Urol* 13 (Suppl 1): 46–47.
19. Walser, T., X. Cui, J. Yanagawa, J. M. Lee, E. Heinrich, G. Lee, S. Sharma, and S. M. Dubinett. 2008. Smoking and lung cancer: The role of inflammation. *Proc Am Thorac Soc* 5 (8): 811–815.
20. Chen, Y. J., J. T. Chang, C. T. Liao, H. M. Wang, T. C. Yen, C. C. Chiu, Y. C. Lu, H. F. Li, and A. J. Cheng. 2008. Head and neck cancer in the betel quid chewing area: Recent advances in molecular carcinogenesis. *Cancer Sci* 99 (8): 1507–1514.
21. Homann, N., I. R. Konig, M. Marks, M. Benesova, F. Stickel, G. Millonig, S. Mueller, and H. K. Seitz. 2009. Alcohol and colorectal cancer: The role of alcohol dehydrogenase 1C polymorphism. *Alcohol Clin Exp Res* 33 (3): 551–556.
22. Genkinger, J. M., D. Spiegelman, K. E. Anderson, L. Bergkvist, L. Bernstein, P. A. van den Brandt, D. R. English, et al. 2009 Alcohol intake and pancreatic cancer risk: A pooled analysis of fourteen cohort studies. *Cancer Epidemiol Biomarkers Prev* 18 (3): 765–776.
23. Crous-Bou, M., M. Porta, T. Lopez, M. Jariod, N. Malats, E. Morales, L. Guarner, J. Rifa, A. Carrato, and F. X. Real. 2009. Lifetime history of alcohol consumption and K-ras mutations in pancreatic ductal adenocarcinoma. *Environ Mol Mutagen* 50 (5): 421–430.
24. McCullough, M. J., and C. S. Farah. 2008. The role of alcohol in oral carcinogenesis with particular reference to alcohol-containing mouthwashes. *Aust Dent J* 53 (4): 302–305.
25. Lof, M., and E. Weiderpass. 2009. Impact of diet on breast cancer risk. *Curr Opin Obstet Gynecol* 21 (1): 80–85.
26. Han, Y. Y., H. Kano, D. L. Davis, A. Niranjan, and L. D. Lunsford. 2009. Cell phone use and acoustic neuroma: The need for standardized questionnaires and access to industry data. *Surg Neurol* 76: 216–222.
27. Kan, P., S. E. Simonsen, J. L. Lyon, and J. R. Kestle. 2008. Cellular phone use and brain tumor: A meta-analysis. *J Neurooncol* 86 (1): 71–78.

28. Hardell, L., and C. Sage. 2008. Biological effects from electromagnetic field exposure and public exposure standards. *Biomed Pharmacother* 62 (2): 104–109.
29. Hardell, L., M. Carlberg, F. Soderqvist, K. H. Mild, and L. L. Morgan. 2007. Long-term use of cellular phones and brain tumours: Increased risk associated with use for > or =10 years. *Occup Environ Med* 64 (9): 626–632.
30. Hardell, L., M. Carlberg, F. Soderqvist, and K. Hansson Mild. 2008. Meta-analysis of long-term mobile phone use and the association with brain tumours. *Int J Oncol* 32 (5): 1097–1103.
31. Takebayashi, T., S. Akiba, Y. Kikuchi, M. Taki, K. Wake, S. Watanabe, and N. Yamaguchi. 2006. Mobile phone use and acoustic neuroma risk in Japan. *Occup Environ Med* 63 (12): 802–807.
32. Croft, R. J., R. J. McKenzie, I. Inyang, G. P. Benke, V. Anderson, and M. J. Abramson. 2008. Mobile phones and brain tumours: A review of epidemiological research. *Australas Phys Eng Sci Med* 31 (4): 255–267.
33. Sadetzki, S., A. Chetrit, A. Jarus-Hakak, E. Cardis, Y. Deutch, S. Duvdevani, A. Zultan, I. Novikov, L. Freedman, and M. Wolf. 2008. Cellular phone use and risk of benign and malignant parotid gland tumors—a nationwide case-control study. *Am J Epidemiol* 167 (4): 457–467.
34. Abdel-Rassoul, G., O. A. El-Fateh, M. A. Salem, A. Michael, F. Farahat, M. El-Batanouny, and E. Salem. 2007. Neurobehavioral effects among inhabitants around mobile phone base stations. *Neurotoxicology* 28 (2): 434–440.
35. Tillmann, T., H. Ernst, S. Ebert, N. Kuster, W. Behnke, S. Rittinghausen, and C. Dasenbrock. 2007. Carcinogenicity study of GSM and DCS wireless communication signals in B6C3F1 mice. *Bioelectromagnetics* 28 (3): 173–187.
36. Kim, J. Y., S. Y. Hong, Y. M. Lee, S. A. Yu, W. S. Koh, J. R. Hong, T. Son, S. K. Chang, and M. Lee. 2008. In vitro assessment of clastogenicity of mobile-phone radiation (835 MHz) using the alkaline comet assay and chromosomal aberration test. *Environ Toxicol* 23 (3): 319–327.
37. Ahern, T. P., T. L. Lash, K. M. Egan, and J. A. Baron. 2009. Lifetime tobacco smoke exposure and breast cancer incidence. *Cancer Causes Control* in press.
38. Duan, L., A. H. Wu, J. Sullivan-Halley, and L. Bernstein. 2009. Passive smoking and risk of oesophageal and gastric adenocarcinomas. *Br J Cancer* 100 (9): 1483–1485.
39. Johnson, K. C., J. Hu, and Y. Mao. 2000. Passive and active smoking and breast cancer risk in Canada, 1994–97. *Cancer Causes Control* 11 (3): 211–221.
40. Johnson, K. C. 2005. Accumulating evidence on passive and active smoking and breast cancer risk. *Int J Cancer* 117 (4): 619–628.
41. Kropp, S., and J. Chang-Claude. 2002. Active and passive smoking and risk of breast cancer by age 50 years among German women. *Am J Epidemiol* 156 (7): 616–626.
42. Theis, R. P., S. M. Dolwick Grieb, D. Burr, T. Siddiqui, and N. R. Asal. 2008. Smoking, environmental tobacco smoke, and risk of renal cell cancer: A population-based case-control study. *BMC Cancer* 8: 387.
43. Hemelt, M., H. Yamamoto, K. K. Cheng, and M. P. Zeegers. 2009. The effect of smoking on the male excess of bladder cancer: A meta-analysis and geographical analyses. *Int J Cancer* 124 (2): 412–419.
44. Montella, M., I. Tramacere, A. Tavani, S. Gallus, A. Crispo, R. Talamini, L. Dal Maso, et al. 2009. Coffee, decaffeinated coffee, tea intake, and risk of renal cell cancer. *Nutr Cancer* 61 (1): 76–80.
45. Ganmaa, D., W. C. Willett, T. Y. Li, D. Feskanich, R. M. van Dam, E. Lopez-Garcia, D. J. Hunter, and M. D. Holmes. 2008. Coffee, tea, caffeine and risk of breast cancer: A 22-year follow-up. *Int J Cancer* 122 (9): 2071–2076.
46. Ishitani, K., J. Lin, J. E. Manson, J. E. Buring, and S. M. Zhang. 2008. Caffeine consumption and the risk of breast cancer in a large prospective cohort of women. *Arch Intern Med* 168 (18): 2022–2031.
47. Tavani, A., S. Gallus, L. Dal Maso, S. Franceschi, M. Montella, E. Conti, and C. La Vecchia. 2001. Coffee and alcohol intake and risk of ovarian cancer: An Italian case-control study. *Nutr Cancer* 39 (1): 29–34.
48. Song, Y. J., A. R. Kristal, K. G. Wicklund, K. L. Cushing-Haugen, and M. A. Rossing. 2008. Coffee, tea, colas, and risk of epithelial ovarian cancer. *Cancer Epidemiol Biomarkers Prev* 17 (3): 712–716.
49. Lueth, N. A., K. E. Anderson, L. J. Harnack, J. A. Fulkerson, and K. Robien. 2008. Coffee and caffeine intake and the risk of ovarian cancer: Rhe Iowa Women's Health Study. *Cancer Causes Control* 19 (10): 1365–1372.
50. Tworoger, S. S., D. M. Gertig, M. A. Gates, J. L. Hecht, and S. E. Hankinson. 2008. Caffeine, alcohol, smoking, and the risk of incident epithelial ovarian cancer. *Cancer* 112 (5): 1169–1177.
51. Kurahashi, N., M. Inoue, M. Iwasaki, S. Sasazuki, and S. Tsugane. 2008. Coffee, green tea, and caffeine consumption and subsequent risk of bladder cancer in relation to smoking status: A prospective study in Japan. *Cancer Sci* in press.

52. Larsson, S. C., and A. Wolk. 2007. Coffee consumption and risk of liver cancer: A meta-analysis. *Gastroenterology* 132 (5): 1740–1745.
53. Tang, N., Y. Wu, J. Ma, B. Wang, and R. Yu. 2009. Coffee consumption and risk of lung cancer: A meta-analysis. *Lung Cancer* 65: 274–283.
54. Ames, B. N. 1983. Dietary carcinogens and anticarcinogens. Oxygen radicals and degenerative diseases. *Science* 221 (4617): 1256–1264.
55. Hogervorst, J. G., L. J. Schouten, E. J. Konings, R. A. Goldbohm, and P. A. van den Brandt. 2009. Lung cancer risk in relation to dietary acrylamide intake. *J Natl Cancer Inst* 101 (9): 651–662.
56. Wogan, G. N., S. S. Hecht, J. S. Felton, A. H. Conney, and L. A. Loeb. 2004. Environmental and chemical carcinogenesis. *Semin Cancer Biol* 14 (6): 473–486.
57. Newmark, H., and W. Mergen. 1981. Application of ascorbic acid and tocopherols as inhibitors of nitrosamine formation and oxidation in food. In *Criteria of Food Acceptance*, ed. J. Solms and R. Hall, 379. Zurich: Forster Publishing.
58. Dion, P. W., E. B. Bright-See, C. C. Smith, and W. R. Bruce. 1982. The effect of dietary ascorbic acid and alpha-tocopherol on fecal mutagenicity. *Mutat Res* 102 (1): 27–37.
59. Duthie, S. J., A. Ma, M. A. Ross, and A. R. Collins. 1996. Antioxidant supplementation decreases oxidative DNA damage in human lymphocytes. *Cancer Res* 56 (6): 1291–1295.
60. Sram, R. J., L. Dobias, A. Pastorkova, P. Rossner, and L. Janca. 1983. Effect of ascorbic acid prophylaxis on the frequency of chromosome aberrations in the peripheral lymphocytes of coal-tar workers. *Mutat Res* 120 (2–3): 181–186.
61. Weitberg, A. B., S. A. Weitzman, E. P. Clark, and T. P. Stossel. 1985. Effects of antioxidants on oxidant-induced sister chromatid exchange formation. *J Clin Invest* 75 (6): 1835–1841.
62. Rao, C. V., and B. S. Reddy. 1993. Modulating effect of amount and types of dietary fat on ornithine decarboxylase, tyrosine protein kinase and prostaglandins production during colon carcinogenesis in male F344 rats. *Carcinogenesis* 14 (7): 1327–1333.
63. Reddy, B. S. 1993. Dietary fat, calories, and fiber in colon cancer. *Prev Med* 22 (5): 738–749.
64. Delafuente, J. C., J. M. Prendergast, and A. Modigh. 1986. Immunologic modulation by vitamin C in the elderly. *Int J Immunopharmacol* 8 (2): 205–211.
65. Ringer, T. V., M. J. DeLoof, G. E. Winterrowd, S. F. Francom, S. K. Gaylor, J. A. Ryan, M. E. Sanders, and G. S. Hughes. 1991. Beta-carotene's effects on serum lipoproteins and immunologic indices in humans. *Am J Clin Nutr* 53 (3): 688–694.
66. Prasad, K. N., and J. Edwards-Prasad. 1982. Effects of tocopherol (vitamin E) acid succinate on morphological alterations and growth inhibition in melanoma cells in culture. *Cancer Res* 42 (2): 550–555.
67. Radner, B. S., and A. R. Kennedy. 1986. Suppression of X-ray induced transformation by vitamin E in mouse C3H/10T1/2 cells. *Cancer Lett* 32 (1): 25–32.
68. Borek, C., A. Ong, H. Mason, L. Donahue, and J. E. Biaglow. 1986. Selenium and vitamin E inhibit radiogenic and chemically induced transformation in vitro via different mechanisms. *Proc Natl Acad Sci U S A* 83 (5): 1490–1494.
69. Pung, A., J. E. Rundhaug, C. N. Yoshizawa, and J. S. Bertram. 1988. Beta-carotene and canthaxanthin inhibit chemically- and physically-induced neoplastic transformation in 10T1/2 cells. *Carcinogenesis* 9 (9): 1533–1539.
70. Kennedy, A. R., and N. I. Krinsky. 1994. Effects of retinoids, beta-carotene, and canthaxanthin on UV- and X-ray–induced transformation of C3H10T1/2 cells in vitro. *Nutr Cancer* 22 (3): 219–232.
71. Venugopal, D., M. Zahid, P. C. Mailander, J. L. Meza, E. G. Rogan, E. L. Cavalieri, and D. Chakravarti. 2008. Reduction of estrogen-induced transformation of mouse mammary epithelial cells by *N*-acetylcysteine. *J Steroid Biochem Mol Biol* 109 (1–2): 22–30.
72. Cohen, M., and H. N. Bhagavan. 1995. Ascorbic acid and gastrointestinal cancer. *J Am Coll Nutr* 14 (6): 565–578.
73. Prasad, K. N., and J. Edwards-Prasad. 1992. Vitamin E and cancer prevention: Recent advances and future potentials. *J Am Coll Nutr* 11 (5): 487–500.
74. Hill, D. L., and C. J. Grubbs. 1982. Retinoids as chemopreventive and anticancer agents intact animals (review). *Anticancer Res* 2 (1–2): 111–124.
75. Krinsky, N. I. 1989. Antioxidant functions of carotenoids. *Free Radic Biol Med* 7 (6): 617–635.
76. Santamaria, L., A. Bianchi, and G. Mobilio. 1988. Cancer prevention by carotenoids. In *Nutrition, Growth and Cancer*, ed. G. P. Tryfiates and K. N. Prasad, 177. New York, NY: Alan R. Liss.
77. Venkateswaran, V., L. H. Klotz, M. Ramani, L. M. Sugar, L. E. Jacob, R. K. Nam, and N. E. Fleshner. 2009. A combination of micronutrients is beneficial in reducing the incidence of prostate cancer and increasing survival in the Lady transgenic model. *Cancer Prev Res (Phila, PA)* 2 (5): 473–483.

78. Lippman, S. M., E. A. Klein, P. J. Goodman, M. S. Lucia, I. M. Thompson, L. G. Ford, H. L. Parnes, et al. 2009. Effect of selenium and vitamin E on risk of prostate cancer and other cancers: The Selenium and Vitamin E Cancer Prevention Trial (SELECT). *JAMA* 301 (1): 39–51.
79. Chen, C. S., J. A. Squire, and P. G. Wells. 2009. Reduced tumorigenesis in p53 knockout mice exposed in utero to low-dose vitamin E. *Cancer* 115 (7): 1563–1575.
80. Wang, Y. J., M. C. Yang, and M. H. Pan. 2008. Dihydrolipoic acid inhibits tetrachlorohydroquinone-induced tumor promotion through prevention of oxidative damage. *Food Chem Toxicol* 46 (12): 3739–3748.
81. Ho, Y. S., C. S. Lai, H. I. Liu, S. Y. Ho, C. Tai, M. H. Pan, and Y. J. Wang. 2007. Dihydrolipoic acid inhibits skin tumor promotion through anti-inflammation and anti-oxidation. *Biochem Pharmacol* 73 (11): 1786–1795.
82. Rossi, C., A. Di Lena, R. La Sorda, R. Lattanzio, L. Antolini, C. Patassini, M. Piantelli, and S. Alberti. 2008. Intestinal tumour chemoprevention with the antioxidant lipoic acid stimulates the growth of breast cancer. *Eur J Cancer* 44 (17): 2696–2704.
83. Reliene, R., and R. H. Schiestl. 2006. Antioxidant N-acetyl cysteine reduces incidence and multiplicity of lymphoma in Atm deficient mice. *DNA Repair* (Amst) 5 (7): 852–859.
84. Balansky, R. M., G. Ganchev, F. D'Agostini, and S. De Flora. 2002. Effects of N-acetylcysteine in an esophageal carcinogenesis model in rats treated with diethylnitrosamine and diethyldithiocarbamate. *Int J Cancer* 98 (4): 493–497.
85. Martin, K. R., C. Trempus, M. Saulnier, F. W. Kari, J. C. Barrett, and J. E. French. 2001. Dietary N-acetyl-L-cysteine modulates benzo[a]pyrene-induced skin tumors in cancer-prone p53 haploinsufficient Tg. AC (v-Ha-*ras*) mice. *Carcinogenesis* 22 (9): 1373–1378.
86. Lubet, R. A., V. E. Steele, I. Eto, M. M. Juliana, G. J. Kelloff, and C. J. Grubbs. 1997. Chemopreventive efficacy of anethole trithione, N-acetyl-L-cysteine, miconazole and phenethylisothiocyanate in the DMBA-induced rat mammary cancer model. *Int J Cancer* 72 (1): 95–101.
87. De Flora, S., G. A. Rossi, and A. De Flora. 1986. Metabolic, desmutagenic and anticarcinogenic effects of N-acetylcysteine. *Respiration* 50 (Suppl 1): 43–49.
88. Hao, J., B. Zhang, B. Liu, M. Lee, X. Hao, K. R. Reuhl, X. Chen, and C. S. Yang. 2009. Effect of alpha-tocopherol, N-acetylcysteine and omeprazole on esophageal adenocarcinoma formation in a rat surgical model. *Int J Cancer* 124 (6): 1270–1275.
89. Sakano, K., M. Takahashi, M. Kitano, T. Sugimura, and K. Wakabayashi. 2006. Suppression of azoxymethane-induced colonic premalignant lesion formation by coenzyme Q_{10} in rats. *Asian Pac J Cancer Prev* 7 (4): 599–603.
90. Toth, B., and K. Patil. 1983. Enhancing effect of vitamin E on murine intestinal tumorigenesis by 1,2-dimethylhydrazine dihydrochloride. *J Natl Cancer Inst* 70 (6): 1107–1111.
91. Fukushima, S., K. Imaida, M. A. Shibata, S. Tamano, Y. Kurata, and T. Shirai. 1988. L-Ascorbic acid amplification of second-stage bladder carcinogenesis promotion by $NaHCO_3$. *Cancer Res* 48 (22): 6317–6320.
92. Hennekens, C. H. 1994. Antioxidant vitamins and cancer. *Am J Med* 97 (3A): 2S–4S; discussion 22S–28S.
93. Buring, J., and C. H. Hennekens. 1995. Antioxidant vitamins in cancer: The Physicians' Health Study and Women's Health Study. In *Nutrients in Cancer Prevention and Treatment*, ed. K. Prasad, L. Santamaria, and R. M. Williams, 223. Totowa, NJ: Humana Press.
94. Koushik, A., D. J. Hunter, D. Spiegelman, K. E. Anderson, A. A. Arslan, W. L. Beeson, P. A. van den Brandt, et al. 2005. Fruits and vegetables and ovarian cancer risk in a pooled analysis of 12 cohort studies. *Cancer Epidemiol Biomarkers Prev* 14 (9): 2160–2167.
95. Kristal, A. R., K. B. Arnold, J. M. Schenk, M. L. Neuhouser, P. Goodman, D. F. Penson, and I. M. Thompson. 2008. Dietary patterns, supplement use, and the risk of symptomatic benign prostatic hyperplasia: Results from the prostate cancer prevention trial. *Am J Epidemiol* 167 (8): 925–934.
96. Rodrigues, M. J., A. Bouyon, and J. Alexandre. 2009. Role of antioxidant complements and supplements in oncology in addition to an equilibrate regimen: A systematic review. *Bull Cancer* 96 (6): 677–684.
97. Jedrychowski, W., and U. Maugeri. 2009. An apple a day may hold colorectal cancer at bay: Recent evidence from a case-control study. *Rev Environ Health* 24 (1): 59–74.
98. Sato, R., K. J. Helzlsouer, A. J. Alberg, S. C. Hoffman, E. P. Norkus, and G. W. Comstock. 2002. Prospective study of carotenoids, tocopherols, and retinoid concentrations and the risk of breast cancer. *Cancer Epidemiol Biomarkers Prev* 11 (5): 451–457.
99. Tamimi, R. M., S. E. Hankinson, H. Campos, D. Spiegelman, S. Zhang, G. A. Colditz, W. C. Willett, and D. J. Hunter. 2005. Plasma carotenoids, retinol, and tocopherols and risk of breast cancer. *Am J Epidemiol* 161 (2): 153–160.

100. Kabat, G. C., M. Kim, L. L. Adams-Campbell, B. J. Caan, R. T. Chlebowski, M. L. Neuhouser, J. M. Shikany, and T. E. Rohan. 2009. Longitudinal study of serum carotenoid, retinol, and tocopherol concentrations in relation to breast cancer risk among postmenopausal women. *Am J Clin Nutr* 90 (1): 162–169.
101. Gallicchio, L., K. Boyd, G. Matanoski, X. G. Tao, L. Chen, T. K. Lam, M. Shiels, et al. 2008. Carotenoids and the risk of developing lung cancer: A systematic review. *Am J Clin Nutr* 88 (2): 372–383.
102. Satia, J. A., A. Littman, C. G. Slatore, J. A. Galanko, and E. White. 2009. Long-term use of beta-carotene, retinol, lycopene, and lutein supplements and lung cancer risk: Results from the VITamins And Lifestyle (VITAL) study. *Am J Epidemiol* 169 (7): 815–828.
103. Ma, E., M. Iwasaki, I. Junko, G. S. Hamada, I. N. Nishimoto, S. M. Carvalho, J. Motola Jr., et al. 2009. Dietary intake of folate, vitamin B_6, and vitamin B_{12}, genetic polymorphism of related enzymes, and risk of breast cancer: A case-control study in Brazilian women. *BMC Cancer* 9: 122.
104. Tang, N. P., B. Zhou, B. Wang, R. B. Yu, and J. Ma. 2009. Flavonoids intake and risk of lung cancer: A meta-analysis. *Jpn J Clin Oncol* 39 (6): 352–359.
105. Wang, L., I. M. Lee, S. M. Zhang, J. B. Blumberg, J. E. Buring, and H. D. Sesso. 2009. Dietary intake of selected flavonols, flavones, and flavonoid-rich foods and risk of cancer in middle-aged and older women. *Am J Clin Nutr* 89 (3): 905–912.
106. Ellinger, S., J. Ellinger, S. C. Muller, and P. Stehle. 2009. Tomatoes and lycopene in prevention and therapy—is there an evidence for prostate diseases? *Aktuelle Urol* 40 (1): 37–43.
107. Thomson, C. A., M. L. Neuhouser, J. M. Shikany, B. J. Caan, B. J. Monk, Y. Mossavar-Rahmani, G. Sarto, L. M. Parker, F. Modugno, and G. L. Anderson. 2008. The role of antioxidants and vitamin A in ovarian cancer: Results from the Women's Health Initiative. *Nutr Cancer* 60 (6): 710–719.
108. Thiebaut, A. C., V. Chajes, M. Gerber, M. C. Boutron-Ruault, V. Joulin, G. Lenoir, F. Berrino, E. Riboli, J. Benichou, and F. Clavel-Chapelon. 2009. Dietary intakes of omega-6 and omega-3 polyunsaturated fatty acids and the risk of breast cancer. *Int J Cancer* 124 (4): 924–931.
109. Anderson, K. E., E. J. Pantuck, A. H. Conney, and A. Kappas. 1985. Nutrient regulation of chemical metabolism in humans. *Fed Proc* 44 (1 Pt 1): 130–133.
110. Conney, A. H., T. Lysz, T. Ferraro, T. F. Abidi, P. S., Manchand, J. D. Laskin, and M. T. Huang. 1991. Inhibitory effect of curcumin and some related dietary compounds on tumor promotion and arachidonic acid metabolism in mouse skin. *Adv Enzyme Regul* 31: 385–396.
111. Albanes, D., O. P. Heinonen, J. K. Huttunen, P. R. Taylor, J. Virtamo, B. K. Edwards, J. Haapakoski, et al. 1995. Effects of alpha-tocopherol and beta-carotene supplements on cancer incidence in the Alpha-Tocopherol Beta-Carotene Cancer Prevention Study. *Am J Clin Nutr* 62 (6 Suppl): 1427S–1430S.
112. The Alpha-Tocopherol, BCCPSG. 1994. The effect of vitamin E and beta carotene on the incidence of lung cancer and other cancers in male smokers. *N Engl J Med* 330 (15): 1029–1035.
113. Omenn, G. S., G. E. Goodman, M. D. Thornquist, J. Balmes, M. R. Cullen, A. Glass, J. P. Keogh, et al. 1996. Effects of a combination of beta carotene and vitamin A on lung cancer and cardiovascular disease. *N Engl J Med* 334 (18): 1150–1155.
114. Hennekens, C. H., J. E. Buring, J. E. Manson, M. Stampfer, B. Rosner, N. R. Cook, C. Belanger, et al. 1996. Lack of effect of long-term supplementation with beta carotene on the incidence of malignant neoplasms and cardiovascular disease. *N Engl J Med* 334 (18): 1145–1149.
115. Van Schooten, F. J., A. Besaratinia, S. De Flora, F. D'Agostini, A. Izzotti, A. Camoirano, A. J. Balm, et al. 2002. Effects of oral administration of N-acetyl-L-cysteine: A multi-biomarker study in smokers. *Cancer Epidemiol Biomarkers Prev* 11 (2): 167–175.
116. van Zandwijk, N., O. Dalesio, U. Pastorino, N. de Vries, and H. van Tinteren. 2000. EUROSCAN, a randomized trial of vitamin A and N-acetylcysteine in patients with head and neck cancer or lung cancer. For the European Organization for Research and Treatment of Cancer Head and Neck and Lung Cancer Cooperative Groups. *J Natl Cancer Inst* 92 (12): 977–986.
117. Kirsh, V. A., R. B. Hayes, S. T. Mayne, N. Chatterjee, A. F. Subar, L. B. Dixon, D. Albanes, G. L. Andriole, D. A. Urban, and U. Peters. 2006. Supplemental and dietary vitamin E, beta-carotene, and vitamin C intakes and prostate cancer risk. *J Natl Cancer Inst* 98 (4): 245–254.
118. Benner, S. E., R. J. Winn, S. M. Lippman, J. Poland, K. S. Hansen, M. A. Luna, and W. K. Hong. 1993. Regression of oral leukoplakia with alpha-tocopherol: A community clinical oncology program chemoprevention study. *J Natl Cancer Inst* 85 (1): 44–47.
119. Garewal, H. 1995. Beta-carotene and antioxidant nutrients in oral cancer prevention. In *Nutrients in Cancer Prevention and Treatment*, ed. K. S. Prasad, L. Santamaria, and R. M. Williams. Totawa, NJ: Humana Press.
120. Hernaandez, J., S. Syed, G. Weiss, G. Fernandes, D. von Merveldt, D. A. Troyer, J. W. Basler, and I. M. Thompson Jr. 2005. The modulation of prostate cancer risk with alpha-tocopherol: A pilot randomized, controlled clinical trial. *J Urol* 174 (2): 519–522.

121. Alkhenizan, A., and K. Hafez. 2007. The role of vitamin E in the prevention of cancer: A meta-analysis of randomized controlled trials. *Ann Saudi Med* 27 (6): 409–414.
122. Weinstein, S. J., M. E. Wright, K. A. Lawson, K. Snyder, S. Mannisto, P. R. Taylor, J. Virtamo, and D. Albanes. 2007. Serum and dietary vitamin E in relation to prostate cancer risk. *Cancer Epidemiol Biomarkers Prev* 16 (6): 1253–1259.
123. Weinstein, S. J., M. E. Wright, P. Pietinen, I. King, C. Tan, P. R. Taylor, J. Virtamo, and D. Albanes. 2005. Serum alpha-tocopherol and gamma-tocopherol in relation to prostate cancer risk in a prospective study. *J Natl Cancer Inst* 97 (5): 396–399.
124. Bairati, I., F. Meyer, M. Gelinas, A. Fortin, A. Nabid, F. Brochet, J. P. Mercier, et al. 2005. Randomized trial of antioxidant vitamins to prevent acute adverse effects of radiation therapy in head and neck cancer patients. *J Clin Oncol* 23 (24): 5805–5813.
125. E. R. Miller 3rd, R. Pastor-Barriuso, D. Dalal, R. A. Riemersma, L. J. Appel, and E. Guallar. 2005. Meta-analysis: High-dosage vitamin E supplementation may increase all-cause mortality. *Ann Intern Med* 142 (1): 37–46.
126. Gerss, J., and W. Kopcke. 2009. The questionable association of vitamin E supplementation and mortality—Inconsistent results of different meta-analytic approaches. *Cell Mol Biol (Noisy-le-grand)* 55 (Suppl): OL1111-20.
127. Mooney, L. A., A. M. Madsen, D. Tang, M. A. Orjuela, W. Y. Tsai, E. R. Garduno, and F. P. Perera. 2005. Antioxidant vitamin supplementation reduces benzo(*a*)pyrene–DNA adducts and potential cancer risk in female smokers. *Cancer Epidemiol Biomarkers Prev* 14 (1): 237–242.
128. Lin, J., N. R. Cook, C. Albert, E. Zaharris, J. M. Gaziano, M. Van Denburgh, J. E. Buring, and J. E. Manson. 2009. Vitamins C and E and beta carotene supplementation and cancer risk: A randomized controlled trial. *J Natl Cancer Inst* 101 (1): 14–23.
129. Stolzenberg-Solomon, R. Z., S. Sheffler-Collins, S. Weinstein, D. H. Garabrant, S. Mannisto, P. Taylor, J. Virtamo, and D. Albanes. 2009. Vitamin E intake, alpha-tocopherol status, and pancreatic cancer in a cohort of male smokers. *Am J Clin Nutr* 89 (2): 584–591.
130. Pastorino, U., M. Infante, M. Maioli, G. Chiesa, M. Buyse, P. Firket, N. Rosmentz, et al. 1993. Adjuvant treatment of stage I lung cancer with high-dose vitamin A. *J Clin Oncol* 11 (7): 1216–1222.
131. Meyskens, F. J. 1995. Role of vitamin A and its derivatives in the treatment of human cancer. In *Nutrients in Cancer Prevention and Treatment*, ed. K. L. Prasad, L. Santamaria, and R. M. Williams. Totawa, NJ: Humana Press.
132. Ingold, K. U., G. W. Burton, D. O. Foster, L. Hughes, D. A. Lindsay, and A. Webb. 1987. Biokinetics of and discrimination between dietary *RRR*- and *SRR*-alpha-tocopherols in the male rat. *Lipids* 22 (3): 163–172.
133. Prasad, K. N., B. Kumar, X. D. Yan, A. J. Hanson, and W. C. Cole. 2003. Alpha-tocopheryl succinate, the most effective form of vitamin E for adjuvant cancer treatment: A review. *J Am Coll Nutr* 22 (2): 108–117.
134. Prasad, K. N. 2003. Antioxidants in cancer care: When and how to use them as an adjunct to standard and experimental therapies. *Expert Rev Anticancer Ther* 3 (6): 903–915.
135. Lamm, D. L., D. R. Riggs, J. S. Shriver, P. F. vanGilder, J. F. Rach, and J. I. DeHaven. 1994. Megadose vitamins in bladder cancer: A double-blind clinical trial. *J Urol* 151 (1): 21–26.
136. Roncucci, L., P. Di Donato, L. Carati, A. Ferrari, M. Perini, G. Bertoni, G. Bedogni, et al. 1993. Antioxidant vitamins or lactulose for the prevention of the recurrence of colorectal adenomas. Colorectal Cancer Study Group of the University of Modena and the Health Care District 16. *Dis Colon Rectum* 36 (3): 227–234.
137. Greenberg, E. R., J. A. Baron, T. D. Tosteson, D. H. Freeman Jr., G. J. Beck, J. H. Bond, T. A. Colacchio, et al. 1994. A clinical trial of antioxidant vitamins to prevent colorectal adenoma. Polyp Prevention Study Group. *N Engl J Med* 331 (3): 141–147.
138. McKeown-Eyssen, G., C. Holloway, V. Jazmaji, E. Bright-See, P. Dion, and W. R. Bruce. 1988. A randomized trial of vitamins C and E in the prevention of recurrence of colorectal polyps. *Cancer Res* 48 (16): 4701–4705.
139. DeCosse, J. J., H. H. Miller, and M. L. Lesser. 1989. Effect of wheat fiber and vitamins C and E on rectal polyps in patients with familial adenomatous polyposis. *J Natl Cancer Inst* 81 (17): 1290–1297.
140. Blot, W. J., J. Y. Li, P. R. Taylor, W. Guo, S. Dawsey, G. Q. Wang, C. S. Yang, et al. 1993. Nutrition intervention trials in Linxian, China: Supplementation with specific vitamin/mineral combinations, cancer incidence, and disease-specific mortality in the general population. *J Natl Cancer Inst* 85 (18): 1483–1492.
141. Qiao, Y. L., S. M. Dawsey, F. Kamangar, J. H. Fan, C. C. Abnet, X. D. Sun, L. L. Johnson, et al. 2009. Total and cancer mortality after supplementation with vitamins and minerals: Follow-up of the Linxian General Population Nutrition Intervention Trial. *J Natl Cancer Inst* 101 (7): 507–518.

142. Biasco, G., and G. M. Paganelli. 1999. European trials on dietary supplementation for cancer prevention. *Ann N Y Acad Sci* 889: 152–156.
143. Hoenjet, K. M., P. C. Dagnelie, K. P. Delaere, N. E. Wijckmans, J. V. Zambon, and G. O. Oosterhof. 2005. Effect of a nutritional supplement containing vitamin E, selenium, vitamin C and coenzyme Q_{10} on serum PSA in patients with hormonally untreated carcinoma of the prostate: A randomised placebo-controlled study. *Eur Urol* 47 (4): 433–439; discussion 439–440.
144. Gorham, E. D., C. F. Garland, F. C. Garland, W. B. Grant, S. B. Mohr, M. Lipkin, H. L. Newmark, E. Giovannucci, M. Wei, and M. F. Holick. 2005. Vitamin D and prevention of colorectal cancer. *J Steroid Biochem Mol Biol* 97 (1–2): 179–194.
145. Gorham, E. D., C. F. Garland, F. C. Garland, W. B. Grant, S. B. Mohr, M. Lipkin, H. L. Newmark, E. Giovannucci, M. Wei, and M. F. Holick. 2007. Optimal vitamin D status for colorectal cancer prevention: A quantitative meta analysis. *Am J Prev Med* 32 (3): 210–216.
146. Wactawski-Wende, J., J. M. Kotchen, G. L. Anderson, A. R. Assaf, R. L. Brunner, M. J. O'Sullivan, K. L. Margolis, et al. 2006. Calcium plus vitamin D supplementation and the risk of colorectal cancer. *N Engl J Med* 354 (7): 684–696.
147. Ding, E. L., S. Mehta, W. W. Fawzi, and E. L. Giovannucci. 2008. Interaction of estrogen therapy with calcium and vitamin D supplementation on colorectal cancer risk: Reanalysis of Women's Health Initiative randomized trial. *Int J Cancer* 122 (8): 1690–1694.
148. Weingarten, M. A., A. Zalmanovici, and J. Yaphe. 2008. Dietary calcium supplementation for preventing colorectal cancer and adenomatous polyps. *Cochrane Database Syst Rev* (1): CD003548.
149. Chlebowski, R. T., K. C. Johnson, C. Kooperberg, M. Pettinger, Wactawski-J. Wende, T. Rohan, J. Rossouw, et al. 2008. Calcium plus vitamin D supplementation and the risk of breast cancer. *J Natl Cancer Inst* 100 (22): 1581–1591.
150. McCullough, M. L., C. Rodriguez, W. R. Diver, H. S. Feigelson, V. L. Stevens, M. J. Thun, and E. E. Calle. 2005. Dairy, calcium, and vitamin D intake and postmenopausal breast cancer risk in the Cancer Prevention Study II Nutrition Cohort. *Cancer Epidemiol Biomarkers Prev* 14 (12): 2898–2904.
151. Martinez, M. E., J. R. Marshall, R. Sampliner, J. Wilkinson, and D. S. Alberts. 2002. Calcium, vitamin D, and risk of adenoma recurrence (United States). *Cancer Causes Control* 13 (3): 213–220.
152. Grau, M. V., J. A. Baron, R. S. Sandler, R. W. Haile, M. L. Beach, T. R. Church, and D. Heber. 2003. Vitamin D, calcium supplementation, and colorectal adenomas: Results of a randomized trial. *J Natl Cancer Inst* 95 (23): 1765–1771.
153. Harnack, L., D. R. Jacobs Jr., K. Nicodemus, D. Lazovich, K. Anderson, and A. R. Folsom. 2002. Relationship of folate, vitamin B-6, vitamin B-12, and methionine intake to incidence of colorectal cancers. *Nutr Cancer* 43 (2): 152–158.
154. Ishihara, J., T. Otani, M. Inoue, M. Iwasaki, S. Sasazuki, and S. Tsugane. 2007. Low intake of vitamin B-6 is associated with increased risk of colorectal cancer in Japanese men. *J Nutr* 137 (7): 1808–1814.
155. Kune, G., and L. Watson. 2006. Colorectal cancer protective effects and the dietary micronutrients folate, methionine, vitamins B_6, B_{12}, C, E, selenium, and lycopene. *Nutr Cancer* 56 (1): 11–21.
156. Lajous, M., E. Lazcano-Ponce, M. Hernandez-Avila, W. Willett, and I. Romieu. 2006. Folate, vitamin B(6), and vitamin B(12) intake and the risk of breast cancer among Mexican women. *Cancer Epidemiol Biomarkers Prev* 15 (3): 443–448.
157. Zhang, S. M. 2004. Role of vitamins in the risk, prevention, and treatment of breast cancer. *Curr Opin Obstet Gynecol* 16 (1): 19–25.
158. Cole, B. F., J. A. Baron, R. S. Sandler, R. W. Haile, D. J. Ahnen, R. S. Bresalier, G. McKeown-Eyssen, et al. 2007. Folic acid for the prevention of colorectal adenomas: A randomized clinical trial. *JAMA* 297 (21): 2351–2359.
159. Logan, R. F., M. J. Grainge, V. C. Shepherd, N. C. Armitage, and K. R. Muir. 2008. Aspirin and folic acid for the prevention of recurrent colorectal adenomas. *Gastroenterology* 134 (1): 29–38.
160. Jaszewski, R., S. Misra, M. Tobi, N. Ullah, J. A. Naumoff, O. Kucuk, E. Levi, B. N. Axelrod, B. B. Patel, and A. P. Majumdar. 2008. Folic acid supplementation inhibits recurrence of colorectal adenomas: A randomized chemoprevention trial. *World J Gastroenterol* 14 (28): 4492–4498.
161. Yang, Q., R. M. Bostick, J. M. Friedman, and W. D. Flanders. 2009. Serum folate and cancer mortality among U.S. adults: Findings from the Third National Health and Nutritional Examination Survey linked mortality file. *Cancer Epidemiol Biomarkers Prev* 18 (5): 1439–1447.
162. Beresford, S. A., K. C. Johnson, C. Ritenbaugh, N. L. Lasser, L. G. Snetselaar, H. R. Black, G. L. Anderson, et al. 2006. Low-fat dietary pattern and risk of colorectal cancer: The Women's Health Initiative Randomized Controlled Dietary Modification Trial. *JAMA* 295 (6): 643–654.

163. Shike, M., L. Latkany, E. Riedel, M. Fleisher, A. Schatzkin, E. Lanza, D. Corle, and C. B. Begg. 2002. Lack of effect of a low-fat, high-fruit, -vegetable, and -fiber diet on serum prostate-specific antigen of men without prostate cancer: Results from a randomized trial. *J Clin Oncol* 20 (17): 3592–3598.
164. Schatzkin, A., E. Lanza, D. Corle, P. Lance, F. Iber, B. Caan, M. Shike, et al. 2000. Lack of effect of a low-fat, high-fiber diet on the recurrence of colorectal adenomas. Polyp Prevention Trial Study Group. *N Engl J Med* 342 (16): 1149–1155.
165. Steck-Scott, S., M. R. Forman, A. Sowell, C. B. Borkowf, P. S. Albert, M. Slattery, B. Brewer, et al. 2004. Carotenoids, vitamin A and risk of adenomatous polyp recurrence in the polyp prevention trial. *Int J Cancer* 112 (2): 295–305.
166. Kant, A. K., A. Schatzkin, B. I. Graubard, and C. Schairer. 2000. A prospective study of diet quality and mortality in women. *JAMA* 283 (16): 2109–2115.
167. Alberts, D. S., M. E. Martinez, D. J. Roe, J. M. Guillen-Rodriguez, J. R. Marshall, J. B. van Leeuwen, M. E. Reid, et al. 2000. Lack of effect of a high-fiber cereal supplement on the recurrence of colorectal adenomas. Phoenix Colon Cancer Prevention Physicians' Network. *N Engl J Med* 342 (16): 1156–1162.
168. Pierce, J. P., L. Natarajan, B. J. Caan, B. A. Parker, E. R. Greenberg, S. W. Flatt, C. L. Rock, et al. 2007. Influence of a diet very high in vegetables, fruit, and fiber and low in fat on prognosis following treatment for breast cancer: The Women's Healthy Eating and Living (WHEL) randomized trial. *JAMA* 298 (3): 289–298.
169. Marnett, L. J. 1992. Aspirin and the potential role of prostaglandins in colon cancer. *Cancer Res* 52 (20): 5575–5589.
170. Slatore, C. G., D. H. Au, A. J. Littman, J. A. Satia, and E. White. 2009. Association of nonsteroidal anti-inflammatory drugs with lung cancer: Results from a large cohort study. *Cancer Epidemiol Biomarkers Prev* 18 (4): 1203–1207.
171. Harris, R. E., J. Beebe-Donk, H. Doss, and D. Burr Doss. 2005. Aspirin, ibuprofen, and other non-steroidal anti-inflammatory drugs in cancer prevention: A critical review of non-selective COX-2 blockade (review). *Oncol Rep* 13 (4): 559–583.
172. Clouser, M. C., D. J. Roe, J. A. Foote, and R. B. Harris. 2009. Effect of non-steroidal anti-inflammatory drugs on non-melanoma skin cancer incidence in the SKICAP-AK trial. *Pharmacoepidemiol Drug Saf* 18 (4): 276–283.
173. Bardia, A., E. A. Platz, S. Yegnasubramanian, A. M. De Marzo, and W. G. Nelson. 2009. Anti-inflammatory drugs, antioxidants, and prostate cancer prevention. *Curr Opin Pharmacol*.
174. Vile, G. F., and C. C. Winterbourn. 1988. Inhibition of adriamycin-promoted microsomal lipid peroxidation by beta-carotene, alpha-tocopherol and retinol at high and low oxygen partial pressures. *FEBS Lett* 238 (2): 353–356.
175. Niki, E. 1987. Interaction of ascorbate and alpha-tocopherol. *Ann N Y Acad Sci* 498: 186–199.
176. Carini, R., G. Poli, M. U. Dianzani, S. P. Maddix, T. F. Slater, and K. H. Cheeseman. 1990. Comparative evaluation of the antioxidant activity of alpha-tocopherol, alpha-tocopherol polyethylene glycol 1000 succinate and alpha-tocopherol succinate in isolated hepatocytes and liver microsomal suspensions. *Biochem Pharmacol* 39 (10): 1597–1601.
177. Sies, H., V. S. Sharov, L. O. Klotz, and K. Briviba. 1997. Glutathione peroxidase protects against peroxynitrite-mediated oxidations. A new function for selenoproteins as peroxynitrite reductase. *J Biol Chem* 272 (44): 27812–27817.
178. Witschi, A., S. Reddy, B. Stofer, and B. H. Lauterburg. 1992. The systemic availability of oral glutathione. *Eur J Clin Pharmacol* 43 (6): 667–669.
179. Niki, E. 1997. Mechanisms and dynamics of antioxidant action of ubiquinol. *Mol Aspects Med* 18 (Suppl): S63–S70.
180. Stoyanovsky, D. A., A. N. Osipov, P. J. Quinn, and V. E. Kagan. 1995. Ubiquinone-dependent recycling of vitamin E radicals by superoxide. *Arch Biochem Biophys* 323 (2): 343–351.
181. Zhang, L. X., R. V. Cooney, and J. S. Bertram. 1992. Carotenoids up-regulate connexin43 gene expression independent of their provitamin A or antioxidant properties. *Cancer Res* 52 (20): 5707–5712.
182. Carter, C. A., M. Pogribny, A. Davidson, C. D. Jackson, L. J. McGarrity, and S. M. Morris. 1996. Effects of retinoic acid on cell differentiation and reversion toward normal in human endometrial adenocarcinoma (RL95-2) cells. *Anticancer Res* 16 (1): 17–24.
183. Prasad, K. N., A. R. Hovland, W. C. Cole, K. C. Prasad, P. Nahreini, J. Edwards-Prasad, and C. P. Andreatta. 2000. Multiple antioxidants in the prevention and treatment of Alzheimer disease: Analysis of biologic rationale. *Clin Neuropharmacol* 23 (1): 2–13.

8 Micronutrients for Improvement of the Standard Therapy in Cancer

INTRODUCTION

Despite extensive research on cancer prevention during the past several decades, the incidence of cancer appears to be on rise. Only a little more than a decade ago, the number of new cases of cancer was about 1.2 million per year. In 2009, it is estimated to be 1.5 million (U.S. Mortality Data, 2005, National Center for Health Statistics, Center for Disease Control and Prevention, 2008).

The U.S. mortality rate from cancer has not changed significantly during the past several decades, despite the development of new treatment modalities. The American Cancer Society has estimated that the death rate in 1950 was about 194 per 100,000 persons; in 2005, this value was about 184, and in 2006 it was 180.7. In 1991, it was estimated to be about 251.1. The cancer death rate data of 1991 may be abnormally high, but there are no data for subsequent or previous years. It appears that cancer deaths were reduced compared to 1991 data, but that they remain the same compared to 1950 data. It is more likely that the cancer death, which was increasing, has been decreased due to advancement of current treatment modalities.

Cancer patients can be divided into three groups: those scheduled to receive standard therapy or experimental therapy; those who become unresponsive to these therapies; and those in remission carrying the risk of recurrence of primary tumors and the development of second new cancers. Except for reducing the risk of recurrence of breast cancer with tamoxifen, there is no effective strategy to reduce the risk of recurrence of the primary tumor or the development of a second new cancer induced by treatment agents. Standard cancer therapy, which includes radiation therapy, chemotherapy, and surgery (whenever feasible and needed), has been useful in producing increased cure rates in certain tumors including Hodgkin's disease, childhood leukemia, and teratocarcinoma. However, the risk of recurrence of the primary tumors and the development of a new cancer and nonneoplastic diseases such as aplastic anemia, retardation of growth in some children, and delayed necrosis in some organs such as the brain, liver, bone, and muscle exist. Acute damage to normal tissue occurs during radiation therapy and/or chemotherapy and, in some instances, such damage becomes the limiting factor for the continuation of therapy.

The efficacy of standard cancer therapy has reached a plateau for most solid tumors despite impressive progress in radiation therapy (e.g., dosimetry and more efficient methods of delivering radiation doses to tumors) and in chemotherapy (e.g., the development of novel drugs with diverse mechanisms of action on cell death and proliferation inhibition). Therefore, additional approaches should be developed to improve the efficacy of standard therapy and to reduce the risk of recurrence of the primary tumor and the development of new cancers among survivors. New approaches should be developed to improve the quality of life of those patients who become unresponsive to all standard and experimental cancer therapies for as long as possible.

Several laboratory experiments and limited clinical studies show that individual antioxidants and their derivatives [vitamin A, retinoids, vitamin C, D-alpha-tocopheryl succinate, natural beta-carotene, selenium, alpha-lipoic acid, and N-acetylcysteine (NAC)], at high doses and after a prolonged treatment period, inhibited the growth of several tumor cells without affecting the normal cells. Thus, these micronutrients could be useful in improving the survival time and quality of life for cancer patients who have become unresponsive to all therapies. These antioxidants at high doses also protected against the toxicity of radiation therapy and chemotherapy without interfering with their efficacy on tumor control. Some experiments have revealed that these antioxidants can increase the growth-inhibitory effects of ionizing radiation and chemotherapeutic agents in a synergistic or an additive manner on cancer cells, in culture and in vivo. Thus, these studies suggest that high-dose antioxidants could increase the efficacy of standard therapy by reducing its toxicity and improving tumor response. Oncologists have failed to appreciate the selective effects of high-dose antioxidants on tumor cells. High-dose antioxidants should be considered as a therapeutic dose.

In contrast to the observations on the selective effects of high-dose antioxidants alone or in combination with standard therapy on tumor cells, low-dose antioxidants can stimulate the growth of some cancer cells and reduce the efficacy of radiation therapy and chemotherapy on cancer cells by protecting them against the cytotoxic effects of therapies. Oncologists use these data on the effects of low-dose antioxidants to strongly discourage patients from using antioxidants during standard therapy. The critical analysis of studies on antioxidants in the prevention or treatment of cancer revealed that, in most treatment studies, preventive doses of antioxidants have been used. Also, most studies utilized a single, low-dose antioxidant.

This chapter will:

- Define the dose range of antioxidants that could be considered as a preventive or a therapeutic dose.
- Present laboratory and clinical studies on the effects of preventive and therapeutic doses of antioxidants, alone or in combination with standard therapeutic agents, on the growth of tumor and normal cells in culture and in vivo.
- Identify the primary reasons for the current controversies regarding the use of antioxidants during standard therapy.
- Propose scientific rationale for preventive and therapeutic micronutrient protocols to be used to reduce the incidence of cancer and improve the efficacy of standard therapy, respectively.

PREVENTIVE AND THERAPEUTIC DOSE RANGES OF ANTIOXIDANTS

Current controversies regarding the value of antioxidants during standard therapy are, in part, due to the fact that no distinction between the effects of preventive and therapeutic doses of antioxidants on cancer cells is made. Therefore, it is essential to define the dose range of preventive and therapeutic doses of antioxidants. Preventive doses may be defined as doses that do not affect the growth of cancer cells or normal cells. Therapeutic doses are defined as doses that inhibit the growth of cancer cells without affecting the growth of normal cells.

In humans, the proposed daily oral preventive dose ranges of antioxidants for adults at high risk for developing cancer are as follows: vitamin A, up to 5000 IU; vitamin C, up to 2 g; vitamin E [alpha-tocopherol, alpha-tocopheryl acetate, or alpha-tocopheryl succinate (alpha-TS)], up to 400 IU; carotenoids (including beta-carotene), up to 25 mg; selenomethionine, up to 200 µg; coenzyme Q_{10}, up to 100 mg; alpha-lipoic acid and NAC, up to 300 mg; and L-carnitine, up to 350 mg. Preventive doses for children would be lower than the doses for adults.

Proposed daily oral therapeutic oral dose ranges of antioxidants for patients undergoing standard therapy or who are unresponsive to all therapies are as follows: vitamin A, 25,000 IU or more; vitamin C, 10 g or more; vitamin E (alpha-tocopherol, alpha-tocopheryl acetate, or alpha-TS), 1600 IU or more; carotenoids (including beta-carotene), 100 mg or more; selenomethionine, 300 µg or more; coenzyme Q_{10}, 400 mg or more; alpha-lipoic acid and NAC, 500 mg or more; and L-carnitine, 500 mg or more. Preventive doses for children would be lower than the doses for adults.

Animals are generally very resistant to most pharmacological and physiological agents, including antioxidants. To observe any growth-inhibitory effects on tumor cells, but not on normal cells, very high doses of antioxidants are needed. Generally, a dose of antioxidants of 100 mg/kg of body weight, or more, is considered a therapeutic dose. The results on therapeutic antioxidant doses in animals cannot be extrapolated to humans. Animal models of cancer may be useful to demonstrate the principle of efficacy of antioxidants in the management of tumors, with or without standard cancer therapeutic agents. They are also useful in demonstrating the mechanisms of action of antioxidants that may or may not be applicable to humans. Nevertheless, doses and dose schedules of micronutrients obtained from animal studies are frequently extrapolated to humans.

Antioxidant doses that inhibit the growth of tumor cells in culture vary from one tumor to another in the same species, from one clone to another for the same tumor type, from one species to another, and from one antioxidant to another. Generally, a dose of an antioxidant that inhibits the growth of tumor cells in culture without affecting the growth of normal cells is considered a therapeutic dose. For example, a dose of 5 µg/ml of D-alpha-tocopheryl succinate is considered a therapeutic dose for murine melanoma cells in culture. For human melanoma, a dose of 20 µg/ml or more is considered a therapeutic dose. A dose of 100 µg/ml of vitamin C is considered a therapeutic dose for human melanoma cells in culture, but 50 µg/ml is considered a preventive dose for the same tumor.

RECOMMENDATION BY ONCOLOGISTS AND USE OF ANTIOXIDANTS BY THEIR PATIENTS

Most oncologists strongly discourage patients from taking antioxidant supplements during radiation therapy, chemotherapy, or experimental therapy, and even after the completion of therapy. A few oncologists may recommend a multiple vitamin preparation containing low doses of antioxidants after the completion of therapy. This recommendation may be harmful because, like normal cells, cancer cells also need certain amounts of micronutrients, including antioxidants, for growth and survival. Low doses of individual dietary antioxidants may stimulate the proliferation of some cancer cells.[1-3] Therefore, it is likely that the use of a multiple micronutrient preparation containing low preventive doses of antioxidants after therapy may increase the risk of recurrence of the primary tumors, possibly due to stimulation of a few residual primary cancer cells that may be present in some cancer patients.

More than 60% of cancer patients use antioxidant supplements, and the majority combine them with standard therapy, mostly without the knowledge of their oncologists.[4] This practice may be harmful, because a multiple vitamin preparation may contain low preventive doses of antioxidants that may interfere with the efficacy of standard therapy. Low doses of antioxidants, such as vitamin E, vitamin C, NAC, selenium, retinol, and beta-carotene[5-10] protect cancer cells against free radical damage produced by chemotherapeutic agents or x-irradiation. Often, neither oncologists nor cancer patients are aware of the potential dangers of taking low preventive doses of antioxidants during radiation or chemotherapy.

When using antioxidants as an adjunct to standard therapy, it is essential that oncologists are aware of the following:

- Tumor cells and cancer cells respond to antioxidant doses differently.
- The effects of therapeutic doses of antioxidants on cancer cells are different from those produced by preventive doses of antioxidants.
- Therapeutic doses of antioxidants not only inhibit the growth of tumor cells, but also enhance the efficacy of standard therapy while reducing its toxicity.
- Preventive doses of antioxidants may stimulate the growth of some cancer cells and reduce the efficacy of standard therapy.
- Multiple antioxidants, rather than a single antioxidant, are more effective.
- Therapeutic doses of antioxidants should be administered twice daily for 3–5 days before the start of standard therapy (radiation therapy or chemotherapy) and should continue for the entire treatment period.

There is a substantial amount of laboratory and animal studies of therapeutic doses and preventive doses of antioxidants, alone or in combination with cancer therapeutic agents, that should convince oncologists to reexamine their current recommendations. All previous clinical studies with antioxidants have utilized a single antioxidant at preventive doses rather than at therapeutic doses. Most cell culture and animal studies have utilized therapeutic doses of primarily a single antioxidant. Therefore, the results obtained from the preventive doses of antioxidants used during therapy should not be utilized for making any recommendation of antioxidant supplements to patients during cancer therapy. In the absence of any clinical study with the therapeutic doses of multiple micronutrients including antioxidants, it is better not to use preventive doses of antioxidants during radiation therapy or chemotherapy.

EFFECTS OF THERAPEUTIC DOSES OF INDIVIDUAL ANTIOXIDANTS ON GROWTH OF CANCER AND NORMAL CELLS

Most laboratory studies on the effects of therapeutic doses (high doses) of antioxidants on the growth and differentiation of cancer cells have utilized a single antioxidant. These studies have provided important mechanistic data that are related to their effects on apoptosis, cell proliferation, and differentiation. Treatment of cancer cells with therapeutic doses of antioxidants markedly alters expression of genes, levels of proteins, translocation of certain proteins from one cellular compartment to another causing differentiation, proliferation inhibition, and apoptosis, depending on the type and form of antioxidant, treatment schedule, and type of tumor cell. The alterations in gene expression and protein levels are directly related to proliferation inhibition and apoptosis. However, the use of a single antioxidant may not the best experimental design to test the efficacy of antioxidants in inhibiting the growth of tumor cells in vivo, because antioxidants interact with each other in an additive or a synergic manner. The use of therapeutic doses of multiple antioxidants would have been a better experimental design, the results of which could have relevance to human cancer treatment. The effects of therapeutic doses of individual or multiple antioxidants on growth, differentiation, and apoptosis of cancer cells are briefly described below.

VITAMIN E AND ITS DERIVATIVES

The notion that all forms of vitamin E have only one function, to scavenge free radicals, and that there is no difference between synthetic and natural forms of vitamin E are incorrect. In 1982, I discovered that alpha-TS induced differentiation, growth inhibition, and cell death in murine melanoma cells in culture, depending on the dose and period of treatment (see Figure 8.1), whereas alpha-tocopherol (alpha-T), alpha-tocopheryl acetate (alpha-TA), and alpha-tocopheryl nicotinate (alpha-TN) were ineffective.[11] Since then, more than 150 studies on the effects of alpha-TS on the growth of several cancer and normal cells in culture and in tumor-bearing animal models have been published.[12–15] The results of these studies showed that alpha-TS selectively inhibited the growth of cancer cells without affecting the growth of normal cells. Alpha-TS also inhibited androgen receptor expression in prostate cancer cells, but not in normal prostate epithelial cells in culture.[16] It also reduced the expression of prostate-specific antigen (PSA) by acting on both the transcription and translation levels.[17] Increased serum levels of alpha-tocopherol were associated with higher prostate cancer survival.[18] Treatment of hormone-resistant human breast cancer cells in culture with alpha-TS makes them sensitive to hormone treatment.[19] These observations on the effect of alpha-TS on hormone-sensitive tumors, if true in vivo, could have enormous impact in the treatment of hormone-resistant endocrine tumors, such as breast cancer and prostate cancer.

Recently, several esterase-resistant analogs of vitamin E have been synthesized. These include alpha-tocopheryl hemisuccinate, alpha-tocopheryl meleamide (alpha-Tam), alpha-tocopheryl malonate (alpha-TM), alpha-tocopheryl oxalate, alpha-tocopheryl oxbutyl sufonic acid, and alpha-tocopheryl oxyacetic acid (alpha-TEA). Some of them are toxic to both normal and cancer cells in culture, but

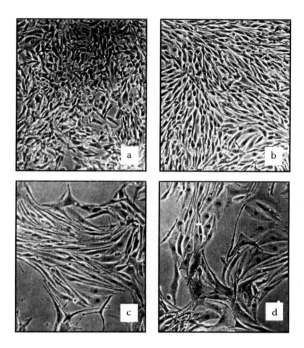

FIGURE 8.1 Melanoma cells (10^5) were plated in tissue culture dishes (60 mm) and D-alpha-tocopheryl succinate (alpha-TS) and sodium succinate, plus ethanol, were added to separate cultures 24 h after plating. Drugs and medium were changed at the second and third days after treatment. Photomicrographs were taken 4 days after treatment. Control cultures showed fibroblastic cells as well as round cells in clumps. Cultures treated with ethanol (1%) and sodium succinate (5–6 µg/ml) also exhibited fibroblastic morphology with fewer round cells (a). Alpha-TS–treated cultures of (b) 6 µg/ml and (c) 8 µg/ml showed a dramatic change in morphology at magnification × 300 (d). (From Prasad, K. N., and J. Edwards-Prasad, *Cancer Res* 42(2), 550–557, 1982.)

they did not show any toxicity in tumor bearing animal models.[20–25] Most studies with vitamin E have primarily utilized an intraperitoneal (IP) route of administration; however, some esterase-resistance vitamin E analogs maintained their effectiveness when administered orally.[21,23,24] The toxicity of these analogs in humans remains uncertain. In addition, these analogs of vitamin E will require FDA approval for human use. Until then, vitamin E succinate, which has been consumed by humans for decades, can be considered the best option for adding to a multiple micronutrient preparation for cancer prevention and improved treatment.

Vitamin C

The role of vitamin C in reducing the growth of cancer cells in humans has become a controversial issue. This may in part be due to the fact that the doses of vitamin C used in the study have varied from preventive to therapeutic doses. The antitumor activity of therapeutic doses of vitamin C is supported by the fact that several laboratory studies revealed that vitamin C at these doses inhibited the growth and migration of several animal and human cancer cell lines in culture and in animal models.[26–31]

Both IP and intravenous (IV) administration of therapeutic doses of vitamin C decreased the growth of murine hepatoma cells, whereas oral administration of the same dose was ineffective.[32] Thus, IV administration of therapeutic doses of vitamin C may be useful in treating human cancer. This route of injection was more effective in raising blood levels of vitamin C to therapeutic concentrations than IP or oral administration in rats.[33,34] The therapeutic doses of vitamin C kill some cancer cells by generating excessive amounts of hydrogen peroxide, but not normal cells in vivo.[34,35] These studies suggest that IV administration of therapeutic doses of vitamin C may produce beneficial effects in cancer patients with a poor prognosis and limited therapeutic options.

COMBINATION OF VITAMIN C OR VITAMIN E WITH OTHER AGENTS

Alpha-TS, in combination with tumor necrosis factor-related apoptosis-inducing ligand (TRAIL) and dendritic cells (stimulates immune function), caused complete tumor regression without causing adverse effects on normal cells.[36] Alpha-TS enhanced the therapeutic efficacy of a tolerated dose of Calcitriol in a prostate cancer xenograft mice model without any evidence of systemic toxicity or hypercalcemia.[37] Vitamin C, in combination with lysine, proline, and green tea extract, reduced the growth of a number of cancer cell lines, in vitro and in vivo, including melanoma cell lines.[38]

VITAMIN A AND CAROTENOIDS

Vitamin A and its derivatives, retinoids and carotenoids, induced differentiation, apoptosis, and growth inhibition on several human and rodent cancer cell lines, in vitro and in vivo, without affecting the growth of normal cells, and type of tumor cell, without producing similar effects on most normal cells in vitro and in vivo. Several reviews and articles have been published on this issue.[39–43] It has been reported that retinoic acid at therapeutic doses inhibited cell proliferation of human squamous cell carcinoma cell lines by decreasing ERK1 activation.[2]

Oral administration of carotenoids, including alpha-carotene and beta-carotene, lycopene, and canthaxanthin reduced the growth of prostate cancer cells and colon cancer cells in culture.[44–48] One of the mechanisms of the antitumor activity of beta-carotene may involve stimulation of T lymphocyte activity.[49]

SELENIUM

Therapeutic doses of selenium compounds (sodium selenite or seleno-L-methionine) inhibited the growth of several human and rodent cancer cells, including breast cancer and prostate cancer, in vitro and in animal models, without affecting the growth of normal cells.[3,50–55] Methyselenic, a metabolite of selenium, is more effective than sodium selenite or seleno-L-methionine.[56,57] The mechanisms of action of therapeutic doses of selenium on tumor growth appear to very complex and involve inhibition of the extracellular-regulated kinase1/2 (ERK1/2) signaling and cellular myelocytomatosis oncogenes (c-*myc*) expression, cyclin D expression, and enhancement of p27Kip1 and c-*jun* NH$_2$-terminal kinase activation, p53 protein expression, and unfolded protein response (UPR) expression.[50,54,56,58] Selenium treatment at therapeutic doses markedly reduced androgen signaling and androgen receptor–mediated gene expression, including PSA in human prostate cancer cells in culture,[59] and estrogen receptor alpha (ERalpha) expression in breast tumor cells in culture.[60]

Selenium, in combination with genistein, was more effective in inducing apoptosis in cancer cells than the individual agents.[61] Treatment of esophageal cancer cells, in culture with sodium selenite plus zinc, enhanced the levels of apoptosis in a synergistic manner.[62] Vitamin E succinate, in combination with methyselenic acid, was more effective in reducing the growth of prostate cancer cells in culture than either of these agents alone, without affecting the growth of normal prostate epithelial cells.[63] Treatment of tamoxifen-sensitive breast cancer cells with methylselenic acid potentiated the growth-inhibitory effects of tamoxifen; however, in tamoxifen-resistance breast cancer cells, treatment with both methyselenic acid and tamoxifen inhibited the growth of cancer cells more than that produced by methyselenic acid alone.[64]

MIXTURE OF DIETARY ANTIOXIDANTS

Individually, carotenoids, retinoic acid (13-*cis* retinoic acid), vitamin C (calcium ascorbate), and vitamin E (D-alpha-tocopheryl succinate) at certain doses did not inhibit the growth of human melanoma cells in culture; however, the mixture of these antioxidants and their derivatives at the same doses reduced the growth of cancer cells by about 50% (see Table 8.1). However, when a dose of vitamin C, which inhibited the growth of cancer cells by about 35%, was added to the mixture, it reduced the growth by about 90%.[65] These results suggest that a mixture of antioxidants should be used in any clinical studies that plan to investigate the efficacy of antioxidants in reducing the growth of tumor cells in humans.

NAC AND ALPHA-LIPOIC ACID

NAC at therapeutic doses reduced the growth of several rodent and human cancer cell lines in culture and in animal models by inducing apoptosis.[66–68] Apoptosis was preceded by increased production of reactive oxygen species (ROS), activation of the tumor suppressor gene, increased expression of Bax, release of cytochrome *c* from mitochondria, caspase activation, induction of proapoptotic signaling (i.e., JNK), and inhibition of antiapoptotic signaling (i.e., PKB/Akt) pathways.[67] NAC treatment also reduced the incidence and multiplicity of lymphoma in AT-mutated-deficient mice and increased their life span.[69] It has been reported that NAC treatment for 8 weeks induced antiangiogenesis by increasing the production of angiostatin, which resulted in endothelial apoptosis and vascular collapse in the tumor.[70] Others have also reported that NAC treatment inhibited angiogenesis and reduced growth of tumor cells in vitro and in animal models.[71] High-dose NAC treatment inhibited tumor growth by increasing the expressions of TNF-alpha on T-cell lymphocytes, and TNF-RI and TNF-RII on tumor cells and on T-cell lymphocytes.[72]

TABLE 8.1
Effect of a Mixture of Four Antioxidant Micronutrients on Growth of Human Melanoma Cells in Culture

Treatment	Cell Number (% of Controls)
Vit C (50 µg/ml)	102 ± 5[a]
PC (10 µg/ml)	96 ± 2
Alpha-TS (10 µg/ml)	102 ± 3
RA (7.5 µg/ml)	103 ± 3
Vit C (50 µg/ml) + PC (10 µg/ml) + Alpha-TS (10 µg/ml) + RA (7.5 µg/ml)	56 ± 3
Vit C (100 µg/ml)	64 ± 3
Vit C (100 µg/ml) + PC (1 µg/ml) + Alpha-TS (10 µg/ml) + RA (7.5 µg/ml)	13 ± 1

Source: Prasad, K. N., C. Hernandez, J. Edwards-Prasad, J. Nelson, T. Borus, and W. A. Robinson, *Nutr Cancer* 22 (3), 233–245, 1994.

Note: Data were summarized from a previous publication.[65]
PC, polar carotenoids, originally referred to as beta-carotene.[180] This is a more soluble fraction of carotenoids without the presence of beta-carotene. Vit C, sodium ascorbate; alpha-TS, alpha-tocopheryl succinate; RA, 13-cis-retinoic acid.

[a] Standard error of the mean.

Alpha-lipoic acid at therapeutic doses induced apoptosis in several cancer cell lines without affecting the normal cells.[67,73–75] The mechanisms of apoptosis involve increased generation of ROS, inhibition of TNF-alpha–induced activation of NF-kappaB, induction of proapoptotic signaling, and inhibition of antiapoptotic signaling.

COENZYME Q_{10}

There are no significant data on the effects of coenzyme Q_{10} alone on growth or survival of tumor cells in culture.

ANTIOXIDANT ENZYMES

Overexpression of Mn-SOD reduced the proliferation and suppressed the malignant phenotype of glioma cells[76] and melanoma cells[77] in culture.

TREATMENT SCHEDULES

Treatment schedule with therapeutic doses of antioxidants is also very important to produce a differential effect on normal and cancer cells. A short exposure time of a few hours, even at therapeutic doses of individual antioxidants, may not cause significant reduction in proliferation or apoptosis of cancer cells. Treatment time of at least 24 h or more is needed to observe a significant reduction in proliferation and apoptosis of cancer cells in culture, without affecting the growth of normal cells.

EFFECTS OF THERAPEUTIC DOSES OF INDIVIDUAL ANTIOXIDANTS ON GENE EXPRESSION PROFILES IN CANCER CELLS

Since therapeutic doses of antioxidants or their derivatives inhibited the growth of cancer cells but not of normal cells, the studies on the expression of genes that are involved in differentiation, growth inhibition, and apoptosis have been investigated only in cancer cells. These studies reveal that retinoids, vitamin E (alpha-TS and alpha-tocopherol), and beta-carotene inhibited as well as stimulated the levels of some cell signaling systems and gene expressions that can lead to decreased cell proliferation rates, increased differentiation, or apoptosis. Some of the changes in gene expression profiles following treatment with therapeutic doses of individual antioxidants include inhibitory as well as stimulatory events. The inhibitory events include decreased expression of c-*myc*, H-*ras*,[78] N-*myc*,[79] mutated p53[80], the activity of protein kinase C activity,[81,82] caspase,[83] tumor necrosis factor,[84] transcriptional factor E2F,[85] and Fas.[86] The stimulatory events include increased expression of wild type p53,[87] p21,[88] transforming growth factor beta (TGF-beta)[13] and the connexin gene.[89] Marked changes in gene expression have been observed as early as 30 min after treatment of neuroblastoma cells with a therapeutic dose of alpha-TS (see Figure 8.2). The changes in gene expression may be one of the major factors that account for the growth-inhibitory effect of alpha-TS on cancer cells.

In addition to changes in gene expression, a novel mechanism of action of alpha-TS has been reported in an animal tumor model. Alpha-TS at therapeutic doses inhibited the growth of tumor cells in vivo without affecting the growth of normal cells. It also reduced the expression of vascular endothelial growth factor (VEGF), and acted as an antiangiogenesis factor at a therapeutic dose that is not toxic to normal cells.[90] It has been reported that NAC at therapeutic doses also induced antiangiogenesis.[70] Others have reported that NAC treatment inhibited angiogenesis and reduced growth of tumor cells in vitro and in animal models.[71] It is unknown whether the therapeutic doses of retinoids, vitamin C, or beta-carotene, which also inhibited the growth of cancer cells, can cause similar effects on angiogenesis in vivo.

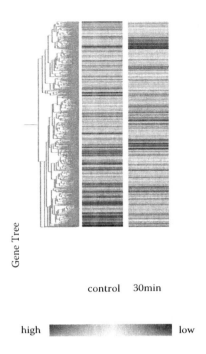

FIGURE 8.2 Hierarchical clustering analysis of gene array data 30 min after treatment with α-TS shows a marked alteration in the levels of gene expression. Lines in the first column represent the relatedness of the overall global gene expression pattern based on measures of gene similarity. (From Prasad, K. N., B. Kumar, X. D. Hanson, and W. C. Cole, *J Am Coll Nutr* 22(2), 108–117, 2003.)

EFFECTS OF PREVENTIVE DOSES OF INDIVIDUAL ANTIOXIDANTS ON CANCER CELL GROWTH

Low preventive doses of vitamin C stimulated the growth of human parotid cell carcinoma in culture.[10] Preventive doses of retinol and beta-carotene stimulated the growth of human pulmonary adenocarcinoma and immortalized human small airway epithelial cells in culture. These effects of micronutrients were associated with an elevated cAMP level and activated cAMP-dependent protein kinase A (PKA).[91] Low preventive doses of selenomethionine stimulated the growth of some cancer cells in vitro.[3] It has been reported that retinoic acid at low preventive doses induced cell proliferation in human squamous cell carcinoma cell lines in vitro by increased EGF signaling.[2]

EFFECTS OF THERAPEUTIC DOSES OF INDIVIDUAL ANTIOXIDANTS ON RADIATION-INDUCED DAMAGE IN CANCER CELLS AND NORMAL CELLS

CELL CULTURE STUDIES

Therapeutic doses of antioxidants or their derivatives enhanced the growth-inhibitory effects (due to apoptosis and proliferation inhibition) of irradiation selectively on cancer cells, while protecting or having no effects on normal cells. Retinoic acid enhanced the effect of irradiation on tumor cells by inhibiting the repair of potentially lethal damage in cancer cells more effectively than in normal fibroblasts.[92] Retinoic acid, in combination with interferon alpha-2a, enhanced radiation-induced damage on neck and head squamous cell carcinoma cells in culture.[93]

We have reported that the inhibitory concentration of vitamin E (alpha-TS) given before and/or after irradiation enhanced the level of radiation-induced decrease in mitotic accumulation[94] and

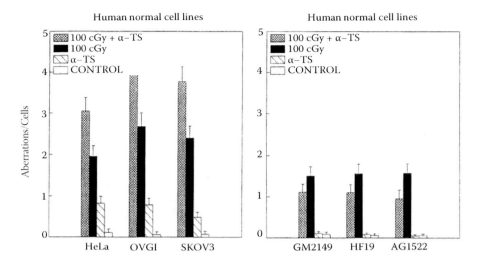

FIGURE 8.3 The effect of D-alpha-tocopheryl succinate (alpha-TS) on the level of radiation-induced chromosomal damage in human cervical cancer (HeLa cells), ovarian carcinoma cell lines (OVG1 and SKOV3), and in normal human skin fibroblasts (GM2149, HF19 and AG1522). Alpha-TS treatment alone increased chromosomal damage in all three cancer cell lines, but not in any normal cell lines. Alpha-TS treatment also enhanced the levels of radiation-induced chromosomal damage in cancer cells but protected normal cells against such damage. The bar is standard error of the mean and the difference between the control and experimental groups in cancer cells, and between the control (irradiation alone) and experimental groups (irradiation plus alpha-TS) is significant at $P < 0.05$. (From Kumar, B., N. Jha, W. C. Cole, J. S. Bedford, and K. N. Prasad, *J Am Coll Nutr* 21(4), 339–343, 2002.)

chromosomal damage[95] in human cervical cancer cells in culture (Figure 8.3). On the other hand, the same dose of alpha-TS did not modify the effect of irradiation on mitotic accumulation in normal cells,[94] but it protected normal cells against radiation-induced chromosomal damage.[95] In another study, we have reported that an aqueous form of vitamin E (alpha-tocopherol) and alpha-TS enhanced the level of radiation-induced growth inhibition in neuroblastoma (NB) cells (Figure 8.4).[12] Alpha-TS enhanced the growth-inhibitory effects of gamma-radiation in Ehrlich Ascites cells and human cervical and breast cancer cells in culture.[96] Vitamin C increased the growth-inhibitory effects of irradiation on NB cells, but not on glioma cells in culture.[11] Dehydroascorbic acid (DHA), the major metabolite of ascorbic acid, acts as a radiosensitizer for hypoxic tumor cells in culture.[97]

Selenomethionine at therapeutic doses enhanced the cell killing effect of ionizing radiation on two human lung cancer cell lines, but not on human diploid lung fibroblasts in culture.[98] This selective effect of selenium on tumor cell response to radiation is similar to those produced by other antioxidants.

ANIMAL STUDIES

Vitamin A (retinyl palmitate) or beta-carotene at therapeutic doses given daily through dietary supplement before x-irradiation and throughout the experimental period enhanced the levels of radiation damage on transplanted breast adenocarcinoma in mice, and protected normal tissue against some of the toxicity of local irradiation (Table 8.2).[99] The administration of vitamin C through drinking water before and after x-irradiation decreased the survival of ascites tumor cells in mice without causing a similar effect on normal cells.[100] The administration of multiple antioxidant micronutrients (vitamins A, C, and E) protected normal cells against damage produced by radio-immunotherapy in mice without protecting cancer cells.[101]

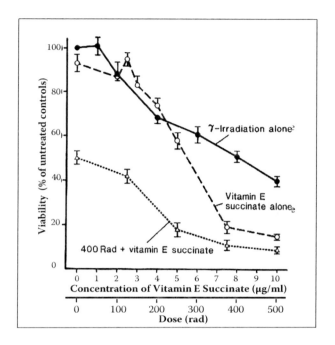

FIGURE 8.4 Vitamin E succinate and x-ray. Neuroblastoma cells (NBP2) were plated in tissue culture dishes (60 mm), and the cells were gamma-irradiated 24 h after plating. Vitamin E succinate and the solvent (ethanol 0.25% and sodium succinate 5 μg/ml) were added immediately before irradiation. The drugs and medium were changed after 2 days of treatment. The number of cells per dish was determined after 3 days of treatment. Each experiment was repeated at least twice involving 3 samples per treatment. The average value ($172 \pm 7 \times 10^4$) of untreated control NB cells was considered to be 100% and the growth in treated cultures was expressed as a percentage of untreated controls. The bar at each point is the standard error of the mean. (From Prasad, K. N., B. Kumar, X. D. Yuan, A. J. Hanson, and W. C. Cole, *J Am Coll Nutr* 22(2), 108–117, 2003.)

TABLE 8.2
Effect of Vitamin A, Beta-Carotene, and Local X-Irradiation on Survival of Mice with Transplanted Breast Adenocarcinoma

Treatment	No. of Mice	1-Year Survival (No. of Mice)
Control	24	0
3000 rads, single dose	24	0
Vitamin A	24	0
Beta-carotene	24	0
Vitamin A + x-ray	24	22
Beta-carotene + x-ray	24	22

Source: Seifter, E., A. Rettura, J. Padawar, S.M. Levenson, In *Vitamins, Nutrition and Cancer*, Karger, Basel, Switzerland, 1984, pp. 1–19.

Note: Diets were supplemented with vitamin A (3000 IU/mouse) and beta-carotene (270 μg/mouse), and these doses were about 10 times greater than the RDA for mice.

Supplementation with therapeutic doses of NAC reduced gamma radiation–induced DNA deletions in yeast, and DNA strand breaks in human lymphoblastic cells, in culture and in mice, but it did not protect against radiation-induced cell death.[102] This study does not reveal the consequence of this nutritional strategy on cancer cells. In view of the fact that cancer cells and normal cells respond differently to therapeutic doses of antioxidants, the results of this study on normal cells cannot be extrapolated to cancer cells.

CLINICAL STUDIES

Retinoic acid and interferon alpha-2a enhanced the efficacy of radiation therapy of locally advanced cervical cancer.[93] Treatment with dietary antioxidants reduced the effect of irradiation on normal tissues in patients with small-cell lung carcinoma.[103,104] Therapeutic doses (100 mg/day) of beta-carotene reduced radiation-induced mucositis without interfering with the efficacy of radiation therapy in patients with cancer of the head and neck.[105] A recent review discussed the pros and cons of using antioxidants in combination with radiation therapy.[106] In a randomized clinical trial involving 91 lung cancer patients, 44 patients received an oral dose of pentoxifylline (PTX) (400 mg, three times a day) and vitamin E (300 mg, twice a day) during the entire period of radiation therapy. These patients further received PTX (400 mg, once a day) and vitamin E (300 mg, once a day) 3 months after radiation therapy. A total of 47 patients were assigned as a control group. The median follow-up period was 13 months (3–28 months). The results showed that radiation-induced lung toxicity was more frequent in the control group than in the antioxidant-treated group.[107]

EFFECTS OF THERAPEUTIC DOSES OF INDIVIDUAL ANTIOXIDANTS ON CHEMOTHERAPEUTIC AGENT-INDUCED DAMAGE IN CANCER CELLS AND NORMAL CELLS

CELL CULTURE STUDIES

The effect of direct interaction between antioxidants and cancer therapeutic agents can initially best be tested on cancer cells in culture, because it is simple, and cost- and time-effective without any interference from complex molecules that are present in vivo. Several studies have revealed that vitamin C, alpha-TS, alpha-TA, vitamin A (including retinoids), and polar carotenoids including beta-carotene at therapeutic doses enhanced the growth-inhibitory effects of most chemotherapeutic agents on some cancer cells in culture.[1] Chemotherapeutic agents used in these studies include 5-FU, vincristine, Adriamycin, bleomycin, 5-(3,3-dimethyl-1-triazeno)-imidazole-4-carboximide (DTIC), cisplatin, tamoxifen, cyclophosphamide, mutamycin, chlorozotocin, and carmustine. The extent of this enhancement depends on the dose and form of the antioxidant, treatment schedule, dose and type of chemotherapeutic agent, and type of tumor cell. Some examples of the antioxidant-induced enhancement of the effect of chemotherapeutic agents are described below.

Vitamin C at therapeutic doses enhanced the effect of 5-fluouracil (5-FU) on neuroblastoma cells in culture (Figure 8.5).[31] Vitamin E succinate increased the effects of sodium butyrate.[108] Vitamin C at therapeutic doses increased the antitumor activity of doxorubicin, cisplatin, and paclitaxel in human breast cancer cells in culture.[109] Vitamin C also increased drug accumulation and reversed vincristine resistance of human non-small-cell lung carcinoma cells.[110] Vitamin C at therapeutic doses enhanced antitumor activity of 5-FU and cisplatin in esophageal cancer cells in culture by inhibiting translocation of NF-kappaB and AP-1.[111]

An aqueous form of vitamin E, alpha-tocopheryl acetate, at therapeutic doses enhanced the effect of vincristine on neuroblastoma cells in culture.[1] Alpha-TS increased the effect of adriamycin on human prostate carcinoma cells in culture.[112] Recently, we have found that alpha-TS increased the effect of adriamycin on human cervical cancer cells (HeLa) without modifying the effect of adriamycin on normal human fibroblasts in culture (our unpublished observation) (Table 8.3). Alpha-TS

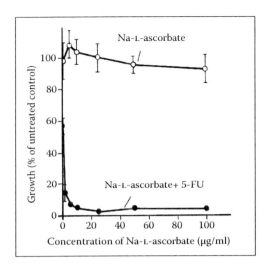

FIGURE 8.5 Effects on growth of P2 mouse neuroblastoma cells by sodium (Na-L) ascorbate with or without 5-FU. Neuroblastoma cells (50,000 per dish) were plated in tissue culture dishes (60 mm), and 5-FU (0.08 μg/ml), plus sodium ascorbate or sodium ascorbate alone, was added 24 h after plating. The drug and medium were changed every day, and the number of cells per dish was determined 3 days after treatment. Each value represents the mean of six to nine samples ± standard deviation. (From Prasad, K. N., P. K. Sinha, M. Ramanujam, and A. Sakamoto, *Proc Natl Acad Sci USA* 76(2), 829–832, 1979.)

also enhanced the effect of carmustine on rat glioma cells in culture (our unpublished observation). Alpha-tocopherol protected cisplatin-induced toxicity without interfering with its antitumor activity in human melanoma transplanted in athymic mice.[113]

Beta-carotene and lycopene at therapeutic doses also enhanced the growth-inhibitory effect of docetaxel on human ER+ MCF-7 breast cancer cells in culture.[114] A mixture of antioxidants

TABLE 8.3
Modification of Adriamycin Effect on Human Cervical Cancer Cells (HeLa) and Human Normal Skin Fibroblasts in Culture by D-Alpha-Tocopheryl Succinate

Treatment	HeLa Cells	Normal Fibroblasts
Solvent control	99 ± 2.6*	104 ± 3.4
Adriamycin (0.1 μg/ml)	57 ± 6.2	77 ± 2.4
Alpha-TS (10 μg/ml)	99 ± 1.6	101 ± 3.7
Adramycin (0.1 μg/ml) + alpha-TS	20 ± 7.9	77 ± 1.7
Adriamycin (0.25 μg/ml)	14 ± 2.9	68 ± 1.0
Adriamycin (0.25 μg/ml) + alpha-TS	5 ± 0.8	62 ± 1.8

Note: Cells (20,000) were plated in a 24-well chamber, and adriamycin and Alpha-tocopheryl succinate (alpha-TS) were added one after another at the same time. Drug, alpha-TS, and fresh growth medium were changed at 2 days after treatment and the viability of cells was determined by MTT assay. Growth in experimental groups was expressed in a percentage of the untreated control. Each experiment was repeated at least twice, and each value represents an average of 6–9 samples ± SEM (our unpublished observation).

[a] Standard error of the mean.

containing retinoic acid, vitamin C, alpha-TS, and polar carotenoids in combination with DTIC, tamoxifen, cisplatin, or interferon-alpha-2a inhibited the proliferation of human melanoma cells in culture more than the growth inhibition produced by the individual agents[65] (Table 8.4). Another study has reported that a mixture of dietary antioxidants (vitamin C, 100 µg/ml; alpha-tocopherol, 10 µg/ml; and beta-carotene, 10 µg/ml) by itself increased cytotoxicity from 4% to 15%, whereas carboplatin (0.5 µg/ml) and paclitaxel (0.05 µmol) increased cytotoxicity to 22% and 87%, respectively. However, the mixture of dietary antioxidants enhanced the apoptotic effect of paclitaxel and carboplatin.[115] The most pronounced effect was observed when the antioxidant mixture was given before treatment with chemotherapeutic agents, followed by paclitaxel treatment for 24 h, and then carboplatin treatment for 24 h (Table 8.5). This suggests that multiple antioxidants are also effective in enhancing the effect of certain chemotherapeutic agents on cancer cells.

Therapeutic doses of selenium compounds (sodium selenite and selenosulfate) reduced cisplatin-induced toxicity without compromising its efficacy on the growth of tumor cells in animal models; however, selenosulfate appeared to be less toxic. In addition, in a highly malignant cancer cell animal model, supplementation with selenosulfate and cisplatin produced a cure rate of 87.5% compared to a 25% cure rate observed in the cisplatin-treated group.[116] Sodium selenite and selenous acid induced growth inhibition in 5-FU–resistant cell lines.[117] Supplementation with selenium enhanced growth-inhibitory effects of taxol and doxorubicin in several tumor cell lines in culture.[118] Selenium nanoparticles enhanced the efficacy of adriamycin on tumor cells.[119] Another selenium compound, diphenylmethylselenocyanate, improved the antitumor activity of cyclophosphamide and, at the same time, reduced its toxicity.[120] There are substantial in vitro studies showing that the selenium compound enhanced the antitumor activity of several types of human and rodent cancer cell lines, while protecting or having no effect on normal cells. However, organic selenium at therapeutic doses (0.2 mg/mouse/day or 10 mg per kg of body weight per day) enhanced the treatment efficacy of some chemotherapeutic agents in athymic mice bearing human squamous cell carcinoma of the

TABLE 8.4
Enhancement of the Effect of Certain Chemotherapeutic Agents by a Mixture of Four Antioxidants on Human Melanoma Cells in Culture

Treatment	Cell Number (% of Controls)
Solvent	101 ± 4[a]
Cisplatin (1 µg/ml)	67 ± 4
Antioxidant mixture	56 ± 3
Cisplatin + antioxidant mixture	38 ± 2
Tamoxifen (2 µg/ml)	81 ± 3
Tamoxifen + antioxidant mixture	30 ± 2
DTIC (100 µg/ml)	71 ± 2
DTIC + antioxidant mixture	38 ± 2
Interferon-alpha2b	82 ± 5
Interferon-alpha2b + antioxidant mixture	29 ± 1

Source: Prasad, K. N., C. Hernandez, J. Edwards-Prasad, J. Nelson, T. Borus, and W. A. Robinson, *Nutr Cancer* 22 (3), 233–245, 1994.

Note: Data were summarized from a previous publication.[65]
Polar carotenoids were originally referred to as beta-carotene.[94]
Vitamin C, 50 µg/ml; polar carotenoids, 10 µg/ml; alpha-tocopheryl succinate, 10 µg/ml; and 13-cis-retinoic acid, 7.5 µg/ml, were added simultaneously.

[a] Standard error of the mean.

TABLE 8.5
Flow-Cytometric Analysis of the Effect of a Combination of the Agents (Paclitaxel, Carboplatin, and Antioxidant Mixture) on Apoptosis in H520 Cells

Serial No.	Treatment of Cells				Apoptosis (% Cells) (Mean ± SE[a]) (Day 5)
	Day 1	Day 2	Day 3	Day 4	
1	Cells plated	–	–	–	20.6 ± 1.2
2	Cells plated	Paclitaxel + carboplatin	–	–	40.3 ± 3.1
3	Cells plated	Paclitaxel	Carboplatin	–	54.3 ± 2.2
4	Cells plated	Vitamins + Paclitaxel	Carboplatin	–	70.11 ± 3.7
5	Cells plated	Vitamins	Paclitaxel	Carboplatin	89.15 ± 4.3

Source: Pathak, A. K., N. Singh, N. Khanna, V. G. Reddy, K. N. Prasad, and V. Kochupillai, *J Am Coll Nutr* 21(5), 416–421, 2002.

Note: Cells were plated on day 1 and flow-cytometry was performed on day 5. Control, serial no. 1. Doses: Paclitaxel, 0.05 μmol/ml; Carboplatin, 0.5 μg/ml; vitamin C, 100 μg/ml; vitamin E, 10 μg/ml; beta-carotene, 10 μg/ml.[115]

[a] SE, standard error. Results are of three separate experiments, each performed in duplicate.

head and neck.[121] The observations could be very exciting if a similar observation is made in human cancer without unacceptable toxicity.

ANIMAL STUDIES

A few in vivo studies support the concept that therapeutic doses of antioxidants selectively enhanced the effect of chemotherapeutic agents on tumor cells by increasing the tumor response. For example, vitamin A (retinyl palmitate) or synthetic beta-carotene at therapeutic doses, which were tenfold higher than the RDA values for these micronutrients, in combination with cyclophosphamide, increased the cure rate from 0% to more than 90% in mice with transplanted adenocarcinoma of the breast.[99] A study using a thiol-containing antioxidant, pyrrolidinedithiocarbamate (PDTC), and a water-soluble vitamin E analog (6-hydroxy-2,5,7,8-tetramethylchroman-2-carboxylic acid; vitamin E), showed that antioxidant treatment enhanced the antitumor effects of 5-FU in athymic mice with human colorectal cancer.[88] The synthetic retinoid (fenretinide) was effective against a human ovarian carcinoma xenograft and potentiated cisplatin activity.[122]

IP administration of NAC (200 mg per kg of body weight) enhanced the cytotoxic effects of 5-FU in athymic mice carrying human colon cancer cells without increasing the toxicity.[123] The IV route of administration of NAC (800 mg/kg of body weight) was effective in reducing cisplatin-induced nephrotoxicity in normal rats, whereas the IP route was ineffective. Oral or IP administration of NAC (400 mg per kg of body weight) was ineffective in protecting against cisplatin-induced renal toxicity, whereas IV administration of 50 mg per kg was effective. Therefore, the neuroprotective effects of NAC are dependent on the dose and route of administration. A study has reported that NAC at a therapeutic dose of 1g per kg of body weight, delivered IP in combination with doxorubicin, reduced tumorigenicity and metastasis following transplantation of B-16 murine melanoma cells in mice.[68]

CLINICAL STUDIES

In a recent analysis of 845 published articles, 19 trials with antioxidants in combination with standard chemotherapy were performed using randomized, controlled experimental designs. Only the results of randomized trials were evaluated. Vitamins A, C, and E, NAC, melatonin, and ellagic acid were used individually. In two of these studies, a mixture of antioxidants was used. The analysis of data revealed that antioxidant supplementation did not reduce the efficacy of chemotherapy. Many of these studies showed that supplementation with antioxidants resulted in increased survival times, increased tumor responses, or both, as well as lower toxicity than controls.[124] The sample size in these studies lacked adequate statistical power. The therapeutic doses were used primarily. Nevertheless, these studies clearly show that the fear of oncologists that antioxidant supplementation might compromise the efficacy of chemotherapy is not justified. The role of individual antioxidants in enhancing the growth-inhibitory effects of cancer therapeutic agents on human tumors is described below.

A review of three studies revealed that vitamin C, in combination with BCG, produced beneficial effects in patients with bladder cancer, and that vitamin, E in combination with omega-3 fatty acids, increased survival in patients with advanced cancer.[125] Analysis of 38 studies showed that vitamin C or vitamin E alone produced some beneficial effects on the survival of cancer patients.[125]

Glutathione-Elevating Agents (NAC and Alpha-Lipoic Acid)

In a randomized, placebo-controlled trial, oral supplementation with 1200 mg NAC as an adjunct to standard chemotherapy (oxaliplatin, 5-fluorouracil, and leucovorin) markedly reduced the incidence of sensory neuropathy (grades 2–4) from 57% (placebo group) to 7% (NAC group) in colon cancer patients with four or more regional lymph nodes metastasis (N2 disease).[126] There were no significant electrophysiological changes in the placebo or NAC group after completion of 12 cycles of chemotherapy. The sample size for this trial is too small to make any conclusive statement, but the results of this pilot clinical study are very impressive.

In a randomized, double-blind, placebo-controlled trial involving 52 cancer patients receiving oxaliplatin-based chemotherapy, infusion of glutathione (1500 mg/m^2) or saline over a 15-min period before administration of oxaliplatin markedly reduced sensory neuropathy. At the end of 12 cycles of chemotherapy, glutathione treatment reduced the incidence of sensory neuropathy (grades 2–4) from 42% (placebo group) to 14% (glutathione group).[127] It is important to point out that this antioxidant treatment did not reduce clinical activity of oxaliplatin. In an open, nonrandomized, clinical study, patients with advanced cancer at different sites were treated with high-dose antioxidants (alpha-lipoic acid orally, NAC IV, and amifostine IV, individually or in combination with vitamin A, vitamin E, and vitamin C) orally for 10 days. The results showed that they reduced serum levels of proinflammatory cytokines, IL-6, and TNF-alpha in these patients.[128]

Patients with advanced terminal pancreatic cancer often lose hope for any chance of prolonged survival with good quality of life. IV administration of therapeutic doses of alpha-lipoic acid, together with a low-dose naltrexone and a healthy lifestyle program, markedly improved the survival time and quality of life of these patients.[129]

In a randomized trial involving 50 patients with cancer of the head and neck, amifostine (300 mg/m^2) was combined with standard radiation therapy and chemotherapy. Amifostine was administered intravenously 15–30 min before radiation for a period of 6 to 7.5 weeks. The results showed that amifostine treatment did not significantly affect clinical outcomes. The amifostine-treated group showed a 90.9% complete response, whereas the control group showed a 78.3% complete response. However, amifostine treatment provided significant reduction in grade 2 xerostomia (4.5%) compared to the control group (30.4%).[130]

Coenzyme Q_{10}

In five patients with breast cancer, an oral supplementation with a therapeutic dose (390 mg/day) of coenzyme Q_{10}, as an adjunct to standard therapy, markedly reduced tumor size and metastasis.[131] A review of six studies, including three randomized and three nonrandomized clinical trials, revealed that an oral administration of coenzyme Q_{10} in combination with anthracyclines (five out of six studies) reduced cardiac and liver toxicity.[132] An oral administration of coenzyme Q_{10} at a therapeutic dose (400 mg/day), in combination with a low dose of recombinant interferon alpha-2b for a period of 3 years, decreased rates of recurrence of tumors in patients with stage I and stage II melanoma after surgical removal.[133] Tamoxifen has been found to increase disease-free time and overall survival of women after primary surgery for breast cancer; however, this drug causes hypertriglyceridemia by reducing the activity of lipolytic enzymes on triglycerides. It also induces angiogenesis and, thereby, causes metastasis. An oral administration of a preventive dose of coenzyme Q_{10} (100 mg/day) and a low dose of tamoxifen to patients with breast cancer reduced angiogenesis and hyperlipidemia.[134] A mixture of micronutrients containing 100 mg coenzyme Q_{10}, 50 mg niacin, and 10 mg riboflavin, when administered orally in combination with tamoxifen daily for 90 days, reduced all lipid and lipoprotein abnormalities to near normal levels.[135] In a randomized clinical trial involving 84 breast cancer patients, the same micronutrient mixture in combination with tamoxifen, when administered orally for a period of 45 and 90 days, decreased the levels of proangiogenic factors and increased the levels of antiangiogenic factors.[136]

In 32 patients with breast cancer, aged 32–81 years with a high-risk classification because of tumor spread to the lymph nodes in the axilla, the effect of a nutritional protocol in combination with standard therapy was evaluated. The nutritional protocol contained 2850 mg vitamin C, 2500 IU vitamin E, 32.5 IU beta-carotene, 387 μg selenium, secondary vitamins and minerals, essential fatty acids (1.2 g gamma linolenic acid and 3.5 g omega-3 fatty acids), and 90 mg coenzyme Q_{10}, and was administered orally. The results showed that none of the patients died during the study period (the expected number was four), no evidence of further metastasis, improved quality of life (no weight loss and reduced use of pain medications), and six patients showed apparent partial remission.[137]

Vitamin E

The effect of high-dose vitamin E (600 mg, orally) on cisplatin-induced peripheral neuropathy was evaluated in a randomized control trial. Fourteen patients received the vitamin E during chemotherapy and 3 months after the cessation of treatment, while 16 patients received no vitamin E during chemotherapy. The incidence of peripheral neuropathy in the vitamin E group was about 21%, whereas it was 68.5% in the control group.[138,139] No adverse effect from the vitamin E was observed in this study. Similar results were obtained with an oral dose of 300 mg vitamin E administered during cisplatin treatment 3 months after the cessation of treatment in another clinical study with 27 cancer patients (13 patients in the vitamin E group and 14 patients in the control group).[140] In a preclinic study, the combination of vitamin E did not interfere with the efficacy of cisplatin in reducing tumor growth. These pilot studies, although not sufficient to make any definitive conclusions, are very encouraging. Supplementation with high-dose vitamin E alone improved immune function in patients with advance colorectal cancer.[141]

Selenium

A review of several clinical studies suggest that supplementation with selenium alone, in combination with radiation therapy, chemotherapy, or surgery did not provide any beneficial effects in reducing toxicity of therapy or improving the quality of life.[142]

Glutamine

In a randomized clinical study involving 86 patients with metastatic colorectal cancer, the efficacy of orally administered glutamine in reducing chemotherapy-induced peripheral neuropathy was evaluated. In this study, 42 patients received glutamine and chemotherapy, and 44 patients received only chemotherapy. Glutamine was administered at a dose of 15 g twice a day for 7 consecutive days every 2 weeks, starting on the day of the oxaliplatin infusion. After completion of therapy, the incidence of peripheral neuropathy in the glutamine group was 11.9%, whereas in the chemotherapy group, it was 31.8%, about a threefold improvement.[143]

MECHANISMS OF ENHANCING THE EFFICACY OF STANDARD THERAPY ON CANCER CELLS BY THERAPEUTIC DOSES OF INDIVIDUAL ANTIOXIDANTS

The exact reasons for the dietary antioxidant-induced enhancement of damage produced by standard therapeutic agents on cancer cells are unknown. We propose that treatment of tumor cells with therapeutic doses of dietary antioxidants before standard therapy can initiate damage in cancer cells, but not in normal cells. Free radicals generated by therapeutic agents, even if completely quenched by antioxidants, become irrelevant because damaged cancer cells suffer further injuries by mechanisms other than free radicals associated with therapeutic agents. The damage to cancer cells is further enhanced by the fact that micronutrients such as retinoic acid can inhibit the repair of radiation damage in cancer cells.[92] It has been reported that alpha-TS–induced apoptosis in cancer cells is independent of p53 and p21,[14] whereas, 5-FU–induced apoptosis is mediated via p53 and p21.[88] Therefore, the combination of two agents may be more effective than the individual agents. High expression of c-*myc* and H-*ras* oncogenes increased the radio-resistance of cancer cells,[144] while the expression of c-*myc* and H-*ras* was reduced by alpha-TS treatment.[12] Therefore, the combination of radiation and alpha-TS caused more cell death than the individual agents alone. Alpha-TS in vivo acts as an antiangiogenesis agent;[90] whereas, radiation or chemotherapeutic agents do not. Therefore, the combination of alpha-TS with these therapeutic agents may be more effective than the individual agents. The effect of therapeutic doses of dietary antioxidants in enhancing the level of damage in cancer cells produced by x-irradiation or chemotherapeutic agents is not due to their antioxidant activity or their differential accumulation in the cells.[95] These dietary antioxidants and their derivatives do not initiate damage in normal cells before standard therapy; therefore, when these cells are treated with radiation or chemotherapeutic agents, they can be protected by antioxidants through their classical antioxidant activity. The exact mechanisms of enhancement of radiation-induced or chemotherapeutic agent–induced damage on cancer cells remain unknown.

CLINICAL STUDIES WITH MULTIPLE DIETARY ANTIOXIDANTS

Eighteen nonrandomized patients with small-cell lung cancer received multiple antioxidant treatments with chemotherapy and/or radiation. The median survival time was markedly enhanced and patients tolerated chemotherapy and irradiation well.[103] Similar observations were made in several private practice settings.[104] A randomized pilot trial (Phase I/II) with high-dose multiple micronutrients including dietary antioxidants and their derivatives (Sevak, a multiple vitamin preparation, 8 g vitamin C as calcium ascorbate, 800 IU vitamin E as alpha-TS, and 60 mg natural beta-carotene, orally, divided into two doses, half in the morning and half in the evening) in patients with 0-III breast cancer receiving radiation therapy has been completed.[145] There were 25 patients in the radiation arm and 22 patients in the combination arm. A follow-up period of 22 months, during which no maintenance supplements were given, show that one patient in the radiation arm developed a new cancer in the contralateral breast, and another in the same arm developed lobular carcinoma in situ (LCIS) in the opposite breast. In the combination arm, no new tumor has developed.

A randomized trial with high-dose multiple antioxidants involving 136 patients of stage IIIb and stage IV non-small-cell lung cancer were conducted to evaluate the efficacy of antioxidants in modifying the response of tumor cells to chemotherapy (paclitaxel and carboplatin). The control arm received only chemotherapy, while the treatment arm received chemotherapy plus high-dose multiple antioxidants (6100 mg vitamin C as ascorbic acid, 1050 mg of vitamin E as DL-alpha tocopheryl succinate, 60 mg synthetic beta-carotene). The preparation of vitamin E also contained selenium, copper sulfate, and zinc sulfate. Antioxidants were administered once a day orally and continued for the entire treatment period. The follow-up period was 2 years. The results showed that 48.6% of patients in the control arm (total 72 patients) completed six cycles of chemotherapy, whereas in the treatment arm (total patients 64), 56.2% completed six cycles of chemotherapy. In the control arm,

TABLE 8.6
Preliminary Results of a Randomized Clinical Trial Using High Dose Multiple Antioxidants as an Adjunct to Chemotherapy

Tumor Response and Survival	Chemotherapy Arm (No. of Patients = 72)	Chemo + Antioxidant (No. of Patients = 64)
Complete response	0	2
Partial response	32%	45%
Overall survival at 1 year	32.9%	39.1%
Overall survival at 1 year	11.1%	15.6%
Median survival time	9 months	11 months

Source: Pathak, A. K., M. Bhutani, R. Guleria, S. Bal, A. Mohan, B. K. Mohanti, A. Sharma, et al., *J Am Coll Nutr* 24(1), 16–21, 2005.

Note: Ascorbic acid, 6100 mg; DL-alpha-tocopheryl succinate, 1050 mg; beta-carotene (synthetic), 60 mg. The vitamin E succinate preparation also contained copper sulfate, manganese sulfate, zinc sulfate, and selenium. The antioxidant was administered daily, orally, 48 h before chemotherapy and continued every day for the entire treatment period.[146]

there was no complete response (CR); however, 2 CRs were observed in the treatment arm. The overall survival in the control arm at 1 and 2 years was 32.9% and 11.1%, respectively, whereas it was 39.1% and 15.6%, respectively, in the treatment arm (Table 8.6). The mean survival time in the control and treatment arms was 9 and 11 months, respectively.[146] There was no difference in toxicity between the two arms. The sample size was small and there was no significant difference on any measures of outcomes. Nevertheless, these results do not support the concern of oncologists that high doses of multiple antioxidants may protect cancer cells from the free radical damage induced by radiation or chemotherapy.

Based on the beneficial effects of multiple antioxidants in combination with standard therapy on two patients with ovarian cancer,[147] Dr. Drisko has started a new trial with multiple antioxidants on ovarian cancers. Cell cultures, animal studies, and limited human studies suggest that a well-designed trial with therapeutic doses of multiple antioxidants, when administered orally before and for the entire treatment period, is urgently needed.

RATIONAL FOR USING MULTIPLE MICRONUTRIENTS

Multiple micronutrients including dietary and endogenous antioxidants are recommended because they are distributed differently in organs and within the same cells, and because their mechanisms of action, in part, different from each other. The combination of two or more antioxidants produced an additive or synergistic effect on growth inhibition of cancer cells. The form and type of vitamin E used are also important to improve its beneficial effects. It is known that various organs of rats selectively absorb the natural form of vitamin E[148] and it has been established that alpha tocopheryl-succinate (alpha-TS) is the most effective form.[12] We have reported that oral ingestion of alpha-TS (800 IU/day) for more than 6 months in humans increased plasma levels of not only alpha-tocopherol, but also of alpha-TS, suggesting that alpha-TS can be absorbed from the intestinal tract without hydrolysis to alpha-tocopherol, provided the pool of alpha-tocopherol in the body has become saturated.[12] The therapeutic doses of selenium inhibited the growth of cancer cells; therefore, they should be added to a multiple micronutrient preparation.

Glutathione represents a potent intracellular antioxidant; however, an oral supplementation with glutathione failed to significantly increase plasma levels of glutathione in human subjects,[149] suggesting that this tripeptide is completely hydrolyzed in the gastrointestinal tract. NAC and alpha-lipoic acid increase the intracellular levels of glutathione and, therefore, can be used in combination to elevate intracellular levels of glutathione. Coenzyme Q_{10} is needed by the mitochondria to generate energy, but at high doses it increased the efficacy of radiation therapy on cancer cells. In addition, B-vitamins and vitamin D should be added for the purpose of general health.

RATIONALE FOR NOT RECOMMENDING ANTIOXIDANT SUPPLEMENTS DURING STANDARD THERAPY

The experimental studies discussed in this section serve as the primary basis for *not* recommending antioxidants during radiation or chemotherapy.

Preventive Doses of Individual Antioxidants Reduce the Efficacy of Cancer Therapeutic Agents

Several studies have shown that preventive doses of antioxidants that do not affect the proliferation of cancer cells, when administered only one time shortly before cancer therapeutic agents, reduced the efficacy of therapeutic agents. Vitamin E (alpha-tocopherol), vitamin C, or NAC, when given in a single, low preventive dose shortly before x-irradiation reduced the effectiveness of irradiation on cancer cells in culture and in vivo models.[5–7,144] Treatment of tumor cells in culture (leukemia and lymphoma cell lines) with low preventive doses of vitamin C reduced the cytotoxicity induced by doxorubicin, cisplatin, vincristine, and methotrexate.[9] Low preventive doses of vitamin C administered before doxorubicin treatment reduced therapeutic efficacy of this chemotherapy in mice with xenogeneic lymphoma tumor.[9] Preventive doses of antioxidants used in these studies do not affect the growth of cancer cells. Alpha-lipoic acid at preventive doses reduced the effectiveness of doxorubicin in murine leukemia.[150] NAC at a preventive dose reduced cisplatin-induced apoptosis from about 31% to about 11% in bladder cancer cells.[8] This is also in contrast to animal studies in which supplementation with a therapeutic dose of NAC enhanced the effectiveness of chemotherapeutic agents. Overexpression of antioxidant enzymes such as mitochondrial manganese-superoxide dismutase (Mn-SOD) in tumor cells decreased their response to radiation.[151,152] Therefore, the use of preventive doses of antioxidants during radiation therapy or chemotherapy may be harmful.

It should be pointed out that rodents exhibit a high degree of resistance to most therapeutic agents. For example, antiangiogenesis drugs, amifostine, and proteasome inhibitors, that were found to be very effective in reducing the growth of tumor cells or enhancing the efficacy of cancer therapeutic agents were found to be toxic in humans and, therefore, their clinical relevance remained limited. Thus, doses of antioxidants that are used in animal studies cannot be extrapolated to calculate the doses that would be relevant for human studies.

Utilization of Data Obtained from the Use of Preventive Doses of Individual Antioxidants in High-Risk Populations

There are no cancer treatment trials indicating that therapeutic doses of multiple antioxidants, when given before therapy and every day thereafter for the entire treatment period, have ever reduced the efficacy of radiation therapy or chemotherapy. Studies often quoted are those that are either epidemiologic studies or intervention trials with one or more antioxidants in high-risk populations, such as heavy tobacco smokers, in which preventive doses of individual antioxidants were used. For example, an oral daily administration of synthetic beta-carotene (25 mg) increased the incidence of lung cancer among male heavy smokers by 17%.[153,154] These studies are often quoted as evidence for not recommending any antioxidants during cancer therapy. Heavy smokers have a high body oxidative environment; therefore, any single antioxidant, including beta-carotene, would be oxidized to form free radicals that can increase the risk of lung cancer. Thus, the increased risk of cancer among male heavy smokers following supplementation with a preventive dose of beta-carotene could have been predicted.

An epidemiologic study[155] analyzed 90 patients with breast cancer who took vitamin and mineral regimens within 180 days of diagnosis and continued for a 2-month period, whether or not they received radiation therapy, chemotherapy, or both. These treatment variables were stratified and, therefore, were not corrected for in data analysis. The follow-up period varied from 20 to 133 months, with a median value of 48 months. No information was provided on whether or not the patients were taking a vitamin and mineral supplement during the follow-up period. The vitamin and mineral doses, number of agents, and the percentage of patients taking the vitamins and minerals were also markedly varied. Beta-carotene doses varied from 0 to 250,000 IU; vitamin B_3 doses varied from 0 to greater than 1 mg; no dose was given for coenzyme Q_{10}; vitamin C doses varied from 1 to 24 g; selenium doses varied from 0 to 1,000 µg; and zinc doses varied from 0 to greater than 50 mg. Among 90 patients, 2% took three agents (no name of agents or doses were mentioned), 23% took four agents (no names of agents or doses mentioned), 56% took five agents (no names of agents or doses mentioned) and 19% took all six agents (no doses were given). These confounding variables were not accounted for while analyzing data. Based on these data, the authors concluded that breast cancer-specific survival and disease-free survival times were not improved by the above vitamin and mineral regimes. Unfortunately, presentation of data without correcting for prognostic and demographic factors alone revealed that patients taking the vitamin and mineral supplements as described in this study produced poor survival and disease-free survival times in comparison to historical controls receiving conventional therapy. The presentation of such data appears to be inconsistent with the author's conclusion and creates a lot of confusion among the public and professionals. Thus, the extrapolation of data obtained from the epidemiologic cancer prevention studies to cancer treatment may be incorrect and misleading.

In a randomized, double-blind, placebo-controlled trial involving 540 patients with stage I or stage II head and neck cancer who received radiation therapy with placebo or radiation therapy with synthetic antioxidants (DL-alpha-tocopherol 400 IU, and beta-carotene 30 mg), and were followed for 3 years. The supplementation with beta-carotene was discontinued after 156 patients were enrolled in the trial because of ethical concerns. The remaining 384 patients continued to receive alpha-tocopherol alone. The results showed that supplementation with vitamin E among smokers enhanced the incidence of recurrence of primary tumors and death due to cancer or from all causes.[156] Several issues can be raised with the design of the experiments. The preventive dose of vitamin E that was used in the cancer prevention trial was used during radiation therapy. Low-dose vitamin E is known to reduce radiation damage in both normal and cancer cells. This is not true with therapeutic doses (high doses) of vitamin E (alpha-TS) or other antioxidants that selectively enhanced the growth-inhibitory effects of radiation on cancer cells, but not on normal cells. Therefore, the conclusion that vitamin E alone and smoking should be strongly discouraged to patients with cancer of the head and neck undergoing radiation therapy would be consistent with the data. Unfortunately, the authors concluded, "Particular attention should be devoted to prevent patients from smoking and taking antioxidant supplements during radiation therapy."[156] This conclusion, with respect to antioxidant supplements, is inaccurate because a preventive dose of vitamin E was used in treatment protocol and, therefore, the results of such a study should not be extrapolated to therapeutic doses of one or multiple antioxidants.

UTILIZATION OF DATA OBTAINED FROM THE USE OF ANTIOXIDANT DEFICIENCY IN COMBINATION WITH THERAPEUTIC AGENTS ON CANCER CELLS

Using transgenic mice with brain tumors, it was reported[157] that a diet deficient in vitamins A and E increased apoptosis by about 5-fold and reduced tumor volume by about 50% after 4 months on the diet in comparison to a standard diet or a diet rich in vitamins A and E (2-fold more than that in standard diet). No evidence of apoptosis was found in spleen, small intestine, or liver. From results such as this, it was inferred that if the deficiency of antioxidants reduces the growth of cancer cells, then an excess of them may stimulate their growth. This inference is not applicable to therapeutic doses of dietary antioxidants that cause proliferation inhibition and/or apoptosis in cancer cells without affecting most normal cells. It should be pointed out that a deficiency in vitamins A and E may induce irreversible neurological and neuromuscular damage, and other toxicities. Furthermore, such an antioxidant-deficient diet before treatment may enhance the effect of x-irradiation or chemotherapeutic agents on both cancer cells and normal cells. Therefore, creating an antioxidant deficiency before standard therapy may not be useful in the management of cancer.

EFFECTS OF THERAPEUTIC DOSES OF INDIVIDUAL ANTIOXIDANTS IN COMBINATION WITH EXPERIMENTAL CANCER THERAPIES ON CANCER CELLS

Hyperthermia

Hyperthermia (43°C to 45°C) alone, or in combination with radiation, is primarily used in the management of local tumors when all other therapeutic modalities have failed. This approach has not been effective for the long-term management of tumors. Therefore, the current treatment approaches must be altered from local hyperthermia at higher temperatures to whole-body hyperthermia at lower temperatures that could be tolerated without the side effects. In addition, nontoxic therapeutic doses of antioxidants could be used to enhance the efficacy of hyperthermia on cancer cells. We have reported[158] that alpha-TS markedly increased the growth-inhibitory effect of low temperature (41°C) and high temperature (43°C) hyperthermia on neuroblastoma cells in culture (Table 8.7). We propose that multiple antioxidants in combination with hyperthermia (local or whole body) may further improve the efficacy of hyperthermia in the treatment of human cancer. Local administration of vitamin C markedly enhanced the efficacy of hyperthermia in reducing the growth of Lewis tumors in mice.[159] Therapeutic doses of vitamin C in combination with hyperthermia increased the survival time of mice carrying Ehrlich ascites tumor cells, compared to untreated controls.[160] Bioflavonoid Quercetin, in combination with hyperthermia, caused synergistic apoptosis in lymphoid cancer cells in culture.[161] Quercetin and tamoxifen together enhanced hyperthermia-induced

TABLE 8.7
Effect of Alpha-TS on Hyperthermia-Induced Growth Inhibition in Neuroblastoma Cells in Culture

Treatment	Cell Number (% of Controls)
Solvent ethanol (0.25%) + sodium succinate (5 µg/ml)	102 ± 3
Alpha-TS (5 µg/ml)	50 ± 3
43°C (20 min)	56 ± 3
Alpha-TS + 43°C	43 ± 1
41°C (45 min)	56 ± 3
Alpha-TS + 41°C	21 ± 2
40°C (8 h)	55 ± 2
Alpha-TS + 40°C	30 ± 2

Source: Rama, B. N., and K. N. Prasad, *Life Sci*, 34 (21), 2089–2097, 1984.

Note: Data were summarized from a previous publication. Values are mean ± SEM.[158]

apoptosis in a synergistic manner in human melanoma cells in culture.[162] Quercetin may also be useful in increasing tumor responses to hyperthermia in combination chemotherapy.[163,164] I propose that a multiple micronutrient protocol may also enhance the efficacy of hyperthermia in the management of human cancer.

SODIUM BUTYRATE AND INTERFERON-ALPHA2B

Butyric acid, a 4-carbon fatty acid, that is a potent inhibitor of histone deacetylase[108,165,166] or its analog, phenylbutyrate,[167,168] induced apoptosis and inhibition of cell proliferation in several rodent and human tumor cell lines in culture. However, clinical studies with these agents produced minimal benefits in cancer patients.[169] Therefore, any agents that can enhance the effect of sodium butyrate or phenylbutyrate would enhance the value of these agents in clinical studies. We have reported that alpha-TS at therapeutic doses enhanced the growth-inhibitory effect of sodium butyrate on certain tumor cells in culture (Figure 8.6).[170] Retinoic acid increased the effect of phenylbutyrate on human prostate cancer cell growth and angiogenesis in athymic mice.[171] Retinoic acid in combination with sodium butyrate also caused a synergistic effect on cell differentiation in poorly differentiated thyroid carcinoma cells in culture; however, in athymic mice carrying the same tumor, the combination of the two agents did not reduce the growth of tumors more than that produced by retinoic acid treatment alone.[172] Antioxidants such as quercetin, curcumin, and ferulic acid enhanced sodium butyrate–induced apoptosis in human erythroleukemic cells in culture.[173]

Alpha-TS[65] and retinoids[93] also enhance the effect of interferon in cell culture and in vivo, respectively. Although treatment of squamous cell carcinoma of the head and neck in culture with retinoic acid, interferon-alpha2a, and alpha-tocopherol, individually or in combinations of two, produced varying degrees of growth inhibition. The combination of three was most effective.[174] The combination of 13-*cis* retinoic acid and interferon-alpha2a enhanced radiation-induced growth inhibition in human cervical carcinoma cells in culture.[175]

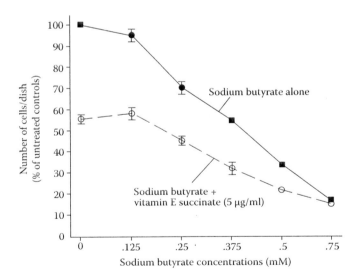

FIGURE 8.6 Effect of D-alpha-tocopheryl succinate (vitamin E succinate) in combination with sodium butyrate on the growth of neuroblastoma cells in culture. Cells (50,000 cells/60 mm dish) were plated in tissue culture dishes, and vitamin E succinate and sodium butyrate were added, one after another, 24 h later. Growth medium and agents were changed at 2 days after treatment and growth was determined at 3 days after treatment. Each value represents an average of six samples. The bar at each point is SEM. (From Rama, B. N., and K. N. Prasad, *Int J Cancer* 34(6) 863–867, 1984.)

Cellular Vaccine

Dendritic cells are potential candidates for the immunotherapy of cancer because they have the ability to process and present antigens to T-cell lymphocytes and stimulate immune responses to kill cancer cells. This therapy has exhibited minimal antitumor activity in established tumors in mice and humans. It has been reported that alpha-TS, administered locally or systemically, enhanced the efficacy of nonmatured dendritic cells, injected intratumorally or subcutaneously, in reducing tumor volume in murine Lewis lung carcinomas.[176] Vesiculated alpha-TS, a more soluble form of alpha-TS, was equally effective in reducing the growth of tumor cells in vitro and in vivo. This form of alpha-TS, in combination with nonmatured dendritic cells or TNF-induced alpha–matured dendritic cells, was more effective in reducing the growth of tumor cells than vesiculated alpha-TS alone.[177] Alpha-TS, in combination with TRAIL and dendritic cells, caused a marked tumor growth inhibition or induced a complete tumor regression.[36]

Gene Therapy

Adenovirus-mediated mda-7 (Ad-mda) gene transfer has been shown to induce apoptosis in various human cancer cells without affecting the growth of normal cells. Alpha-TS also produced similar effects on normal and cancer cells. Treatment of human ovarian cells in culture with Ad-mda and alpha-TS induce apoptosis more than that produced by the individual agents; however, it did not affect the growth of normal cells.[178]

PROPOSED MICRONUTRIENT PROTOCOLS

Based on the studies with therapeutic and preventive doses of primarily individual antioxidants alone or in combination with radiation therapy and/or chemotherapy presented in this chapter, I propose two distinct micronutrient protocols. One is to be used during standard therapy and in those cancer patients who have become unresponsive to all therapies [active micronutrient treatment protocol (AMTP)], and the other is to be used after completion of therapy.

AMTP Using Therapeutic Doses of Multiple Antioxidants

Based on new laboratory and clinical studies, I propose a modification of an earlier protocol used in one clinical study.[145] The modified formulation of AMTP contains vitamin A, 25,000 IU; vitamin C, 10 g; D-alpha-tocopheryl succinate, 1600 IU; natural carotenoids, 100 mg; selenium, 300 μg; coenzyme Q_{10}, 400 mg; omega-3, fatty acids 4 g; glutamine, 5 g; vitamin D, 1000 IU; B-vitamins (two to three times higher than the RDA), and appropriate minerals; but no iron, copper, or manganese. This formulation can be administered orally in two divided doses, one-half dose in the morning and one-half dose in the evening. The rationale for taking antioxidants twice a day is that the biological half-lives of micronutrients markedly vary. AMTPs should be started at least 3 days before standard or experimental therapies and should be continued for 1 month after completion of therapy. This protocol is expected to improve the efficacy of radiation therapy and chemotherapy by increasing tumor response and decreasing toxicity. This protocol should not be used before surgery, because high doses of vitamin E may interfere with the clotting mechanism; however, it can be started 3 days after surgery to stimulate the healing processes. This protocol can also be used for those patients who have become refractory to all therapies to improve the survival time and quality of life. A Phase-I study is needed to determine the safety of the proposed micronutrient protocol, followed by a well-designed clinical study. The results obtained from these studies would settle the current controversies, and if positive, may markedly enhance the efficacy of cancer therapies and reduce their toxicities.

Preventive Micronutrient Protocol Using Preventive Doses of Multiple Antioxidants

A month after completion of standard therapy, the preventive micronutrient protocol can be started. The formulation for this protocol contains vitamin A; 3000 IU; vitamin C, 1 g; vitamin E 400 IU (D-alpha-tocopheryl succinate, 300 IU and D-alpha-tocopheryl acetate, 100 IU); natural carotenoids, 15 mg; selenium, 100 µg; coenzyme Q_{10}; 100 mg; omega-3, fatty acids 2 g; alpha-lipoic acid, 250 mg; NAC, 250 mg; L-carnitine, 100 mg; vitamin D, 800 IU; B-vitamins (two to three times higher than the RDA); and appropriate minerals; but no iron, copper or manganese.

This formulation is expected to reduce the recurrence of the primary tumor, improve the quality of life, and reduce the risk of developing a second new primary tumor.

A well-designed clinical study should be initiated in cancer patients after therapy, as well as in high-risk populations such as heavy cigarette smokers. The results obtained from these studies would settle the current controversies regarding the value of antioxidants in cancer prevention and, if positive, may contribute to decreasing the incidence of cancer in high-risk populations.

RECOMMENDATIONS FOR DIET AND LIFESTYLE MODIFICATIONS

Modifications in diet and lifestyle are equally important to improve the efficacy of the proposed micronutrient protocols. Recommended changes include a low-fat, high-fiber diet, rich in fruits and vegetables. Recommended modifications in lifestyle include no tobacco products, reduced physical and mental stress, moderate daily exercise, and avoidance of excessive consumption of caffeine and alcohol beverages.

CONCLUSIONS

The incidence of cancer is on the rise and overall cancer mortality remains the same as in 1950. Cancer patients can be divided into three groups: those receiving standard or experimental therapy; those who become unresponsive to these therapies; and those in remission carrying the risk of recurrence of the primary tumors and the development of second new primary cancer. While impressive progress in standard cancer therapy has been made, the value of this therapy in the management of solid tumors may have reached a plateau and adverse serious side effects remain the major concern of patients. At present, there is no strategy to reduce the risk of recurrence of the primary tumors or the development of a second primary cancer among survivors. Patients unresponsive to standard or experimental therapies have few options other than a poor quality of life for the remainder of their life. Therefore, additional approaches should be developed to improve the efficacy of current therapeutic approaches to cancer. At present, oncologists do not recommend antioxidant supplements during radiation therapy or chemotherapy, fearing that they may reduce the effectiveness of the therapy. On the other hand, many cancer patients take antioxidant supplements during therapy without the knowledge of their oncologists. There is a great deal of controversy, not only between patients and oncologists, but also between nutritional oncology researchers and clinicians. The resolution of this controversy should benefit both researchers and cancer patients.

This chapter presented experimental and clinical data on the effects of antioxidants, alone or in combination with ionizing radiation and chemotherapeutic agents. From the critical analysis of these data, it appears that high doses (therapeutic doses) of individual antioxidants that inhibited the growth of cancer cells without affecting the growth of normal cells increased the growth-inhibitory effects of cancer therapeutic agents selectively on cancer cells. On the other hand, low doses (preventive doses) of individual antioxidants either had no effect or stimulated the growth of cancer cells, and reduced the growth-inhibitory effects of the cancer therapeutic agents. The clinical studies that have used preventive doses of antioxidant during radiation or chemotherapy have reported adverse effects; those using therapeutic doses of antioxidant have observed beneficial effects. The failure to distinguish between the effects of therapeutic doses and preventive doses of antioxidants is contributing to current controversies. The use of a single antioxidant in cell culture models or animal models may be justified, but this may not yield optimal results in humans. The rationale for using multiple antioxidants has been presented in this chapter.

I have proposed an AMTP that can be used as an adjunct to radiation therapy, chemotherapy, or experimental therapy. It is expected that introduction of this protocol may improve the efficacy of standard cancer therapy by increasing tumor response and decreasing toxicity. This micronutrient protocol can also be used when patients become unresponsive to all therapies in order to improve the survival time and quality of life. I have also proposed a preventive micronutrient protocol that can be used after completion of standard therapy. This protocol is expected to reduce the risk of recurrence of the primary tumors and the development of second primary cancers. Well-designed clinical studies to test the efficacy of these two protocols should be initiated to settle the current controversies regarding the value of antioxidant supplements during and after cancer therapies.

REFERENCES

1. Prasad, K. N., A. Kumar, V. Kochupillai, and W. C. Cole. 1999. High doses of multiple antioxidant vitamins: Essential ingredients in improving the efficacy of standard cancer therapy. *J Am Coll Nutr* 18 (1): 13–25.
2. Crowe, D. L., R. Kim, and R. A. Chandraratna. 2003. Retinoic acid differentially regulates cancer cell proliferation via dose-dependent modulation of the mitogen-activated protein kinase pathway. *Mol Cancer Res* 1 (7): 532–540.
3. Verma, A., M. J. Atten, B. M. Attar, and O. Holian. 2004. Selenomethionine stimulates MAPK (ERK) phosphorylation, protein oxidation, and DNA synthesis in gastric cancer cells. *Nutr Cancer* 49 (2): 184–190.
4. Richardson, M. A., T. Sanders, J. L. Palmer, A. Greisinger, and S. E. Singletary. 2000. Complementary/alternative medicine use in a comprehensive cancer center and the implications for oncology. *J Clin Oncol* 18 (13): 2505–2514.
5. Salganik, R. I. 2001. The benefits and hazards of antioxidants: Controlling apoptosis and other protective mechanisms in cancer patients and the human population. *J Am Coll Nutr* 20 (5 Suppl): 464S–472S; discussion 473S–475S.
6. Labriola, D., and R. Livingston. 1999. Possible interactions between dietary antioxidants and chemotherapy. *Oncology* (Williston Park) 13 (7): 1003–1008; discussion 1008, 1011–1012.
7. Witenberg, B., Y. Kletter, H. H. Kalir, Z. Raviv, E. Fenig, A. Nagler, D. Halperin, and I. Fabian. 1999. Ascorbic acid inhibits apoptosis induced by x irradiation in HL60 myeloid leukemia cells. *Radiat Res* 152 (5): 468–478.
8. Miyajima, A., J. Nakashima, M. Tachibana, K. Nakamura, M. Hayakawa, and M. Murai. 1999. *N*-Acetylcysteine modifies *cis*-dichlorodiammineplatinum-induced effects in bladder cancer cells. *Jpn J Cancer Res* 90 (5): 565–570.
9. Heaney, M. L., J. R. Gardner, N. Karasavvas, D. W. Golde, D. A. Scheinberg, E. A. Smith, and O. A. O'Connor. 2008. Vitamin C antagonizes the cytotoxic effects of antineoplastic drugs. *Cancer Res* 68 (19): 8031–8038.
10. Prasad, K. N., and R. Kumar. 1996. Effect of individual and multiple antioxidant vitamins on growth and morphology of human nontumorigenic and tumorigenic parotid acinar cells in culture. *Nutr Cancer* 26 (1): 11–19.
11. Prasad, K. N., and J. Edwards-Prasad. 1982. Effects of tocopherol (vitamin E) acid succinate on morphological alterations and growth inhibition in melanoma cells in culture. *Cancer Res* 42 (2): 550–555.
12. Prasad, K. N., B. Kumar, X. D. Yan, A. J. Hanson, and W. C. Cole. 2003. alpha-Tocopheryl succinate, the most effective form of vitamin E for adjuvant cancer treatment: A review. *J Am Coll Nutr* 22 (2): 108–117.
13. Kline, K., W. Yu, and B. G. Sanders. 2001. Vitamin E: Mechanisms of action as tumor cell growth inhibitors. *J Nutr* 131 (1): 161S–163S.
14. Neuzil, J., T. Weber, N. Gellert, and C. Weber. 2001. Selective cancer cell killing by alpha-tocopheryl succinate. *Br J Cancer* 84 (1): 87–89.

15. Wu, X. X., Y. Kakehi, X. H. Jin, M. Inui, and M. Sugimoto. 2009. Induction of apoptosis in human renal cell carcinoma cells by vitamin E succinate in caspase-independent manner. *Urology* 73 (1): 193–199.
16. Huang, P. H., D. Wang, H. C. Chuang, S. Wei, S. K. Kulp, and C. S. Chen. 2009. alpha-Tocopheryl succinate and derivatives mediate the transcriptional repression of androgen receptor in prostate cancer cells by targeting the PP2A-JNK-Sp1-signaling axis. *Carcinogenesis* 30 (7): 1125–1131.
17. Zhang, Y., J. Ni, E. M. Messing, E. Chang, C. R. Yang, and S. Yeh. 2002. Vitamin E succinate inhibits the function of androgen receptor and the expression of prostate-specific antigen in prostate cancer cells. *Proc Natl Acad Sci USA* 99 (11): 7408–7413.
18. Watters, J. L., M. H. Gail, S. J. Weinstein, J. Virtamo, and D. Albanes. 2009. Associations between alpha-tocopherol, beta-carotene, and retinol and prostate cancer survival. *Cancer Res* 69 (9): 3833–3841.
19. Israel, K., W. Yu, B. G. Sanders, and K. Kline. 2000. Vitamin E succinate induces apoptosis in human prostate cancer cells: Role for Fas in vitamin E succinate-triggered apoptosis. *Nutr Cancer* 36 (1): 90–100.
20. Turanek, J., X. F. Wang, P. Knotigova, S. Koudelka, L. F. Dong, E. Vrublova, E. Mahdavian, et al. 2009. Liposomal formulation of alpha-tocopheryl maleamide: In vitro and in vivo toxicological profile and anticancer effect against spontaneous breast carcinomas in mice. *Toxicol Appl Pharmacol* 237 (3): 249–257.
21. Hahn, T., K. Fried, L. H. Hurley, and E. T. Akporiaye. 2009. Orally active alpha-tocopheryloxyacetic acid suppresses tumor growth and multiplicity of spontaneous murine breast cancer. *Mol Cancer Ther* 8 (6): 1570–1578.
22. Kogure, K., S. Manabe, I. Suzuki, A. Tokumura, and K. Fukuzawa. 2005. Cytotoxicity of alpha-tocopheryl succinate, malonate and oxalate in normal and cancer cells in vitro and their anti-cancer effects on mouse melanoma in vivo. *J Nutr Sci Vitaminol (Tokyo)* 51 (6): 392–397.
23. Lawson, K. A., K. Anderson, M. Simmons-Menchaca, J. Atkinson, L. Sun, B. G. Sanders, and K. Kline. 2004. Comparison of vitamin E derivatives alpha-TEA and VES in reduction of mouse mammary tumor burden and metastasis. *Exp Biol Med (Maywood)* 229 (9): 954–963.
24. Ni, J., T. Mai, S. T. Pang, I. Haque, K. Huang, M. A. DiMaggio, S. Xie, N. S. James, D. Kasi, S. R. Chemler, and S. Yeh. 2009. In vitro and in vivo anticancer effects of the novel vitamin E ether analogue *RRR*-alpha-tocopheryloxybutyl sulfonic acid in prostate cancer. *Clin Cancer Res* 15 (3): 898–906.
25. Fariss, M. W., M. B. Fortuna, C. K. Everett, J. D. Smith, D. F. Trent, and Z. Djuric. 1994. The selective antiproliferative effects of alpha-tocopheryl hemisuccinate and cholesteryl hemisuccinate on murine leukemia cells result from the action of the intact compounds. *Cancer Res* 54 (13): 3346–3351.
26. Lee, S. K., J. S. Kang, J. Jung da, D. Y. Hur, J. E. Kim, E. Hahm, S. Bae, et al. 2008. Vitamin C suppresses proliferation of the human melanoma cell SK-MEL-2 through the inhibition of cyclooxygenase-2 (COX-2) expression and the modulation of insulin-like growth factor II (IGF-II) production. *J Cell Physiol* 216 (1): 180–188.
27. Wybieralska, E., M. Koza, J. Sroka, J. Czyz, and Z. Madeja. 2008. Ascorbic acid inhibits the migration of Walker 256 carcinosarcoma cells. *Cell Mol Biol Lett* 13 (1): 103–111.
28. Hong, S. W., D. H. Jin, E. S. Hahm, S. H. Yim, J. S. Lim, K. I. Kim, Y. Yang, et al. 2007. Ascorbate (vitamin C) induces cell death through the apoptosis-inducing factor in human breast cancer cells. *Oncol Rep* 18 (4): 811–815.
29. Sun, Y. X., Q. S. Zheng, G. Li, D. A. Guo, and Z. R. Wang. 2006. Mechanism of ascorbic acid–induced reversion against malignant phenotype in human gastric cancer cells. *Biomed Environ Sci* 19 (5): 385–391.
30. Gonzalez, M. J., J. R. Miranda-Massari, E. M. Mora, A. Guzman, N. H. Riordan, H. D. Riordan, J. J. Casciari, J. A. Jackson, and A. Roman-Franco. 2005. Orthomolecular oncology review: Ascorbic acid and cancer 25 years later. *Integr Cancer Ther* 4 (1): 32–44.
31. Prasad, K. N., P. K. Sinha, M. Ramanujam, and A. Sakamoto. 1979. Sodium ascorbate potentiates the growth inhibitory effect of certain agents on neuroblastoma cells in culture. *Proc Natl Acad Sci USA* 76 (2): 829–832.
32. Verrax, J., and P. B. Calderon. 2009. Pharmacologic concentrations of ascorbate are achieved by parenteral administration and exhibit antitumoral effects. *Free Radic Biol Med* 47 (1): 32–40.
33. Chen, Q., M. G. Espey, A. Y. Sun, J. H. Lee, M. C. Krishna, E. Shacter, P. L. Choyke, et al. 2007. Ascorbate in pharmacologic concentrations selectively generates ascorbate radical and hydrogen peroxide in extracellular fluid in vivo. *Proc Natl Acad Sci USA* 104 (21): 8749–8754.
34. Chen, Q., M. G. Espey, M. C. Krishna, J. B. Mitchell, C. P. Corpe, G. R. Buettner, E. Shacter, and M. Levine. 2005. Pharmacologic ascorbic acid concentrations selectively kill cancer cells: Action as a pro-drug to deliver hydrogen peroxide to tissues. *Proc Natl Acad Sci USA* 102 (38): 13604–13609.

35. Chen, Q., M. G. Espey, A. Y. Sun, C. Pooput, K. L. Kirk, M. C. Krishna, D. B. Khosh, J. Drisko, and M. Levine. 2008. Pharmacologic doses of ascorbate act as a prooxidant and decrease growth of aggressive tumor xenografts in mice. *Proc Natl Acad Sci USA* 105 (32): 11105–11109.
36. Tomasetti, M., and J. Neuzil. 2007. Vitamin E analogues and immune response in cancer treatment. *Vitam Horm* 76: 463–491.
37. Yin, Y., J. Ni, M. Chen, Y. Guo, and S. Yeh. 2009. *RRR*-alpha-Vitamin E succinate potentiates the antitumor effect of calcitriol in prostate cancer without overt side effects. *Clin Cancer Res* 15 (1): 190–200.
38. Roomi, M. W., T. Kalinovsky, N. W. Roomi, J. Monterrery, M. Rath, and A. Niedzwiecki. 2008. A nutrient mixture suppresses hepatic metastasis in athymic nude mice injected with murine B16FO melanoma cells. *Biofactors* 33 (3): 181–189.
39. Meyskens, F. L., Jr. 1995. Role of vitamin A and its derivatives in the treatment of human cancer. In *Nutrients in Cancer Prevention and Treatment*, ed. K. N. Prasad, L. Santamaria, and R. M. Williams, 349–362. Totowa, NJ: Humana Press.
40. Garewal, H. 1995. Beta-carotene and antioxidant nutrients in oral cancer prevention. In *Nutrients in Cancer Prevention and Treatment*, ed. K. N. Prasad, L. Santamaria, and R. M. Williams, 235–247. Totowa, NJ: Humana Press.
41. Prakash, P., N. I. Krinsky, and R. M. Russell. 2000. Retinoids, carotenoids, and human breast cancer cell cultures: A review of differential effects. *Nutr Rev* 58 (6): 170–176.
42. Simeone, A. M., and A. M. Tari. 2004. How retinoids regulate breast cancer cell proliferation and apoptosis. *Cell Mol Life Sci* 61 (12): 1475–1484.
43. Murakami, C., M. Takemura, Y. Sugiyama, S. Kamisuki, H. Asahara, M. Kawasaki, T. Ishidoh, et al. 2002. Vitamin A–related compounds, all-*trans* retinal and retinoic acids, selectively inhibit activities of mammalian replicative DNA polymerases. *Biochim Biophys Acta* 1574 (1): 85–92.
44. Onogi, N., M. Okuno, R. Matsushima-Nishiwaki, Y. Fukutomi, H. Moriwaki, Y. Muto, and S. Kojima. 1998. Antiproliferative effect of carotenoids on human colon cancer cells without conversion to retinoic acid. *Nutr Cancer* 32 (1): 20–24.
45. Williams, A. W., T. W. Boileau, J. R. Zhou, S. K. Clinton, and J. W. Erdman Jr. 2000. Beta-carotene modulates human prostate cancer cell growth and may undergo intracellular metabolism to retinol. *J Nutr* 130 (4): 728–732.
46. Briviba, K., K. Schnabele, E. Schwertle, M. Blockhaus, and G. Rechkemmer. 2001. Beta-carotene inhibits growth of human colon carcinoma cells in vitro by induction of apoptosis. *Biol Chem* 382 (12): 1663–1668.
47. Hwang, E. S., and P. E. Bowen. 2004. Cell cycle arrest and induction of apoptosis by lycopene in LNCaP human prostate cancer cells. *J Med Food* 7 (3): 284–289.
48. van Breemen, R. B., and N. Pajkovic. 2008. Multitargeted therapy of cancer by lycopene. *Cancer Lett* 269 (2): 339–351.
49. Tomita, Y., K. Himeno, K. Nomoto, H. Endo, and T. Hirohata. 1987. Augmentation of tumor immunity against syngeneic tumors in mice by beta-carotene. *J Natl Cancer Inst* 78 (4): 679–681.
50. Jiang, W., C. Jiang, H. Pei, L. Wang, J. Zhang, H. Hu, and J. Lu. 2009. In vivo molecular mediators of cancer growth suppression and apoptosis by selenium in mammary and prostate models: Lack of involvement of gadd genes. *Mol Cancer Ther* 8 (3): 682–691.
51. Sanmartin, C., D. Plano, and J. A. Palop. 2008. Selenium compounds and apoptotic modulation: A new perspective in cancer therapy. *Mini Rev Med Chem* 8 (10): 1020–1031.
52. Rooprai, H. K., I. Kyriazis, R. K. Nuttall, D. R. Edwards, D. Zicha, D. Aubyn, D. Davies, R. Gullan, and G. J. Pilkington. 2007. Inhibition of invasion and induction of apoptosis by selenium in human malignant brain tumour cells in vitro. *Int J Oncol* 30 (5): 1263–1271.
53. Cao, T. M., F. Y. Hua, C. M. Xu, B. S. Han, H. Dong, L. Zuo, X. Wang, Y. Yang, H. Z. Pan, and Z. N. Zhang. 2006. Distinct effects of different concentrations of sodium selenite on apoptosis, cell cycle, and gene expression profile in acute promyeloytic leukemia-derived NB4 cells. *Ann Hematol* 85 (7): 434–442.
54. Goel, A., F. Fuerst, E. Hotchkiss, and C. R. Boland. 2006. Selenomethionine induces p53 mediated cell cycle arrest and apoptosis in human colon cancer cells. *Cancer Biol Ther* 5 (5): 529–535.
55. Husbeck, B., L. Nonn, D. M. Peehl, and S. J. Knox. 2006. Tumor-selective killing by selenite in patient-matched pairs of normal and malignant prostate cells. *Prostate* 66 (2): 218–225.
56. Zeng, H., M. Wu, and J. H. Botnen. 2009. Methylselenol, a selenium metabolite, induces cell cycle arrest in G1 phase and apoptosis via the extracellular-regulated kinase 1/2 pathway and other cancer signaling genes. *J Nutr* 139: 1613–1618.

57. Li, G. X., H. J. Lee, Z. Wang, H. Hu, J. D. Liao, J. C. Watts, G. F. Combs, Jr., and J. Lu. 2008. Superior in vivo inhibitory efficacy of methylseleninic acid against human prostate cancer over selenomethionine or selenite. *Carcinogenesis* 29 (5): 1005–1012.
58. Zu, K., T. Bihani, A. Lin, Y. M. Park, K. Mori, and C. Ip. 2006. Enhanced selenium effect on growth arrest by BiP/GRP78 knockdown in p53-null human prostate cancer cells, *Oncogene* 25 (4): 546–554.
59. Chun, J. Y., N. Nadiminty, S. O. Lee, S. A. Onate, W. Lou, and A. C. Gao. 2006. Mechanisms of selenium down-regulation of androgen receptor signaling in prostate cancer. *Mol Cancer Ther* 5 (4): 913–918.
60. Shah, Y. M., A. Kaul, Y. Dong, C. Ip, and B. G. Rowan. 2005. Attenuation of estrogen receptor alpha (ERalpha) signaling by selenium in breast cancer cells via downregulation of ERalpha gene expression. *Breast Cancer Res Treat* 92 (3): 239–250.
61. Zhao, R., N. Xiang, F. E. Domann, and W. Zhong. 2009. Effects of selenite and genistein on G2/M cell cycle arrest and apoptosis in human prostate cancer cells. *Nutr Cancer* 61 (3): 397–407.
62. Xiao, H. J., C. Y. Huang, H. Y. Wang, and M. Li. 2008. Effect of selenium and zinc on the proliferation of human esophageal cancer Eca109 cell line in vitro. *Nan Fang Yi Ke Da Xue Xue Bao* 28 (12): 2117–2120.
63. Reagan-Shaw, S., M. Nihal, H. Ahsan, H. Mukhtar, and N. Ahmad. 2008. Combination of vitamin E and selenium causes an induction of apoptosis of human prostate cancer cells by enhancing Bax/Bcl-2 ratio. *Prostate* 68 (15): 1624–1634.
64. Shah, Y. M., M. Al-Dhaheri, Y. Dong, C. Ip, F. E. Jones, and B. G. Rowan. 2005. Selenium disrupts estrogen receptor (alpha) signaling and potentiates tamoxifen antagonism in endometrial cancer cells and tamoxifen-resistant breast cancer cells. *Mol Cancer Ther* 4 (8): 1239–1249.
65. Prasad, K. N., C. Hernandez, J. Edwards-Prasad, J. Nelson, T. Borus, and W. A. Robinson. 1994. Modification of the effect of tamoxifen, cis-platin, DTIC, and interferon-alpha 2b on human melanoma cells in culture by a mixture of vitamins. *Nutr Cancer* 22 (3): 233–245.
66. Li, J., H. J. Tu, G. Dai, Y. C. Dai, Q. Wu, Q. Z. Shi, Q. Cao, and Z. J. Li. 2007. N-Acetyl cysteine inhibits human signet ring cell gastric cancer cell line (SJ-89) cell growth by inducing apoptosis and DNA synthesis arrest. *Eur J Gastroenterol Hepatol* 19 (9): 769–774.
67. Simbula, G., A. Columbano, G. M. Ledda-Columbano, L. Sanna, M. Deidda, A. Diana, and M. Pibiri. 2007. Increased ROS generation and p53 activation in alpha-lipoic acid–induced apoptosis of hepatoma cells. *Apoptosis* 12 (1): 113–123.
68. De Flora, S., F. D'Agostini, L. Masiello, D. Giunciuglio, and A. Albini. 1996. Synergism between N-acetylcysteine and doxorubicin in the prevention of tumorigenicity and metastasis in murine models. *Int J Cancer* 67 (6): 842–848.
69. Reliene, R., and R. H. Schiestl. 2006. Antioxidant N-acetyl cysteine reduces incidence and multiplicity of lymphoma in Atm deficient mice. *DNA Repair (Amst)* 5 (7): 852–859.
70. Agarwal, A., U. Munoz-Najar, U. Klueh, S. C. Shih, and K. P. Claffey. 2004. N-Acetyl-cysteine promotes angiostatin production and vascular collapse in an orthotopic model of breast cancer. *Am J Pathol* 164 (5): 1683–1696.
71. Albini, A., M. Morini, F. D'Agostini, N. Ferrari, F. Campelli, G. Arena, D. M. Noonan, C. Pesce, and S. De Flora. 2001. Inhibition of angiogenesis-driven Kaposi's sarcoma tumor growth in nude mice by oral N-acetylcysteine. *Cancer Res* 61 (22): 8171–8178.
72. Delneste, Y., P. Jeannin, L. Potier, P. Romero, and J. Y. Bonnefoy. 1997. N-Acetyl-L-cysteine exhibits antitumoral activity by increasing tumor necrosis factor alpha-dependent T-cell cytotoxicity. *Blood* 90 (3): 1124–1132.
73. Shi, D. Y., H. L. Liu, J. S. Stern, P. Z. Yu, and S. L. Liu. 2008. Alpha-lipoic acid induces apoptosis in hepatoma cells via the PTEN/Akt pathway. *FEBS Lett* 582 (12): 1667–1671.
74. Vig-Varga, E., E. A. Benson, T. L. Limbil, B. M. Allison, M. G. Goebl, and M. A. Harrington. 2006. Alpha-lipoic acid modulates ovarian surface epithelial cell growth. *Gynecol Oncol* 103 (1): 45–52.
75. Wenzel, U., A. Nickel, and H. Daniel. 2005. alpha-Lipoic acid induces apoptosis in human colon cancer cells by increasing mitochondrial respiration with a concomitant O2-*-generation. *Apoptosis* 10 (2): 359–368.
76. Zhong, W., L. W. Oberley, T. D. Oberley, and D. K. St Clair. 1997. Suppression of the malignant phenotype of human glioma cells by overexpression of manganese superoxide dismutase. *Oncogene* 14 (4): 481–490.
77. Church, S. L., J. W. Grant, L. A. Ridnour, L. W. Oberley, P. E. Swanson, P. S. Meltzer, and J. M. Trent. 1993. Increased manganese superoxide dismutase expression suppresses the malignant phenotype of human melanoma cells. *Proc Natl Acad Sci USA* 90 (7): 3113–3117.

78. Prasad, K. N., R. J. Cohrs, and O. K. Sharma. 1990. Decreased expressions of c-*myc* and H-*ras* oncogenes in vitamin E succinate induced morphologically differentiated murine B-16 melanoma cells in culture. *Biochem Cell Biol* 68 (11): 1250–1255.
79. Thiele, C. J., C. P. Reynolds, and M. A. Israel. 1985. Decreased expression of N-*myc* precedes retinoic acid-induced morphological differentiation of human neuroblastoma. *Nature* 313 (6001): 404–406.
80. Schwartz, J. R. 1995. Molecular and biochemical control of tumor growth following treatment with carotenoids or tocopherols. In *Nutrients in Cancer Prevention and Treatment*, ed. K. N. Prasad, L. Santamaria, and R. M. Williams, 287–316. Totawa, NJ: Humana Press.
81. Gopalakrishna, R., U. Gundimeda, and Z. Chen. 1995. Vitamin E succinate inhibits protein kinase C: Correlation with its unique inhibitory effects on cell growth and transformation. In *Nutrients in Cancer Prevention and Treatment*, ed. K. N. Prasad, L. Santamaria, and R. M. Williams, 21–37. Totawa, NJ: Humana Press.
82. Mahoney, C. W., and A. Azzi. 1988. Vitamin E inhibits protein kinase C activity. *Biochem Biophys Res Commun* 154 (2): 694–697.
83. Neuzil, J., I. Svensson, T. Weber, C. Weber, and U. T. Brunk. 1999. Alpha-tocopheryl succinate-induced apoptosis in Jurkat T cells involves caspase-3 activation, and both lysosomal and mitochondrial destabilisation. *FEBS Lett* 445 (2–3): 295–300.
84. Nakamura, T., M. Goto, A. Matsumoto, and I. Tanaka. 1998. Inhibition of NF-kappa B transcriptional activity by alpha-tocopheryl succinate. *Biofactors* 7 (1–2), 21–30.
85. Turley, J. M., F. W. Ruscetti, S. J. Kim, T. Fu, F. V. Gou, and M. C. Birchenall-Roberts. 1997. Vitamin E succinate inhibits proliferation of BT-20 human breast cancer cells: Increased binding of cyclin A negatively regulates E2F transactivation activity. *Cancer Res* 57 (13): 2668–2675.
86. Turley, J. M., T. Fu, F. W. Ruscetti, J. A. Mikovits, D. C. Bertolette 3rd, and M. C. Birchenall-Roberts. 1997. Vitamin E succinate induces Fas-mediated apoptosis in estrogen receptor-negative human breast cancer cells. *Cancer Res* 57 (5): 881–890.
87. Schwartz, J. L. 1995. Molecular and biochemical control of tumor growth following treatment with carotenoids or tocopherols. In *Nutrients in Cancer Prevention and Treatment*, ed. K. N. Prasad, L. Santamaria, and R. M. Williams, 287–316. Totawa, NJ: Humana Press.
88. Chinery, R., J. A. Brockman, M. O. Peeler, Y. Shyr, R. D. Beauchamp, and R. J. Coffey. 1997. Antioxidants enhance the cytotoxicity of chemotherapeutic agents in colorectal cancer: A p53-independent induction of p21WAF1/CIP1 via C/EBPbeta. *Nat Med* 3 (11): 1233–1241.
89. Zhang, L. X., R. V. Cooney, and J. S. Bertram. 1992. Carotenoids up-regulate connexin43 gene expression independent of their provitamin A or antioxidant properties. *Cancer Res* 52 (20): 5707–5712.
90. Barnett, K. T., F. D. Fokum, and M. P. Malafa. 2002. Vitamin E succinate inhibits colon cancer liver metastases. *J Surg Res* 106 (2): 292–298.
91. Al-Wadei, H. A., T. Takahashi, and H. M. Schuller. 2006. Growth stimulation of human pulmonary adenocarcinoma cells and small airway epithelial cells by beta-carotene via activation of cAMP, PKA, CREB and ERK1/2. *Int J Cancer* 118 (6): 1370–1380.
92. Rutz, H. P., and J. B. Little. 1989. Modification of radiosensitivity and recovery from X ray damage in vitro by retinoic acid. *Int J Radiat Oncol Biol Phys* 16 (5): 1285–1288.
93. Lippman, S. M., J. J. Kavanagh, M. Paredes-Espinoza, F. Delgadillo-Madrueno, P. Paredes-Casillas, W. K. Hong, E. Holdener, and I. H. Krakoff. 1992. 13-*cis*-Retinoic acid plus interferon alpha-2a: Highly active systemic therapy for squamous cell carcinoma of the cervix. *J Natl Cancer Inst* 84 (4): 241–245.
94. Jha, M. N., J. S. Bedford, W. C. Cole, J. Edward-Prasad, and K. N. Prasad. 1999. Vitamin E (D-alpha-tocopheryl succinate) decreases mitotic accumulation in gamma-irradiated human tumor, but not in normal, cells. *Nutr Cancer* 35 (2): 189–194.
95. Kumar, B., M. N. Jha, W. C. Cole, J. S. Bedford, and K. N. Prasad. 2002. D-alpha-Tocopheryl succinate (vitamin E) enhances radiation-induced chromosomal damage levels in human cancer cells, but reduces it in normal cells. *J Am Coll Nutr* 21 (4): 339–343.
96. Girdhani, S., S. M. Bhosle, S. A. Thulsidas, A. Kumar, and K. P. Mishra. 2005. Potential of radiosensitizing agents in cancer chemo-radiotherapy. *J Cancer Res Ther* 1 (3), 129–131.
97. Koch, C. J., and J. E. Biaglow. 1978. Toxicity, radiation sensitivity modification, and metabolic effects of dehydroascorbate and ascorbate in mammalian cells. *J Cell Physiol* 94 (3): 299–306.
98. Shin, S. H., M. J. Yoon, M. Kim, J. I. Kim, S. J. Lee, Y. S. Lee, and S. Bae. 2007. Enhanced lung cancer cell killing by the combination of selenium and ionizing radiation. *Oncol Rep* 17 (1): 209–216.
99. Seifter, E., A. Rettura, J. Padawar, and S. M. Levenson. 1984. Vitamin A and beta-carotene as adjunctive therapy to tumor excision, radiation therapy and chemotherapy. In *Vitamins, Nutrition and Cancer*, ed. K. N. Prasad, 1–19. Basel, Switzerland: Karger.

100. Tewfik, F. A., H. H. Tewfik, and E. F. Riley. 1982. The influence of ascorbic acid on the growth of solid tumors in mice and on tumor control by X-irradiation. *Int J Vitam Nutr Res Suppl* 23, 257–263.
101. Blumenthal, R. D., W. Lew, A. Reising, D. Soyne, L. Osorio, Z. Ying, and D. M. Goldenberg. 2000. Antioxidant vitamins reduce normal tissue toxicity induced by radio-immunotherapy. *Int J Cancer* 86 (2): 276–280.
102. Reliene, R., J. M. Pollard, Z. Sobol, B. Trouiller, R. A.c Gatti, and R. H. Schiestl. 2009. *N*-Acetyl cysteine protects against ionizing radiation-induced DNA damage but not against cell killing in yeast and mammals. *Mutat Res* 665 (1–2), 37–43.
103. Jaakkola, K., P. Lahteenmaki, J. Laakso, E. Harju, H. Tykka, and K. Mahlberg. 1992. Treatment with antioxidant and other nutrients in combination with chemotherapy and irradiation in patients with small-cell lung cancer. *Anticancer Res* 12 (3): 599–606.
104. Lamson, D. W., and M. S. Brignall. 1999. Antioxidants in cancer therapy; their actions and interactions with oncologic therapies. *Altern Med Rev* 4 (5): 304–329.
105. Mills, E. E. 1988. The modifying effect of beta-carotene on radiation and chemotherapy induced oral mucositis. *Br J Cancer* 57 (4): 416–417.
106. Prasad, K. N., W. C. Cole, B. Kumar, and K. Che Prasad. 2002. Pros and cons of antioxidant use during radiation therapy. *Cancer Treat Rev* 28 (2): 79–91.
107. Misirlioglu, C. H., T. Demirkasimoglu, B. Kucukplakci, E. Sanri, and K. Altundag. 2007. Pentoxifylline and alpha-tocopherol in prevention of radiation-induced lung toxicity in patients with lung cancer. *Med Oncol* 24 (3): 308–311.
108. Prasad, K. N., and P. K. Sinha. 1976. Effect of sodium butyrate on mammalian cells in culture: A review. *In Vitro* 12 (2): 125–132.
109. Kurbacher, C. M., U. Wagner, B. Kolster, P. E. Andreotti, D. Krebs, and H. W. Bruckner. 1996. Ascorbic acid (vitamin C) improves the antineoplastic activity of doxorubicin, cisplatin, and paclitaxel in human breast carcinoma cells in vitro. *Cancer Lett* 103 (2): 183–189.
110. Chiang, C. D., E. J. Song, V. C. Yang, and C. C. Chao. 1994. Ascorbic acid increases drug accumulation and reverses vincristine resistance of human non-small-cell lung-cancer cells. *Biochem J* 301 (Pt 3): 759–764.
111. Abdel-Latif, M. M., A. A. Raouf, K. Sabra, D. Kelleher, and J. V. Reynolds. 2005. Vitamin C enhances chemosensitization of esophageal cancer cells in vitro. *J Chemother* 17 (5): 539–549.
112. Ripoll, E. A., B. N. Rama, and M. M. Webber. 1986. Vitamin E enhances the chemotherapeutic effects of adriamycin on human prostatic carcinoma cells in vitro. *J Urol* 136 (2): 529–531.
113. Leonetti, C., A. Biroccio, C. Gabellini, M. Scarsella, V. Maresca, E. Flori, L. Bove, et al. 2003. Alpha-tocopherol protects against cisplatin-induced toxicity without interfering with antitumor efficacy. *Int J Cancer* 104 (2): 243–250.
114. Czeczuga-Semeniuk, E., D. Lemancewicz, and S. Wolczynski. 2007. Can vitamin A modify the activity of docetaxel in MCF-7 breast cancer cells? *Folia Histochem Cytobiol* 45 (Suppl 1): S169–S174.
115. Pathak, A. K., N. Singh, N. Khanna, V. G. Reddy, K. N. Prasad, and V. Kochupillai. 2002. Potentiation of the effect of paclitaxel and carboplatin by antioxidant mixture on human lung cancer h520 cells. *J Am Coll Nutr* 21 (5): 416–421.
116. Zhang, J., D. Peng, H. Lu, and Q. Liu. 2008. Attenuating the toxicity of cisplatin by using selenosulfate with reduced risk of selenium toxicity as compared with selenite. *Toxicol Appl Pharmacol* 226 (3): 251–259.
117. Thant, A. A., Wu, Y., Lee, J., Mishra, D. K., Garcia, H., Koeffler, H. P., and Vadgama, J. V. 2008. Role of caspases in 5-FU and selenium-induced growth inhibition of colorectal cancer cells. *Anticancer Res* 28 (6A): 3579–3592.
118. Vadgama, J. V., Y. Wu, D. Shen, S. Hsia, and J. Block. 2000. Effect of selenium in combination with Adriamycin or Taxol on several different cancer cells. *Anticancer Res* 20 (3A): 1391–1414.
119. Tan, L., X. Jia, X. Jiang, Y. Zhang, H. Tang, S. Yao, and Q. Xie. 2009. In vitro study on the individual and synergistic cytotoxicity of adriamycin and selenium nanoparticles against Bel7402 cells with a quartz crystal microbalance. *Biosens Bioelectron* 24 (7): 2268–2272.
120. Chakraborty, P., U. H. Sk, and S. Bhattacharya. 2009. Chemoprotection and enhancement of cancer chemotherapeutic efficacy of cyclophosphamide in mice bearing Ehrlich ascites carcinoma by diphenyl-methyl selenocyanate. *Cancer Chemother Pharmacol* 64: 971–980.
121. Cao, S., F. A. Durrani, and Y. M. Rustum. 2004. Selective modulation of the therapeutic efficacy of anticancer drugs by selenium containing compounds against human tumor xenografts. *Clin Cancer Res* 10 (7): 2561–2569.

122. Formelli, F., and L. Cleris. 1993. Synthetic retinoid fenretinide is effective against a human ovarian carcinoma xenograft and potentiates cisplatin activity. *Cancer Res* 53 (22): 5374–5376.
123. Bach, S. P., S. E. Williamson, E. Marshman, S. Kumar, S. T. O'Dwyer, C. S. Potten, and A. J. Watson. 2001. The antioxidant N-acetylcysteine increases 5-fluorouracil activity against colorectal cancer xenografts in nude mice. *J Gastrointest Surg* 5 (1): 91–97.
124. Block, K. I., A. C. Koch, M. N. Mead, P. K. Tothy, R. A. Newman, and C. Gyllenhaal. 2007. Impact of antioxidant supplementation on chemotherapeutic efficacy: A systematic review of the evidence from randomized controlled trials. *Cancer Treat Rev* 33 (5): 407–418.
125. Coulter, I. D., M. L. Hardy, S. C. Morton, L. G. Hilton, W. Tu, D. Valentine, and P. G. Shekelle. 2006. Antioxidants vitamin C and vitamin e for the prevention and treatment of cancer. *J Gen Intern Med* 21 (7): 735–744.
126. Lin, P. C., M. Y. Lee, W. S. Wang, C. C. Yen, T. C. Chao, L. T. Hsiao, M. H. Yang, P. M. Chen, K. P. Lin, and T. J. Chiou. 2006. N-Acetylcysteine has neuroprotective effects against oxaliplatin-based adjuvant chemotherapy in colon cancer patients: Preliminary data. *Support Care Cancer* 14 (5): 484–487.
127. Cascinu, S., V. Catalano, L. Cordella, R. Labianca, P. Giordani, A. M. Baldelli, G. D. Beretta, E. Ubiali, and G. Catalano. 2002. Neuroprotective effect of reduced glutathione on oxaliplatin-based chemotherapy in advanced colorectal cancer: A randomized, double-blind, placebo-controlled trial. *J Clin Oncol* 20 (16): 3478–3483.
128. Mantovani, G., A. Maccio, C. Madeddu, L. Mura, E. Massa, G. Gramignano, M. R. Lusso, V. Murgia, P. Camboni, and L. Ferreli. 2003. Reactive oxygen species, antioxidant mechanisms, and serum cytokine levels in cancer patients: Impact of an antioxidant treatment. *J Environ Pathol Toxicol Oncol* 22 (1): 17–28.
129. Berkson, B. M., D. M. Rubin, and A. J. Berkson. 2006. The long-term survival of a patient with pancreatic cancer with metastases to the liver after treatment with the intravenous alpha-lipoic acid/low-dose naltrexone protocol. *Integr Cancer Ther* 5 (1): 83–89.
130. Antonadou, D., M. Pepelassi, M. Synodinou, M. Puglisi, and N. Throuvalas. 2002. Prophylactic use of amifostine to prevent radiochemotherapy-induced mucositis and xerostomia in head-and-neck cancer. *Int J Radiat Oncol Biol Phys* 52 (3): 739–747.
131. Lockwood, K., S. Moesgaard, T. Yamamoto, and K. Folkers. 1995. Progress on therapy of breast cancer with vitamin Q10 and the regression of metastases. *Biochem Biophys Res Commun* 212 (1): 172–177.
132. Roffe, L., K. Schmidt, and E. Ernst. 2004. Efficacy of coenzyme Q10 for improved tolerability of cancer treatments: A systematic review. *J Clin Oncol* 22 (21): 4418–4424.
133. Rusciani, L., I. Proietti, A. Paradisi, A. Rusciani, G. Guerriero, A. Mammone, A. De Gaetano, and S. Lippa. 2007. Recombinant interferon alpha-2b and coenzyme Q10 as a postsurgical adjuvant therapy for melanoma: A 3-year trial with recombinant interferon-alpha and 5-year follow-up. *Melanoma Res* 17 (3): 177–183.
134. Sachdanandam, P. 2008. Antiangiogenic and hypolipidemic activity of coenzyme Q10 supplementation to breast cancer patients undergoing Tamoxifen therapy. *Biofactors* 32 (1–4): 151–159.
135. Yuvaraj, S., V. G. Premkumar, K. Vijayasarathy, S. G. Gangadaran, and P. Sachdanandam. 2007. Ameliorating effect of coenzyme Q10, riboflavin and niacin in tamoxifen-treated postmenopausal breast cancer patients with special reference to lipids and lipoproteins. *Clin Biochem* 40 (9–10): 623–628.
136. Premkumar, V. G., S. Yuvaraj, S. Sathish, P. Shanthi, and P. Sachdanandam. 2008. Anti-angiogenic potential of coenzyme Q10, riboflavin and niacin in breast cancer patients undergoing tamoxifen therapy. *Vascul Pharmacol* 48 (4–6): 191–201.
137. Lockwood, K., S. Moesgaard, T. Hanioka, and K. Folkers. 1994. Apparent partial remission of breast cancer in "high risk" patients supplemented with nutritional antioxidants, essential fatty acids and coenzyme Q10. *Mol Aspects Med* 15 (Suppl): s231–s240.
138. Argyriou, A. A., E. Chroni, A. Koutras, G. Iconomou, S. Papapetropoulos, P. Polychronopoulos, and H. P. Kalofonos. 2006. A randomized controlled trial evaluating the efficacy and safety of vitamin E supplementation for protection against cisplatin-induced peripheral neuropathy: Final results. *Support Care Cancer* 14 (11): 1134–1140.
139. Argyriou, A. A., E. Chroni, A. Koutras, J. Ellul, S. Papapetropoulos, G. Katsoulas, G. Iconomou, and H. P. Kalofonos. 2005. Vitamin E for prophylaxis against chemotherapy-induced neuropathy: A randomized controlled trial. *Neurology* 64 (1): 26–31.
140. Pace, A., A. Savarese, M. Picardo, V. Maresca, U. Pacetti, G. Del Monte, A. Biroccio, et al. 2003. Neuroprotective effect of vitamin E supplementation in patients treated with cisplatin chemotherapy. *J Clin Oncol* 21 (5): 927–931.

141. Malmberg, K. J., R. Lenkei, M. Petersson, T. Ohlum, F. Ichihara, B. Glimelius, J. E. Frodin, G. Masucci, and R. Kiessling. 2002. A short-term dietary supplementation of high doses of vitamin E increases T helper 1 cytokine production in patients with advanced colorectal cancer. *Clin Cancer Res* 8 (6): 1772–1778.
142. Dennert, G., and M. Horneber. 2006. Selenium for alleviating the side effects of chemotherapy, radiotherapy and surgery in cancer patients. *Cochrane Database Syst Rev* 3: CD005037.
143. Wang, W. S., J. K. Lin, T. C. Lin, W. S. Chen, J. K. Jiang, H. S. Wang, T. J. Chiou, J. H. Liu, C. C. Yen, and P. M. Chen. 2007. Oral glutamine is effective for preventing oxaliplatin-induced neuropathy in colorectal cancer patients. *Oncologist* 12 (3): 312–319.
144. Prasad, K. N. 1995. *Handbook of Radiobiology*, Boca Raton, FL: CRC Press.
145. Walker, E. M., D. Ross, J. Pegg, G. Devine, K. N. Prasad, J. H. Kim. 2002. Nutritional and high dose antioxidant interventions during radiation therapy for cancer of the breast. International Conference on Nutrition and Cancer, Montevideo, Uruguay, July 2002.
146. Pathak, A. K., M. Bhutani, R. Guleria, S. Bal, A. Mohan, B. K. Mohanti, A. Sharma, et al. 2005. Chemotherapy alone vs. chemotherapy plus high dose multiple antioxidants in patients with advanced non small cell lung cancer. *J Am Coll Nutr* 24 (1): 16–21.
147. Drisko, J. A., J. Chapman, and V. J. Hunter. 2003. The use of antioxidants with first-line chemotherapy in two cases of ovarian cancer. *J Am Coll Nutr* 22 (2): 118–123.
148. Ingold, K. U., G. W. Burton, D. O. Foster, L. Hughes, D. A. Lindsay, and A. Webb. 1987. Biokinetics of and discrimination between dietary *RRR*- and *SRR*-alpha-tocopherols in the male rat. *Lipids* 22 (3): 163–172.
149. Witschi, A., S. Reddy, B. Stofer, and B. H. Lauterburg. 1992. The systemic availability of oral glutathione. *Eur J Clin Pharmacol* 43 (6): 667–669.
150. Dovinova, I., L. Novotny, P. Rauko, and P. Kvasnicka. 1999. Combined effect of lipoic acid and doxorubicin in murine leukemia. *Neoplasma* 46 (4): 237–241.
151. Hirose, K., D. L. Longo, J. J. Oppenheim, and K. Matsushima. 1993. Overexpression of mitochondrial manganese superoxide dismutase promotes the survival of tumor cells exposed to interleukin-1, tumor necrosis factor, selected anticancer drugs, and ionizing radiation. *FASEB J* 7 (2): 361–368.
152. Sun, J., Y. Chen, M. Li, and Z. Ge. 1998. Role of antioxidant enzymes on ionizing radiation resistance. *Free Radic Biol Med* 24 (4): 586–593.
153. Omenn, G. S., G. E. Goodman, M. D. Thornquist, J. Balmes, M. R. Cullen, A. Glass, J. P. Keogh, et al. 1996. Effects of a combination of beta carotene and vitamin A on lung cancer and cardiovascular disease. *N Engl J Med* 334 (18): 1150–1155.
154. Albanes, D., O. P. Heinonen, J. K. Huttunen, P. R. Taylor, J. Virtamo, B. K. Edwards, J. Haapakoski, et al. 1995. Effects of alpha-tocopherol and beta-carotene supplements on cancer incidence in the Alpha-Tocopherol Beta-Carotene Cancer Prevention Study. *Am J Clin Nutr* 62 (6 Suppl): 1427S–1430S.
155. Seifried, H. E., S. S. McDonald, D. E. Anderson, P. Greenwald, and J. A. Milner. 2003. The antioxidant conundrum in cancer. *Cancer Res* 63 (15): 4295–4298.
156. Meyer, F., I. Bairati, A. Fortin, M. Gelinas, A. Nabid, F. Brochet, and B. Tetu. 2008. Interaction between antioxidant vitamin supplementation and cigarette smoking during radiation therapy in relation to long-term effects on recurrence and mortality: A randomized trial among head and neck cancer patients. *Int J Cancer* 122 (7): 1679–1683.
157. Salganik, R. I., C. D. Albright, J. Rodgers, J. Kim, S. H. Zeisel, M. S. Sivashinskiy, and T. A. Van Dyke. 2000. Dietary antioxidant depletion: Enhancement of tumor apoptosis and inhibition of brain tumor growth in transgenic mice. *Carcinogenesis* 21 (5): 909–914.
158. Rama, B. N., and K. N. Prasad. 1984. Effect of hyperthermia in combination with vitamin E and cyclic AMP on neuroblastoma cells in culture. *Life Sci* 34 (21): 2089–2097.
159. Yang, T. N., C. F. Ren, H. Q. Pan, J. L. Wang, Z. Y. Zhang, and C. H. Su. 1987. Effect of vitamin C (V.C) on thermal sensitivity of Lewis tumor. *Zhonghua Zhong Liu Za Zhi* 9 (6): 421–423, 23.
160. Kageyama, K., Y. Onoyama, S. Otani, I. Matsui-Yuasa, N. Nagao, and N. Miwa. 1995. Enhanced inhibitory effects of hyperthermia combined with ascorbic acid on DNA synthesis in Ehrlich ascites tumor cells grown at a low cell density. *Cancer Biochem Biophys* 14 (4): 273–280.
161. Fujita, M., M. Nagai, M. Murata, K. Kawakami, S. Irino, and J. Takahara. 1997. Synergistic cytotoxic effect of quercetin and heat treatment in a lymphoid cell line (OZ) with low HSP70 expression. *Leuk Res* 21 (2): 139–145.
162. Piantelli, M., D. Tatone, G. Castrilli, F. Savini, N. Maggiano, L. M. Larocca, F. O. Ranelletti, and P. G. Natali. 2001. Quercetin and tamoxifen sensitize human melanoma cells to hyperthermia. *Melanoma Res* 11 (5): 469–476.

163. Debes, A., M. Oerding, R. Willers, U. Gobel, and R. Wessalowski. 2003. Sensitization of human Ewing's tumor cells to chemotherapy and heat treatment by the bioflavonoid quercetin. *Anticancer Res* 23 (4): 3359–3366.
164. Shen, J., W. Zhang, J. Wu, and Y. Zhu. 2008. The synergistic reversal effect of multidrug resistance by quercetin and hyperthermia in doxorubicin-resistant human myelogenous leukemia cells. *Int J Hyperthermia* 24 (2): 151–159.
165. Louis, M., R. R. Rosato, L. Brault, S. Osbild, E. Battaglia, X. H. Yang, S. Grant, and D. Bagrel. 2004. The histone deacetylase inhibitor sodium butyrate induces breast cancer cell apoptosis through diverse cytotoxic actions including glutathione depletion and oxidative stress. *Int J Oncol* 25 (6): 1701–1711.
166. Li, F., H. S. Luo, Y. J. Ding, and X. Li. 2004. Influence of sodium butyrate on growth of HT-29 colon carcinoma cells and expression of inducible nitric oxide synthase (iNOS), *Ai Zheng* 23 (4): 416–420.
167. Samid, D., S. Shack, and L. T. Sherman. 1992. Phenylacetate: A novel nontoxic inducer of tumor cell differentiation. *Cancer Res* 52 (7): 1988–1992.
168. Melchior, S. W., L. G. Brown, W. D. Figg, J. E. Quinn, R. A. Santucci, J. Brunner, J. W. Thuroff, P. H. Lange, and R. L. Vessella. 1999. Effects of phenylbutyrate on proliferation and apoptosis in human prostate cancer cells in vitro and in vivo. *Int J Oncol* 14 (3): 501–508.
169. Thibault, A., D. Samid, M. R. Cooper, W. D. Figg, A. C. Tompkins, N. Patronas, D. J. Headlee, D. R. Kohler, D. J. Venzon, and C. E. Myers. 1995. Phase I study of phenylacetate administered twice daily to patients with cancer. *Cancer* 75 (12): 2932–2938.
170. Rama, B. N., and K. N. Prasad. 1986. Modification of the hyperthermic response on neuroblastoma cells by cAMP and sodium butyrate. *Cancer* 58 (7): 1448–1452.
171. Pili, R., M. P. Kruszewski, B. W. Hager, J. Lantz, and M. A. Carducci. 2001. Combination of phenylbutyrate and 13-*cis* retinoic acid inhibits prostate tumor growth and angiogenesis. *Cancer Res* 61 (4): 1477–1485.
172. Massart, C., A. Denais, and J. Gibassier. 2006. Effect of all-*trans* retinoic acid and sodium butyrate in vitro and in vivo on thyroid carcinoma xenografts. *Anticancer Drugs* 17 (5): 559–563.
173. Indap, M. A., and M. S. Barkume. 2003. Efficacies of plant phenolic compounds on sodium butyrate induced anti-tumour activity. *Indian J Exp Biol* 41 (8): 861–864.
174. Zhang, X., Z. G. Chen, F. R. Khuri, and D. M. Shin. 2007. Induction of cell cycle arrest and apoptosis by a combined treatment with 13-*cis*-retinoic acid, interferon-alpha2a, and alpha-tocopherol in squamous cell carcinoma of the head and neck. *Head Neck* 29 (4): 351–361.
175. Ryu, S., O. B. Kim, S. H. Kim, S. Q. He, and J. H. Kim. 1998. In vitro radiosensitization of human cervical carcinoma cells by combined use of 13-*cis*-retinoic acid and interferon-alpha2a. *Int J Radiat Oncol Biol Phys* 41 (4): 869–873.
176. Ramanathapuram, L. V., J. J. Kobie, D. Bearss, C. M. Payne, K. T. Trevor, and E. T. Akporiaye. 2004. alpha-Tocopheryl succinate sensitizes established tumors to vaccination with nonmatured dendritic cells. *Cancer Immunol Immunother* 53 (7): 580–588.
177. Ramanathapuram, L. V., T. Hahn, M. W. Graner, E. Katsanis, and E. T. Akporiaye. 2006. Vesiculated alpha-tocopheryl succinate enhances the anti-tumor effect of dendritic cell vaccines. *Cancer Immunol Immunother* 55 (2): 166–177.
178. Shanker, M., B. Gopalan, S. Patel, D. Bocangel, S. Chada, and R. Ramesh. 2007. Vitamin E succinate in combination with mda-7 results in enhanced human ovarian tumor cell killing through modulation of extrinsic and intrinsic apoptotic pathways. *Cancer Lett* 254 (2): 217–226.
179. Rama, B. N., and K. N. Prasad. 1984. Effects of DL-alpha-tocopheryl succinate in combination with sodium butyrate and cAMP stimulating agent on neuroblastoma cells in culture. *Int J Cancer* 34 (6): 863–867.

9 Micronutrients in the Prevention and Improvement of the Standard Therapy for Alzheimer's Disease

INTRODUCTION

The Alzheimer Association has estimated that Alzheimer's disease (AD) affects about 5.3 million Americans. More than half of AD patients receive treatment and specialized care. AD accounts for 50–70% percent of dementia cases. Other types of dementia include vascular dementia, mixed dementia, and dementia with Lewy bodies. In western Norway, the analysis of dementia cases from 2005 to 2007 revealed that 65% had AD dementia, 20% had dementia with Lewy bodies, 5.6% had vascular dementia, 5.6% had Parkinson's disease with dementia, 2% had frontotemporal dementia, and 1.5% had alcoholic dementia.[1]

In recent years, significant advances have been made in the biochemical and genetic bases of this disease. Despite these advances in our understanding of this disease, no evidenced-based strategy has been proposed to reduce the risk of AD, and no effective therapy for this disease exists at this time. This may be due to the fact that the major biological events, increased oxidative stress and chronic inflammation, responsible for the initiation and progression of AD are not being addressed by standard medications. Antioxidants can neutralize free radicals and reduce chronic inflammation; therefore, supplementation with antioxidants alone may reduce the risk of AD, and, when used in combination with standard therapy, they may enhance its efficacy. We have published two reviews in which the importance of multiple micronutrients, including dietary and endogenous antioxidants, in reducing the risk of AD and in improving the efficacy of the current therapy for the treatment of neurodegenerative diseases, including AD, has been emphasized.[2,3] This chapter briefly discusses the following topics:

- Incidence and cost
- Etiology and neuropathology
- Increased oxidative stress and chronic inflammation
- Amyloid fragment-induced neurodegeneration
- Proteasome-inhibition-induced neurotoxicity
- Generation of beta amyloid induced by high cholesterol levels
- Gene mutations in familial AD
- Laboratory and clinical studies with antioxidants
- Role of nonsteroidal anti-inflammatory drugs in prevention and treatment
- Current therapies
- Rationale for using multiple micronutrients, including dietary and endogenous antioxidants, for prevention and improved treatment, in combination with standard therapy
- Recommended multiple micronutrients and low-dose aspirin for prevention and, in combination with standard therapy, for improved treatment

INCIDENCE AND COST

The incidence of AD and other dementia doubles every 5 years beyond the age of 65, and about 50% of the U.S. population 85 years or older have symptoms of AD.[4-6] Only about 5–10% of AD is due to hereditary factors and appears at an early age. The remaining cases are considered to be idiopathic or sporadic, and appear at a late age. In view of the fact that about 33 million Americans are age 65 and older, this number is predicted to increase to 51 million by the year 2025.[4] Thus, AD is a major medical concern. The annual economic cost of AD health care expenses and lost wages (for both AD patients and their caregivers) is estimated to be $80–100 billion.[4]

ETIOLOGY OF AD

Studies on the environmental, dietary, and lifestyle-related, or biochemical-related, etiology of AD are important in order to identify targets for the development of new drugs or agents for the prevention and the treatment of this disease. Among environmental factors, high consumption of aluminum from drinking water may increase the risk of developing dementia.[7] It has been reported that high dietary intake of vitamin C and vitamin E may reduce the risk of AD, and among current smokers the intake of beta-carotene and flavonoids may also decrease the risk of AD.[8] Vitamin D deficiency appears to be associated with both AD and Parkinson disease.[9]

The major biochemical-related etiological factors that increase the risk of AD include increased oxidative stress caused by increased production of free radicals derived from oxygen and nitrogen, and proinflammatory cytokines released from chronic inflammatory reactions. Even beta-amyloid fragments that play a dominant role in the pathogenesis of AD mediate their toxic effect via free radicals.[10-12] Other biochemical etiological factors that increase the risk of dementia include high cholesterol levels[13,14] and proteosome inhibition.[15,16] These etiological factors provide useful targets to develop a rational strategy for prevention and improved treatment of AD.

NEUROPATHOLOGY OF AD

The diagnosis of AD is made by postmortem analysis of the brains of patients with dementia. The presence of intracellular neurofibrillary tangles (NFTs) containing hyperphosphorylated tau protein and apolipoprotein E,[17-19] and extracellular senile (neuritic) plaques containing many proteins, including alpha-synuclein, beta-amyloid, ubiquitin, apolipoprotein E, presenilins, and alpha antichymotrypsin, are considered hallmarks of AD.[20-25] Interestingly, a recent study has shown that Lewy bodies are present in the brains of about 60% of AD cases.[26] The mechanisms of formation and dissolution of these cytoplasmic inclusions are under extensive investigation in order to develop novel drugs for the treatment of AD.

INCREASED OXIDATIVE STRESS IN AD

SOURCES OF FREE RADICALS IN NORMAL BRAIN

Before discussing the role of increased oxidative stress in AD, it is essential to describe briefly the sources of free radicals in a normal brain. The brain utilizes about 25% of respired oxygen even though it represents only 5% of the body weight. Free radicals are generated in the brain during the normal intake of oxygen, during infection, and during the normal oxidative metabolism of certain substrates. During normal aerobic respiration, the mitochondria of one rat nerve cell will process about 10^{12} oxygen molecules and reduce them to water. During this process, superoxide anion ($O_2^{\cdot -}$), hydrogen peroxide (H_2O_2), and hydroxyl ($OH^{\cdot}$) are produced. Partially reduced oxygen, which represents about 2% of consumed oxygen, leaks out from the mitochondria and generates about 20 billion molecules of $O_2^{\cdot -}$ and H_2O_2 per cell per day.[27,28] During bacterial or viral infection, phagocytic cells generate high levels of nitric oxide (NO), $O_2^{\cdot-}$, and H_2O_2 to kill infective agents; however, these radicals can also damage normal cells.[29] During degradation of fatty acids and other molecules by peroxisomes, H_2O_2 is produced as a byproduct. During oxidative metabolism of ingested toxins, free radicals are also generated.

Some brain enzymes such as monoamine oxidase (MAO), tyrosine hydroxylase, and L-amino acid oxidase produce H_2O_2 as a normal byproduct of their activity.[30] Furthermore, auto-oxidation of ascorbate and catecholamines generates H_2O_2.[31] Oxidative stress can also be generated by Ca^{2+}-mediated activation of glutamate receptors. The Ca^{2+}-dependent activation of phospholipase A_2 by N-methyl-D-aspartate (NMDA) releases arachidonic acid, which then liberates $O^{2\cdot-}$ during the biosynthesis of eicosanoids.[32] Another radical, NO, is formed by nitric oxide synthase stimulated by Ca^{2+}. NO can react with $O^{2\cdot-}$ to form peroxynitrite anions that can form $OH^{\cdot}$, the highly reactive hydroxyl radical. NMDA receptor stimulation produces marked elevations in $O^{2\cdot-}$ and $OH^{\cdot}$ levels.[33] Some enzymes, such as xanthine oxidase and flavoprotein oxidase (e.g., aldehyde oxidase), also form superoxide anions during metabolism of their respective substrates. Oxidation of hydroquinone and thiol and the synthesis of uric acid from purines form superoxide anions.

Certain external agents can increase oxidative stress. For example, cigarette smoking increases the level of NO by about 1000 ppm[34,35] and depletes antioxidant levels.[36,37] Free iron and copper can increase the free radical levels.[38] Some plants ingested as food contain large amounts of phenolic compounds such as chlorogenic and caffeic acid, which can be oxidized to form radicals.[39,40] These studies suggest that the brain generates high levels of reactive oxygen species (ROS) and reactive nitrogen species (RNS) every day. The brain has the highest levels of unsaturated fatty acids, which are easily oxidizable by free radicals. Paradoxically, the brain is least prepared to handle this excessive load of free radicals. It has low levels of both antioxidant enzyme systems and dietary antioxidants. These inherent biological features make the brain very vulnerable to increased oxidative stress. Despite this, the risk of idiopathic AD becomes significant only after the age of 65. This is due to the fact that neurons exhibit a high degree of plasticity in maintaining normal brain functions. The fact that clinical symptoms of neurological diseases including AD appear only when a significant number of neurons are lost supports the value of plasticity of the neurons in maintaining normal brain function.

FORMATION OF FREE RADICALS DERIVED FROM OXYGEN AND NITROGEN

The brain utilizes 3.5 ml oxygen/100 g of brain tissue per minute.[41] About 2% of the oxygen consumed becomes ROS.[28] The formation of some of these ROS is described below.

When molecular oxygen (O_2) acquires an electron, the superoxide anion, ($O^{2\cdot-}$) is formed:

$$O^2 + e^- = O^{2\cdot-}$$

Superoxide dismutase (SOD) and H^+ can react with $O^{2\cdot-}$ to form hydrogen peroxide, H_2O_2:

$$2O^{2\cdot-} + 2H + SOD \rightarrow H_2O_2 + O_2$$

$$O^{2\cdot-} + H^+ \rightarrow HO_2^{\cdot} \text{ (hydroperoxy radical)}$$

$$2HO_2^{\cdot} \rightarrow H_2O_2 + O_2$$

Ferric and ferrous forms of iron can react with superoxide anion and hydrogen peroxide to produce molecular oxygen and hydroxyl radical ($OH^{\cdot}$), respectively:

$$Fe^{3+} + O^{2\cdot-} \rightarrow Fe^{2+} + O_2$$

$$Fe^{2+} + H_2O_2 \rightarrow Fe^{3+} + OH^{\bullet} + OH^- \text{ (Fenton reaction)}$$

The hydroxyl radical can also be formed from superoxide anion by the Haber–Weiss reaction:

$$O^{2\bullet-} + H_2O_2 \rightarrow O_2 + OH^- + OH^{\bullet}$$

Both the Fenton and Haber–Weiss reactions require a transition metal such as copper or iron. Among ROS, $OH^{\bullet}$ is the most damaging free radical and is very short-lived. The hydroxyl radical is very reactive with a variety of organic compounds, leading to the production of more radical compounds:

$$RH \text{ (organic compound)} + OH^{\bullet} \rightarrow R^{\bullet} \text{ (organic radical)} + H_2O$$

$$R^{\bullet} + O_2 \rightarrow RO_2^{\bullet} \text{ (peroxy radical)}$$

Catalase detoxifies hydrogen peroxide to form water and molecular oxygen:

$$H_2O_2 + \text{catalase} \rightarrow H_2O \text{ and } O_2$$

RNS are represented by nitric oxide ($NO^{\bullet}$). $NO^{\bullet}$ is synthesized by the enzyme nitric oxide synthase from L-arginine and, in the brain, it acts both as a neurotransmitter and, in excessive amounts, acts as a neurotoxin. $NO^{\bullet}$ can combine with superoxide anion to form peroxynitrite, a powerful oxidant.

$$NO^{\bullet} + O^{2\bullet-} \rightarrow ONOO^- \text{ (peroxynitrite)}$$

When protonated (likely at physiological pH), peroxynitrite spontaneously decomposes to reactive nitric dioxide and hydroxyl radicals:

$$ONOO^- + H^+ \rightarrow {}^{\bullet}NO_2 + OH^{\bullet}$$

SOD can also enhance the peroxynitrite-mediated nitration of tyrosine residues on critical proteins, presumably via a species similar to the nitronium cation (NO_2^+):

$$ONOO^- + SOD \rightarrow NO_2^+ \rightarrow \text{Nitration of tyrosine}$$

These data reveal that several different types of radicals are constantly formed in the brain. Their levels can be increased by enhanced turnover of catecholamines, increased levels of free iron, impaired mitochondrial functions, decreased glutathione levels, etc. Antioxidant enzymes, which can protect cells against the damaging effects of these free radicals include catalase, SOD, and glutathione peroxidase. Therefore, decreased levels of catalase, glutathione peroxidase, or SOD can also enhance the amounts of free radicals. Natural dietary antioxidants include vitamins A, C, and E, carotenoids, flavonoids, and polyphenols. Some biosynthetic antioxidants include coenzyme Q_{10}, alpha-lipoic acid, glutathione, the reduced form of nucleotide adenine dehydrogenase (NADH), and urates. Consumption of a diet low in antioxidants may also increase the levels of free radicals. Thus, maintenance of a balance in favor of antioxidants is essential for the protection of brain function. When this balance is shifted in favor of oxidants, the epigenetic components of neurons suffer damage, and slow accumulation of such damage may initiate degeneration and eventually cause death of neurons.

OXIDATIVE STRESS–INDUCED MITOCHONDRIAL DAMAGE IN AD

Mitochondria may be one of the most sensitive primary targets of oxidative stress in adult neurons.[42] This may be due to the fact that mitochondrial DNA (mtDNA) does not encode for any repair enzymes, and, unlike nuclear DNA, it is not shielded by protective histones. Additionally, mtDNA is in close proximity to the site where free radicals are generated during oxidative phosphorylation.[42] Indeed, an increased frequency of mutations in mtDNA has been found in autopsy samples of AD brains,[43] and several studies have implicated mitochondrial defects in the pathogenesis of AD.[42–46] Because the onset of AD coincides with older age, it is reasonable to suggest that damaged mtDNA, which is normally removed during mitochondrial turnover, accumulates in neurons due to the slowing down of this process in older individuals. Thus, the number of defective mitochondria may accumulate with age and this could lead to reduced production of ATP that could then initiate slow degenerative processes in neurons. Reduced ATP levels result in decreased energy metabolism. For example, decreased glucose uptake coupled with reduced activity of cytochrome oxidase (complex IV) leads to increased production of ROS by mitochondria.[41,45] This could then constitute a continuous cycle of production of increased levels of free radicals and enhanced mitochondrial dysfunction. A defect in energy production may also increase the sensitivity of neurons to excitatory amino acids.[47] Impaired mitochondria may alter metabolism of APP, leading to decreased secretion of APP, and increased generation of potentially amyloidogenic derivatives (11.5 kDa COOH-terminal derivative, which contains the full-length amyloid sequence) that are intermediate metabolites in the production of beta–amyloid.[48] An excess of free Zn is found in the autopsied brain of AD patients,[49] and increased free Zn can impair mitochondrial function.[50] Thus, mitochondria appear to be one of the major targets of oxidative damage that mediate neurodegeneration in AD. Because of increased production of free radicals, reduced levels of antioxidants, and high levels of unsaturated fatty acids that are easily damaged by free radicals, the brain is particularly sensitive to oxidative stress.[28,41,45,46] Indeed, increased oxidative stress has been implicated in the loss of neurons associated with AD.[51–57] A number of observations substantiate the presence of high levels of oxidative stress in AD brains; for example, (1) the serum levels of vitamins A, E, and beta-carotene were lower in well-nourished patients with AD than in control patients[58]; (2) higher expression of heme oxygenase is found in the brains of AD patients[59,60]; (3) increased consumption of oxygen is found in AD patients[61]; (4) increased activity of glucose-6-phosphate dehydrogenase is found in the AD brain[62]; and (5) activation of calcium-dependent neural proteinase (calpain) is found in AD brains,[63] which may trigger events leading to the formation of free radicals.[64] The increased levels of lipofuscin formation in a small number of degenerating neurons probably results in a marked progressive increase in superoxide radicals and H_2O_2 formation and reduced production of ATP, which overwhelms the endogenous antioxidant systems that protect against free radical-induced damage.[65] The fibroblasts obtained from familial AD patients were more sensitive to oxidative stress than those obtained from age-matched normal controls.[66] Alpha-ketoglutarate dehydrogenase complex (KGDHC), a mitochondrial enzyme, is decreased in the brains of AD patients.[67] It is interesting to note that in AD patients who carry the ApoE4 allele of the ApoE gene, the Clinical Dementia Rating (CDR) correlated better with KGDHC activity than with densities of neuritic plaques and NTFs; however, in patients without the ApoE4, the CDR correlated better with plaques and NTFs than with KGDHC activity.[67] This suggests that mitochondrial dysfunctions may be more important for the development of AD in patients who carry the ApoE4 allele than in those who do not.

Additional evidence for the increased oxidative stress in AD brains include the following: (1) homogenates of the frontal cortex from AD brains obtained at autopsy revealed a 22% higher production of free radicals and, in the presence of iron, a 50% higher production of free radicals than those of age-matched normal controls[68]; (2) peroxynitrite also exacerbates the pathogenesis of AD[69]; (3) increased neuronal nitric oxide synthase (nNOS) expression in reactive astrocytes correlated with apoptosis in hippocampal neurons of AD brains[70]; (4) glutamine synthetase, a highly sensitive enzyme to oxidative stress, showed decreased activity in AD brains[69]; (5) the level of glutathione transferase is decreased in ventricular CSF and in AD brains compared to brains from age-matched controls[71]; and (6) increased levels of oxidized proteins are found in the blood of both AD patients and their relatives when compared with non-AD controls.[72] Taken together, these data strongly suggest that increased oxidative stress represents one of the major biochemical events that plays an important role in initiation and progression of AD.

BETA-AMYLOID MEDIATES ITS NEUROTOXIC EFFECTS THROUGH FREE RADICALS IN AD

It is now established that beta-amyloid fragments (1–42) generated by cleavage of the amyloid precursor protein (APP) play a central role in the pathogenesis of AD.[20–22,73] There are two pathways of processing APP in neurons. The predominant pathway of APP processing consists of successive cleavages by alpha- and gamma-secretases, whereas the other pathway involves sequential cleavage of APP by beta- and gamma-secretases. It is the latter pathway that generates neurotoxic beta-amyloid. Normally, alpha-secretase cleaves inside the beta-amyloid sequence of APP, releasing the soluble N-terminal domain of APP that exhibits neurotrophic and neuroprotective properties. In patients with AD, a decrease in alpha-secretase–mediated processing of APP has been found in autopsied brain samples.[74] It is not certain whether a decrease in alpha-secretase-mediated processing of APP is associated with an increase in processing of APP by beta- and gamma-secretases.

It has been shown that aggregates of beta-amyloid fragments are toxic to neurons in culture[12,75,76] and can cause cell death by apoptosis[77] or necrosis.[10] Several agents can enhance the aggregation of beta-amyloid. They include excess amounts of free Zn and Cu,[78] iron, and aluminum[79] and complement proteins.[80] The aggregated form of beta-amyloid participates in the formation of senile plaque, which can serve as a chronic source of inflammatory reactions, the products of which can enhance the progression of degeneration in nerve cells.

Increased oxidative stress may enhance intracellular accumulation of beta-amyloid in neurons.[81] Studies show that membranes containing oxidatively damaged phospholipids accumulated beta-amyloid faster than membranes containing only unoxidized saturated phospholipids.[82] It has been proposed that one of the mechanisms of action of beta-amyloid-induced neurotoxicity is mediated by free radicals.[10–12] This is supported by the fact that vitamin E protects neuronal cells in culture against beta-amyloid–induced toxicity.[83] It has been shown that methionine in the 35th position of beta-amyloid may be responsible for generating free radicals.[84] This was confirmed by a series of studies on substitutions of amino acids[84] and by prevention of beta-amyloid-induced toxicity with vitamin E.[83] Experiments on a transgenic mouse model of AD support the concept that beta-amyloid-induced neurotoxicity is mediated by oxidative stress. For example, it has been reported[85] that Cu/Zn SOD, and hemoxygenase-1 (HO-1), markers of oxidative stress, were elevated in aged transgenic mice.

It has been shown that an increase in beta-amyloid fragments precedes tau pathology (formation of NTFs) in the frontal cortex.[86] This suggests that tau pathology, which requires at least two steps, hyperphosphorylation and accumulation of hyperphosphorylated tau, occurs later than increased generation of beat-amyloid fragments. Hyperphosphorylation of tau can result from increased PKA activity and/or decreased phosphatase activity. Proteasome inhibition may also reduce degradation of hyperphosphorylated tau proteins, causing them to slowly accumulate and lead to the formation of NFTs within the cells.

CHOLESTEROL-INDUCED GENERATION OF BETA-AMYLOID

Epidemiologic studies have found that hypercholesterolemia may be a risk factor in the development of AD.[13,14] This was confirmed in the transgenic animal model of AD.[14] This study revealed that high dietary cholesterol increases beta-amyloid accumulation and, thereby, accelerates AD-related pathology in animals.[87] The accumulation of beta-amyloid can be reversed by removing cholesterol from the rabbit's diet.[87] Inhibitors of HMG CoA reductase decrease production of beta-amyloid in rabbit[14] and in fetal rat hippocampal neurons in culture.[88] An epidemiologic study has shown that lovastatin, an inhibitor of HMG CoA reductase, reduced the risk of AD in hypercholesterolemic patients.[89] In a recent epidemiologic study, the use of statins, but not of nonstatin cholesterol-lowering drugs, was associated with a reduced incidence of AD in comparison to those who never took statins.[90] These results suggest that lower levels of cholesterol may reduce the risk of AD and that some of the effects of high cholesterol levels are primarily mediated via beta-amyloid.

Statins (cholesterol-lowering drugs) can be divided into two distinct groups, those with a closed-ring structure (lovastatin, Simvastatin, mevastatin) and those with an open-ring structure (pravastatin and fluvastatin). Statins with a closed-ring structure are metabolized in vivo to an open-ring structure, which then inhibits HMG CoA reductase activity. However, a small amount of the drug could be maintained in a closed-ring structure, which can inhibit proteasome activity.[91] We have demonstrated that mevastatin with a closed-ring structure caused rapid degeneration of differentiated neuroblastoma (NB) cells in culture, whereas, pravastatin with an open-ring structure did not.[92] Mevastatin inhibited proteasome activity in differentiated NB, whereas, pravastatin did not. Differentiated NB cells did not convert any portion of mevastatin into an open-ring structure. This is in sharp contrast to the observation made in vivo where most mevastatin is converted to an open-ring structure by the liver enzyme. These results suggest that mevastatin-induced degeneration of differentiated NB cells may be related to inhibition of proteasome activity.[92] The studies discussed in this section reveal that lowering cholesterol levels could reduce the risk of AD, whereas, the presence of increased amounts of unmetabolized statin with a closed-ring structure could increase the risk of AD. A careful study on the effects of statins with a closed-ring and an open-ring structure on neuroprotection and neurodegeneration should be evaluated by laboratory experiments and epidemiologic studies before their relevance in AD can be determined.

PROTEASOME INHIBITION INDUCED NEURODEGENERATION IN AD

Proteasome play an important role in regulating certain transcriptional factors by splicing inactive peptide fragments into active ones. Proteasomes also play a crucial role in the degradation of ubiquitin-conjugated abnormal proteins that could be toxic to neurons. Therefore, inhibition of proteasome in neurons can initiate and promote neurodegeneration. Indeed, the role of proteasome inhibition has been proposed for the degeneration of neurons in AD brains.[15,93,94] In our study, inhibition of proteasome by lactacystin causes rapid degeneration of neuronal cells in culture.[95] Several factors can inhibit proteasome activity. They include increased oxidative stress, defects in ubiquitin-conjugated enzymes,[16] mutation in ubiquitin,[96] and beta-amyloid.[93] The exact mechanisms of proteasome inhibition in AD neurons are unknown, but they could involve more than one mechanism.

GENETIC DEFECTS IN IDIOPATHIC AD

There is no solid evidence for nuclear gene defects that increase the risk of idiopathic AD, although varying degrees of association between certain gene defects and onset of this disease exist. Several studies have suggested that persons who are homozygous for the apolipoprotein E (ApoE), E4 allele, develop AD 10 to 20 years earlier than those who have E2 or E3 alleles.[97,98] Even persons who are heterozygous for E4 allele, develop AD 5 to 10 years earlier than those who have E2 or E3 alleles.[99] About 40% of idiopathic AD is associated with the presence of E4 allele, and it is present in the senile plaque.[17,99] These data suggest that the presence of E4 allele could be an important risk factor for AD. However, it has been shown that this allele is neither essential nor specific to the development of AD.[99] Thus, the role of this ApoE allele in neurodegeneration remains uncertain. It has been reported that E4 allele binds to NFTs and beta-amyloid.[17] This property of ApoE4 is not sufficient to have any direct role in neurodegeneration associated with AD. However, a recent study has reported that in patients who carry ApoE4, the clinical dementia rating was correlated better with decreased alpha-ketoglutarate dehydrogenase complex, a mitochondrial enzyme, than with the plaques or NFTs.[67] This suggests that in some cases of AD, ApoE4 may have some role in the propagation of degenerative processes. A study has reported that mutation in the alpha2-macroglobulin gene is present in about 30% of idiopathic AD[100]; however, another study found no such association between alpha2-macroglobulin mutation and risk of AD.[101] Recent studies have identified two gene defects in idiopathic AD. Mutation in the ubiquitin gene and down-regulation of PS-2 were observed in AD brains.[102,103] We have shown that differentiated neuronal cells in culture over expressing human APP become sensitive to neurotoxin including oxidative stress.[104]

The genetic polymorphisms play an important role in determining the risk of AD in some populations.[105,106] The levels of beta-secretase, a rate-limiting enzyme in formation of beta-amyloid, were elevated in the autopsied samples of AD brain.[107,108] It appears that amyloid plaque induces beta-secretase in surrounding neurons. In addition, transforming growth factor-beta (TGF-beta) enhances beta-amyloid production in human astrocytes, but not in neurons.[109] This could contribute to the formation of NFT.

MUTATED GENES MEDIATE THEIR EFFECTS THROUGH INCREASED PRODUCTION OF BETA-AMYLOID IN FAMILIAL AD

In some familial AD, mutations (about seven) in the APP gene have been reported, all of which increase the production of beta-amyloid[110]; however, this accounts for less than 1% of all familial AD. Mutations (about 50) in presenilin-I gene have been found in about 50% of familial AD,[110] whereas, mutations in presenilin-II have been observed in less than 1% of familial AD.[110,111] Presenilin-I is present in senile plaques and NTFs of AD brains.[110] Mutations in APP and presenilin-1 (PS-1) increase the production of beta-amyloid-42, which causes neuronal death via increasing oxidative stress in primary neuronal cultures obtained from knock-in mice expressing mutant human APP and PS-1 compared to those obtained from wild-type mice.[112] The levels of oxidative damage as a function of age was more pronounced in knock-in mice expressing mutant human APP and PS-1 genes in comparison to those observed in wild-type mice.[113] This effect was independent of dietary cholesterol.[114] It has been reported that mutations in PS-1 may increase neuronal sensitivity to apoptosis by decreasing the levels of beta-catenin, which is involved in regulation of apoptosis.[115] In addition, PS-1 mutation may also impair proteolytic release and nuclear translocation of Notch-1 intracellular domain, an essential step in activating Notch-1 signaling.[116] Mutation in PS-1 increased the activity of gamma-secretase activity that increases the production of beta-amyloid.[117]

Mutation in gamma secretase results in rare forms of early onset of AD due to production of increased amounts of beta-amyloid.[118] The activity of gamma secretase increases as a function of age in female mice[118] and that may be, in part, responsible for the relatively increased incidence of AD commonly observed in women.

The nature of the interaction between APP and presenilins in causing neuronal damage is not well understood. It has been postulated[23] that APP interacts specifically and transcellularly with either PS-1 or PS-2. This complex is incorporated into intracellular vesicles, which fuse with multivesicular bodies that contain proteases. Beta-amyloid is then produced by proteolysis of APP and released by the usual intracellular traffic between the lysosomal compartment and the plasma membrane into the extracellular spaces where it forms senile (neuritic) plaques.

These studies suggest that mutations in both APP and PS-1 increase the rate of production of beta-amyloid. Excessive production of beta-amyloid can generate more free radicals, inhibit proteasome activity, and contribute to the formation of senile plaques, all of which contribute to progressive neurodegeneration in the AD brain.

INCREASED LEVELS OF MARKERS OF CHRONIC INFLAMMATION IN AD

Evidence of chronic inflammatory reactions in autopsied brains from patients with AD was first observed by Dr. Alois Alzheimer himself. The role of chronic inflammation in AD pathogenesis is supported by the epidemiologic studies that show that rheumatoid arthritis patients, who were on high doses of non-steroidal anti-inflammatory drugs (NSAIDs), had a reduced incidence of AD.[119–122] The direct evidence came from the studies in which it was demonstrated that the mediators and products of inflammatory reaction, such as cytokines,[123,124] complement proteins,[80,125–127] free radicals,[51–54] adhesion molecules,[128–130] and prostaglandins[57,131] were toxic in experimental models of neurons.

Increased levels of proinflammatory cytokines such as IL-1 beta and TNF-alpha are found in autopsied samples of brains of AD patients.[132] There appears to be close interaction between beta-amyloid and proinflammatory cytokines with respect to the production and levels of beta-amyloid and beta-amyloid-induced neurotoxicity. Beta-amyloid-induced inflammatory responses and vascular disruption in AD brains are mediated through TNF-alpha and IL-1 beta.[133,134] In wild-type mice, the levels of beta-amyloid can be enhanced by INF-gamma and TNF-alpha through suppression of degradation of beta-amyloid. TNF-alpha also enhanced the levels of beta-amyloid by stimulating the activity of beta-secretase, a rate-limiting enzyme in the production of beta-amyloid.[134] The combination of INF-gamma and TNF-alpha increased the production of beta-amyloid and reduced the secretion of nontoxic soluble APP fragments in human neuronal cells in culture.[135] Beta-amyloid-induced toxicity can be enhanced by IL-1 beta and TNF-alpha.[133,136] Interferon-gamma, IL-1beta, and TNF-alpha increase the gamma-secretase activity and production of beta-amyloid via JNK-dependent mitogen-activated protein kinase pathways.[137]

Both beta-amyloid and NMDA interact with each other in causing neuronal damage. Individually, beta-amyloid and NMDA produced neuronal damage, whereas IL-6, a proinflammatory cytokine, did not.[138] The combination of beta-amyloid and NMDA was more effective than the individual agents. However, the combination of three (beta-amyloid, NMDA, and IL-6) was most effective in causing damage to neurons.[138] It appears that the combination of beta-amyloid and NMDA causes increased production of ROS in cortical neurons through activation of NADPH oxidase,[139] suggesting the involvement of an NMDA receptor subtype in the mechanisms of damage produced by beta-amyloid.

The role of inflammatory reactions in AD pathogenesis was further supported by clinical studies in which administration of NSAIDs reduced the rate of deterioration of cognitive function in moderate to advanced AD patients.[140–143] However, a recent clinical study with new NSAIDs (celecoxib or naproxen) in men and women aged 70 years or more with a familial history of AD revealed that these drugs did not improve cognitive function, but a detrimental effect of naproxen was observed.[144] In another clinical trial, the effect of ibuprofen on sources of resting electroencephalographic (EEG) rhythms in mild AD patients was evaluated. The results showed that in the placebo group, amplitude of delta sources was globally greater at follow-up than baseline; however, amplitude of delta sources remained stable or decreased in the majority of patients receiving ibuprofen.[145] It has been reported that NSAIDs such as ibuprofen, aspirin, indomethacin, and naproxen inhibit to a varying degree formation of beta-amyloid fibrils from beta-amyloid and destabilize preformed beta-amyloid fibrils in vitro.[146] Ibuprofen reduced the levels of beta-amyloid and hyperphosphorylated tau protein, and improved memory deficits in AD transgenic mice.[147]

There appears to be strong evidence to suggest that increased oxidative stress and chronic inflammation play an important role in the pathogenesis of idiopathic AD; however, in familial AD, chronic inflammation may play a minor role in the progression of AD. This is due to the fact that mutations in APP, PS-1, or PS-2 that are found in familial AD increase production of beta-amyloid, which mediates its action through free radicals.[110,111–114,117,118] Most studies with NSAIDs on patients with idiopathic AD reported beneficial effects.[140–143,145] However, a recent study with NSAIDs on patients with familial AD reported no beneficial effect.[144] This result may not be surprising because, in familial AD, excessive production of beta-amyloid fragments that mediate their action through free radicals causes neurodegeneration. Therefore, the data obtained from the use of NSAIDs in familial AD should not be extrapolated to idiopathic AD. It is possible that the use of free radical scavengers such as antioxidants would have been more useful in reducing the progression of familial AD patients than NSAIDs alone. The combination of the two may be more effective than the individual agents.

NEUROGLOBIN IN AD

Neuroglobin (Ngb) is an O_2-binding heme protein related to hemoglobin and myoglobin. It is widely and specifically located in neurons of central and peripheral nervous system of vertebrates. It reversibly binds with oxygen with a high affinity. Expression of Ngb increases in response to neuronal hypoxia and protects neurons from damage caused by hypoxia in vitro and in vivo.[148–150] It also protects the brain from experimental stroke in vivo.[151] Age-dependent loss of Ngb was found in rat cerebral neocortex, hippocampus, caudate-putamen, and cerebellum.[152,153]

Overexpression of wild-type Ngb, but not mutant Ngb, in neuronal cells in culture (PC-12 cell line) decreased H_2O_2-induced free radical accumulation and lipid peroxidation without changing the levels of antioxidant enzymes.[154] It also reduced H_2O_2-induced mitochondrial dysfunction and improved the survival of cells. It has been reported that Ngb also protected neurons against beta-amyloid-induced toxicity in the PC-12 neuronal cell line[155] and in the murine cortical neurons in culture.[156] Ngb also attenuates the AD phenotype of transgenic mice.[157] These studies suggest that Ngb reduces oxidative stress in neurons by acting as an antioxidant. It has been observed that Ngb expression is reduced with increasing age, and it is lower in women than in men.[157] The latter may, in part, account for the increased risk of AD in women. Furthermore, the expression of Ngb is up-regulated in the autopsied samples of temporal lobes of AD patients, which may be a protective response to the disease process. Therefore, it is possible that the decrease in levels of Ngb may increase the risk of AD.

CURRENT TREATMENTS OF AD

In randomized, double-blind, parallel-group clinical trials, all acetylcholinesterase inhibitors (AChEIs) have shown varying degrees of efficacy over placebos in improving cognitive function in patients with mild to moderate AD. Among donepezil, galantamine, and rivastigmine, donepezil was found to be slightly more effective than others,[158] but others have reported no such difference between these drugs.[159] In the Hispanic population, the safety and beneficial effects of donepezil on cognitive function were similar to those found in the general population.[160] The annual cost of donepezil, galantamine, and rivastigmine was not significantly different.[161]

The beneficial effects of AChEIs on cognitive function depend upon the viability of cholinergic neurons in the brain of AD patients. They increase the levels of acetylcholine in the neurons. These drugs do not affect the level of oxidative stress or chronic inflammation primarily responsible for neurodegeneration in AD brains; therefore, their efficacy does not last for a long period. The progression of the disease continues to occur because of oxidative-stress- and chronic-inflammation–induced progressive neuronal death. The addition of agents that can reduce oxidative stress and chronic inflammation to the current therapeutic modalities may prolong the effectiveness of AChEI in improving cognitive function in AD patients. Therefore, we propose that antioxidants that neutralize free radicals and reduce inflammation and an NSAID that reduces inflammation should be utilized in combination with standard therapy in order to improve the current management of AD.

LABORATORY AND CLINICAL STUDIES WITH ANTIOXIDANTS IN AD

The studies discussed in this chapter show that increased production of free radicals derived from oxygen and nitrogen and products of chronic inflammation such as proinflammatory cytokines play a central role in the initiation and progression of neurodegeneration associated with AD. Therefore, it appears rational to propose that antioxidants would be beneficial in the prevention of AD and as an adjunct to standard therapy in the treatment of AD. Since antioxidants such as vitamin E, in combination with aspirin, inhibit cyclooxygenase activity in a synergistic manner, the addition of low-dose aspirin in combination with multiple antioxidants may be useful in reducing the incidence of AD in high-risk populations such as those with a family history of AD and those who are 65 years or older. Such a strategy may also be effective when combined with the standard therapy in improving treatment outcomes in patients with mild to moderate AD. Although laboratory studies with individual dietary or endogenous antioxidants in animal and cell culture models have consistently produced protective effects on neurons from damage produced by oxidative stress and chronic inflammation, limited clinical studies with an individual dietary or endogenous antioxidant have produced inconsistent results in patients with mild to moderate AD. These studies are described in the following subsections.

ALPHA-LIPOIC ACID

In an open-label study involving 43 patients with mild to moderate AD receiving standard therapy and a follow-up period of 48 months, it was observed that the addition of alpha-lipoic acid to the treatment protocol reduced the progression of the disease.[162] This effect was more pronounced in patients with mild AD than in those with moderate AD. The fibroblasts from AD patients exhibited the highest levels of oxidative damage markers in comparison to fibroblasts from age-matched and young controls; however, treatment with alpha-lipoic acid and n-acetylcysteine individually reduced the levels of markers of oxidative damage, but the combination of the two was more effective than the individual agents.[163] Alpha-lipoic acid also reduced beta-amyloid-induced toxicity on neuronal cells in culture.[164] The natural form of alpha-lipoic acid (R-LA) is more effective than the synthetic form (Rac-LA); however, the salt form of alpha-lipoic acid is absorbed better than R-LA or Rac-LA.[165] Orally administered alpha-lipoic acid does cross the blood–brain barrier in rats.[166] In a mouse model of AD, administration of R-LA through diet reduced oxidative damage, but did not improve cognitive performance or the levels of beta-amyloid.[167] Chronic administration of alpha-lipoic acid through diet reduced hippocampal-dependent memory deficits of a transgenic mice model of cerebral amyloidosis associated with AD.[168] Dietary supplementation with a combination of alpha-lipoic acid, acetyl-L-carnitine, glycerophosphocoline, docosahexaenoic acid, and phosphatidylserine reduced oxidative damage to the murine brain and improved cognitive performance.[169]

The proposed mechanisms of alpha-lipoic acid include the following: (1) increase in acetylcholine production by activation of choline acetyltransferase; (2) chelation of redox active transient metals; (3) scavenging of free radicals; and (4) increase in glutathione levels.[170] In addition, alpha-lipoic acid also reduced the expression of proinflammatory cytokines such as TNF-alpha and inducible nitric oxide synthase (NOSi).[171] The protective effect of alpha-lipoic acid may also be mediated through activation of PKB/Akt signaling pathways.[164] These studies suggest that treatment with alpha-lipoic acid alone does not produce consistent results in patients with AD.

COENZYME Q_{10} AND MELATONIN

Coenzyme Q_{10} reduced beta-amyloid overproduction and intracellular deposit of beta-amyloid in the cortex of the AD transgenic mice.[172] Coenzyme Q_{10} treatment decreased malondialdehyde (MDA) level and enhanced the activity of SOD in these mice. Coenzyme Q_{10} also prevented the formation of beta-amyloid fibrils and destabilized preformed beta-amyloid.[173] It decreased beta-amyloid-induced mitochondrial dysfunction in vitro.[174] Serum levels of coenzyme Q_{10} did not change in patients with AD.[175] It has been reported that supplementation with both coenzyme Q_{10} and alpha-tocopheryl acetate improved age-related learning deficits in mice.[176]

Melatonin treatment prevented increased the levels of thiobarbituric acid reactive substances (TBARS), SOD activity, decreased glutathione levels, and up-regulated apoptotic-related factors such as BAX, caspase-3, and prostate apoptosis response-4 (Par-4) in AD transgenic mice.[177] Long-term melatonin treatment improves cognitive function in AD transgenic mice. The mechanisms of this protection by melatonin involve preventing aggregation of beta-amyloid and reducing the levels of proinflammatory cytokines and oxidative stress.[178] Patients with AD often exhibit both agitated behavior and poor sleep patterns. In a clinical study, supplementation with melatonin failed to affect these abnormal symptoms in AD patients compared to the placebo group.[179] However, melatonin in combination with standard therapy produced more beneficial effects on cognitive function and depression than produced by standard therapy alone.[180] These studies suggest that treatment with coenzyme Q_{10} or melatonin alone does not produce consistent results in patients with AD.

NICOTINAMIDE, NICOTINAMIDE ADENINE DINUCLEOTIDE (NAD+), AND NICOTINAMIDE ADENINE DINUCLEOTIDE DEHYDROGENASE (NADH)

It has been reported that the administration of NADH (10 mg/day) improved cognitive function in AD patients.[181] In old rats, administration of NADH improved cognitive function.[182] However, further clinical studies with NADH in patients with AD did not improve cognitive function, but did not allow progressive cognitive deterioration compared to placebo control. NADH-treated patients showed significantly better performance on measures of verbal fluency, visual-constructional ability, and abstract verbal reasoning.[183] In another study, supplementation with NADH had no effect on cognitive function in patients with mild to moderate AD.[184]

Histone deacetylase inhibitors increase histone acetylation and enhance memory and neuronal plasticity. Nicotinamide, a competitive inhibitor of Class III NAD+-dependent histone deacetylase activity, restored memory deficits in AD transgenic mice.[185] It also selectively reduced a specific phospho-species of tau protein (Thr231) that is associated with microtubule depolymerization. The overexpression of a Thr231-phospho-mimic tau in neuronal cells in culture increased clearance and decreased accumulation of tau compared with wild-type tau. Nicotinamide, a precursor of NAD+ also attenuated glutamate-induced toxicity and preserved cellular levels of NAD+ to support the activity of SIRT-1.[186] These preclinical data suggest that oral supplementation with nicotinamide may be safe and useful in the treatment of AD and other taupathies. Caloric restriction up-regulated NAD+-dependent SIRT1 in the mouse brain[186] and this may be one of the mechanism of protection against amyloid neuropathology.[187] A 30% caloric restriction reduced levels of beta-amyloid, but increased the level of SRT1 in the brain of squirrel monkeys.[188] The addition of NAD+ or nicotinamide to the preparation of a multiple micronutrient preparation may be necessary to improve the efficacy of standard therapy.

VITAMIN A, VITAMIN E, AND VITAMIN C

Vitamin A and beta-carotene inhibited formation of beta-amyloid fibrils in a dose-dependent manner. They also destabilized preformed beta-amyloid fibrils in vitro.[189] Retinoic acid treatment decreased activation of microglia and astrocytes, reduced degeneration of neurons, and improved spatial learning and memory in AD transgenic mice, compared with the vehicle-control.[190] It also down-regulated the activity of cyclin-dependent kinase 5, a major kinase, involved in both APP and tau phosphorylation. Vitamin E treatment protected cortical synaptosomal membranes and hippocampal neurons[84] and other neurons[83] in culture against beta-amyloid-induced toxicity. Like vitamin A and beta-carotene, curcumin also inhibited formation of beta-amyloid fibrils and destabilized preformed beta-amyloid fibrils in vitro in a dose-dependent manner.[189] Vitamin E and pycnogenol protected neuronal cells in culture against beta-amyloid-induced apoptosis by attenuating caspase-3 activation, DNA fragmentation, and cleavage of poly (ADP-ribose) polymerase (PARP).[191]

A recent analysis of clinical studies revealed that vitamin E alone may not be useful in the prevention or treatment of AD.[192] However, a controlled clinical trial with DL-alpha-tocopherol (synthetic form; 2000 IU/day) in patients with moderately severe impairment from AD showed some beneficial effects with respect to the rate of deterioration of cognitive function.[193] In certain counties of North Carolina, analysis of older African-American and white individuals from 1986 to 2000 revealed that the supplemental use of vitamins was low; however, supplementation with vitamin C and/or vitamin E did not delay the incidence of AD or dementia in these populations.[194] In a prospective cohort study performed by Group Health Cooperative, Seattle, Washington, it was found that supplementation with vitamin E and vitamin C, individually or in combination, did not reduce the risk of AD or overall dementia over the 5.5-year observation period.[195] In a cross-sectional and prospective study in elderly (65 years and older) patients with dementia, it was found that use of vitamin C and vitamin E in combination was associated with reduced prevalence and incidence of AD.[196] In AD transgenic mice, it was shown that vitamin E supplementation reduced the levels and deposits of amyloid in the brain; however, vitamin E supplementation was ineffective at decreasing the levels and deposit of amyloid in older mice.[197] In a transgenic model of Down's syndrome, supplementation with vitamin E alone delays onset of cognitive dysfunction and pathological changes in the basal forebrain.[198] These studies suggest that treatment with one or two dietary antioxidants alone does not produce consistent results in patients with AD.

Serum Levels of Dietary Antioxidants

To determine the antioxidant status in patients with AD, serum and cerebrospinal fluid (CSF) levels of dietary antioxidants were analyzed. The results showed that serum levels of vitamin E and beta-carotene were lower in patients with AD and multi-infarct dementia compared to controls.[58] In another study, serum levels of beta-carotene and vitamin A were lower in AD patients compared to control; however, the level of alpha-carotene did not change.[199] The average CSF and serum level of vitamin E was lower in patients with AD than controls.[200] The plasma levels of dietary antioxidants (vitamin C, vitamin A, vitamin E, and carotenoids including beta-carotene, alpha-carotene, lutein, zeaxanthin, lycopene, SOD, and glutathione peroxidase) were lower in patients with AD, as well as in elderly subjects with mild cognitive impairment compared to control subjects.[201] In another study, plasma vitamin C levels were lowered in subjects with dementia compared to controls, which was not explained by their dietary intake of vitamin C.[202]

B-Vitamins

In most studies, the serum levels of vitamin B_{12} in AD patients were significantly lower than the controls, and this may, in part, contribute to degeneration of neurons.[203,204] Indeed, vitamin B_{12} supplementation increased choline acetyl transferase activity in cholinergic neurons in cats[205] and improved cognitive functions in AD patients.[206] A recent analysis of published data revealed that there was no adequate benefit from folic acid supplementation, with or without vitamin B_{12}, on the cognitive function or mood of healthy elderly people[207]; however, in a group of healthy elderly people with high homocysteine levels, supplementation with folic acid for a period of 3 years was associated with significant improvement in global functioning, memory storage, and information processing speed. In a pilot study, it was observed that, in patients with AD, supplementation with folic improved the efficacy of the cholinesterase inhibitor.[207] In another multicenter clinical study, supplementation with folic acid, vitamin B_6, and vitamin B_{12} did not show any beneficial effects on cognitive function decline in individuals with mild to moderated AD.[208] Supplementation with vitamin B_{12} alone did not benefit cognitive or psychiatric symptoms in the vast majority of elderly patients with dementia having low serum vitamin-12 levels.[209] These studies suggest that treatment with one or more B-vitamins alone does not produce consistent results in patients with AD.

Resveratrol

Several epidemiologic studies suggest that the moderate consumption of red wine is associated with a lower incidence of AD and dementia in the general population and that resveratrol, a major polyphenol in red wine, exhibits neuroprotective effects in vitro and in animal models.[210,211] Consumption of three servings of wine daily was associated with a lower risk of AD in elderly individuals without the APOE epsilon-4-allele.[212] Resveratrol protects neuronal cells in culture against beta-amyloid-induced toxicity. This effect is mediated through enhancing the intracellular levels of glutathione, an important antioxidant within the cells.[213] It also lowered intracellular levels of beta-amyloid in different neuronal cell lines.[214] This effect of resveratrol was due to increased degradation of beta-amyloid by proteasome. This mechanism of resveratrol was supported by the fact that a resveratrol-induced decrease in beta-amyloid was prevented by several selective inhibitors of proteasome and by siRNA-directed silencing of proteasome subunit beta5 activity.[214] Resveratrol treatment also up-regulated SIRT1 gene, a mammalian homologue of yeast silent information regulator-2 gene (SIR-2), that attenuated neuronal degeneration and death in an animal model of AD.[215,216] These studies suggest that treatment with resveratrol alone does not produce consistent results in patients with AD.

GINKGO BILOBA AND OMEGA-3 FATTY ACIDS

A randomized, double-blind, placebo-controlled clinical trial in a community of volunteers aged 75 years and older with normal cognition revealed that the administration of *G. biloba* was not effective in reducing the incidence of AD or overall dementia.[217] Long-term consumption of *G. biloba* extract through diet lowered human APP levels by 50% compared to controls in the cortex, but not in the hippocampal regions of the brain of AD transgenic mice.[218]

In a similarly designed study in patients with mild to moderate AD, supplementation with omega-3 fatty acids (1.7 g of docosahexaenoic acid and 0.6 g of eicosapentaenoic acid) did not delay the rate cognitive decline; however, beneficial effects were observed in a small group of patients with very mild AD.[219] Analysis of published observational studies and clinical trials suggests that omega-3 fatty acids may slow down cognitive decline in elderly individuals without dementia, but it is ineffective in reducing the incidence of AD or dementia.[220] In the Canadian Study of Health and Aging (CSHA), there was no association between omega-3 fatty acids and the risk of dementia.[221] In a randomized, double-blind, placebo-controlled trial, supplementation with omega-3 fatty acids showed significant improvement in Alzheimer's Disease Assessment Scale (ADAS-cog) compared to placebo control in individuals with mild cognitive impairment; however, there was no significant difference in patients with AD.[222] These studies suggest that treatment with *G. biloba* or omega-3 fatty acids alone does not produce consistent results in patients with AD.

GREEN TEA EPIGALLOCATECHIN-3-GALLATE AND CAFFEINE

Treatment of AD transgenic mice with green tea epigallocatechin-3-gallate (EGCG) improved cognitive function and reduced the levels of beta-amyloid and phosphorylated tau isoforms.[223] Long-term caffeine treatment decreased the production of beta-amyloid and improved cognitive function in AD transgenic mice; therefore it was suggested that daily moderate consumption of caffeine may reduce the risk of AD.[224] These studies are not sufficient to recommend either EGCG or caffeine for reduction in the risk of developing AD.

PROBLEMS WITH USING A SINGLE NUTRIENT IN AD

Based on the consistency of laboratory data on the beneficial effects of the individual dietary and endogenous antioxidants or B-vitamins alone, it is tempting to suggest that a similar beneficial effect of these dietary antioxidants can be obtained when used individually in human populations at high risk of developing AD or in patients with mild to moderate AD. The fact that the high-risk populations for most chronic diseases, including AD, and patients with chronic diseases have a high internal oxidative environment suggests that administration of vitamin E or vitamin C alone can result in the oxidation of these antioxidants in such an oxidative environment. It is well-known that an oxidized antioxidant acts as a pro-oxidant that is likely to increase the risk of chronic diseases. Therefore, the temptation to extrapolate laboratory results on antioxidants and chronic diseases should be resisted. Nevertheless, many clinical studies with beta-carotene alone in heavy tobacco smokers, vitamin E alone in heart disease, and AD were initiated and, as expected, they all produced inconsistent results varying from no effect, to beneficial effects, to even harmful effects. Because of the failure to obtain consistent beneficial effects with individual micronutrients in patients with mild to moderate AD or those at high risk of developing AD, I recommend the use of multiple micronutrients including dietary and endogenous antioxidants and B-vitamins for reducing the risk of AD, and for improving the efficacy of standard therapy in AD.

RATIONALE FOR USING MULTIPLE MICRONUTRIENTS IN AD

High-risk populations include persons older than 65 years and persons with a family history of AD. Because of the potential for increased levels of oxidative stress and/or enhanced sensitivity of neurons to oxidative stress in the brains of patients of this population, oral supplementation with appropriate micronutrients appears to be one of the rational choices for the prevention and/or delayed onset of AD. Conventional experimental designs for prevention of AD have utilized only one or two antioxidants or B-vitamins. These designs are not suitable for determining the maximal efficacy of micronutrient therapy due to their varied mechanisms of action and distribution, varied environments at the cellular and organ level (oxygenation, aqueous and lipid components), and the varied types of free radicals. The biological rational for using multiple micronutrients for the prevention or improved treatment of AD is described below.

Almost all antioxidants can act as pro-oxidants when oxidized. Therefore, the use of single antioxidants in clinical trials cannot be considered rational for improving disease outcome. For example, beta-carotene (BC) is more effective in quenching oxygen radicals than most other antioxidants.[225] BC can perform certain biological functions that cannot be produced by its metabolite vitamin A, and vice versa.[226,227] It has been reported that BC treatment enhances the expression of the connexin gene, which codes for a gap junction protein in mammalian fibroblasts in culture, whereas vitamin A treatment does not produce such an effect.[227] Vitamin A can induce differentiation in certain normal and cancer cells, whereas BC and other carotenoids do not.[228,229] Thus, BC and vitamin A have, in part, different biological functions. The gradient of oxygen pressure varies within cells. Some antioxidants, such as vitamin E, are more effective as quenchers of free radicals in reduced oxygen pressure, whereas BC and vitamin A are more effective in higher atmospheric pressures.[230] Vitamin C is necessary to protect cellular components in aqueous environments, whereas carotenoids and vitamins A and E protect cellular components in lipid environments. In addition, vitamin C is necessary for the activity of tyrosine hydroxylase, which is the rate-limiting enzyme in the synthesis of catecholamines. Oxidized forms of vitamin C and vitamin E can also act as radicals; therefore, excessive amounts of any one of these forms, when used as a single agent, could be harmful over a long period. Vitamin C also plays an important role in maintaining cellular levels of vitamin E by recycling vitamin E radicals (oxidized) to the reduced (antioxidant) form.[231] Also, oxidative DNA damage produced by the high levels of vitamin C could be protected by vitamin E.

The form of vitamin E used is also important in any clinical trial. It has been established that D-alpha-tocopheryl succinate (alpha-TS) is the most effective form of vitamin both in vitro and in vivo.[232,233] This form of vitamin E is more soluble than alpha-tocopherol and enters cells more readily. Therefore, it is expected to cross the blood-brain barrier in greater amounts than alpha-tocopherol. However, this has not yet been demonstrated in animals or humans. We have reported that an oral ingestion of alpha-TS (800 IU/day) in humans increased plasma levels of not only alpha–tocopherol, but also alpha-TS, suggesting that a portion of alpha-TS can be absorbed from the intestinal tract before hydrolysis.[234] This observation is important because the conventional assumption based on rodents has been that esterified forms of vitamin E, such as alpha-TS, alpha-tocopheryl nicotinate, and alpha-tocopheryl acetate, can be absorbed from the intestinal tract only after they are hydrolyzed to alpha-tocopherol. Our preliminary data shows that this assumption may not be true for the absorption of alpha-TS in humans.

An endogenous antioxidant, glutathione, is effective in catabolizing H_2O_2 and anions. However, oral supplementation with glutathione failed to significantly increase plasma levels of glutathione in human subjects,[235] suggesting that this tripeptide is completely hydrolyzed in the gastrointestinal tract. Therefore, we propose to utilize N-acetylcysteine and alpha-lipoic acid, which increase the cellular levels of glutathione by different mechanisms in a multiple micronutrient preparation.

Other endogenous antioxidants, such as coenzyme Q_{10}, may have some potential value in the prevention and improved treatment of AD. Since mitochondrial dysfunction is associated with AD, and since coenzyme Q_{10} is needed for the generation of ATP by mitochondria, it is essential to add this antioxidant to a multiple micronutrient preparation. A study has shown that Ubiquinol (coenzyme Q_{10}) scavenges peroxy radicals faster than alpha–tocopherol[236] and, like vitamin C, can regenerate vitamin E in a redox cycle.[237] However, it is a weaker antioxidant than alpha-tocopherol. Coenzyme Q_{10} administration has been shown to improve clinical symptoms in patients with mitochondrial encephalomyopathies.[238] Nicotinamide, a precursor of NAD^+ also attenuated glutamate-induced toxicity and preserved cellular levels of NAD^+ to support the activity of SIRT-1.[186] It is also a competitive inhibitor of histone deacetylase activity and restores memory deficits in AD transgenic mice.[185] These preclinical data suggest that oral supplementation with nicotinamide may be safe and useful in the prevention and improved treatment of AD. Recent clinical studies with NADH revealed that NAD treatment did not improve cognitive functions in AD patients. Selenium is a cofactor of glutathione peroxidase, and Se-glutathione peroxidase acts as an antioxidant by increasing the intracellular level of glutathione. There may be some other mechanisms of selenium. Therefore, these agents should be added to a multiple micronutrient preparation for the prevention and improved treatment of AD in combination with standard therapy.

In addition to dietary and endogenous antioxidants, B-vitamins should be added to a multiple micronutrient preparation. Although the role of folic acid, with or without vitamin B_{12}, in the management of AD remains controversial, B-vitamins are essential for normal health.

RATIONALE FOR USING NSAIDS IN AD PREVENTION

Since inflammatory reactions represent one of the major factors that initiate and promote neurodegeneration in AD brains, the use of NSAIDs in the prevention and treatment of AD appears rational. Laboratory, epidemiological, and clinical studies support this recommendation. Laboratory data have shown that products of inflammatory reactions such as prostaglandins,[57,131] cytokines,[123,124] complement proteins,[80,125–127,239] adhesion molecules,[128–130] and free radicals[53,65,240] are neurotoxic. Epidemiological studies have revealed that rheumatoid arthritis patients who are on high doses of NSAIDs have a reduced incidence of AD.[119–122,241–243] NSAIDs also reduce the rate of deterioration of cognitive functions in AD patients.[50,141–143] However, the administration of prednisone, a powerful anti-inflammatory agent, was not useful in patients with AD.[244] Treatment with a mixed Cox-1/Cox-2 inhibitor and a PGE2 analog failed to produce any significant benefit on cognitive function.[245] A specific inhibitor of Cox-2 was also not useful in improving cognitive function.[246] Therefore, it was suggested that the Cox-2 enzyme may not be the appropriate target for AD treatment.[247] This is supported by the following additional evidence: (1) the brains of nondemented elderly people taking NSAIDs had fewer activated microglia, suggesting a reduced anti-inflammatory environment[248]; and (2) chronic administration of ibuprofen reduced inflammation, dystrophic neurite formation, and beta-amyloid deposition in a transgenic AD model.[249] Thus, the use of NSAIDs for the prevention and the reduction of progression of AD remains one of the viable options.[2,3,247,250] These drugs do not improve the function of surviving neurons or protect neurons from further damage caused by oxidative and nitrosylative stress that is generated by mechanisms other than inflammatory reactions.

RECOMMENDED MICRONUTRIENTS IN COMBINATION WITH LOW-DOSES OF NSAIDS FOR PREVENTION OF AD IN HIGH-RISK POPULATIONS

The high-risk populations include those with a family history of AD and those aged 65 years and older. A micronutrient supplement may include vitamin A (retinyl palmitate), vitamin E (both D- alpha-tocopherol and D-alpha-TS), natural mixed carotenoids, vitamin C (calcium ascorbate), vitamin D, B-vitamins, selenium, zinc, and chromium. No iron, copper, or manganese would be included because these trace minerals are known to interact with vitamin C to produce free radicals. These trace minerals are absorbed from the intestinal tract more in the presence of antioxidants than in their absence, which could result in increased body stores of free forms of these minerals.

Increased iron stores have been linked to increased risk of several chronic diseases including AD.[251] A low-dose aspirin is recommended because of its anti-inflammatory effect and because, in combination with vitamin E, it produced a syngerstic effect on the inhibition of cyclooxygenase activity[252]; therefore, the combination of the two may be more effective in reducing the levels of chronic inflammation than the individual agents. Indeed, consumption of vitamin E and vitamin C together in combination with NSAIDs was associated with reduced cognitive decline over time in elderly individuals with an APOE-epsilon-4-allele.[253] The efficacy of the proposed recommendation of micronutrients in combination with aspirin remains to be tested by clinical studies in high-risk populations; however, they have been used in humans for several decades and, therefore, they should be considered safe. Meanwhile, the proposed recommendations can be adopted in consultation with physicians and health professionals in order to reduce the risk of AD in high-risk populations.

RATIONALE FOR USING ACETYLCHOLINESTERASE INHIBITORS IN THE TREATMENT OF AD

It has been proposed that the gradual loss of cognitive functions in AD is due to the loss of cholinergic neurons; therefore, cholinergic drugs (acetylcholinesterase inhibitors) are used to improve the function of surviving neurons in AD patients. However, these agents do not protect cholinergic neurons against the damaging effects of oxidative and nitrosylative stress and other neurotoxins. Consequently, neurons continue to die and the beneficial effects of cholinergic drugs do not last long.

RECOMMENDED MICRONUTRIENTS AND LOW-DOSE NSAIDS WITH STANDARD THERAPY IN PATIENTS WITH DEMENTIA

It has been proposed that the gradual loss of cognitive functions in AD is due to the progressive loss of cholinergic neurons. The presence of some viable cholinergic neurons in patients with mild to moderate dementia, with or without AD, allows the use of drugs that inhibit acetylcholinesterase activity to increase acetylcholine levels. These drugs improved cognitive function by enhancing the activity of surviving cholinergic neurons in AD patients. However, these drugs do not protect cholinergic neurons against the damaging effects of oxidative and nitrosylative stress and other neurotoxins. Consequently, neurons continue to die in spite of this treatment, and thus, beneficial effects of cholinergic drugs last as long as neurons are alive. Therefore, the addition of a multiple micronutrient preparation and a low-dose aspirin in combination with standard therapy may prolong the beneficial effects of current drugs in patients with dementia, with or without AD, by protecting the surviving neurons from oxidative-stress- and inflammation-induced death.

The recommended multiple micronutrient preparation should be taken orally and divided into two doses: half in the morning, and the other half in the evening with a meal. This is because the biological half-lives of micronutrients are highly variable; this can create high levels of fluctuations in the tissue levels of micronutrients. A twofold difference in the levels of certain micronutrients such as alpha-TS can cause a marked difference in the expression of gene profiles. To maintain relatively consistent levels of micronutrients in the brain, the proposed micronutrients must be taken twice a day.

DIET AND LIFESTYLE RECOMMENDATIONS FOR AD

Even though there is no direct link between diet- and lifestyle-related factors and the initiation or progression of AD, it is always useful to include a balanced, low-fat, high-fiber diet that contains plenty of fruits and vegetables. A low-calorie diet also appears to be useful in improving memory. Among fruits, blueberries and raspberries are particularly important because of their protective role against oxidative injuries in the brain. Lifestyle recommendations include daily moderate exercise, reduced stress, and no tobacco smoking.

CONCLUSIONS

The results of many studies presented in this chapter suggest that increased oxidative stress and chronic inflammation play a dominant role in the initiation and progression of dementia with or without AD. Therefore, supplementation with multiple micronutrients including dietary and endogenous antioxidants in combination with low-dose NSAIDs such as aspirin would be useful in reducing the risk of dementia in high-risk populations (persons with a family history of AD or aged 65 years and older). The efficacy of current drugs depends upon the viability of cholinergic neurons. These drugs do not address the issues of increased oxidative stress and chronic inflammation, which are responsible for neuronal degeneration. Therefore, the same micronutrient preparation and a low-dose aspirin in combination with currently used acetylcholinesterase inhibitors may prolong their beneficial effects by reducing the rate of degeneration of cholinergic neurons in patients with dementia, with or without AD. Dietary recommendations include a low-calorie diet. Clinical studies using the proposed recommendations for prevention and for improved treatment in combination with standard therapy should be initiated. Meanwhile, those interested in the proposed micronutrient approach to prevention or management of dementia, with or without AD, may like to adopt these recommendations in consultation with their physicians or health professionals.

REFERENCES

1. Aarsland, D., A. Rongve, S. P. Nore, R. Skogseth, S. Skulstad, U. Ehrt, D. Hoprekstad, and C. Ballard. 2008. Frequency and case identification of dementia with Lewy bodies using the revised consensus criteria. *Dement Geriatr Cogn Disord* 26 (5): 445–452.
2. Prasad, K. N., A. R. Hovland, W. C. Cole, K. C. Prasad, P. Nahreini, J. Edwards-Prasad, and C. P. Andreatta. 2000. Multiple antioxidants in the prevention and treatment of Alzheimer disease: Analysis of biologic rationale. *Clin Neuropharmacol* 23 (1): 2–13.
3. Prasad, K. N., W. C. Cole, and K. C. Prasad. 2002. Risk factors for Alzheimer's disease: Role of multiple antioxidants, non-steroidal anti-inflammatory and cholinergic agents alone or in combination in prevention and treatment. *J Am Coll Nutr* 21 (6): 506–522.
4. NIA. 1997. *Progress Report on Alzheimer's Disease*. Bethesda, MD: National Institute of Health.
5. Schoenberg, B. S., E. Kokmen, and H. Okazaki. 1987. Alzheimer's disease and other dementing illnesses in a defined United States population: Incidence rates and clinical features. *Ann Neurol* 22 (6): 724–729.
6. Evans, D. A., H. H. Funkenstein, M. S. Albert, P. A. Scherr, N. R. Cook, M. J. Chown, L. E. Hebert, C. H. Hennekens, and J. O. Taylor. 1989. Prevalence of Alzheimer's disease in a community population of older persons higher than previously reported. *JAMA* 262 (18): 2551–2556.
7. Rondeau, V., H. Jacqmin-Gadda, D. Commenges, C. Helmer, and J. F. Dartigues. 2009. Aluminum and silica in drinking water and the risk of Alzheimer's disease or cognitive decline: Findings from 15-year follow-up of the PAQUID cohort. *Am J Epidemiol* 169 (4): 489–496.
8. Engelhart, M. J., M. I. Geerlings, A. Ruitenberg, J. C. van Swieten, A. Hofman, J. C. Witteman, and M. M. Breteler. 2002. Dietary intake of antioxidants and risk of Alzheimer disease. *JAMA* 287 (24): 3223–3229.

9. Evatt, M. L., M. R. Delong, N. Khazai, A. Rosen, S. Triche, and V. Tangpricha. 2008. Prevalence of vitamin d insufficiency in patients with Parkinson disease and Alzheimer disease. *Arch Neurol* 65 (10): 1348–1352.
10. Behl, C., J. B. Davis, R. Lesley, and D. Schubert. 1994. Hydrogen peroxide mediates amyloid beta protein toxicity. *Cell* 77 (6): 817–827.
11. Butterfield, D. A., K. Hensley, M. Harris, M. Mattson, and J. Carney. 1994. beta-Amyloid peptide free radical fragments initiate synaptosomal lipoperoxidation in a sequence-specific fashion: Implications to Alzheimer's disease. *Biochem Biophys Res Commun* 200 (2): 710–715.
12. Schubert, D., C. Behl, R. Lesley, A. Brack, R. Dargusch, Y. Sagara, and H. Kimura. 1995. Amyloid peptides are toxic via a common oxidative mechanism. *Proc Natl Acad Sci U S A* 92 (6): 1989–1893.
13. Wolozin, B., W. Kellman, P. Ruosseau, G. G. Celesia, and G. Siegel. 2000. Decreased prevalence of Alzheimer disease associated with 3-hydroxy-3-methyglutaryl coenzyme A reductase inhibitors. *Arch Neurol* 57 (10): 1439–1443.
14. Sparks, D. L., T. A. Martin, D. R. Gross, and J. C. Hunsaker 3rd. 2000. Link between heart disease, cholesterol, and Alzheimer's disease: A review. *Microsc Res Tech* 50 (4): 287–290.
15. Checler, F., C. A. da Costa, K. Ancolio, N. Chevallier, E. Lopez-Perez, and P. Marambaud. 2000. Role of the proteasome in Alzheimer's disease. *Biochim Biophys Acta* 1502 (1): 133–138.
16. Lopez Salon, M., L. Morelli, E. M. Castano, E. F. Soto, and J. M. Pasquini. 2000. Defective ubiquitination of cerebral proteins in Alzheimer's disease. *J Neurosci Res* 62 (2): 302–310.
17. Martin, J. B. 1999. Molecular basis of the neurodegenerative disorders. *N Engl J Med* 340 (25): 1970–1980.
18. Goedert, M., R. Jakes, R. A. Crowther, J. Six, U. Lubke, M. Vandermeeren, P. Cras, J. Q. Trojanowski, and V. M. Lee. 1993. The abnormal phosphorylation of tau protein at Ser-202 in Alzheimer disease recapitulates phosphorylation during development. *Proc Natl Acad Sci U S A* 90 (11): 5066–5070.
19. Grundke-Iqbal, I., K. Iqbal, Y. C. Tung, M. Quinlan, H. M. Wisniewski, and L. I. Binder. 1986. Abnormal phosphorylation of the microtubule-associated protein tau (tau) in Alzheimer cytoskeletal pathology. *Proc Natl Acad Sci U S A* 83 (13): 4913–4917.
20. Yankner, B. A., and M. M. Mesulam. 1991. Seminars in medicine of the Beth Israel Hospital, Boston. beta-Amyloid and the pathogenesis of Alzheimer's disease. *N Engl J Med* 325 (26): 1849–1857.
21. Hardy, J., and D. Allsop. 1991. Amyloid deposition as the central event in the aetiology of Alzheimer's disease. *Trends Pharmacol Sci* 12 (10): 383–388.
22. Selkoe, D. J. 1994. Cell biology of the amyloid beta-protein precursor and the mechanism of Alzheimer's disease. *Annu Rev Cell Biol* 10: 373–403.
23. Dewji, N. N., and S. J. Singer. 1996. Genetic clues to Alzheimer's disease. *Science* 271 (5246): 159–160.
24. Wang, G. P., S. Khatoon, K. Iqbal, and I. Grundke-Iqbal. 1991. Brain ubiquitin is markedly elevated in Alzheimer disease. *Brain Res* 566 (1–2): 146–151.
25. Kudo, T., K. Iqbal, R. Ravid, D. F. Swaab, and I. Grundke-Iqbal. 1994. Alzheimer disease: Correlation of cerebro-spinal fluid and brain ubiquitin levels. *Brain Res* 639 (1): 1–7.
26. Hamilton, R. L. 2000. Lewy bodies in Alzheimer's disease: A neuropathological review of 145 cases using alpha-synuclein immunohistochemistry. *Brain Pathol* 10 (3): 378–384.
27. Ames, B. N., M. K. Shigenaga, and T. M. Hagen. 1993. Oxidants, antioxidants, and the degenerative diseases of aging. *Proc Natl Acad Sci U S A* 90 (17): 7915–7922.
28. Boveris, A., and B. Chance. 1973. The mitochondrial generation of hydrogen peroxide. General properties and effect of hyperbaric oxygen. *Biochem J* 134 (3): 707–716.
29. Ames, B. N., W. E. Durston, E. Yamasaki, and F. D. Lee. 1973. Carcinogens are mutagens: A simple test system combining liver homogenates for activation and bacteria for detection. *Proc Natl Acad Sci U S A* 70 (8): 2281–2285.
30. Coyle, J. T., and P. Puttfarcken. 1993. Oxidative stress, glutamate, and neurodegenerative disorders. *Science* 262 (5134): 689–695.
31. Graham, D. G. 1978. Oxidative pathways for catecholamines in the genesis of neuromelanin and cytotoxic quinones. *Mol Pharmacol* 14 (4): 633–643.
32. Chan, P. H., and R. A. Fishman. 1980. Transient formation of superoxide radicals in polyunsaturated fatty acid-induced brain swelling. *J Neurochem* 35 (4): 1004–1007.
33. Lafon-Cazal, M., S. Pietri, M. Culcasi, and J. Bockaert. 1993. NMDA-dependent superoxide production and neurotoxicity. *Nature* 364 (6437): 535–537.
34. Kiyosawa, H., M. Suko, H. Okudaira, K. Murata, T. Miyamoto, M. H. Chung, H. Kasai, and S. Nishimura. 1990. Cigarette smoking induces formation of 8-hydroxydeoxyguanosine, one of the oxidative DNA damages in human peripheral leukocytes. *Free Radic Res Commun* 11 (1–3): 23–27.

35. Reznick, A. Z., C. E. Cross, M. L. Hu, Y. J. Suzuki, S. Khwaja, A. Safadi, P. A. Motchnik, L. Packer, and B. Halliwell. 1992. Modification of plasma proteins by cigarette smoke as measured by protein carbonyl formation. *Biochem J* 286 (Pt 2): 607–611.
36. Schectman, G., J. C. Byrd, and R. Hoffmann. 1991. Ascorbic acid requirements for smokers: Analysis of a population survey. *Am J Clin Nutr* 53 (6): 1466–1470.
37. Duthie, G. G., J. R. Arthur, and W. P. James. 1991. Effects of smoking and vitamin E on blood antioxidant status. *Am J Clin Nutr* 53 (4 Suppl): 1061S–1063S.
38. Winterbourn, C. C. 1995. Toxicity of iron and hydrogen peroxide: The Fenton reaction. *Toxicol Lett* 82–83: 969–974.
39. Ames, B. N., M. Profet, and L. S. Gold. 1990. Dietary pesticides (99.99% all natural). *Proc Natl Acad Sci U S A* 87 (19): 7777–7781.
40. Gold, L. S., T. H. Slone, B. R. Stern, N. B. Manley, and B. N. Ames. 1992. Rodent carcinogens: Setting priorities. *Science* 258 (5080): 261–265.
41. Guyton, A. C. 1971. Blood flow through special areas of the body. In *Textbook of Medical Physiology*, 4th ed., ed. A. C. Guyton, 367–378. Philadelphia, PA: WB Saunders.
42. Wallace, D. C. 1992. Mitochondrial genetics: A paradigm for aging and degenerative diseases? *Science* 256 (5057): 628–632.
43. Shoffner, J. M., M. D. Brown, A. Torroni, M. T. Lott, M. F. Cabell, S. S. Mirra, M. F. Beal, et al. 1993. Mitochondrial DNA variants observed in Alzheimer disease and Parkinson disease patients. *Genomics* 17 (1): 171–184.
44. Saraiva, A. A., M. M. Borges, M. D. Madeira, M. A. Tavares, and M. M. Paula-Barbosa. 1985. Mitochondrial abnormalities in cortical dendrites from patients with Alzheimer's disease. *J Submicrosc Cytol* 17 (3): 459–464.
45. Kish, S. J., C. Bergeron, A. Rajput, S. Dozic, F. Mastrogiacomo, L. J. Chang, J. M. Wilson, L. M. DiStefano, and J. N. Nobrega. 1992. Brain cytochrome oxidase in Alzheimer's disease. *J Neurochem* 59 (2): 776–779.
46. Mutisya, E. M., A. C. Bowling, and M. F. Beal. 1994. Cortical cytochrome oxidase activity is reduced in Alzheimer's disease. *J Neurochem* 63 (6): 2179–2184.
47. Mattson, M. P. 1994. Calcium and neuronal injury in Alzheimer's disease. Contributions of beta-amyloid precursor protein mismetabolism, free radicals, and metabolic compromise. *Ann N Y Acad Sci* 747: 50–76.
48. Gabuzda, D., J. Busciglio, L. B. Chen, P. Matsudaira, and B. A. Yankner. 1994. Inhibition of energy metabolism alters the processing of amyloid precursor protein and induces a potentially amyloidogenic derivative. *J Biol Chem* 269 (18): 13623–13628.
49. Cuajungco, M. P., and G. J. Lees. 1998. Nitric oxide generators produce accumulation of chelatable zinc in hippocampal neuronal perikarya. *Brain Res* 799 (1): 118–129.
50. Brown, A. M., B. S. Kristal, M. S. Effron, A. I. Shestopalov, P. A. Ullucci, K. F. Sheu, J. P. Blass, and A. J. Cooper. 2000. Zn^{2+} inhibits alpha-ketoglutarate–stimulated mitochondrial respiration and the isolated alpha-ketoglutarate dehydrogenase complex. *J Biol Chem* 275 (18): 13441–13447.
51. Chen, L., J. S. Richardson, J. E. Caldwell, and L. C. Ang. 1994. Regional brain activity of free radical defense enzymes in autopsy samples from patients with Alzheimer's disease and from nondemented controls. *Int J Neurosci* 75 (1–2): 83–90.
52. Richardson, J. S., K. V. Subbarao, and L. C. Ang. 1992. On the possible role of iron-induced free radical peroxidation in neural degeneration in Alzheimer's disease. *Ann N Y Acad Sci* 648: 326–327.
53. Smith, M. A., L. M. Sayre, V. M. Monnier, and G. Perry. 1995. Radical ageing in Alzheimer's disease. *Trends Neurosci* 18 (4): 172–176.
54. Harman, D. A. 1996. Hypothesis on the pathogenesis of Alzheimer's disease. *Ann N Y Acad Sci* 786: 152–168.
55. McIntosh, L. J., M. A. Trush, and J. C. Troncoso. 1997. Increased susceptibility of Alzheimer's disease temporal cortex to oxygen free radical-mediated processes. *Free Radic Biol Med* 23 (2): 183–190.
56. Smith, M. A., P. L. Richey Harris, L. M. Sayre, J. S. Beckman, and G. Perry. 1997. Widespread peroxynitrite-mediated damage in Alzheimer's disease. *J Neurosci* 17 (8): 2653–2657.
57. Prasad, K. N., A. R. Hovland, F. G. La Rosa, and P. G. Hovland. 1998. Prostaglandins as putative neurotoxins in Alzheimer's disease. *Proc Soc Exp Biol Med* 219 (2): 120–125.
58. Zaman, Z., S. Roche, P. Fielden, P. G. Frost, D. C. Niriella, and A. C. Cayley. 1992. Plasma concentrations of vitamins A and E and carotenoids in Alzheimer's disease. *Age Ageing* 21 (2): 91–94.
59. Schipper, H. M., S. Cisse, and E. G. Stopa. 1995. Expression of heme oxygenase-1 in the senescent and Alzheimer-diseased brain. *Ann Neurol* 37 (6): 758–768.

60. Smith, M. A., R. K. Kutty, P. L. Richey, S. D. Yan, D. Stern, G. J. Chader, B. Wiggert, R. B. Petersen, and G. Perry. 1994. Heme oxygenase-1 is associated with the neurofibrillary pathology of Alzheimer's disease. *Am J Pathol* 145 (1): 42–47.
61. Sims, N. R., D. M. Bowen, D. Neary, and A. N. Davison. 1983. Metabolic processes in Alzheimer's disease: Adenine nucleotide content and production of 14CO2 from [U-14C]glucose in vitro in human neocortex. *J Neurochem* 41 (5): 1329–1334.
62. Martins, R. N., C. G. Harper, G. B. Stokes, and C. L. Masters. 1986. Increased cerebral glucose-6-phosphate dehydrogenase activity in Alzheimer's disease may reflect oxidative stress. *J Neurochem* 46 (4): 1042–1045.
63. Saito, K., J. S. Elce, J. E. Hamos, and R. A. Nixon. 1993. Widespread activation of calcium-activated neutral proteinase (calpain) in the brain in Alzheimer disease: A potential molecular basis for neuronal degeneration. *Proc Natl Acad Sci U S A* 90 (7): 2628–2632.
64. Nixon, R. A., and A. M. Cataldo. 1994. Free radicals, proteolysis, and the degeneration of neurons in Alzheimer disease: How essential is the beta-amyloid link? *Neurobiol Aging* 15 (4): 463–469; discussion 473.
65. Harman, D. 1992. Free radical theory of aging. *Mutat Res* 275 (3–6): 257–266.
66. Tesco, G., S. Latorraca, P. Piersanti, S. Piacentini, L. Amaducci, and S. Sorbi. 1992. Alzheimer skin fibroblasts show increased susceptibility to free radicals. *Mech Ageing Dev* 66 (2): 117–120.
67. Gibson, G. E., V. Haroutunian, H. Zhang, L. C. Park, Q. Shi, M. Lesser, R. C. Mohs, R. K. Sheu, and J. P. Blass. 2000. Mitochondrial damage in Alzheimer's disease varies with apolipoprotein E genotype. *Ann Neurol* 48 (3): 297–303.
68. Zhou, Y., J. S. Richardson, M. J. Mombourquette, and J. A. Weil. 1995. Free radical formation in autopsy samples of Alzheimer and control cortex. *Neurosci Lett* 195 (2): 89–92.
69. Koppal, T. 1998. Peroxynitrite-mediated damage to brain membrane alterations in Alzheimer's disease (AD). *Soc Neurosci* 24: 1217a.
70. Simic, G., P. J. Lucassen, Z. Krsnik, B. Kruslin, I. Kostovic, B. Winblad, and N. Bogdanovi. 2000. nNOS expression in reactive astrocytes correlates with increased cell death related DNA damage in the hippocampus and entorhinal cortex in Alzheimer's disease. *Exp Neurol* 165 (1): 12–26.
71. Lovell, M. A., C. Xie, and W. R. Markesbery. 1998. Decreased glutathione transferase activity in brain and ventricular fluid in Alzheimer's disease. *Neurology* 51 (6): 1562–1566.
72. Conrad, C. C., P. L. Marshall, J. M. Talent, C. A. Malakowsky, J. Choi, and R. W. Gracy. 2000. Oxidized proteins in Alzheimer's plasma. *Biochem Biophys Res Commun* 275 (2): 678–681.
73. Joachim, C. L., and D. J. Selkoe. 1992. The seminal role of beta-amyloid in the pathogenesis of Alzheimer disease. *Alzheimer Dis Assoc Disord* 6 (1): 7–34.
74. Postina, R. A. 2008. Closer look at alpha-secretase. *Curr Alzheimer Res* 5 (2): 179–186.
75. Simmons, L. K., P. C. May, K. J. Tomaselli, R. E. Rydel, K. S. Fuson, E. F. Brigham, S. Wright, et al. 1994. Secondary structure of amyloid beta peptide correlates with neurotoxic activity in vitro. *Mol Pharmacol* 45 (3): 373–379.
76. Lorenzo, A., and B. A. Yankner. 1994. beta-Amyloid neurotoxicity requires fibril formation and is inhibited by congo red. *Proc Natl Acad Sci U S A* 91 (25): 12243–12247.
77. Loo, G. 2003. Redox-sensitive mechanisms of phytochemical-mediated inhibition of cancer cell proliferation (review). *J Nutr Biochem* 14 (2): 64–73.
78. Koh, J. Y., S. W. Suh, B. J. Gwag, Y. Y. He, C. Y. Hsu, and D. W. Choi. 1996. The role of zinc in selective neuronal death after transient global cerebral ischemia. *Science* 272 (5264): 1013–1016.
79. Bondy, S. C., and A. Truong. 1999. Potentiation of beta-folding of beta-amyloid peptide 25–35 by aluminum salts. *Neurosci Lett* 267 (1): 25–28.
80. Eikelenboom, P., and F. C. Stam. 1982. Immunoglobulins and complement factors in senile plaques. An immunoperoxidase study. *Acta Neuropathol (Berl)* 57 (2–3): 239–242.
81. Misonou, H., M. Morishima-Kawashima, and Y. Ihara. 2000. Oxidative stress induces intracellular accumulation of amyloid beta-protein (Abeta) in human neuroblastoma cells. *Biochemistry* 39 (23): 6951–6959.
82. Koppaka, V., and P. H. Axelsen. 2000. Accelerated accumulation of amyloid beta proteins on oxidatively damaged lipid membranes. *Biochemistry* 39 (32): 10011–10016.
83. Behl, C., J. Davis, G. M. Cole, and D. Schubert. 1992. Vitamin E protects nerve cells from amyloid beta protein toxicity. *Biochem Biophys Res Commun* 186 (2): 944–950.
84. Varadarajan, S., S. Yatin, J. Kanski, F. Jahanshahi, and D. A. Butterfield. 1999. Methionine residue 35 is important in amyloid beta-peptide–associated free radical oxidative stress. *Brain Res Bull* 50 (2): 133–141.

85. Pappolla, M. A., Y. J. Chyan, R. A. Omar, K. Hsiao, G. Perry, M. A. Smith, and P. Bozner. 1998. Evidence of oxidative stress and in vivo neurotoxicity of beta-amyloid in a transgenic mouse model of Alzheimer's disease: A chronic oxidative paradigm for testing antioxidant therapies in vivo. *Am J Pathol* 152 (4): 871–877.
86. Naslund, J., V. Haroutunian, R. Mohs, K. L. Davis, P. Davies, P. Greengard, and J. D. Buxbaum. 2000. Correlation between elevated levels of amyloid beta-peptide in the brain and cognitive decline. *JAMA* 283 (12): 1571–1577.
87. Refolo, L. M., B. Malester, J. LaFrancois, T. Bryant-Thomas, R. Wang, G. S. Tint, K. Sambamurti, K. Duff, and M. A. Pappolla. 2000. Hypercholesterolemia accelerates the Alzheimer's amyloid pathology in a transgenic mouse model. *Neurobiol Dis* 7 (4): 321–331.
88. Simons, M., P. Keller, B. De Strooper, K. Beyreuther, C. G. Dotti, and K. Simons. 1998. Cholesterol depletion inhibits the generation of beta-amyloid in hippocampal neurons. *Proc Natl Acad Sci U S A* 95 (11): 6460–6464.
89. Jick, H., G. L. Zornberg, S. S. Jick, S. Seshadri, and D. A. Drachman. 2000. Statins and the risk of dementia. *Lancet* 356 (9242): 1627–1631.
90. Haag, M. D., A. Hofman, P. J. Koudstaal, B. H. Stricker, and M. M. Breteler. 2009. Statins are associated with a reduced risk of Alzheimer disease regardless of lipophilicity. The Rotterdam Study. *J Neurol Neurosurg Psychiatry* 80 (1): 13–17.
91. Rao, S., D. C. Porter, X. Chen, T. Herliczek, M. Lowe, and K. Keyomarsi. 1999. Lovastatin-mediated G1 arrest is through inhibition of the proteasome, independent of hydroxymethyl glutaryl-CoA reductase. *Proc Natl Acad Sci U S A* 96 (14): 7797–7802.
92. Kumar, B., C. Andreatta, W. T. Koustas, W. C. Cole, J. Edwards-Prasad, and K. N. Prasad. 2002. Mevastatin induces degeneration and decreases viability of cAMP-induced differentiated neuroblastoma cells in culture by inhibiting proteasome activity, and mevalonic acid lactone prevents these effects. *J Neurosci Res* 68 (5): 627–635.
93. Gregori, L., J. F. Hainfeld, M. N. Simon, and D. Goldgaber. 1997. Binding of amyloid beta protein to the 20S proteasome. *J Biol Chem* 272 (1): 58–62.
94. Rockwell, P., H. Yuan, R. Magnusson, and M. E. Figueiredo-Pereira. 2000. Proteasome inhibition in neuronal cells induces a proinflammatory response manifested by upregulation of cyclooxygenase-2, its accumulation as ubiquitin conjugates, and production of the prostaglandin PGE(2). *Arch Biochem Biophys* 374 (2): 325–333.
95. Nahreini, P., C. Andreatta, and K. N. Prasad. 2001. Proteasome activity is critical for the cAMP-induced differentiation of neuroblastoma cells. *Cell Mol Neurobiol* 21 (5): 509–521.
96. Lam, Y. A., C. M. Pickart, A. Alban, M. Landon, C. Jamieson, R. Ramage, R. J. Mayer, and R. Layfield. 2000. Inhibition of the ubiquitin–proteasome system in Alzheimer's disease. *Proc Natl Acad Sci U S A* 97 (18): 9902–9906.
97. Farrer, L. A., L. A. Cupples, J. L. Haines, B. Hyman, W. A. Kukull, R. Mayeux, R. H. Myers, M. A. Pericak-Vance, N. Risch, and C. M. van Duijn. 1997. Effects of age, sex, and ethnicity on the association between apolipoprotein E genotype and Alzheimer disease. A meta-analysis. APOE and Alzheimer Disease Meta Analysis Consortium. *JAMA* 278 (16): 1349–1356.
98. Marx, J. 1998. New gene tied to common form of Alzheimer's disease. *Science* 281 (5376): 507, 509.
99. McConnell, L. M., B. A. Koenig, H. T. Greely, and T. A. Raffin. 1998. Genetic testing and Alzheimer disease: Has the time come? Alzheimer Disease Working Group of the Stanford Program in Genomics, Ethics & Society. *Nat Med* 4 (7): 757–759.
100. Blacker, D., M. A. Wilcox, N. M. Laird, L. Rodes, S. M. Horvath, R. C. Go, R. Perry, et al. 1998. Alpha-2 macroglobulin is genetically associated with Alzheimer disease. *Nat Genet* 19 (4): 357–360.
101. Kehoe, P., F. Wavrant-De Vrieze, R. Crook, W. S. Wu, P. Holmans, I. Fenton, G. Spurlock, et al. 1999. A full genome scan for late onset Alzheimer's disease. *Hum Mol Genet* 8 (2): 237–245.
102. McMillan, P. J., J. B. Leverenz, and D. M. Dorsa. 2000. Specific downregulation of presenilin 2 gene expression is prominent during early stages of sporadic late-onset Alzheimer's disease. *Brain Res Mol Brain Res* 78 (1–2): 138–145.
103. Cruts, M., and C. Van Broeckhoven. 1998. Molecular genetics of Alzheimer's disease. *Ann Med* 30 (6): 560–565.
104. Hanson, A. J., J. E. Prasad, P. Nahreini, C. Andreatta, B. Kumar, X. D. Yan, and K. N. Prasad. 2003. Overexpression of amyloid precursor protein is associated with degeneration, decreased viability, and increased damage caused by neurotoxins (prostaglandins A1 and E2, hydrogen peroxide, and nitric oxide) in differentiated neuroblastoma cells. *J Neurosci Res* 74 (1): 148–159.

105. Candore, G., C. R. Balistreri, M. P. Grimaldi, S. Vasto, F. Listi, M. Chiappelli, F. Licastro, D. Lio, and C. Caruso. 2006. Age-related inflammatory diseases: Role of genetics and gender in the pathophysiology of Alzheimer's disease. *Ann N Y Acad Sci* 1089: 472–486.
106. Candore, G., C. R. Balistreri, M. P. Grimaldi, F. Listi, S. Vasto, M. Chiappelli, F. Licastro, G. Colonna-Romano, D. Lio, and C. Caruso. 2007. Polymorphisms of pro-inflammatory genes and Alzheimer's disease risk: A pharmacogenomic approach. *Mech Ageing Dev* 128 (1): 67–75.
107. Zhao, J., Y. Fu, M. Yasvoina, P. Shao, B. Hitt, T. O'Connor, S. Logan, et al. 2007. Beta-site amyloid precursor protein cleaving enzyme 1 levels become elevated in neurons around amyloid plaques: Implications for Alzheimer's disease pathogenesis. *J Neurosci* 27 (14): 3639–3649.
108. Velliquette, R. A., T. O'Connor, and R. Vassar. 2005. Energy inhibition elevates beta-secretase levels and activity and is potentially amyloidogenic in APP transgenic mice: Possible early events in Alzheimer's disease pathogenesis. *J Neurosci* 25 (47): 10874–10883.
109. Lesne, S., F. Docagne, C. Gabriel, G. Liot, D. K. Lahiri, L. Buee, L. Plawinski, et al. 2003. Transforming growth factor-beta 1 potentiates amyloid-beta generation in astrocytes and in transgenic mice. *J Biol Chem* 278 (20): 18408–18418.
110. Sherrington, R., E. I. Rogaev, Y. Liang, E. A. Rogaeva, G. Levesque, M. Ikeda, H. Chi, et al. 1995. Cloning of a gene bearing missense mutations in early-onset familial Alzheimer's disease. *Nature* 375 (6534): 754–760.
111. Busciglio, J., H. Hartmann, A. Lorenzo, C. Wong, K. Baumann, B. Sommer, M. Staufenbiel, and B. A. Yankner. 1997. Neuronal localization of presenilin-1 and association with amyloid plaques and neurofibrillary tangles in Alzheimer's disease. *J Neurosci* 17 (13): 5101–5107.
112. Mohmmad Abdul, H., R. Sultana, J. N. Keller, D. K. St Clair, W. R. Markesbery, and D. A. Butterfield. 2006. Mutations in amyloid precursor protein and presenilin-1 genes increase the basal oxidative stress in murine neuronal cells and lead to increased sensitivity to oxidative stress mediated by amyloid beta-peptide (1–42), HO and kainic acid: Implications for Alzheimer's disease. *J Neurochem* 96 (5): 1322–1335.
113. Abdul, H. M., R. Sultana, D. K. St Clair, W. R. Markesbery, and D. A. Butterfield. 2008. Oxidative damage in brain from human mutant APP/PS-1 double knock-in mice as a function of age. *Free Radic Biol Med* 45 (10): 1420–1425.
114. Mohmmad Abdul, H., G. L. Wenk, M. Gramling, B. Hauss-Wegrzyniak, and D. A. Butterfield. 2004. APP and PS-1 mutations induce brain oxidative stress independent of dietary cholesterol: Implications for Alzheimer's disease. *Neurosci Lett* 368 (2): 148–150.
115. Zhang, Z., H. Hartmann, V. M. Do, D. Abramowski, C. Sturchler-Pierrat, M. Staufenbiel, B. Sommer, et al. 1998. Destabilization of beta-catenin by mutations in presenilin-1 potentiates neuronal apoptosis. *Nature* 395 (6703): 698–6702.
116. Song, W., P. Nadeau, M. Yuan, X. Yang, J. Shen, and B. A. Yankner. 1999. Proteolytic release and nuclear translocation of Notch-1 are induced by presenilin-1 and impaired by pathogenic presenilin-1 mutations. *Proc Natl Acad Sci U S A* 96 (12): 6959–6963.
117. Tabaton, M., and E. Tamagno. 2007. The molecular link between beta- and gamma-secretase activity on the amyloid beta precursor protein. *Cell Mol Life Sci* 64 (17): 2211–2218.
118. Placanica, L., L. Tarassishin, G. Yang, E. Peethumnongsin, S. H. Kim, H. Zheng, S. S. Sisodia, and Y. M. Li. 2009. Pen2 and presenilin-1 modulate the dynamic equilibrium of presenilin-1 and presenilin-2 gamma-secretase complexes. *J Biol Chem* 284 (5): 2967–2977.
119. Jenkinson, M. L., M. R. Bliss, A. T. Brain, and D. L. Scott. 1989. Rheumatoid arthritis and senile dementia of the Alzheimer's type. *Br J Rheumatol* 28 (1): 86–88.
120. Breitner, J. C., B. A. Gau, K. A. Welsh, B. L. Plassman, W. M. McDonald, M. J. Helms, and J. C. Anthony. 1994. Inverse association of anti-inflammatory treatments and Alzheimer's disease: Initial results of a co-twin control study. *Neurology* 44 (2): 227–232.
121. McGeer, P. L., M. Schulzer, and E. G. McGeer. 1996. Arthritis and anti-inflammatory agents as possible protective factors for Alzheimer's disease: A review of 17 epidemiologic studies. *Neurology* 47 (2): 425–432.
122. McGeer, E. G., and P. L. McGeer. 1998. The importance of inflammatory mechanisms in Alzheimer disease. *Exp Gerontol* 33 (5): 371–378.
123. Shalit, F., B. Sredni, L. Stern, E. Kott, and M. Huberman. 1994. Elevated interleukin-6 secretion levels by mononuclear cells of Alzheimer's patients. *Neurosci Lett* 174 (2): 130–132.
124. Sharif, S. F., R. J. Hariri, V. A. Chang, P. S. Barie, R. S. Wang, and J. B. Ghajar. 1993. Human astrocyte production of tumour necrosis factor-alpha, interleukin-1 beta, and interleukin-6 following exposure to lipopolysaccharide endotoxin. *Neurol Res* 15 (2): 109–112.

125. Rogers, J., N. R. Cooper, S. Webster, J. Schultz, P. L. McGeer, S. D. Styren, W. Civin, et al. 1992. Complement activation by beta-amyloid in Alzheimer disease. *Proc Natl Acad Sci U S A* 89 (21): 10016–10020.
126. Rogers, J., L.-F. Lue, L. Brachova, S. Webster, and J. Schultz. 1995. Inflammation as a response and a cause of Alzheimer's pathophysiology. *Dementia* 9: 133–138.
127. Webster, S., S. O'Barr, and J. Rogers. 1994. Enhanced aggregation and beta structure of amyloid beta peptide after coincubation with C1q. *J Neurosci Res* 39 (4): 448–456.
128. Frohman, E. M., T. C. Frohman, S. Gupta, A. de Fougerolles, and S. van den Noort. 1991. Expression of intercellular adhesion molecule 1 (ICAM-1) in Alzheimer's disease. *J Neurol Sci* 106 (1): 105–111.
129. Verbeek, M. M., I. Otte-Holler, J. R. Westphal, P. Wesseling, D. J. Ruiter, and R. M. de Waal. 1994. Accumulation of intercellular adhesion molecule-1 in senile plaques in brain tissue of patients with Alzheimer's disease. *Am J Pathol* 144 (1): 104–116.
130. Rozemuller, J. M., P. Eikelenboom, S. T. Pals, and F. C. Stam. 1989. Microglial cells around amyloid plaques in Alzheimer's disease express leucocyte adhesion molecules of the LFA-1 family. *Neurosci Lett* 101 (3): 288–292.
131. Prasad, K. N., F. G. La Rosa, and J. E. Prasad. 1998. Prostaglandins act as neurotoxin for differentiated neuroblastoma cells in culture and increase levels of ubiquitin and beta-amyloid. *In Vitro Cell Dev Biol Anim* 34 (3): 265–274.
132. Sutton, E. T., T. Thomas, M. W. Bryant, C. S. Landon, C. A. Newton, and J. A. Rhodin. 1999. Amyloid-beta peptide induced inflammatory reaction is mediated by the cytokines tumor necrosis factor and interleukin-1. *J Submicrosc Cytol Pathol* 31 (3): 313–323.
133. Ramirez, G., S. Rey, and R. von Bernhardi. 2008. Proinflammatory stimuli are needed for induction of microglial cell-mediated AbetaPP_{244-C} and Abeta-neurotoxicity in hippocampal cultures. *J Alzheimers Dis* 15 (1): 45–59.
134. Yamamoto, M., T. Kiyota, M. Horiba, J. L. Buescher, S. M. Walsh, H. E. Gendelman, and T. Ikezu. 2007. Interferon-gamma and tumor necrosis factor-alpha regulate amyloid-beta plaque deposition and beta-secretase expression in Swedish mutant APP transgenic mice. *Am J Pathol* 170 (2): 680–692.
135. Blasko, I., F. Marx, E. Steiner, T. Hartmann, and B. Grubeck-Loebenstein. 1999. TNFalpha plus IFNgamma induce the production of Alzheimer beta-amyloid peptides and decrease the secretion of APPs. *FASEB J* 13 (1): 63–68.
136. Patel, J. R., and G. J. Brewer. 2008. Age-related changes to tumor necrosis factor receptors affect neuron survival in the presence of beta-amyloid. *J Neurosci Res* 86 (10): 2303–2313.
137. Liao, Y. F., B. J. Wang, H. T. Cheng, L. H. Kuo, and M. S. Wolfe. 2004. Tumor necrosis factor-alpha, interleukin-1beta, and interferon-gamma stimulate gamma-secretase–mediated cleavage of amyloid precursor protein through a JNK-dependent MAPK pathway. *J Biol Chem* 279 (47): 49523–49532.
138. Qiu, Z., and D. L. Gruol. 2003. Interleukin-6, beta-amyloid peptide and NMDA interactions in rat cortical neurons. *J Neuroimmunol* 139 (1–2): 51–57.
139. Shelat, P. B., M. Chalimoniuk, J. H. Wang, J. B. Strosznajder, J. C. Lee, A. Y. Sun, A. Simonyi, and G. Y. Sun. 2008. Amyloid beta peptide and NMDA induce ROS from NADPH oxidase and AA release from cytosolic phospholipase A2 in cortical neurons. *J Neurochem* 106 (1): 45–55.
140. Rich, J. B., D. X. Rasmusson, M. F. Folstein, K. A. Carson, C. Kawas, and J. Brandt. 1995. Nonsteroidal anti-inflammatory drugs in Alzheimer's disease. *Neurology* 45 (1): 51–55.
141. McGeer, P. L., E. McGeer, J. Rogers, and J. Sibley. 1990. Anti-inflammatory drugs and Alzheimer disease. *Lancet* 335 (8696): 1037.
142. Lucca, U., M. Tettamanti, G. Forloni, and A. Spagnoli. 1994. Nonsteroidal antiinflammatory drug use in Alzheimer's disease. *Biol Psychiatry* 36 (12): 854–856.
143. Rogers, J., L. C. Kirby, S. R. Hempelman, D. L. Berry, P. L. McGeer, A. W. Kaszniak, J. Zalinski, et al. 1993. Clinical trial of indomethacin in Alzheimer's disease. *Neurology* 43 (8): 1609–1611.
144. Martin, B. K., C. Szekely, J. Brandt, S. Piantadosi, J. C. Breitner, S. Craft, D. Evans, R. Green, and M. Mullan. 2008. Cognitive function over time in the Alzheimer's Disease Anti-inflammatory Prevention Trial (ADAPT): Results of a randomized, controlled trial of naproxen and celecoxib. *Arch Neurol* 65 (7): 896–905.
145. Babiloni, C., G. B. Frisoni, C. Del Percio, O. Zanetti, C. Bonomini, E. Cassetta, P. Pasqualetti, et al. 2009. Ibuprofen treatment modifies cortical sources of EEG rhythms in mild Alzheimer's disease. *Clin Neurophysiol* 120 (4): 709–718.
146. Hirohata, M., K. Ono, H. Naiki, and M. Yamada. 2005. Non-steroidal anti-inflammatory drugs have anti-amyloidogenic effects for Alzheimer's beta-amyloid fibrils in vitro. *Neuropharmacology* 49 (7): 1088–1099.

147. McKee, A. C., I. Carreras, L. Hossain, H. Ryu, W. L. Klein, S. Oddo, F. M. LaFerla, B. G. Jenkins, N. W. Kowall, and A. Dedeoglu. 2008. Ibuprofen reduces Abeta, hyperphosphorylated tau and memory deficits in Alzheimer mice. *Brain Res* 1207: 225–236.
148. Wakasugi, K., C. Kitatsuji, and I. Morishima. 2005. Possible neuroprotective mechanism of human neuroglobin. *Ann N Y Acad Sci* 1053: 220–230.
149. Liu, J., Z. Yu, S. Guo, S. R. Lee, C. Xing, C. Zhang, Y. Gao, D. G. Nicholls, E. H. Lo, and X. Wang. 2009. Effects of neuroglobin overexpression on mitochondrial function and oxidative stress following hypoxia/reoxygenation in cultured neurons. *J Neurosci Res* 87 (1): 164–170.
150. Yu, Z., J. Liu, S. Guo, C. Xing, X. Fan, M. Ning, J. C. Yuan, E. H. Lo, and X. Wang. 2009. Neuroglobin-overexpression alters hypoxic response gene expression in primary neuron culture following oxygen glucose deprivation. *Neuroscience* 162 (2): 396–403.
151. Sun, Y., K. Jin, A. Peel, X. O. Mao, L. Xie, and D. A. Greenberg. 2003. Neuroglobin protects the brain from experimental stroke in vivo. *Proc Natl Acad Sci U S A* 100 (6): 3497–3500.
152. Sun, Y., K. Jin, X. O. Mao, L. Xie, A. Peel, J. T. Childs, A. Logvinova, X. Wang, and D. A. Greenberg. 2005. Effect of aging on neuroglobin expression in rodent brain. *Neurobiol Aging* 26 (2): 275–278.
153. Greenberg, D. A., K. Jin, and A. A. Khan. 2008. Neuroglobin: An endogenous neuroprotectant. *Curr Opin Pharmacol* 8 (1): 20–24.
154. Li, R. C., M. W. Morris, S. K. Lee, F. Pouranfar, Y. Wang, and D. Gozal. 2008. Neuroglobin protects PC12 cells against oxidative stress. *Brain Res* 1190: 159–166.
155. Li, R. C., F. Pouranfar, S. K. Lee, M. W. Morris, Y. Wang, and D. Gozal. 2008. Neuroglobin protects PC12 cells against beta-amyloid–induced cell injury. *Neurobiol Aging* 29 (12): 1815–1822.
156. Khan, A. A., X. O. Mao, S. Banwait, K. Jin, and D. A. Greenberg. 2007. Neuroglobin attenuates beta-amyloid neurotoxicity in vitro and transgenic Alzheimer phenotype in vivo. *Proc Natl Acad Sci U S A* 104 (48): 19114–19119.
157. Szymanski, M., R. Wang, M. D. Fallin, S. S. Bassett, and D. Avramopoulos. 2008. Neuroglobin and Alzheimer's dementia: Genetic association and gene expression changes. *Neurobiol Aging* in press.
158. Lopez-Pousa, S., A. Turon-Estrada, J. Garre-Olmo, I. Pericot-Nierga, M. Lozano-Gallego, M. Vilalta-Franch, M. Hernandez-Ferrandiz, et al. 2005. Differential efficacy of treatment with acetylcholinesterase inhibitors in patients with mild and moderate Alzheimer's disease over a 6-month period. *Dement Geriatr Cogn Disord* 19 (4): 189–195.
159. Birks, J., and L. Flicker. 2006. Donepezil for mild cognitive impairment. *Cochrane Database Syst Rev* 3: CD006104.
160. Lopez, O. L., J. A. Mackell, Y. Sun, L. M. Kassalow, Y. Xu, T. McRae, and H. Li. 2008. Effectiveness and safety of donepezil in Hispanic patients with Alzheimer's disease: A 12-week open-label study. *J Natl Med Assoc* 100 (11): 1350–1358.
161. Mucha, L., S. Shaohung, B. Cuffel, T. McRae, T. L. Mark, and M. Del Valle. 2008. Comparison of cholinesterase inhibitor utilization patterns and associated health care costs in Alzheimer's disease. *J Manag Care Pharm* 14 (5): 451–461.
162. Hager, K., M. Kenklies, J. McAfoose, J. Engel, and G. Munch. 2007. Alpha-lipoic acid as a new treatment option for Alzheimer's disease—a 48 months follow-up analysis. *J Neural Transm Suppl* (72): 189–193.
163. Moreira, P. I., P. L. Harris, X. Zhu, M. S. Santos, C. R. Oliveira, M. A. Smith, and G. Perry. 2007. Lipoic acid and N-acetyl cysteine decrease mitochondrial-related oxidative stress in Alzheimer disease patient fibroblasts. *J Alzheimers Dis* 12 (2): 195–206.
164. Zhang, L., G. Q. Xing, J. L. Barker, Y. Chang, D. Maric, W. Ma, B. S. Li, and D. R. Rubinow. 2001. Alpha-lipoic acid protects rat cortical neurons against cell death induced by amyloid and hydrogen peroxide through the Akt signalling pathway. *Neurosci Lett* 312 (3): 125–128.
165. Carlson, D. A., A. R. Smith, S. J. Fischer, K. L. Young, and L. Packer. 2007. The plasma pharmacokinetics of R-(+)-lipoic acid administered as sodium R-(+)-lipoate to healthy human subjects. *Altern Med Rev* 12 (4): 343–351.
166. Chng, H. T., L. S. New, A. H. Neo, C. W. Goh, E. R. Browne, and E. C. Chan. 2009. Distribution study of orally administered lipoic acid in rat brain tissues. *Brain Res* 1251: 80–86.
167. Siedlak, S. L., G. Casadesus, K. M. Webber, M. A. Pappolla, C. S. Atwood, M. A. Smith, and G. Perry. 2009. Chronic antioxidant therapy reduces oxidative stress in a mouse model of Alzheimer's disease. *Free Radic Res* 43 (2): 156–164.
168. Quinn, J. F., J. R. Bussiere, R. S. Hammond, T. J. Montine, E. Henson, R. E. Jones, and R. W. Stackman Jr. 2007. Chronic dietary alpha-lipoic acid reduces deficits in hippocampal memory of aged Tg2576 mice. *Neurobiol Aging* 28 (2): 213–225.

169. Suchy, J., A. Chan, and T. B. Shea. 2009. Dietary supplementation with a combination of alpha-lipoic acid, acetyl-l-carnitine, glycerophosphocoline, docosahexaenoic acid, and phosphatidylserine reduces oxidative damage to murine brain and improves cognitive performance. *Nutr Res* 29 (1): 70–74.
170. Holmquist, L., G. Stuchbury, K. Berbaum, S. Muscat, S. Young, K. Hager, J. Engel, and G. Munch. 2007. Lipoic acid as a novel treatment for Alzheimer's disease and related dementias. *Pharmacol Ther* 113 (1): 154–164.
171. Maczurek, A., K. Hager, M. Kenklies, M. Sharman, R. Martins, J. Engel, D. A. Carlson, and G. Munch. 2008. Lipoic acid as an anti-inflammatory and neuroprotective treatment for Alzheimer's disease. *Adv Drug Deliv Rev* 60 (13–14): 1463–1470.
172. Yang, X., Y. Yang, G. Li, J. Wang, and E. S. Yang. 2008. Coenzyme Q10 attenuates beta-amyloid pathology in the aged transgenic mice with Alzheimer presenilin 1 mutation. *J Mol Neurosci* 34 (2): 165–171.
173. Ono, K., K. Hasegawa, H. Naiki, and M. Yamada. 2005. Preformed beta-amyloid fibrils are destabilized by coenzyme Q10 in vitro. *Biochem Biophys Res Commun* 330 (1): 111–116.
174. Moreira, P. I., M. S. Santos, C. Sena, E. Nunes, R. Seica, and C. R. Oliveira. 2005. CoQ10 therapy attenuates amyloid beta-peptide toxicity in brain mitochondria isolated from aged diabetic rats. *Exp Neurol* 196 (1): 112–119.
175. de Bustos, F., J. A. Molina, F. J. Jimenez-Jimenez, A. Garcia-Redondo, C. Gomez-Escalonilla, J. Porta-Etessam, A. Berbel, et al. 2000. Serum levels of coenzyme Q10 in patients with Alzheimer's disease. *J Neural Transm* 107 (2): 233–239.
176. McDonald, S. R., R. S. Sohal, and M. J. Forster. 2005. Concurrent administration of coenzyme Q10 and alpha-tocopherol improves learning in aged mice. *Free Radic Biol Med* 38 (6): 729–736.
177. Feng, Z., C. Qin, Y. Chang, and J. T. Zhang. 2006. Early melatonin supplementation alleviates oxidative stress in a transgenic mouse model of Alzheimer's disease. *Free Radic Biol Med* 40 (1): 101–109.
178. Olcese, J. M., C. Cao, T. Mori, M. B. Mamcarz, A. Maxwell, M. J. Runfeldt, L. Wang, et al. 2009. Protection against cognitive deficits and markers of neurodegeneration by long-term oral administration of melatonin in a transgenic model of Alzheimer disease. *J Pineal Res* 47 (1): 82–96.
179. Gehrman, P. R., D. J. Connor, J. L. Martin, T. Shochat, J. Corey-Bloom, and S. Ancoli-Israel. 2009. Melatonin fails to improve sleep or agitation in double-blind randomized placebo-controlled trial of institutionalized patients with Alzheimer disease. *Am J Geriatr Psychiatry* 17 (2): 166–169.
180. Furio, A. M., L. I. Brusco, and D. P. Cardinali. 2007. Possible therapeutic value of melatonin in mild cognitive impairment: A retrospective study. *J Pineal Res* 43 (4): 404–409.
181. Birkmayer, J. G. 1996. Coenzyme nicotinamide adenine dinucleotide: New therapeutic approach for improving dementia of the Alzheimer type. *Ann Clin Lab Sci* 26 (1): 1–9.
182. Rex, A., M. Spychalla, and H. Fink. 2004. Treatment with reduced nicotinamide adenine dinucleotide (NADH) improves water maze performance in old Wistar rats. *Behav Brain Res* 154 (1): 149–153.
183. Demarin, V., S. S. Podobnik, D. Storga-Tomic, and G. Kay. 2004. Treatment of Alzheimer's disease with stabilized oral nicotinamide adenine dinucleotide: A randomized, double-blind study. *Drugs Exp Clin Res* 30 (1): 27–33.
184. Rainer, M., E. Kraxberger, M. Haushofer, H. A. Mucke, and K. A. Jellinger. 2000. No evidence for cognitive improvement from oral nicotinamide adenine dinucleotide (NADH) in dementia. *J Neural Transm* 107 (12): 1475–1481.
185. Green, K. N., J. S. Steffan, H. Martinez-Coria, X. Sun, S. S. Schreiber, L. M. Thompson, and F. M. LaFerla. 2008. Nicotinamide restores cognition in Alzheimer's disease transgenic mice via a mechanism involving sirtuin inhibition and selective reduction of Thr231-phosphotau. *J Neurosci* 28 (45): 11500–11510.
186. Liu, D., M. Pitta, and M. P. Mattson. 2008. Preventing NAD(+) depletion protects neurons against excitotoxicity: Bioenergetic effects of mild mitochondrial uncoupling and caloric restriction. *Ann N Y Acad Sci* 1147: 275–282.
187. Qin, W., T. Yang, L. Ho, Z. Zhao, J. Wang, L. Chen, W. Zhao, M. Thiyagarajan, et al. 2006. Neuronal SIRT1 activation as a novel mechanism underlying the prevention of Alzheimer disease amyloid neuropathology by calorie restriction. *J Biol Chem* 281 (31): 21745–21754.
188. Qin, W., M. Chachich, M. Lane, G. Roth, M. Bryant, R. de Cabo, M. A. Ottinger, et al. 2006. Calorie restriction attenuates Alzheimer's disease type brain amyloidosis in squirrel monkeys (*Saimiri sciureus*). *J Alzheimers Dis* 10 (4): 417–422.
189. Ono, K., Y. Yoshiike, A. Takashima, K. Hasegawa, H. Naiki, and M. Yamada. 2004. Vitamin A exhibits potent antiamyloidogenic and fibril-destabilizing effects in vitro. *Exp Neurol* 189 (2): 380–392.
190. Ding, Y., A. Qiao, Z. Wang, J. S. Goodwin, E. S. Lee, M. L. Block, M. Allsbrook, M. P. McDonald, and G. H. Fan. 2008. Retinoic acid attenuates beta-amyloid deposition and rescues memory deficits in an Alzheimer's disease transgenic mouse model. *J Neurosci* 28 (45): 11622–11634.

191. Peng, Q. L., A. R. Buz'Zard, and B. H. Lau. 2002. Pycnogenol protects neurons from amyloid-beta peptide–induced apoptosis. *Brain Res Mol Brain Res* 104 (1): 55–65.
192. Isaac, M. G., R. Quinn, and N. Tabet. 2008. Vitamin E for Alzheimer's disease and mild cognitive impairment. *Cochrane Database Syst Rev* (3): CD002854.
193. Sano, M., C. Ernesto, R. G. Thomas, M. R. Klauber, K. Schafer, M. Grundman, P. Woodbury, et al. 1997. A controlled trial of selegiline, alpha-tocopherol, or both as treatment for Alzheimer's disease. The Alzheimer's Disease Cooperative Study. *N Engl J Med* 336 (17): 1216–1222.
194. Fillenbaum, G. G., M. N. Kuchibhatla, J. T. Hanlon, M. B. Artz, C. F. Pieper, K. E. Schmader, M. W. Dysken, and S. L. Gray. 2005. Dementia and Alzheimer's disease in community-dwelling elders taking vitamin C and/or vitamin E. *Ann Pharmacother* 39 (12): 2009–2014.
195. Gray, S. L., M. L. Anderson, P. K. Crane, J. C. Breitner, W. McCormick, J. D. Bowen, L. Teri, and E. Larson. 2008. Antioxidant vitamin supplement use and risk of dementia or Alzheimer's disease in older adults. *J Am Geriatr Soc* 56 (2): 291–295.
196. Zandi, P. P., J. C. Anthony, A. S. Khachaturian, S. V. Stone, D. Gustafson, J. T. Tschanz, M. C. Norton, K. A. Welsh-Bohmer, and J. C. Breitner. 2004. Reduced risk of Alzheimer disease in users of antioxidant vitamin supplements: The Cache County Study. *Arch Neurol* 61 (1): 82–88.
197. Sung, S., Y. Yao, K. Uryu, H. Yang, V. M. Lee, J. Q. Trojanowski, and D. Pratico. 2004. Early vitamin E supplementation in young but not aged mice reduces Abeta levels and amyloid deposition in a transgenic model of Alzheimer's disease. *FASEB J* 18 (2): 323–325.
198. Lockrow, J., A. Prakasam, P. Huang, H. Bimonte-Nelson, K. Sambamurti, and A. C. Granholm. 2009. Cholinergic degeneration and memory loss delayed by vitamin E in a Down syndrome mouse model. *Exp Neurol* 216 (2): 278–289.
199. Jimenez-Jimenez, F. J., J. A. Molina, F. de Bustos, M. Orti-Pareja, J. Benito-Leon, A. Tallon-Barranco, T. Gasalla, J. Porta, and J. Arenas. 1999. Serum levels of beta-carotene, alpha-carotene and vitamin A in patients with Alzheimer's disease. *Eur J Neurol* 6 (4): 495–497.
200. Jimenez-Jimenez, F. J., F. de Bustos, J. A. Molina, J. Benito-Leon, A. Tallon-Barranco, T. Gasalla, M. Orti-Pareja, et al. 1997. Cerebrospinal fluid levels of alpha-tocopherol (vitamin E) in Alzheimer's disease. *J Neural Transm* 104 (6–7): 703–710.
201. Rinaldi, P., M. C. Polidori, A. Metastasio, E. Mariani, P. Mattioli, A. Cherubini, M. Catani, R. Cecchetti, U. Senin, and P. Mecocci. 2003. Plasma antioxidants are similarly depleted in mild cognitive impairment and in Alzheimer's disease. *Neurobiol Aging* 24 (7): 915–919.
202. Charlton, K. E., T. L. Rabinowitz, L. N. Geffen, and M. A. Dhansay. 2004. Lowered plasma vitamin C, but not vitamin E, concentrations in dementia patients. *J Nutr Health Aging* 8 (2): 99–107.
203. Cole, M. G., and J. F. Prchal. 1984. Low serum vitamin B_{12} in Alzheimer-type dementia. *Age Ageing* 13 (2): 101–105.
204. Regland, B., C. G. Gottfries, and L. Oreland. 1991. Vitamin B_{12}-induced reduction of platelet monoamine oxidase activity in patients with dementia and pernicious anaemia. *Eur Arch Psychiatry Clin Neurosci* 240 (4–5): 288–291.
205. Nadeau, A., and A. G. Roberge. 1988. Effects of vitamin B_{12} supplementation on choline acetyltransferase activity in cat brain. *Int J Vitam Nutr Res* 58 (4): 402–406.
206. Ikeda, T., K. Yamamoto, K. Takahashi, Y. Kaku, M. Uchiyama, K. Sugiyama, and M. Yamada. 1992. Treatment of Alzheimer-type dementia with intravenous mecobalamin. *Clin Ther* 14 (3): 426–437.
207. Malouf, R., and J. Grimley Evans. 2008. Folic acid with or without vitamin B12 for the prevention and treatment of healthy elderly and demented people. *Cochrane Database Syst Rev* (4): CD004514.
208. Aisen, P. S., L. S. Schneider, M. Sano, R. Diaz-Arrastia, C. H. van Dyck, M. F. Weiner, T. Bottiglieri, et al. 2008. High-dose B vitamin supplementation and cognitive decline in Alzheimer disease: A randomized controlled trial. *JAMA* 300 (15): 1774–1783.
209. van Dyck, C. H., J. M. Lyness, R. M. Rohrbaugh, and A. P. Siegal. 2009. Cognitive and psychiatric effects of vitamin B12 replacement in dementia with low serum B12 levels: A nursing home study. *Int Psychogeriatr* 21 (1): 138–147.
210. Vingtdeux, V., U. Dreses-Werringloer, H. Zhao, P. Davies, and P. Marambaud. 2008. Therapeutic potential of resveratrol in Alzheimer's disease. *BMC Neurosci* 9 (Suppl 2): S6.
211. Wang, J., L. Ho, Z. Zhao, I. Seror, N. Humala, D. L. Dickstein, M. Thiyagarajan, S. S. Percival, S. T. Talcott, and G. M. Pasinetti. 2006. Moderate consumption of Cabernet Sauvignon attenuates Abeta neuropathology in a mouse model of Alzheimer's disease. *FASEB J* 20 (13): 2313–2320.
212. Luchsinger, J. A., M. X. Tang, M. Siddiqui, S. Shea, and R. Mayeux. 2004. Alcohol intake and risk of dementia. *J Am Geriatr Soc* 52 (4): 540–546.

213. Savaskan, E., G. Olivieri, F. Meier, E. Seifritz, A. Wirz-Justice, and F. Muller-Spahn. 2003. Red wine ingredient resveratrol protects from beta-amyloid neurotoxicity. *Gerontology* 49 (6): 380–383.
214. Marambaud, P., H. Zhao, and P. Davies. 2005. Resveratrol promotes clearance of Alzheimer's disease amyloid-beta peptides. *J Biol Chem* 280 (45): 37377–37382.
215. Anekonda, T. S. 2006. Resveratrol—a boon for treating Alzheimer's disease? *Brain Res Rev* 52 (2): 316–226.
216. Tang, B. L., and C. E. Chua. 2008. SIRT1 and neuronal diseases. *Mol Aspects Med* 29 (3): 187–200.
217. DeKosky, S. T., J. D. Williamson, A. L. Fitzpatrick, R. A. Kronmal, D. G. Ives, J. A. Saxton, O. L. Lopez, et al. 2008. Ginkgo biloba for prevention of dementia: A randomized controlled trial. *JAMA* 300 (19): 2253–2262.
218. Augustin, S., G. Rimbach, K. Augustin, R. Schliebs, S. Wolffram, and R. Cermak. 2009. Effect of a short- and long-term treatment with *Ginkgo biloba* extract on amyloid precursor protein levels in a transgenic mouse model relevant to Alzheimer's disease. *Arch Biochem Biophys* 481 (2): 177–182.
219. Freund-Levi, Y., M. Eriksdotter-Jonhagen, T. Cederholm, H. Basun, G. Faxen-Irving, A. Garlind, I. Vedin, B. Vessby, L. O. Wahlund, and J. Palmblad. 2006. Omega-3 fatty acid treatment in 174 patients with mild to moderate Alzheimer disease: OmegAD study: A randomized double-blind trial. *Arch Neurol* 63 (10): 1402–1408.
220. Fotuhi, M., P. Mohassel, and K. Yaffe. 2009. Fish consumption, long-chain omega-3 fatty acids and risk of cognitive decline or Alzheimer disease: A complex association. *Nat Clin Pract Neurol* 5 (3): 140–152.
221. Kroger, E., R. Verreault, P. H. Carmichael, J. Lindsay, P. Julien, E. Dewailly, P. Ayotte, and D. Laurin. 2009. Omega-3 fatty acids and risk of dementia: The Canadian Study of Health and Aging. *Am J Clin Nutr* 90 (1): 184–192.
222. Chiu, C. C., K. P. Su, T. C. Cheng, H. C. Liu, C. J. Chang, M. E. Dewey, R. Stewart, and S. Y. Huang. 2008. The effects of omega-3 fatty acids monotherapy in Alzheimer's disease and mild cognitive impairment: A preliminary randomized double-blind placebo-controlled study. *Prog Neuropsychopharmacol Biol Psychiatry* 32 (6): 1538–1544.
223. Rezai-Zadeh, K., G. W. Arendash, H. Hou, F. Fernandez, M. Jensen, M. Runfeldt, R. D. Shytle, and J. Tan. 2008. Green tea epigallocatechin-3-gallate (EGCG) reduces beta-amyloid mediated cognitive impairment and modulates tau pathology in Alzheimer transgenic mice. *Brain Res* 1214: 177–187.
224. Arendash, G. W., W. Schleif, K. Rezai-Zadeh, E. K. Jackson, L. C. Zacharia, J. R. Cracchiolo, D. Shippy, and J. Tan. 2006. Caffeine protects Alzheimer's mice against cognitive impairment and reduces brain beta-amyloid production. *Neuroscience* 142 (4): 941–952.
225. Krinsky, N. I. 1989. Antioxidant functions of carotenoids. *Free Radic Biol Med* 7 (6): 617–635.
226. Hazuka, M. B., J. Edwards-Prasad, F. Newman, J. J. Kinzie, and K. N. Prasad. 1990. Beta-carotene induces morphological differentiation and decreases adenylate cyclase activity in melanoma cells in culture. *J Am Coll Nutr* 9 (2): 143–149.
227. Zhang, L. X., R. V. Cooney, and J. S. Bertram. 1992. Carotenoids up-regulate connexin43 gene expression independent of their provitamin A or antioxidant properties. *Cancer Res* 52 (20): 5707–5712.
228. Carter, C. A., M. Pogribny, A. Davidson, C. D. Jackson, L. J. McGarrity, and S. M. Morris. 1996. Effects of retinoic acid on cell differentiation and reversion toward normal in human endometrial adenocarcinoma (RL95-2) cells. *Anticancer Res* 16 (1): 17–24.
229. F. L. Meyskens Jr. 1995. Role of vitamin A and its derivatives in the treatment of human cancer. In *Nutrients in Cancer Prevention and Treatment*, ed. K. N. Prasad, L. Santamaria, and R. M. Williams, 349–362. Totowa, NJ: Humana Press.
230. Vile, G. F., and C. C. Winterbourn. 1988. Inhibition of adriamycin-promoted microsomal lipid peroxidation by beta-carotene, alpha-tocopherol and retinol at high and low oxygen partial pressures. *FEBS Lett* 238 (2): 353–356.
231. McCay, P. B. 1985. Vitamin E: Interactions with free radicals and ascorbate. *Annu Rev Nutr* 5: 323–40.
232. Prasad, K. N., B. Kumar, X. D. Yan, A. J. Hanson, and W. C. Cole. 2003. alpha-Tocopheryl succinate, the most effective form of vitamin E for adjuvant cancer treatment: A review. *J Am Coll Nutr* 22 (2): 108–117.
233. Schwartz, J. L. 1995. Molecular and biochemical control of tumor growth following treatment with carotenoids or tocopherols. In *Nutrients in Cancer Prevention and Treatment*, ed. K. N. Prasad, L. Santamaria, and R. M. Williams, 287–316. Totowa, NJ: Humana Press.
234. Prasad, K. N., and J. Edwards-Prasad. 1992. Vitamin E and cancer prevention: Recent advances and future potentials. *J Am Coll Nutr* 11 (5): 487–500.

235. Witschi, A., S. Reddy, B. Stofer, and B. H. Lauterburg. 1992. The systemic availability of oral glutathione. *Eur J Clin Pharmacol* 43 (6): 667–669.
236. Niki, E. 1997. Mechanisms and dynamics of antioxidant action of ubiquinol. *Mol Aspects Med* 18 (Suppl): S63–S70.
237. Hiramatsu, M., R. D. Velasco, D. S. Wilson, and L. Packer. 1991. Ubiquinone protects against loss of tocopherol in rat liver microsomes and mitochondrial membranes. *Res Commun Chem Pathol Pharmacol* 72 (2): 231–241.
238. Chen, R. S., C. C. Huang, and N. S. Chu. 1997. Coenzyme Q10 treatment in mitochondrial encephalomyopathies. Short-term double-blind, crossover study. *Eur Neurol* 37 (4): 212–218.
239. Eikelenboom, P., J. M. Rozemuller, G. Kraal, F. C. Stam, P. A. McBride, M. E. Bruce, and H. Fraser. 1991. Cerebral amyloid plaques in Alzheimer's disease but not in scrapie-affected mice are closely associated with a local inflammatory process. *Virchows Arch B Cell Pathol Incl Mol Pathol* 60 (5): 329–336.
240. Anderton, B. 1994. Free radicals on the mind. Hydrogen peroxide mediates amyloid beta protein toxicity. *Hum Exp Toxicol* 13 (10): 719.
241. Myllykangas-Luosujarvi, R., and H. Isomaki. 1994. Alzheimer's disease and rheumatoid arthritis. *Br J Rheumatol* 33 (5): 501–502.
242. Breitner, J. C., K. A. Welsh, M. J. Helms, P. C. Gaskell, B. A. Gau, A. D. Roses, M. A. Pericak-Vance, and A. M. Saunders. 1995. Delayed onset of Alzheimer's disease with nonsteroidal anti-inflammatory and histamine H_2 blocking drugs. *Neurobiol Aging* 16 (4): 523–530.
243. Andersen, K., L. J. Launer, A. Ott, A. W. Hoes, M. M. Breteler, and A. Hofman. 1995. Do nonsteroidal anti-inflammatory drugs decrease the risk for Alzheimer's disease? The Rotterdam Study. *Neurology* 45 (8): 1441–1445.
244. Aisen, P. S., K. L. Davis, J. D. Berg, K. Schafer, K. Campbell, R. G. Thomas, M. F. Weiner, et al. 2000. A randomized controlled trial of prednisone in Alzheimer's disease. Alzheimer's Disease Cooperative Study. *Neurology* 54 (3): 588–593.
245. Scharf, S., A. Mander, A. Ugoni, F. Vajda, and N. Christophidis. 1999. A double-blind, placebo-controlled trial of diclofenac/misoprostol in Alzheimer's disease. *Neurology* 53 (1): 197–201.
246. Sainati, S., D. Ingram, and S. Talwalker. 2000. Results of a double-blind, placebo-controlled study of Celecoxib in the treatment of progression of Alzheimer's disease. 6th International Stockholm–Spingfield Symposium of Advances in Alzheimer's Therapy, Stockholm.
247. McGeer, P. L. 2000. Cyclo-oxygenase-2 inhibitors: Rationale and therapeutic potential for Alzheimer's disease. *Drugs Aging* 17 (1): 1–11.
248. Mackenzie, I. R., and D. G. Munoz. 1998. Nonsteroidal anti-inflammatory drug use and Alzheimer-type pathology in aging. *Neurology* 50 (4): 986–990.
249. Lim, G. P., F. Yang, T. Chu, P. Chen, W. Beech, B. Teter, T. Tran, et al. 2000. Ibuprofen suppresses plaque pathology and inflammation in a mouse model for Alzheimer's disease. *J Neurosci* 20 (15): 5709–5714.
250. O'Banion, M. K. 2000. The potential of cyclooxygenase inhibitors in treatment and prevention of Alzheimer's disease. *Curr Opin Anti-Inflamm Immunomod Invest Drugs* 2: 186.
251. Olanow, C. W., and G. W. Arendash. 1994. Metals and free radicals in neurodegeneration. *Curr Opin Neurol* 7 (6): 548–558.
252. Abate, A., G. Yang, P. A. Dennery, S. Oberle, and H. Schroder. 2000. Synergistic inhibition of cyclooxygenase-2 expression by vitamin E and aspirin. *Free Radic Biol Med* 29 (11): 1135–1142.
253. Fotuhi, M., P. P. Zandi, K. M. Hayden, A. S. Khachaturian, C. A. Szekely, H. Wengreen, R. G. Munger, et al. 2008. Better cognitive performance in elderly taking antioxidant vitamins E and C supplements in combination with nonsteroidal anti-inflammatory drugs: The Cache County Study. *Alzheimers Dement* 4 (3): 223–227.

10 Micronutrients for the Prevention and Improvement of the Standard Therapy for Parkinson's Disease

INTRODUCTION

Parkinson's disease (PD) is a slow, progressive neurological disorder of the central nervous system.[1] In 1917, Dr. James Parkinson, a British physician, published an article on *The Shaky Palsy* describing the major symptoms of the disease that would later bear his name. Since then, pathologists and neurologists have repeatedly reported that loss of dopamine (DA)-producing nerve cells (DA neurons) from the substantia nigra region of the brain is primarily responsible for most of the motor control abnormalities observed in PD patients, although other cells are also affected in this disease. It is estimated that in normal individuals about 3–5% of DA neurons are lost every decade; however, in PD patients, the rate of loss is greater than that found in normal individuals.[2] The analysis of autopsied samples of PD brains revealed that about 70–75% of DA neurons are lost by the time the disease becomes detectable.[2] This suggests that DA neurons possess a high degree of functional plasticity.

The major environmental-, dietary- or lifestyle-related factors that initiate or promote the progression of degeneration of DA neurons associated with PD are not known. However, the research of the past several decades has identified several biological mechanisms that may be contributing factors. Among them, increased oxidative stress, inflammation, and mitochondrial defects are most important in sporadic PD. Even in familial PD, in which some genetic defects have been identified, these biological mechanisms play a central role in the initiation and progression of PD. Thus, they could serve as a biological basis for developing preventive treatments and improving current treatment strategies for both sporadic and familial PD. At present, there is no effective strategy for reducing the incidence or progression of PD in high-risk populations (familial cases, early stage PD, and individuals over the age of 65 years). The current drug and surgical treatments are very effective at improving the major symptoms of PD; but the efficacy of these treatments only lasts for as long as DA neurons remain viable. Additionally, the severe side-effects of levodopa, a gold standard therapy, are observed after some time, possibly mediated via increased oxidative stress and chronic inflammation. It is known that auto-oxidation of L-dopa and DA generates excessive amounts of free radicals that could damage not only DA neurons, but neurons in other regions of the brain. The toxic side-effects become a limiting factor for the continuation of levodopa therapy. None of the current treatments with drugs or surgical procedures affect the levels of oxidative stress and inflammation that are major contributors to the degeneration of DA neurons. Antioxidants that have potential to reduce the rate of degeneration of DA neurons by reducing oxidative stress and inflammation have not been utilized on the basis of a scientific rationale in all clinical studies published thus far. The clinical trials to evaluate the role of antioxidants in the progression of PD have utilized only one dietary antioxidant, primarily vitamin E, which may not be adequate to reduce both oxidative stress and chronic inflammation in the brain. Therefore, additional clinical studies should be initiated, using a formulation of multiple micronutrients containing both dietary and endogenous antioxidants at appropriate doses and dose schedule for reducing the risk and progression of PD, and improving the efficacy of standard therapy in PD patients.

This chapter briefly describes the incidence, cost, etiology, neuropathology, genetic defects, and current treatment and discusses the role of oxidative stress, chronic inflammation, and mitochondrial dysfunction in the degeneration of DA neurons associated with PD. It also describes the scientific rationale and evidence for using the proposed micronutrients for reducing the risk and progression of PD, and for improving the efficacy of the standard therapy in patients with PD by well-designed clinical trials.

INCIDENCE AND COST

At present, PD affects about 500,000 Americans,[3] and about 50,000 new cases are diagnosed annually. From 1994 to 1995, the incidence of PD was evaluated by gender, age, and race/ethnicity.[4] The overall annual incidence rate was 12.3 per 100,000; but this increased to 44.0 per 100,000. The age-adjusted incidence rate for men was 19.0 per 100,000, and for women it was 9.9 per 100,000, suggesting that men may be more sensitive to this disease than women. The age- and gender-adjusted annual incidence rates in ethnic groups were highest among Hispanics, followed by non-Hispanic Whites, Asians, and Blacks. The incidence rates among non-Hispanic Whites and Asians were 13.6 and 11.3 per 100,000, respectively; among Hispanics and Asians, the incidence rates were 16.6 and 11.3 per 100,000, respectively. The incidence rates among non-Hispanic Whites and Blacks were 13.6 and 10.2 per 100,000, respectively. In all groups other than Asians, the incidence of PD among men was about twofold higher than women. Among Asians, the incidence of PD was slightly lower among men than women.

In 1992, the total direct and indirect cost of PD was estimated to be $6 billion. This cost is likely to increase in the future, because the disease occurs primarily in older people, and because the average age of Americans will increase.[3]

ETIOLOGY

Age is a risk factor for most idiopathic (sporadic) neurological diseases including PD. A sustained adverse interaction between environmental toxins and internal toxins such as increased oxidative stress and chronic inflammation products, and genetic (nuclear genes) and epigenetic (mitochondria, membranes, microfilaments, proteins) components of neurons could initiate and promote the progression of degeneration of DA neurons. An exposure to excessive amounts of manganese such as observed among manganese miners increased the incidence of PD-like disease.[5] This is because increased brain levels of free manganese can enhance production of free radicals, which then gradually cause damage to DA neurons. In 1980, increased incidence of a PD-like disease was seen among users of the designer drug, meperidene, which contains 1-methyl-4-phenyl 1,2,3,6-tetrahydropyridine (MPTP), a neurotoxic byproduct formed during the synthesis of this drug.[6] At least one of the mechanisms of action of MPTP-induced degeneration of DA neurons is mediated by free radicals.[6]

In an effort to identify other external agents as risk factors, several epidemiologic studies were performed.[7-11] The results of these studies revealed some potential risk factors such as rural living, well-water consumption, and exposure to herbicides and pesticides (e.g., dieldrin and dithiocarbamates). Although no particular dietary risk factors for PD were identified, the consumption of nuts and salad oil (pressed from seeds) appeared to be of protective value.[8] Vitamin E consumption was found to be lower among patients with PD than among the normal controls.[11]

NEUROPATHOLOGY AND SYMPTOMS

The degeneration of DA neurons of the substantia nigra is a characteristic feature of PD. Surviving neurons contain Lewy bodies, a pathological hallmark of PD. The Lewy bodies are present in other areas of the brain, particularly brain stem areas like the locus ceruleus that sends out processes throughout the brain. Thus, PD is not just a disease of the substantia nigra DA neurons alone. The incidence of Lewy bodies in 139 autopsied brain samples of elderly individuals with normal cognitive function and without any type of movement disorders was evaluated. The results showed that about 23% of the samples contained Lewy bodies in various regions of the brains. The most common regions involved were medulla (26%), amygdala (24%), Pons (20%), and midbrain (20%).[12] Lewy bodies contain predominantly neurofilaments that are important components of the neuronal cytoskeleton and ubiquitin that degrades abnormal proteins. Lewy bodies also contain high levels of alpha-synuclein. More recently, the presence of another protein, FOXO3 (a transcriptional activator that can trigger neuronal death upon oxidative stress), was demonstrated in Lewy bodies in the autopsied brain samples of PD as well as in the Lewy body dementia.[13] Lewy bodies are considered consequences of neuronal damage. They can be transferred from one neuron to another by endocytosis. This was demonstrated by the fact that Lewy bodies were present in the neurons grafted in patients with PD and in a transgenic animal model of PD.[14] In vitro studies showed that extracellular alpha-synuclein oligomers can induce intracellular alpha-synuclein aggregation in neurons.

The major symptoms of PD include tremor, muscle rigidity, postural problems, gait disorders, speaking difficulties, cognitive dysfunction, and immobility that ultimately lead to total disability and death. Genetic, oxidative damage, chronic inflammation, and mitochondrial dysfunction play a central role in the pathogenesis of PD. One of the consequences of genetic defects results in mitochondrial dysfunction that accelerates the production of free radicals.

GENETICS OF PD

Mutations in six genes have been identified in familial PD, and their actions in degeneration of DA neurons have been elucidated. Mutations in alpha-synuclein (SNCA), PARKIN, PTEN-induced kinase 1 (PINK1), DJ-1, and leucin-rich repeat kinase 2 (LRRK2) are associated with familial PD,[15–18] and account for about 2–3% of all cases of PD. The levels of the ATP13A2 gene that encodes lysosomal ATPase increased in the brains of patients with sporadic or idiopathic PD.[19] The transgenic animal models confirm the role of these mutations in the pathology of PD.[20,21] Among familial PD, mutations in the PARKIN gene account for about 50%, PINK1 8–15%, and DJ-1 about 1% of cases.[22] The mutation in the LRRK2 gene is involved not only in familial PD, but also in some sporadic PD. Several variants in LRRK2 and SNCA have been associated with an increased risk of sporadic PD.[23] There appears to be interaction between the PARKIN, PINK1, and DJ-1genes. It was demonstrated that these genes formed a complex referred to as PPD complex to promote ubiquitination and degradation of PARKIN substrates, including PRKIN itself in neuroblastoma cells in culture and human brain lysates.[24] Genetic ablation of either PINK1 or DJ-1 reduced ubiquitination of endogenous PARKIN and decreased degradation of aberrantly expressed PRKIN substrates. Expression of PINK1 increased PARKIN-mediated degradation of heat-shock-induced misfolded protein. However, mutations in PARKIN and PINK1 reduced degradation of PARKIN substrates by impairing ubiquitin E3 ligase activity.[24]

DJ-1 GENE

DJ-1, originally identified as an oncogene, is a ubiquitous redox-responsive protein with diverse biological functions, including protection against oxidative stress. It acts as a transcriptional regulator of antioxidant-mediated gene expression.[25] DJ-1 is very sensitive to oxidative stress and the oxidized form is considered a biomarker for neurodegenerative diseases, including sporadic PD.[26] Overexpression of wild-type DJ-1 made cells more resistant to oxidative stress induced by H_2O_2,[27] protected neurons against DA- and 6-hydroxydopamine (6-OHDA)-induced toxicity, and reduced intracellular levels of reactive oxygen species (ROS).[28,29] The levels of wild-type DJ-1 can be upregulated by antioxidant treatment in rats.[30] Mutations in DJ-1 and PARKIN genes make animals more sensitive to oxidative stress and mitochondrial toxins implicated in sporadic PD. Mutated DJ-1 makes DA neurons more vulnerable to oxidative stress-induced apoptosis.[31] Inactivated forms of DJ-1 may also promote aggregation of alpha-synuclein that impairs mitochondrial function causing DA neurons to degenerate slowly.[32]

The plasma levels of mutated DJ-1 protein in sporadic PD were higher than those in control subjects. Additionally, the plasma levels in advanced stages of PD were higher than those in early stages, suggesting that the plasma level of mutated DJ-1 protein could be considered as a biomarker for determining the severity of the disease.[33]

Alpha-Synuclein Gene

A family of homologous proteins, alpha- and beta-synuclein, is located primarily in the presynaptic regions of brain neurons, whereas gamma-synuclein is present in the peripheral nervous system and retina.[34] Lewy bodies, hallmarks of PD, contain predominantly alpha-synuclein in aggregated form, which has been implicated in the pathogenesis of PD. The overexpression of wild-type alpha-synuclein caused degenerative changes in human DA neurons in culture,[35] and in transgenic rat DA neurons.[36,37] The overexpression of human wild-type alpha-synuclein in differentiated neuroblastoma cells decreased their viability and increased their sensitivity to oxidative stress and neurotoxins such as H_2O_2, nitric oxide, and prostaglandin E2.[38] Increased oxidative stress, proteasome inhibition, and endoplasmic reticulum stress up-regulated wild-type alpha-synuclein expression in fibroblasts obtained from patients with PD, compared to those obtained from normal subjects.[39] The overexpression of wild-type alpha-synuclein is associated with the degeneration of DA neurons. Increased oxidative stress also causes aggregation of alpha-synuclein that is toxic to DA neurons. The mechanisms of action of alpha-synuclein are not well understood; however, it has been suggested that alpha-synuclein-induced neurotoxicity is related to the increased oxidative stress[40,41] that are caused by impaired mitochondria. Alpha-synuclein enters mitochondria through import receptors located in both the outer and inner mitochondrial membranes[42] and excessive accumulation of alpha-synuclein causes mitochondrial dysfunction. This is due to the fact that overexpression of alpha-synuclein causes nitration of mitochondrial proteins and the release of cytochrome c from the mitochondria.[43] These biological events that are related to increased oxidative stress may initiate degeneration of DA neurons. The overexpression of human wild-type or mutant (A53T or A30P) alpha-synuclein in human neuroblastoma cells in culture enhanced aggregation of alpha-synuclein.[44] Mutant alpha-synuclein (A53T) transfected mice developed intraneuronal Lewy bodies-like inclusions, mitochondrial dysfunction, and apoptotic death in neocortical, brain stem, and motor neurons.[45] The role of dysfunctional mitochondria in the pathogenesis of PD is further substantiated by the fact that chronic inhibition of complex I activity by rotenone-induced neurodegeneration characteristics of PD in rats. This effect of rotenone caused accumulation and aggregation of alpha-synuclein and ubiquitin, progressive oxidative damage, and caspase-dependent death in human neuroblastoma cells in culture.[46] DA metabolite 3- and 4-dihydroxyphenylacetaldehyde, interacts with alpha-synuclein proteins causing them to aggregate.[37]

The aggregated form of alpha-synuclein plays an important role in the pathogenesis of PD.[47] Mitochondrial dysfunction can also induce alpha-synuclein oligomerization through increased protein oxidation and microtubule depolymerization.[48] Alpha-synuclein-knockout mice developed without gross abnormality but are resistant to MPTP-induced degeneration of DA neurons. Genetic ablation of alpha-synuclein also protected neuronal cells in culture against oxidative stress,[47] increased the resistance of human DA neuron-like cells to 1-methyl-4-phenylpyridine (MPP+).[49,50] Conversely, overexpression of wild-type alpha-synuclein or mutant alpha-synuclein (A53T) increased the sensitivity of neurons to MPP+, which induced mitochondrial dysfunction, and 6-OHDA, which increased oxidative stress in human neuroblastoma cells in culture.[51] Antioxidants such as Edaravone protected only against MPP+-induced toxicity, and epigallocatechin-3-o-gallate protected only against 6-OHDA-induced neurodegeneration.[51] This study suggests that one type of antioxidant is not sufficient to affect neurodegeneration induced by diverse groups of toxins. Mutant alpha-synuclein (A53T), but not other variants such as A30P, induced adult onset of PD in transgenic mice, and this effect was associated with abnormal accumulation of detergent insoluble alpha-synuclein protein.[52] Overexpression of wild-type alpha-synuclein or mutated alpha-synuclein had no effect on proteasome activity in neuronal cells, in culture or in transgenic mice,[53,54] although alpha-synuclein directly inhibited the activity of purified 20S sub-units of proteasome reversibly in vitro.[54] The inhibition of proteasome in human neuroblastoma cells in culture failed to induce alpha-synuclein aggregation.[54] These results suggest that proteasome inhibition and overexpression of alpha-synuclein that are associated with PD are not related. It is likely that the increased oxidative stress that up-regulates alpha-synuclein and inhibits proteasome activity is a primary event in the pathogenesis of PD. Since alpha-synuclein is degraded by proteasome and by autophagic pathways,[55,56] any defects in one or both pathways can lead to an accumulation of alpha-synuclein in neurons. Whether or not a protein forms aggregation depends on the cellular concentration of the protein and the thermodynamic properties inherent to each protein. Therefore, an increase in the cellular concentration of alpha-synuclein can lead to aggregation. Oxidation of alpha-synuclein can also cause aggregation. Tyrosinase, a rate-limiting enzyme in the synthesis of melanin, in combination with alpha-synuclein, allows aggregation of alpha-synuclein.[57] The abnormal aggregation of alpha-synuclein plays a central role in the degeneration of DA neurons.[55] The interaction between alpha-synuclein and PARKIN resulted in decreased PARKIN and alpha-tubulin ubiquitation, accumulation of insoluble PARKIN, and cytoskeletal alterations, with reduced neurite outgrowth.[58]

PTEN-INDUCED PUTATIVE KINASE 1

PINK1, a mitochondrial Ser/Thr kinase, is a ubiquitous protein expressed throughout the human brain, and is primarily located in the mitochondrial membrane and the cytosol. One of the functions of wild-type PINK1 is to protect mitochondria against a variety of stress-signaling pathways. Genetic ablation of wild-type PINK1 caused a loss of mitochondrial membrane potential and a decrease in ATP synthesis, complex IV activity, and mitochondrial electron transport chain function.[59] Impairment of the mitochondrial electron transport chain and an increased frequency of deletions of mitochondrial DNA, which codes some of the subunits of the mitochondrial electron transport chain, have been found in the autopsied samples of the substantia nigra of PD brains. PINK1 is also present in Lewy bodies.[60] Like mutated alpha-synuclein, mutated PINK1 also impairs mitochondrial function. Mutant PINK1 (W437X) enhanced the levels of mutant synuclein (A53T)-induced mitochondrial dysfunction. This effect was associated with increased intracellular calcium levels.[61] Coexpression of mutated PINK1 and alpha-synuclein altered mitochondrial structure and neurite growth, which were totally blocked by the inhibitor of mitochondrial calcium flux.[61] Mutant PINK1 or PNK1 knockdown reduced mitochondrial respiration and ATP synthesis, inhibited proteasome activity, and increased alpha-synuclein aggregation in neuronal cells in culture.[62]

The wild-type PARKIN is considered one of the most important factors that improve mitochondrial dysfunction.[63] PINK1 and PARKIN play a central role in the regulation of mitochondrial dynamics and function (fission, fusion, and migration and energy generation); therefore, mutations in these genes can impair mitochondrial function and dynamics.[24] Mitochondrial dysfunction interferes with the generation of energy and produces more free radicals that initiate degeneration of DA neurons, eventually causing neuronal death. Mutated PINK1 increased oxidative damage in the fibroblasts obtained from PD patients as well as up-regulated wild-type alpha-synuclein expression in fibroblasts obtained from normal subjects.[39]

INCREASED OXIDATIVE STRESS IN PD

Several studies have demonstrated the presence of high levels of oxidative stress in autopsied brain samples of PD patients. The normal brain has the highest concentration of unsaturated fatty acids of all organs, and these fatty acids are very susceptible to lipid peroxidation. Indeed, high levels of oxidative damage have been observed in the autopsied samples of the substantia nigra of PD brains.[64–67] Autopsied samples of the substantia nigra of PD brains contained reduced levels of antioxidant enzymes[68,69] and antioxidants.[70–72] More recent studies confirmed and extended these earlier observations in PD brains.

The levels of markers of oxidative damage and vitamin E were measured in 211 patients with PD and 135 healthy controls. The results showed that leukocyte 8-hydroxyguanosine and plasma malondialdehyde (MDA) were elevated, while erythrocyte glutathione peroxidase and plasma vitamin E levels were reduced in PD patients compared to the control subjects.[73,74] Reduced glutathione levels were observed in the substantia nigra of the autopsied brain samples of PD patients indicating the presence of high oxidative stress.[75–77] Reduced glutathione can impair mitochondrial function. Isofurans are products of lipid peroxidation and their formation is favored in the presence of high oxygen tension. The levels of isofurans, but not F2-isoprostane, are elevated in the autopsied samples of the substantia nigra of PD patients.[78] Heme oxygenase-1 (HO-1) is a cellular stress protein expressed in the brain and other tissues, which becomes elevated in response to increased oxidative stress. The expression of HO-1 is up-regulated in the autopsied samples of the substantia nigra of PD brains.[79] The antioxidant capacity in the autopsied substantia nigra of PD brains was lower than control subjects.[80] It has been reported that the NADH dehydrogenase activity in the platelets of PD patients was lower compared to healthy age- and gender–matched controls, whereas the activity of succinate dehydrogenase was similar in both groups.[81]

The serum levels of vitamin A, vitamin E, and vitamin C in PD patients did not differ from controls[82–85]; however, plasma levels of vitamin C and vitamin E were decreased in patients with vascular PD.[85] These data suggest that the serum and plasma levels of vitamin A, vitamin C, and vitamin E do not play any significant roles in the pathogenesis of PD, because they do not reflect the brain levels of antioxidants. Thus, brain tissue levels of antioxidants, rather than the blood levels of antioxidants, may play significant roles in the initiation and progression of both sporadic and familial PD.

Several studies have confirmed that PD is associated with a significant increase in free iron in the degenerating substantia nigra.[86–88] The effects of iron on the degeneration of DA neurons are via increased oxidative stress. The mechanisms of accumulation of iron in the substantia nigra are unknown; however, isoforms of the divalent metal transporter-1 (DMT1) are elevated in the substantia nigra of PD brains.[89] Using an MPTP model of rat PD, it was demonstrated that the expression of DMT1 and the levels of iron increased in treated animals. These two biological events were associated with increased oxidative stress and neuronal death.[89] The mutation in DMT1 protected rats against toxicity produced by MPTP or 6-OHDA. Manganese enhanced DA-induced apoptosis in mesencephalic neurons.[90] The effect of manganese is mediated by induction of NF-kappaB and activation of nitric oxide synthase that generates increased amounts of free radicals.

It has been reported that the neuromelanin granules accumulate in the substantia nigra of PD patients. Neuromelanin are formed from auto-oxidation of catecholamines in the substantia nigra of PD brains, and contain significant amounts of iron.[91,92] Neuromelanin can cause degeneration in DA neurons by generating H_2O_2 when it is intact, or by releasing redox active metals such as iron if it is impaired. In addition, dying DA neurons can release melanin that can initiate chronic inflammatory responses by activating microglia cells. Excessive production of NO by treatment with MPTP plays a significant role in the degeneration of DA neurons because NO oxide can be oxidized to form peroxynitrite, a form of nitrogen-derived free radical that is highly neurotoxic. Therefore, the involvement of NO in the pathophysiology of PD has been proposed.[93] Thus, antioxidants that are known to neutralize free radicals should be useful in protecting DA neurons from dying.

Glutamate is a major excitatory transmitter in the mammalian central nervous system, and is neurotoxic when present in excess at the synapses. With the depletion of nigrostriatal DA neurons, the glutamatergic projections from the subthalamic nucleus to the basal ganglia output nuclei become overactive.[94] The glutamatergic activity also increased in the striatal region of the PD brain.

In the animal model of PD, inhibitors of glutamate receptors ameliorated abnormality in motor movements.[95,96] Increased glutamate signaling in the substantia nigra played an important role in the mechanisms of neuronal death induced by chronic treatment of mice with MPTP.[97] Thus, increased glutamatergic activity may play an important role in the pathogenesis and symptoms of PD. Antioxidants that can block the toxic effects of glutamate[98,99] should be useful in improving some of the symptoms of PD, and in protecting neurons from glutamate-induced toxicity.

INCREASED INFLAMMATION IN PD

Microglia-initiated chronic inflammation responses also play important roles in the mechanism of degeneration of DA neurons in PD.[100,101] Aggregated or nitrated alpha-synuclein activates microglia, which contributes to the degeneration of DA neurons by releasing proinflammatory cytokines and other neurotoxic factors.[102–104] It has been reported that nitric oxide and superoxide released by activated microglia may promote inflammation, as well as abnormal alpha-synuclein (excessive amounts or a mutated form) to cause degeneration of DA neurons in transgenic mice models of PD.[105] In autopsied brain samples of PD brains, the number of activated microglia cells increased in the substantia nigra during the progression of PD. The levels of proinflammatory cytokines IL-6 and TNF-alpha increased in both PD and Lewy body disease.[106] The analysis of neuronal loss in autopsied samples of substantia nigra suggests that neurons containing melanin are primarily lost.[107] Indeed, pathologists have consistently observed depigmentation of the substantia nigra in the autopsied samples of PD brains. The addition of human neuromelanin to microglia cell cultures induced chemotactic effects and activated the proinflammatory transcription factor NF-kappaB.[107] This treatment of microglia cells also up-regulated TNF-alpha, IL-6, and nitric oxide. These results suggest that the presence of extracellular neuromelanin serves as a chronic source of inflammation that aggravates the rate of degeneration of DA neurons. Although the inflammatory response is considered a protective response, chronic activation of microglia cells may produce excessive amounts of proinflammatory cytokines, compliment proteins, adhesion molecules, and ROS—all of which are neurotoxic. It has been reported that cyclooxygenase (COX) is the rate-limiting enzyme in the synthesis of prostaglandins that are neurotoxic in excessive amounts.[108] The inducible isoform COX-2 is up-regulated in the DA neurons in autopsied brain samples of PD patients, and in neurotoxin-induced animal PD models. The overexpression of COX-2 in human neuroblastoma cells facilitated oxidation of DA, and proteins including alpha-synuclein.[109] The studies presented in this section clearly show that chronic inflammation plays an important role in the degeneration and apoptosis of DA neurons in PD. Therefore, agents such as high-dose antioxidants and a low-dose nonsteroidal anti-inflammatory drug (NSAID) such as aspirin that inhibits chronic inflammation may help in reducing the incidence of PD in high-risk populations. When used as an adjunctive therapy, they may improve the efficacy of standard therapy in the treatment of PD.

MITOCHONDRIAL DYSFUNCTION IN PD

Mitochondrial dysfunction plays a central role in most neurodegenerative diseases including PD,[110,111] but can be considered as a secondary event in the initiation and progression of PD, because mitochondrial dysfunctions can be induced by diverse groups of external and internal agents. External agents include MPTP and insecticides and pesticides, whereas internal agents include increased oxidative stress, chronic inflammation, and mutated or aggregated alpha-synuclein, mutated PINK1, DJ-1, and PARKIN genes.[18,112,113] The mitochondrial dysfunctions include impaired electron transport chain, mitochondrial DNA defects, impaired calcium buffering, reduced ATP synthesis, anomalies of morphology, and dynamics of mitochondria.[114,115] The consequences of mitochondrial dysfunction include increased oxidative stress, release of cytochrome c, activation of caspase, release of calcium, up-regulation of Bax expression and its translocation to mitochondria, and proteasome inhibition—all of which contribute to the degeneration of DA neurons and eventually their death.[110,116,117] Thus, reducing oxidative stress by antioxidants should protect mitochondria, and thereby, reduce the risk of PD.

LABORATORY AND HUMAN STUDIES IN PD WITH ANTIOXIDANTS

Several in vitro and animal studies suggest that supplementation with individual antioxidants should be useful in reducing the risk and progression of PD; however, clinical studies with individual antioxidants have produced inconsistent results varying from no effect to minimal beneficial effects.

IN VITRO STUDIES

Alpha-synuclein fibrils are considered toxic to DA neurons. It has been reported that certain antioxidants such as vitamin A, beta-carotene (BC), and coenzyme Q_{10} inhibited formation of alpha-synuclein fibrils in a dose-dependent manner, whereas vitamin B_2, vitamin B_6, vitamin C, and vitamin E were ineffective in vitro.[118] In addition, vitamin A, BC, and coenzyme Q_{10} destabilized preformed alpha-synuclein fibrils in a dose-dependent manner. The results of these studies cannot be extrapolated to human PD, but they would suggest that supplementation with these antioxidants may help to reduce the risk of PD by preventing the aggregation of alpha-synuclein and by destabilizing the preformed alpha-synuclein fibrils.

DA is known to induce apoptosis in several lines of neuronal cells in culture by increasing oxidative stress. The viability of DA-treated human melanocytes significantly decreased in a dose-dependent manner, whereas keratinocytes exhibited less sensitivity to DA treatment. *N*-Acetylcysteine (NAC) or glutathione protected against DA-induced toxicity in normal human melanocytes, whereas other antioxidants such as vitamin C, vitamin E, trolox, and quercetin were ineffective.[119] Melatonin, deprenyl, and vitamin E inhibited auto-oxidation of DA in a dose-dependent manner, whereas vitamin C was ineffective.[120] These studies further confirmed that only certain antioxidants could protect DA neurons against free radicals generated by auto-oxidation of DA. Glutamate-depleted mesencephalic neurons become very sensitive to neurotoxins; however, treatment with ascorbate completely prevented the neurotoxin-induced degeneration in both normal and glutamate-depleted neurons in culture.[121] Glutamate, an excitatory neurotransmitter, is toxic in excessive amounts to DA neurons by causing increase in oxidative stress. This effect of glutamate can be blocked by an analog of NAC (*N*-acetylcysteine amide),[122] vitamin E,[98] and coenzyme Q_{10}.[99]

STUDIES IN ANIMAL MODELS OF PD

Some neurological abnormalities of PD in rodents similar to those observed in humans were induced by 6-OHDA, or MPTP. Therefore, they have been used to evaluate the efficacy of antioxidants in reducing drug-induced neurological abnormalities. Pretreatment of rats with D-alpha tocopherol or DL-alpha-tocopherol significantly reduced 6-OHDA–induced behavior and biochemical abnormalities.[123,124] Intramuscular administration of D-alpha-tocopheryl succinate, the most effective form of vitamin E,[125] protected against 6-OHDA-induced death of locus coeruleus neurons as well as behavioral and biochemical changes in rats.[126,127] Black tea extract, which exhibits antioxidant activity, also reduced 6-OHDA-induced degeneration of the nigrostriatal dopaminergic system, and improved motor and neurochemical deficits.[128]

Melatonin, a neurohormone secreted by the pineal gland, exhibits antioxidant activity. Melatonin and deprenyl prevent auto-oxidation of DA in a synergistic manner. Melatonin, but not deprenyl, prevented MPTP-induced inhibition of mitochondrial complex I activity and oxidative damage in nigrostriatal neuron.[129] Deprenyl significantly restored MPTP-induced decreases in DA levels and tyrosine hydroxylase (TH) activity; however, the combination of melatonin and deprenyl was more effective than the individual agents.[129] Quinolinic acid, an excitotoxin and free radical precursor, and 3-nitropropionic acid, a mitochondrial toxin, induced oxidative damage, and behavioral alterations. Administration of levocarnitine (L-CAR) at micromolar concentrations reduced neurotoxin-induced oxidative damage and behavior abnormalities.[130] Analysis of laboratory studies revealed that L-carnitine, coenzyme Q_{10}, lipoic acid, vitamin E, and resveratrol reduced damage to neurons induced by diverse groups of neurotoxins such as MPTP, rotenone, and 3-nitropropionic acid.[131] A green tea phenolic compound, epigallocatechin-3-gallate, which exhibits antioxidant properties, reduced MPTP-induced PD in mice through inhibition of nitric oxide synthase activity.[132] In collaboration with Dr. Clive Charlton of Meharry Medical College, Nashville, TN, we have found that both curcumin and a mixture of dietary and endogenous antioxidants (a gift from Premier Micronutrient Corporation, Nashville, TN) reduced the incidence of death and hypokinesia induced by MPTP treatment in mice. Although both curcumin and an antioxidant mixture markedly blocked MPTP-induced depletion of TH activity, only the antioxidant mixture enhanced the TH activity. This suggests that an antioxidant mixture treatment was more effective than the curcumin treatment in reducing the adverse effects of MPTP in mice.

It has been proposed that nicotinamide, also called niacin (vitamin B_3)-derived NDA(P)H is an antioxidant and a cofactor of enzymes. It can inhibit oxidative damage and improve mitochondrial function and, thus, can protect against neurodegeneration and improve motor function. Treatment of human neuroblastoma cells in culture with a relatively high dose of nicotinamide protected from MPP^+-induced cellular toxicity, and decrease in complex I and alpha-ketoglutarate dehydrogenase activity, and an increase in ROS, and oxidation of DNA and protein.[133] In addition, in the Drosophila model of PD (an alpha-synuclein transgenic fly), nicotinamide treatment significantly improved motor dysfunction (climbing ability). In a cellular model of PD (rotenone treatment for 4 weeks), pretreatment with B-vitamins for a period of 4 weeks prevented rotenone-induced mitochondrial dysfunction, oxidative stress, accumulation of alpha-synuclein, and poly-ubiquitin.[134] These studies also revealed that the presence of B-vitamins is essential for producing beneficial effects in experimental models of PD.

Nicotinamide, a precursor of nicotinamide adenine dinucleotide (NAD^+), also attenuated glutamate-induced toxicity and preserved cellular levels of NAD^+ to support the activity of SIRT-1.[135] It is also a competitive inhibitor of histone deacetylase activity, and restores memory deficits in AD transgenic mice.[136]

The sirtuin family of deacetylase enzymes consists of seven proteins (SIRT1-7) that are dependent on NAD^+ for their activities exhibit different biological functions. Three proteins are located in the nucleus, three in the mitochondria, and one in the cytoplasm.[137] SIRT1 is a regulator of mitochondrial biogenesis. Resveratrol, an activator of SIRT1, stimulated mitochondrial biogenesis in mice, which may reduce production of ROS.[138] There is compelling evidence that SIRT3 is localized in the mitochondria and appears to be responsible for the majority of protein deacetylation in this organelle.[139] A potent inhibitor of silent information regulator-2 (SIRT2) that prevents formation of alpha-synuclein fibrils may be useful in PD treatment.[137] It protected DA neurons from induced death and improved symptoms of PD in a Drosophila model of PD.[140] This suggests that SIRT2 promotes formation of alpha-synuclein fibrils. Thus, different isoforms of SIRT have different biological functions in the brain.

STUDIES IN HUMAN PD

Most clinical trials utilized a single antioxidant, primarily vitamin E, and that may have contributed to the inconsistent results. Deprenyl and Tocopherol Antioxidative Therapy of Parkinsonism (DATATOP), a randomized, double-blind, placebo-controlled, multicenter clinical trial, was initiated in 1989 to evaluate the efficacy of deprenyl (10 mg/day) and DL-tocopherol (2000 IU/day), individually and in combination, in patients with early stage PD when no therapy was required. The primary outcome was prolongation of the time needed before levodopa therapy. After a follow-up period of 8.2 years, deprenyl significantly delayed the need for levodopa therapy, but alpha tocopherol was ineffective.[141,142] The use of a single dietary antioxidant vitamin E was a major flaw in this study design, in view of the fact that glutathione deficiency in the brain is a consistent finding in most neurodegenerative diseases including PD; therefore, the addition of a glutathione-elevating agent such as alpha-lipoic acid and NAC would have been useful. Mitochondrial dysfunction is also commonly observed in PD and other neurodegenerative diseases; therefore, the addition of coenzyme Q_{10} and L-carnitine, which improve the function of mitochondria, would have been useful. There was another flaw in the DATATOP study design with an antioxidant. A multiple vitamin preparation (One-a-day™) was allowed for all individuals who wished to take it. It was argued that the effect of 30 IU vitamin E, which was present in the multiple vitamin preparation, would not significantly contribute to the effect of 2000 IU vitamin E. This argument may not be valid, since it has been shown that antioxidants used individually had no effect on growth of mammalian cancer cells in culture, but when they are combined at the same doses produced pronounced effect on growth inhibition, suggesting they may interact with each other in a synergistic manner.[143,144] Therefore, the impact of 30 IU vitamin E in a multiple vitamin preparation would be more pronounced than that produced by 30 IU vitamin E alone. Hence, the consumption of a multiple vitamin preparation containing a low dose of vitamin E by control subjects is likely to create an unacceptable variable while evaluating the efficacy of a high dose of vitamin E alone in early PD patients, especially when both experimental and placebo group were allowed to have a multiple vitamin preparation in an uncontrolled fashion. The patients with PD have a high oxidative environment in the brain. It is known that individual antioxidants when oxidized act as pro-oxidants. Therefore, the conclusion of the DATATOP study that antioxidants are not useful in reducing the progression of PD is not valid.

In an open-labeled clinical trial, the efficacy of high doses of alpha-tocopherol and ascorbate was tested in early PD patients. Patients were allowed to receive amantadine and anticholinergics, but not levodopa or a DA agonist. The primary outcome was a delay of the necessity of levodopa therapy. The results showed that these antioxidants extended the time before levodopa therapy was needed by 2.5 years.[145] This study shows that a mixture of antioxidants may be a better approach for extending the time before levodopa therapy is necessary than a single antioxidant in patients with early-stage PD.

In a multicenter, randomized, double-blind, placebo-controlled trial involving 80 early-stage PD patients who did not require any therapy, the efficacy of coenzyme Q_{10} at doses of 300, 600, or 1200 mg/day was evaluated. The primary outcome was Unified Parkinson Disease Rating Score (UPDRS), and the patients were followed-up for 16 months or until their disability required levodopa therapy. The results showed that coenzyme Q_{10} at the highest dose of 1200 mg/day was safe and well tolerated by patients. The results also revealed that less disability developed in patients receiving coenzyme Q_{10} compared to placebo controls; the benefit was greater in patients receiving the highest dosage.[146] Reviews of several open and controlled clinical studies revealed that daily supplementation with coenzyme Q_{10} either had no effect or had minimal benefit in early-stage PD patients.[147,148]

In a randomized, double-blind, placebo-controlled trial involving 35 patients with tardive dyskinesia (17 patients received vitamin E and 18 patients received a placebo), the efficacy of vitamin E alone at a dose of 800 IU/day was evaluated. Twenty-nine of these patients had a diagnosis of schizophrenia and 6 had a diagnosis of mood disorder. They were followed up for 2 months. Patients were assessed using modified Abnormal Involuntary Movement Scale (mAIMS), Simpson-Angus Scale for Extrapyramidal Side Effects, Brief Psychiatric Rating Scale, and dyskinesia. The results showed that vitamin E supplementation reduced the severity of tardive dyskinesia in patients who had this disease for 5 years or less.[149]

The efficacy of reduced nicotinamide adenine dinucleotide (NADH) in the treatment of PD patients has become controversial. This is consistent with the fact that most clinical studies with a single antioxidant have yielded inconsistent results. In an open label clinical study involving 885 PD patients, the efficacy of orally or intravenously administered NADH was evaluated.[150] The results showed that about 80% of the patients had beneficial clinical effects. However, younger patients and patients with a shorter duration of the disease exhibited more clinical benefits compared to older patients and patients with a longer duration of the disease. An oral administration of NADH was as effective as an intravenous one. Another clinical study evaluated the efficacy of intravenously administered NADH over a period of 7 days in combination with levodopa in 11 patients with PD.[151] These patients showed a significant response on the criterion of the Unified Parkinson's Disease Rating Scale. NADH treatment also significantly increased the bioavailability of levodopa in these patients. In contrast, a short-term (4 days IV, and 2 and 4 weeks IM) treatment of five patients with NADH did not produce any clinical benefit.[152] A review of the clinical efficacy of NADH has concluded that it is premature to recommend NADH alone for the treatment of PD.[153]

Several epidemiologic studies suggest that a diet rich in vitamin E may reduce the risk of PD.[11,154,155] These epidemiologic studies with vitamin E conflict with the results obtained from the intervention trials. It is possible that the diet contains antioxidants other than vitamin E and, therefore, its interaction with other antioxidants may have contributed to the beneficial effect on reducing the risk of PD. Thus, epidemiologic studies would favor the use of multiple antioxidants in any clinical study on PD. This is in contrast to in vitro and animal studies in which a single antioxidant consistently protected DA neurons against neurotoxin-induced degeneration.

PROBLEMS OF USING A SINGLE ANTIOXIDANT IN PD

Laboratory studies consistently showed that supplementation with individual antioxidants may reduce the symptoms and improve neurochemical changes in animal models of PD. Although epidemiologic studies revealed that a diet rich in vitamin E may reduce the risk of PD, the clinical trials with individual antioxidants have been inconsistent, producing minimal benefit at best. In PD patients, the levels of oxidative stress in the brain are high. Administration of a single antioxidant in such patients may not be effective, because this antioxidant may be oxidized in the presence of a high oxidative environment and then act as a pro-oxidant. In addition, the dose requirement of a single antioxidant to produce any beneficial effect in PD patients may be so high that it can cause toxicity after long-term consumption. Because of the failure to obtain consistent beneficial effects with individual antioxidants in patients with early PD, I recommend the use of multiple micronutrients including dietary and endogenous antioxidants and B-vitamins for reducing the risk of PD, and for improving the efficacy of standard therapy. Additional rationales for using multiple micronutrients in patients with PD are described below.

RATIONALE FOR USING MULTIPLE MICRONUTRIENTS IN PD

High-risk populations include persons aged 65 years and older, persons with a family history of PD, or persons with early stage PD where no therapy is yet required. Because of the potential for increased levels of oxidative stress, chronic inflammation, and enhanced sensitivity of neurons to oxidative stress in the brains of individuals of these populations, oral supplementation with appropriate micronutrients appears to be a rational choice for the prevention of PD in high-risk populations. It extends the time before levodopa therapy is needed in early-stage PD patients. Experimental designs of most clinical studies in early-stage PD have utilized only one antioxidant for reducing the rate of progression of PD. These designs are not suitable for determining the efficacy of micronutrient therapy because individual antioxidants can act as pro-oxidants when oxidized. In addition, their mechanisms of action and distribution at cellular and organ levels differ, their internal cellular and organ environments (oxygenation, aqueous, and lipid components) differ, and their affinity for various types of free radicals differ. For example, BC is more effective in quenching oxygen radicals than most other antioxidants.[156] BC can perform certain biological functions that cannot be produced by its metabolite vitamin A, and vice versa.[157,158] It has been reported that BC treatment enhances the expression of the connexin gene, which codes for a gap junction protein in mammalian fibroblasts in culture, whereas vitamin A treatment does not produce such an effect.[158] Vitamin A can induce differentiation in certain normal and cancer cells, whereas BC and other carotenoids do not.[159,160] Thus, BC and vitamin A have, in part, different biological functions.

The gradient of oxygen pressure varies within the cells. Some antioxidants, such as vitamin E, are more effective as quenchers of free radicals in reduced oxygen pressure, whereas BC and vitamin A are more effective in higher atmospheric pressures.[161] Vitamin C is necessary to protect cellular components in aqueous environments, whereas carotenoids and vitamins A and E protect cellular components in lipid environments. Additionally, vitamin C is necessary for the activity of TH, which is the rate-limiting enzyme in the synthesis of catecholamines. Vitamin C also plays an important role in maintaining cellular levels of vitamin E by recycling vitamin E radical (oxidized) to the reduced (antioxidant) form.[162] Also, oxidative DNA damage produced by high levels of vitamin C could be protected by vitamin E. Oxidized forms of vitamin C and vitamin E can also act as radicals; therefore, excessive amounts of any one of these forms, when used as a single agent, could be harmful over a long period of time.

The form of vitamin E used is also important in any clinical trial. It has been established that D-alpha-tocopheryl succinate (alpha-TS) is the most effective form of vitamin E both in vitro and in vivo.[125,163] This form of vitamin E is more soluble than alpha-tocopherol and enters cells more readily. Therefore, it is expected to cross the blood–brain barrier in greater amounts than alpha-tocopherol. However, this has not yet been demonstrated in animals or humans. We have reported that an oral ingestion of alpha-TS (800 IU/day) in humans increased plasma levels of not only alpha-tocopherol, but also alpha-TS, suggesting that a portion of alpha-TS can be absorbed from the intestinal tract before hydrolysis.[164] This observation is important because the conventional assumption based on the rodent studies has been that esterified forms of vitamin E such as alpha-TS, alpha-tocopheryl nicotinate, or alpha-tocopheryl acetate can be absorbed from the intestinal tract only after they are hydrolyzed to alpha-tocopherol. Our preliminary data showed that this assumption may not be true for the absorption of alpha-TS in humans.

The levels of an endogenous antioxidants glutathione are significantly reduced during early phases of PD, which may increase oxidative stress, and eventually neuronal death in the substantia nigra.[165] Glutathione is effective in catabolizing H_2O_2 and anions. However, an oral supplementation with glutathione failed to significantly increase plasma levels of glutathione in human subjects,[166] suggesting that this tripeptide is completely hydrolyzed in the GI tract. Therefore, I propose to utilize NAC and alpha-lipoic acid, which increase the cellular levels of glutathione by different mechanisms, in a multiple micronutrient preparation. In addition, R-alpha-lipoic acid and acetyl-L-carnitine together promoted mitochondrial biogenesis in murine adipocytes in culture; however, no effect was observed when these antioxidants were used individually.[167] These types of studies further emphasized the value of using more than one antioxidant in any clinical or laboratory studies involving PD.

Other endogenous antioxidants, such as coenzyme Q_{10}, may also have some potential value in prevention and improved treatment of PD. Since mitochondrial dysfunction is associated with PD and since coenzyme Q_{10} is needed for the generation of ATP by mitochondria, it is essential to add this antioxidant in multiple micronutrient preparations in order to improve the function of mitochondria. A study has shown that ubiquinol (coenzyme Q_{10}) scavenges peroxy radicals faster than alpha–tocopherol[168] and, like vitamin C, can regenerate vitamin E in a redox cycle.[169] However, it is a weaker antioxidant than alpha-tocopherol. Coenzyme Q_{10} administration has been shown to improve clinical symptoms in patients with mitochondrial encephalomyopathies[170] and has shown minimal benefit in early stage PD patients.[147,148]

Selenium is a cofactor of glutathione peroxidase and Se-glutathione peroxidase increases the intracellular level of glutathione, which is a powerful antioxidant. There may be some other mechanisms of action of selenium. Therefore, selenium and coenzyme Q_{10} should be added to a multiple micronutrient preparation for prevention and improved treatment of PD. Because of the biology of antioxidants discussed earlier, the use of single antioxidants in clinical trials cannot be considered rational for improving disease outcomes in patients with PD.

The preclinical data on nicotinamide suggests that oral supplementation with vitamin B_3 may be safe and useful in reducing the progression and improving the treatment of PD. Therefore, in addition to dietary and endogenous antioxidants, B-vitamins, which are necessary for general health, should be added to a multiple micronutrient preparation for reducing the incidence or improving treatment of PD.

RATIONALE FOR USING AN NSAID IN PD PREVENTION

Since inflammatory reactions represent one of the major factors that initiate and promote degeneration of DA neurons in PD brains, the use of an NSAID for the prevention and treatment of PD appears rational. Laboratory data have shown that products of inflammatory reactions such as prostaglandins,[108,171] cytokines,[172,173] complement proteins,[174–178] adhesion molecules,[179–181] and free radicals[182–184] are neurotoxic. Thus, the use of low-dose NSAIDs for preventing PD or reducing the progression of PD remains one of the viable options. These drugs do not improve the function of surviving neurons or protect neurons from further damage caused by oxidative and nitrosylative stress that is generated by mechanisms other than chronic inflammatory reactions.

RECOMMENDED MICRONUTRIENT SUPPLEMENT FOR USE IN COMBINATION WITH A LOW-DOSE NSAID FOR THE PREVENTION OF PD IN HIGH-RISK POPULATIONS

The high-risk populations include those with a family history of PD and those aged 65 years and older. A formulation of multiple micronutrients may include vitamin A (retinyl palmitate), vitamin E (both D-alpha-tocopherol and D-TS), natural mixed carotenoids, vitamin C (calcium ascorbate), coenzyme Q_{10}, R-alpha-lipoic acid, NAC, L-carnitine, vitamin D, B-vitamins, selenium, zinc, and chromium. No iron, copper, or manganese would be included because these trace minerals are known to interact with vitamin C to produce free radicals. More of these trace minerals are absorbed from the intestinal tract in the presence of antioxidants than in their absence, which could result in increased body stores of these minerals. Increased free iron stores have been linked to increased risk of several chronic diseases including PD.[185] Low-dose aspirin is recommended because of its anti-inflammatory effect and because, in combination with vitamin E, it produces a synergistic effect on the inhibition of COX activity[186]; therefore, the combination of multiple micronutrients and aspirin may be more effective in reducing the levels of chronic inflammation than the individual agents. The efficacy of the proposed micronutrient formulation in combination with aspirin remains to be tested in high-risk populations or in patients with early-stage PD, but they have been used in humans for several decades without significant reported toxicity. Meanwhile, the proposed micronutrient and aspirin recommendations may be adopted by the individuals among high-risk populations and those with early-stage PD, in consultation with their physicians or health professionals. It is expected that the proposed recommendations would reduce the risk of PD in high-risk populations and the rate of progression of the disease in patients with an early stage PD.

The recommended micronutrient supplements should be taken orally and divided into two doses, half in the morning and the other half in the evening with a meal. This is because the biological half-lives of micronutrients are highly variable, which can create high levels of fluctuations in the tissue levels of micronutrients. A twofold difference in the levels of certain micronutrients such as alpha-TS can cause a marked difference in the expression of gene profiles (our unpublished data). To maintain relatively consistent levels of micronutrients in the brain, the proposed micronutrients should be taken twice a day.

RECOMMENDED MICRONUTRIENT SUPPLEMENT FOR USE IN COMBINATION WITH A LOW-DOSE NSAID FOR REDUCING THE RATE OF PROGRESSION OF PD IN EARLY-STAGE PATIENTS

The patients with early-stage PD provide an excellent opportunity to study the efficacy of multiple micronutrients on reducing the rate of progression of PD. The micronutrients listed in the preceding section can also be used for this population.

CURRENT TREATMENTS OF PD

The current treatment strategies involve increasing the function of surviving DA neurons by maintaining adequate levels of DA. To accomplish this, L-dopa, a precursor of DA, and DA-receptor agonists are used. Deprenyl and catechol-*o*-methyl transferase (COMT) inhibitor are used to prevent degradation of DA. In some cases, acetylcholinesterase inhibitor is utilized to balance between two neurotransmitters, DA and acetylcholine, by reducing the levels of acetylcholine. In cases where drug therapy becomes ineffective, highly effective surgical methods to relieve some of the symptoms of PD, such as tremors, are available. None of these treatments prevents DA neurons from dying due to increased oxidative stress and chronic inflammation.

RATIONALE FOR USING A MICRONUTRIENT SUPPLEMENT AND AN NSAID IN COMBINATION WITH STANDARD THERAPY IN PD PATIENTS

Increased oxidative stress, chronic inflammation, and mitochondrial dysfunction play an important role in the progression of PD. Levodopa therapy is considered the gold standard for the treatment of PD, but its toxicity becomes a limiting factor, and the treatment is discontinued after about 5 years. The reasons for this effect of levodopa are unknown. In vitro studies have suggested that treatment of neuronal cells in culture with L-dopa is very toxic. This is due to the fact that L-dopa generates excessive amounts of free radicals during auto-oxidation as well as during oxidative metabolism of its product, DA; however, from animal studies it appears that there is no evidence of similar effects of L-dopa in vivo.[187] In a randomized, double-blind, placebo-controlled trial involving 361 patients with early-stage PD, the effects of various doses of levodopa for a period of 40 weeks were investigated.[188] The results showed that the patients receiving the highest dose of levodopa had significantly more dyskinesia, hypertonia, infection, headache, and nausea than those receiving a placebo. The clinical data showed that levodopa treatment either slowed the progression of PD or improved the symptoms of the disease. However, neuroimaging data suggests that levodopa treatment increased the rate of loss of nigrostriatal DA nerve terminals and reduced the levels of the DA transporter more than the placebo treatment. A further investigation of this issue revealed that the dose of levodopa is a factor in producing motor complications of dyskinesia and in wearing-off, and these can develop as early as 5 to 6 months at high levodopa doses.[189] Since L-dopa has a potential to cause increased oxidative damage peripherally and/or centrally, it appears rational to propose that supplementation with multiple antioxidants, in combination with levodopa therapy, may improve the efficacy of this therapy by reducing the side-effects. This would then allow levodopa treatment to be effective for a period longer than that currently expected. Furthermore, the oxidation of L-dopa is reduced by antioxidants; it could then be possible to reduce the dosage of levodopa without sacrificing its efficacy.

In a rat PD model (induced by rotenone), the efficacy of oral L-dopa therapy, with or without various doses of coenzyme Q_{10}, was evaluated.[190] The results showed that L-dopa therapy improved the symptoms and restored striatal DA levels, but it did not show any significant effect on striatal mitochondrial complex I activity, ATP levels, or the expression of Bcl2. Administration of coenzyme Q_{10} at a high dose with L-dopa increased striatal complex I activity, ATP levels, DA levels, and Bcl2 expression compared to coenzyme Q_{10} treatment at low doses with L-dopa.

RECOMMENDED MICRONUTRIENT SUPPLEMENT AND LOW-DOSE NSAID IN COMBINATION WITH STANDARD THERAPY IN PD PATIENTS

Levodopa therapy is considered the gold standard for the treatment of PD. The severe side-effects develop after varying periods of treatment, depending on the dose. These drugs improved the symptoms of PD by enhancing the functions of surviving DA neurons in PD patients. However, none of the drugs used for the treatment of PD protects DA neurons against the damaging effects of oxidative and nitrosylative stresses and products of chronic inflammation. Consequently, neurons continue to die in spite of standard treatment and, thus, the beneficial effects of levodopa or other drugs last as long as the DA neurons are alive. Therefore, the addition of a formulation of multiple micronutrients and a low-dose aspirin such as described in the previous section on PD prevention may improve the efficacy of standard therapy. The efficacy of this proposed strategy, in combination with standard therapy, should be tested in well-designed clinical trials. Meanwhile, the proposed micronutrient and aspirin recommendations may be adopted by PD patients who are receiving standard therapy in consultation with their physicians or health professionals. It is expected that the proposed recommendations would enhance the efficacy of standard therapy.

DIET AND LIFESTYLE RECOMMENDATIONS FOR PD

Even though there is no direct link between diet- and lifestyle-related factors and the initiation or progression of PD, it is always useful to include a balanced, low-fat diet that contains plenty of fruits and vegetables. Among fruits, blueberries and raspberries are particularly important because of their protective role against oxidative injuries in the brain. Lifestyle recommendations include daily moderate exercise, reduced stress, and no tobacco smoking or drug use.

CONCLUSIONS

The results of many studies presented in this review suggest that increased oxidative stress, chronic inflammation, and mitochondrial dysfunction play a dominant role in the initiation and progression of sporadic PD. Even in familial PD, these biological events play a crucial role in the pathogenesis of PD. Mitochondria are very sensitive to increased oxidative stress that can induce mitochondrial dysfunction. Therefore, supplementation with a formulation of multiple micronutrients, including dietary and endogenous antioxidants, in combination with a low-dose NSAID such as aspirin, would be useful in reducing the risk of PD in high-risk populations (persons with a family history of PD and those 65 years and older), and the rate of progression of the disease in patients with early-stage PD. The efficacy of standard therapy including levodopa depends on the viability of DA neurons. However, the drugs used in the standard therapy do not address the issues of increased oxidative stress and chronic inflammation that are responsible for neuronal degeneration. Therefore, the same formulation of multiple micronutrients and a low-dose aspirin in combination with standard therapy may improve the efficacy of this therapy by reducing the rate of degeneration of DA neurons in PD patients. Dietary recommendations include a diet rich in antioxidants, low in fat, and high in fiber. Lifestyle recommendations include daily moderate exercise, reduced stress, and no tobacco smoking or drug use. The clinical studies using the proposed micronutrient formulation should be initiated for reducing the risk of PD in high-risk populations (familial PD and individuals over the age of 65 years) and the rate of progression of the disease in patients with early-stage PD, and for improving the efficacy of standard therapy. Meanwhile, those PD individuals interested in a micronutrient approach to reducing the risk or the rate of progression of the disease, or improving the efficacy of standard therapy in the treatment of PD, may like to adopt these recommendations in consultation with their physicians or health professionals.

REFERENCES

1. Olanow, C. W., and M. B. Youdim. 1996. *Neurodegeneration and Neuroprotection in Parkinson's Disease.* New York, NY: Academic Press.
2. Mandel, S., E. Grunblatt, P. Riederer, M. Gerlach, Y. Levites, and M. B. Youdim. 2003. Neuroprotective strategies in Parkinson's disease: An update on progress. *CNS Drugs* 17 (10): 729–762.
3. NINDS. 2008. Parkinson's Disease: A Research Planning Workshop, National Instutute of Health, Bethesda, MD.

4. Van Den Eeden, S. K., C. M. Tanner, A. L. Bernstein, R. D. Fross, A. Leimpeter, D. A. Bloch, and L. M. Nelson. 2003. Incidence of Parkinson's disease: Variation by age, gender, and race/ethnicity. *Am J Epidemiol* 157 (11), 1015–1022.
5. Mena, I., K. Horiuchi, K. Burke, and C. G. Cotzias. 1969. Chronic manganese poisoning. Individual susceptibility and absorption of iron. *Neurology* 19 (10), 1000–1006.
6. Ballard, P. A., J. W. Tetrud, and J. W. Langston. 1985. Permanent human parkinsonism due to 1-methyl-4-phenyl-1,2,3,6-tetrahydropyridine (MPTP): Seven cases. *Neurology* 35 (7), 949–956.
7. Langston, J. W. 1998. Epidemiology versus genetics in Parkinson's disease: Progress in resolving an age-old debate. *Ann Neurol* 44 (3 Suppl 1), S45–S52.
8. Golbe, L. I., T. M. Farrell, and P. H. Davis. 1988. Case-control study of early life dietary factors in Parkinson's disease. *Arch Neurol* 45 (12), 1350–1353.
9. Seidler, A., W. Hellenbrand, B. P. Robra, P. Vieregge, P. Nischan, J. Joerg, W. H. Oertel, G. Ulm, and E. Schneider. 1996. Possible environmental, occupational, and other etiologic factors for Parkinson's disease: A case-control study in Germany. *Neurology* 46 (5), 1275–1284.
10. Zhang, Z. X., D. W. Anderson, L. Lavine, and N. Mantel. 1990. Patterns of acquiring parkinsonism–Dementia complex on Guam. 1944 through 1985. *Arch Neurol* 47 (9), 1019–1024.
11. de Rijk, M. C., M. M. Breteler, J. H. den Breeijen, L. J. Launer, D. E. Grobbee, F. G. van der Meche, and A. Hofman. 1997. Dietary antioxidants and Parkinson disease. The Rotterdam Study. *Arch Neurol* 54 (6), 762–765.
12. Markesbery, W. R., G. A. Jicha, H. Liu, and F. A. Schmitt. 2009. Lewy body pathology in normal elderly subjects. *J Neuropathol Exp Neurol* 68 (7), 816–822.
13. Su, B., H. Liu, X. Wang, S. G. Chen, S. L. Siedlak, E. Kondo, R. Choi, et al. 2009. Ectopic localization of FOXO3a protein in Lewy bodies in Lewy body dementia and Parkinson's disease. *Mol Neurodegener* 4, 32.
14. Desplats, P., H. J. Lee, E. J. Bae, C. Patrick, E. Rockenstein, L. Crews, B. Spencer, E. Masliah, and S. J. Lee. 2009. Inclusion formation and neuronal cell death through neuron-to-neuron transmission of alpha-synuclein. *Proc Natl Acad Sci USA* 106 (31), 13010–13015.
15. Gandhi, P. N., S. G. Chen, and A. L. Wilson-Delfosse. 2009. Leucine-rich repeat kinase 2 (LRRK2): A key player in the pathogenesis of Parkinson's disease. *J Neurosci Res* 87 (6), 1283–1295.
16. Giaime, E., C. Sunyach, C. Druon, S. Scarzello, G. Robert, S. Grosso, P. Auberger, et al. 2009. Loss of function of DJ-1 triggered by Parkinson's disease-associated mutation is due to proteolytic resistance to caspase-6. *Cell Death Differ* 17, 158–169.
17. Fitzgerald, J. C., and H. Plun-Favreau. 2008. Emerging pathways in genetic Parkinson's disease: Autosomal-recessive genes in Parkinson's disease—A common pathway? *FEBS J* 275 (23), 5758–5766.
18. Dodson, M. W., and M. Guo. 2007. Pink1, Parkin, DJ-1 and mitochondrial dysfunction in Parkinson's disease. *Curr Opin Neurobiol* 17 (3), 331–337.
19. Klein, C., and K. Lohmann-Hedrich. 2007. Impact of recent genetic findings in Parkinson's disease. *Curr Opin Neurol* 20 (4), 453–464.
20. Li, Y., W. Liu, T. F. Oo, L. Wang, Y. Tang, V. Jackson-Lewis, C. Zhou, et al. 2009. Mutant LRRK2(R1441G) BAC transgenic mice recapitulate cardinal features of Parkinson's disease. *Nat Neurosci* 12 (7), 826–828.
21. Giasson, B. I., and V. M. Van Deerlin. 2008. Mutations in LRRK2 as a cause of Parkinson's disease. *Neurosignals* 16 (1), 99–105.
22. da Costa, C. A. 2007. DJ-1: A newcomer in Parkinson's disease pathology. *Curr Mol Med* 7 (7), 650–657.
23. Wider, C., and Z. K. Wszolek. 2007. Clinical genetics of Parkinson's disease and related disorders. *Parkinsonism Relat Disord* 13 Suppl 3, S229–S232.
24. Bueler, H. 2009. Impaired mitochondrial dynamics and function in the pathogenesis of Parkinson's disease. *Exp Neurol* 218 (2), 235–246.
25. Kahle, P. J., J. Waak, and T. Gasser. 2009. DJ-1 and prevention of oxidative stress in Parkinson's disease and other age-related disorders. *Free Radic Biol Med* 47, 1354–1361.
26. Bandopadhyay, R., A. E. Kingsbury, M. R. Cookson, A. R. Reid, I. M. Evans, A. D. Hope, A. M. Pittman, et al. 2004. The expression of DJ-1 (PARK7) in normal human CNS and idiopathic Parkinson's disease. *Brain* 127 (Pt 2), 420–430, 2004.
27. Gu, L., T. Cui, C. Fan, H. Zhao, C. Zhao, L. Lu, and H. Yang. 2009. Involvement of ERK1/2 signaling pathway in DJ-1–induced neuroprotection against oxidative stress. *Biochem Biophys Res Commun* 383 (4), 469–474.

28. Lev, N., D. Ickowicz, Y. Barhum, S. Lev, E. Melamed, and D. Offen. 2009. DJ-1 protects against dopamine toxicity. *J Neural Transm* 116 (2), 151–160.
29. Lev, N., D. Ickowicz, E. Melamed, and D. Offen. 2008. Oxidative insults induce DJ-1 upregulation and redistribution: implications for neuroprotection. *Neurotoxicology* 29 (3), 397–405.
30. Nunome, K., S. Miyazaki, M. Nakano, S. Iguchi-Ariga, and H. Ariga. 2008. Pyrroloquinoline quinone prevents oxidative stress–induced neuronal death probably through changes in oxidative status of DJ-1. *Biol Pharm Bull* 31 (7), 1321–1326.
31. Xu, J., N. Zhong, H. Wang, J. E. Elias, C. Y. Kim, I. Woldman, C. Pifl, S. P. Gygi, C. Geula, and B. A. Yankner. 2005. The Parkinson's disease-associated DJ-1 protein is a transcriptional co-activator that protects against neuronal apoptosis. *Hum Mol Genet* 14 (9), 1231–1241.
32. Batelli, S., D. Albani, R. Rametta, L. Polito, F. Prato, M. Pesaresi, A. Negro, and G. Forloni. 2008. DJ-1 modulates alpha-synuclein aggregation state in a cellular model of oxidative stress: Relevance for Parkinson's disease and involvement of HSP70. *PLoS One* 3 (4), e1884.
33. Waragai, M., M. Nakai, J. Wei, M. Fujita, H. Mizuno, G. Ho, E. Masliah, H. Akatsu, F. Yokochi, and M. Hashimoto. 2007. Plasma levels of DJ-1 as a possible marker for progression of sporadic Parkinson's disease. *Neurosci Lett* 425 (1), 18–22.
34. Duda, J. E., U. Shah, S. E. Arnold, V. M. Lee, and J. Q. Trojanowski. 1999. The expression of alpha-, beta-, and gamma-synucleins in olfactory mucosa from patients with and without neurodegenerative diseases. *Exp Neurol* 160 (2), 515–522.
35. Zhou, W., J. Schaack, W. M. Zawada, and C. R. Freed. 2002. Overexpression of human alpha-synuclein causes dopamine neuron death in primary human mesencephalic culture. *Brain Res* 926 (1–2), 42–50.
36. Lo Bianco, C., J. L. Ridet, B. L. Schneider, N. Deglon, and P. Aebischer. 2002. alpha-Synucleinopathy and selective dopaminergic neuron loss in a rat lentiviral-based model of Parkinson's disease. *Proc Natl Acad Sci USA* 99 (16), 10813–10818.
37. Galvin, J. E. 2006. Interaction of alpha-synuclein and dopamine metabolites in the pathogenesis of Parkinson's disease: A case for the selective vulnerability of the substantia nigra. *Acta Neuropathol* 112 (2), 115–126.
38. Prasad, J. E., B. Kumar, C. Andreatta, P. Nahreini, A. J. Hanson, X. D. Yan, and K. N. Prasad. 2004. Overexpression of alpha-synuclein decreased viability and enhanced sensitivity to prostaglandin E(2), hydrogen peroxide, and a nitric oxide donor in differentiated neuroblastoma cells. *J Neurosci Res* 76 (3), 415–422.
39. Hoepken, H. H., S. Gispert, M. Azizov, M. Klinkenberg, F. Ricciardi, A. Kurz, B. Morales-Gordo, et al. 2008. Parkinson patient fibroblasts show increased alpha-synuclein expression. *Exp Neurol* 212 (2), 307–313.
40. Lucking, C. B., and A. Brice. 2000. Alpha-synuclein and Parkinson's disease. *Cell Mol Life Sci* 57 (13–14), 1894–1908.
41. el-Agnaf, O. M., and G. B. Irvine. 2002. Aggregation and neurotoxicity of alpha-synuclein and related peptides. *Biochem Soc Trans* 30 (4), 559–565.
42. Devi, L., and H. K. Anandatheerthavarada. 2009. Mitochondrial trafficking of APP and alpha synuclein: Relevance to mitochondrial dysfunction in Alzheimer's and Parkinson's diseases. *Biochim Biophys Acta* 1802, 11–19.
43. Parihar, M. S., A. Parihar, M. Fujita, M. Hashimoto, and P. Ghafourifar. 2008. Mitochondrial association of alpha-synuclein causes oxidative stress. *Cell Mol Life Sci* 65 (7–8), 1272–1284.
44. Parihar, M. S., A. Parihar, M. Fujita, M. Hashimoto, and P. Ghafourifar. 2009. Alpha-synuclein overexpression and aggregation exacerbates impairment of mitochondrial functions by augmenting oxidative stress in human neuroblastoma cells. *Int J Biochem Cell Biol* 41, 2015–2024.
45. Martin, L. J., Y. Pan, A. C. Price, W. Sterling, N. G. Copeland, N. A. Jenkins, D. L. Price, and M. K. Lee. 2006. Parkinson's disease alpha-synuclein transgenic mice develop neuronal mitochondrial degeneration and cell death. *J Neurosci* 26 (1), 41–50.
46. Sherer, T. B., R. Betarbet, A. K. Stout, S. Lund, M. Baptista, A. V. Panov, M. R. Cookson, and J. T. Greenamyre. 2002. An in vitro model of Parkinson's disease: Linking mitochondrial impairment to altered alpha-synuclein metabolism and oxidative damage. *J Neurosci* 22 (16), 7006–7015.
47. Junn, E., K. W. Lee, B. S. Jeong, T. W. Chan, J. Y. Im, and M. M. Mouradian. 2009. Repression of alpha-synuclein expression and toxicity by microRNA-7. *Proc Natl Acad Sci USA* 106 (31), 13052–13057.
48. Esteves, A. R., D. M. Arduino, R. H. Swerdlow, C. R. Oliveira, and S. M. Cardoso. 2009. Oxidative Stress involvement in alpha-synuclein oligomerization in Parkinsons disease cybrids. *Antioxid Redox Signal* 11, 439–448.

49. Fountaine, T. M., L. L. Venda, N. Warrick, H. C. Christian, P. Brundin, K. M. Channon, and R. Wade-Martins. 2008. The effect of alpha-synuclein knockdown on MPP+ toxicity in models of human neurons. *Eur J Neurosci* 28 (12), 2459–2473.
50. Wu, F., W. S. Poon, G. Lu, A. Wang, H. Meng, L. Feng, Z. Li, and S. Liu. 2009. alpha-Synuclein knockdown attenuates MPP(+) induced mitochondrial dysfunction of SH-SY5Y cells. *Brain Res* 1292, 173–179.
51. Ma, L., T. T. Cao, G. Kandpal, L. Warren, J. Fred Hess, G. R. Seabrook, and W. J. Ray. 2009. Genome-wide microarray analysis of the differential neuroprotective effects of antioxidants in neuroblastoma cells overexpressing the familial Parkinson's disease alpha-synuclein A53T mutation. *Neurochem Res* 35, 130–142.
52. Lee, M. K., W. Stirling, Y. Xu, X. Xu, D. Qui, A. S. Mandir, T. M. Dawson, N. G. Copeland, N. A. Jenkins, and D. L. Price. 2002. Human alpha-synuclein-harboring familial Parkinson's disease-linked Ala-53 → Thr mutation causes neurodegenerative disease with alpha-synuclein aggregation in transgenic mice. *Proc Natl Acad Sci USA* 99 (13), 8968–8973.
53. Martin-Clemente, B., B. Alvarez-Castelao, I. Mayo, A. B. Sierra, V. Diaz, M. Milan, I. Farinas, T. Gomez-Isla, I. Ferrer, and J. G. Castano. 2004. alpha-Synuclein expression levels do not significantly affect proteasome function and expression in mice and stably transfected PC12 cell lines. *J Biol Chem* 279 (51), 52984–52990.
54. Dyllick-Brenzinger, M., C. A. D'Souza, B. Dahlmann, P. M. Kloetzel, and A. Tandon. 2009. Reciprocal effects of alpha-synuclein overexpression and proteasome inhibition in neuronal cells and tissue. *Neurotox Res* 17, 215–227.
55. Kim, C., and S. J. Lee. 2008. Controlling the mass action of alpha-synuclein in Parkinson's disease. *J Neurochem* 107 (2): 303–316.
56. Xilouri, M., T. Vogiatzi, K. Vekrellis, and L. Stefanis. 2008. alpha-Synuclein degradation by autophagic pathways: A potential key to Parkinson's disease pathogenesis. *Autophagy* 4 (7), 917–919.
57. Tessari, I., M. Bisaglia, F. Valle, B. Samori, E. Bergantino, S. Mammi, and L. Bubacco. 2008. The reaction of alpha-synuclein with tyrosinase: Possible implications for Parkinson disease. *J Biol Chem* 283 (24), 16808–16817.
58. Kawahara, K., M. Hashimoto, P. Bar-On, G. J. Ho, L. Crews, H. Mizuno, E. Rockenstein, S. Z. Imam, and E. Masliah. 2008. alpha-Synuclein aggregates interfere with Parkin solubility and distribution: Role in the pathogenesis of Parkinson disease. *J Biol Chem* 283 (11), 6979–6987.
59. Gegg, M. E., J. M. Cooper, A. H. Schapira, and J. W. Taanman. 2009. Silencing of PINK1 expression affects mitochondrial DNA and oxidative phosphorylation in dopaminergic cells. *PLoS One* 4 (3), e4756.
60. Gandhi, S., M. M. Muqit, L. Stanyer, D. G. Healy, P. M. Abou-Sleiman, I. Hargreaves, S. Heales, M. Ganguly, et al. 2006. PINK1 protein in normal human brain and Parkinson's disease. *Brain* 129 (Pt 7), 1720–1731.
61. Marongiu, R., B. Spencer, L. Crews, A. Adame, C. Patrick, M. Trejo, B. Dallapiccola, E. M. Valente, and E. Masliah. 2009. Mutant Pink1 induces mitochondrial dysfunction in a neuronal cell model of Parkinson's disease by disturbing calcium flux. *J Neurochem* 108 (6), 1561–1574.
62. Liu, W., C. Vives-Bauza, R. Acin-Perez, A. Yamamoto, Y. Tan, Y. Li, J. Magrane, et al. 2009. PINK1 defect causes mitochondrial dysfunction, proteasomal deficit and alpha-synuclein aggregation in cell culture models of Parkinson's disease. *PLoS One* 4 (2), e4597.
63. Mitsui, T., Y. Kuroda, and R. Kaji. 2008. Parkin and mitochondria. *Brain Nerve* 60 (8), 923–929.
64. Dexter, D. T., A. E. Holley, W. D. Flitter, T. F. Slater, F. R. Wells, S. E. Daniel, A. J. Lees, P. Jenner, and C. D. Marsden. 1994. Increased levels of lipid hydroperoxides in the parkinsonian substantia nigra: An HPLC and ESR study. *Mov Disord* 9 (1), 92–97.
65. Dexter, D. T., C. J. Carter, F. R. Wells, F. Javoy-Agid, Y. Agid, A. Lees, P. Jenner, and C. D. Marsden. 1989. Basal lipid peroxidation in substantia nigra is increased in Parkinson's disease. *J Neurochem* 52 (2), 381–389.
66. Sanchez-Ramos, J., E. Overvik, and B. Ames. 1994. A marker of oxyradical-mediated DNA damage (8-hydroxy-2'-deoxyguanosine) is increased in nigro-striatum of Parkinson's disease brain. *Neurodegeneration* 3, 197–204.
67. Ebadi, M., S. K. Srinivasan, and M. D. Baxi. 1996. Oxidative stress and antioxidant therapy in Parkinson's disease. *Prog Neurobiol* 48 (1), 1–19.
68. Ambani, L. M., M. H. Van Woert, and S. Murphy. 1975. Brain peroxidase and catalase in Parkinson disease. *Arch Neurol* 32 (2), 114–118.

69. Kish, S. J., C. Morito, and O. Hornykiewicz. 1985. Glutathione peroxidase activity in Parkinson's disease brain. *Neurosci Lett* 58 (3), 343–346.
70. Riederer, P., E. Sofic, W. D. Rausch, B. Schmidt, G. P. Reynolds, K. Jellinger, and M. B. Youdim. 1989. Transition metals, ferritin, glutathione, and ascorbic acid in parkinsonian brains, *J Neurochem* 52 (2), 515–520.
71. Perry, T. L., D. V. Godin, and S. Hansen. 1982. Parkinson's disease: A disorder due to nigral glutathione deficiency? *Neurosci Lett* 33 (3), 305–310.
72. Sofic, E., K. W. Lange, K. Jellinger, and P. Riederer. 1992. Reduced and oxidized glutathione in the substantia nigra of patients with Parkinson's disease. *Neurosci Lett* 142 (2), 128–130.
73. Chen, C. M., J. L. Liu, Y. R. Wu, Y. C. Chen, H. S. Cheng, M. L. Cheng, and D. T. Chiu. 2009. Increased oxidative damage in peripheral blood correlates with severity of Parkinson's disease. *Neurobiol Dis* 33 (3), 429–435.
74. Sanyal, J., S. K. Bandyopadhyay, T. K. Banerjee, S. C. Mukherjee, D. P. Chakraborty, B. C. Ray, and V. R. Rao. 2009. Plasma levels of lipid peroxides in patients with Parkinson's disease. *Eur Rev Med Pharmacol Sci* 13 (2), 129–132.
75. Sian, J., D. T. Dexter, A. J. Lees, S. Daniel, Y. Agid, F. Javoy-Agid, P. Jenner, and C. D. Marsden. 1994. Alterations in glutathione levels in Parkinson's disease and other neurodegenerative disorders affecting basal ganglia. *Ann Neurol* 36 (3), 348–355.
76. Jenner, P. 1998. Oxidative mechanisms in nigral cell death in Parkinson's disease. *Mov Disord* 13 Suppl 1, 24–34.
77. Fitzmaurice, P. S., L. Ang, M. Guttman, A. H. Rajput, Y. Furukawa, and S. J. Kish. 2003. Nigral glutathione deficiency is not specific for idiopathic Parkinson's disease. *Mov Disord* 18 (9), 969–976.
78. Fessel, J. P., C. Hulette, S. Powell, L. J. Roberts, 2nd, and J. Zhang. 2003. Isofurans, but not F2-isoprostanes, are increased in the substantia nigra of patients with Parkinson's disease and with dementia with Lewy body disease. *J Neurochem* 85 (3), 645–650.
79. Schipper, H. M., A. Liberman, and E. G. Stopa. 1998. Neural heme oxygenase-1 expression in idiopathic Parkinson's disease. *Exp Neurol* 150 (1), 60–68.
80. Sofic, E., A. Sapcanin, I. Tahirovic, I. Gavrankapetanovic, K. Jellinger, G. P. Reynolds, T. Tatschner, and P. Riederer. 2006. Antioxidant capacity in postmortem brain tissues of Parkinson's and Alzheimer's diseases. *J Neural Transm Suppl* (71), 39–43.
81. Varghese, M., M. Pandey, A. Samanta, P. K. Gangopadhyay, and K. P. Mohanakumar. 2009. Reduced NADH coenzyme Q dehydrogenase activity in platelets of Parkinson's disease, but not Parkinson plus patients, from an Indian population. *J Neurol Sci* 279 (1–2), 39–42.
82. Fernandez-Calle, P., F. J. Jimenez-Jimenez, J. A. Molina, F. Cabrera-Valdivia, A. Vazquez, D. Garcia Urra, F. Bermejo, M. Cruz Matallana, and R. Codoceo. 1993. Serum levels of ascorbic acid (vitamin C) in patients with Parkinson's disease. *J Neurol Sci* 118 (1), 25–28.
83. Fernandez-Calle, P., J. A. Molina, F. J. Jimenez-Jimenez, A. Vazquez, M. Pondal, P. J. Garcia-Ruiz, D. G. Urra, J. Domingo, and R. Codoceo. 1992. Serum levels of alpha-tocopherol (vitamin E) in Parkinson's disease. *Neurology* 42 (5), 1064–1066.
84. King, D., J. R. Playfer, and N. B. Roberts. 1992. Concentrations of vitamins A, C and E in elderly patients with Parkinson's disease. *Postgrad Med J* 68 (802), 634–637.
85. Paraskevas, G. P., E. Kapaki, O. Petropoulou, M. Anagnostouli, V. Vagenas, and C. Papageorgiou. 2003. Plasma levels of antioxidant vitamins C and E are decreased in vascular parkinsonism. *J Neurol Sci* 215 (1–2), 51–55.
86. Double, K. L., M. Gerlach, M. B. Youdim, and P. Riederer. 2000. Impaired iron homeostasis in Parkinson's disease. *J Neural Transm Suppl* (60), 37–58.
87. Graham, J. M., M. N. Paley, R. A. Grunewald, N. Hoggard, and P. D. Griffiths. 2000. Brain iron deposition in Parkinson's disease imaged using the PRIME magnetic resonance sequence. *Brain* 123 (Pt 12): 2423–2431.
88. Andersen, J. K. 2004. Iron dysregulation and Parkinson's disease. *J Alzheimers Dis* 6 (6 Suppl), S47–S52.
89. Salazar, J., N. Mena, S. Hunot, A. Prigent, D. Alvarez-Fischer, M. Arredondo, C. Duyckaerts, V. Sazdovitch, et al. 2008. Divalent metal transporter 1 (DMT1) contributes to neurodegeneration in animal models of Parkinson's disease. *Proc Natl Acad Sci USA* 105 (47), 18578–18583.
90. Prabhakaran, K., D. Ghosh, G. D. Chapman, and P. G. Gunasekar. 2008. Molecular mechanism of manganese exposure-induced dopaminergic toxicity. *Brain Res Bull* 76 (4), 361–367.

91. Enochs, W. S., T. Sarna, L. Zecca, P. A. Riley, and H. M. Swartz. 1994. The roles of neuromelanin, binding of metal ions, and oxidative cytotoxicity in the pathogenesis of Parkinson's disease: A hypothesis. *J Neural Transm Park Dis Dement Sect* 7 (2), 83–100.
92. Good, P. F., C. W. Olanow, and D. P. Perl. 1992. Neuromelanin-containing neurons of the substantia nigra accumulate iron and aluminum in Parkinson's disease: A LAMMA study. *Brain Res* 593 (2), 343–346.
93. Ebadi, M., and S. K. Sharma. 2003. Peroxynitrite and mitochondrial dysfunction in the pathogenesis of Parkinson's disease. *Antioxid Redox Signal* 5 (3), 319–335.
94. Blandini, F., R. H. Porter, and J. T. Greenamyre. 1996. Glutamate and Parkinson's disease. *Mol Neurobiol* 12 (1), 73–94.
95. Bonsi, P., D. Cuomo, B. Picconi, G. Sciamanna, A. Tscherter, M. Tolu, G. Bernardi, P. Calabresi, and A. Pisani. 2007. Striatal metabotropic glutamate receptors as a target for pharmacotherapy in Parkinson's disease. *Amino Acids* 32 (2), 189–195.
96. Ossowska, K., J. Konieczny, J. Wardas, M. Pietraszek, K. Kuter, S. Wolfarth, and A. Pilc. 2007. An influence of ligands of metabotropic glutamate receptor subtypes on parkinsonian-like symptoms and the striatopallidal pathway in rats. *Amino Acids* 32 (2), 179–188.
97. Meredith, G. E., S. Totterdell, M. Beales, and C. K. Meshul. 2009. Impaired glutamate homeostasis and programmed cell death in a chronic MPTP mouse model of Parkinson's disease. *Exp Neurol* 219 (1), 334–340.
98. Schubert, D., H. Kimura, and P. Maher. 1992. Growth factors and vitamin E modify neuronal glutamate toxicity. *Proc Natl Acad Sci U S A* 89 (17), 8264–8267.
99. Sandhu, J. K., S. Pandey, M. Ribecco-Lutkiewicz, R. Monette, H. Borowy-Borowski, P. R. Walker, and M. Sikorska. 2003. Molecular mechanisms of glutamate neurotoxicity in mixed cultures of NT2-derived neurons and astrocytes: Protective effects of coenzyme Q10. *J Neurosci Res* 72 (6), 691–703.
100. Whitton, P. S. 2007. Inflammation as a causative factor in the aetiology of Parkinson's disease. *Br J Pharmacol* 150 (8), 963–976.
101. McGeer, P. L., and E. G. McGeer. 2008. Glial reactions in Parkinson's disease. *Mov Disord* 23 (4), 474–483.
102. Reynolds, A. D., J. G. Glanzer, I. Kadiu, M. Ricardo-Dukelow, A. Chaudhuri, P. Ciborowski, R. Cerny, et al. 2008. Nitrated alpha-synuclein–activated microglial profiling for Parkinson's disease. *J Neurochem* 104 (6), 1504–1525.
103. Zhang, W., T. Wang, Z. Pei, D. S. Miller, X. Wu, M. L. Block, B. Wilson, Y. Zhou, J. S. Hong, and J. Zhang. 2005. Aggregated alpha-synuclein activates microglia: A process leading to disease progression in Parkinson's disease. *FASEB J* 19 (6), 533–542.
104. Roodveldt, C., J. Christodoulou, and C. M. Dobson. 2008. Immunological features of alpha-synuclein in Parkinson's disease. *J Cell Mol Med* 12 (5B), 1820–1829.
105. Gao, H. M., P. T. Kotzbauer, K. Uryu, S. Leight, J. Q. Trojanowski, and V. M. Lee. 2008. Neuroinflammation and oxidation/nitration of alpha-synuclein linked to dopaminergic neurodegeneration. *J Neurosci* 28 (30), 7687–7698.
106. Sawada, M., K. Imamura, and T. Nagatsu. 2006. Role of cytokines in inflammatory process in Parkinson's disease. *J Neural Transm Suppl* (70), 373–381.
107. Wilms, H., L. Zecca, P. Rosenstiel, J. Sievers, G. Deuschl, and R. Lucius. 2007. Inflammation in Parkinson's diseases and other neurodegenerative diseases: cause and therapeutic implications. *Curr Pharm Des* 13 (18), 1925–1928.
108. Prasad, K. N., A. R. Hovland, F. G. La Rosa, and P. G. Hovland. 1998. Prostaglandins as putative neurotoxins in Alzheimer's disease. *Proc Soc Exp Biol Med* 219 (2), 120–125.
109. Chae, S. W., B. Y. Kang, O. Hwang, and H. J. Choi. 2008. Cyclooxygenase-2 is involved in oxidative damage and alpha-synuclein accumulation in dopaminergic cells. *Neurosci Lett* 436 (2), 205–209.
110. Arduino, D. M., A. R. Esteves, S. M. Cardoso, and C. R. Oliveira. 2009. Endoplasmic reticulum and mitochondria interplay mediates apoptotic cell death: Relevance to Parkinson's disease. *Neurochem Int* 55 (5), 341–348.
111. Gubellini, P., B. Picconi, M. Di Filippo, and P. Calabresi. 2009. Downstream mechanisms triggered by mitochondrial dysfunction in the basal ganglia: From experimental models to neurodegenerative diseases. *Biochim Biophys Acta* 1802, 151–161.
112. Gautier, C. A., T. Kitada, and J. Shen. 2008. Loss of PINK1 causes mitochondrial functional defects and increased sensitivity to oxidative stress. *Proc Natl Acad Sci U S A* 105 (32), 11364–11369.
113. Lee, S. J. 2003. Alpha-synuclein aggregation: A link between mitochondrial defects and Parkinson's disease? *Antioxid Redox Signal* 5 (3), 337–348.

114. Banerjee, R., A. A. Starkov, M. F. Beal, and B. Thomas. 2009. Mitochondrial dysfunction in the limelight of Parkinson's disease pathogenesis. *Biochim Biophys Acta* 1792 (7), 651–663.
115. Yang, J. L., L. Weissman, V. A. Bohr, and M. P. Mattson. 2008. Mitochondrial DNA damage and repair in neurodegenerative disorders. *DNA Repair (Amst)* 7 (7), 1110–1120.
116. Perier, C., J. Bove, D. C. Wu, B. Dehay, D. K. Choi, V. Jackson-Lewis, S. Rathke-Hartlieb, et al. 2007. Two molecular pathways initiate mitochondria-dependent dopaminergic neurodegeneration in experimental Parkinson's disease. *Proc Natl Acad Sci U S A* 104 (19), 8161–8166.
117. Domingues, A. F., D. M. Arduino, A. R. Esteves, R. H. Swerdlow, C. R. Oliveira, and S. M. Cardoso. 2008. Mitochondria and ubiquitin–proteasomal system interplay: Relevance to Parkinson's disease. *Free Radic Biol Med* 45 (6), 820–825.
118. Ono, K., and M. Yamada. 2007. Vitamin A potently destabilizes preformed alpha-synuclein fibrils in vitro: Implications for Lewy body diseases. *Neurobiol Dis* 25 (2), 446–454.
119. Park, E. S., S. Y. Kim, J. I. Na, H. S. Ryu, S. W. Youn, D. S. Kim, H. Y. Yun, and K. C. Park. 2007. Glutathione prevented dopamine-induced apoptosis of melanocytes and its signaling. *J Dermatol Sci* 47 (2), 141–149.
120. Khaldy, H., G. Escames, J. Leon, F. Vives, J. D. Luna, and D. Acuna-Castroviejo. 2000. Comparative effects of melatonin, l-deprenyl, Trolox and ascorbate in the suppression of hydroxyl radical formation during dopamine autoxidation in vitro. *J Pineal Res* 29 (2), 100–107.
121. Ehrhart, J., and G. D. Zeevalk. 2003. Cooperative interaction between ascorbate and glutathione during mitochondrial impairment in mesencephalic cultures. *J Neurochem* 86 (6), 1487–1497.
122. Penugonda, S., S. Mare, G. Goldstein, W. A. Banks, and N. Ercal. 2005. Effects of N-acetylcysteine amide (NACA), a novel thiol antioxidant against glutamate-induced cytotoxicity in neuronal cell line PC12. *Brain Res* 1056 (2), 132–238.
123. Cadet, J. L., M. Katz, V. Jackson-Lewis, and S. Fahn. 1989. Vitamin E attenuates the toxic effects of intrastriatal injection of 6-hydroxydopamine (6-OHDA) in rats: Behavioral and biochemical evidence. *Brain Res* 476 (1), 10–15.
124. Heim, C., W. Kolasiewicz, T. Kurz, and K. H. Sontag. 2001. Behavioral alterations after unilateral 6-hydroxydopamine lesions of the striatum. Effect of alpha-tocopherol. *Pol J Pharmacol* 53 (5), 435–448.
125. Prasad, K. N., B. Kumar, X. D. Yan, A. J. Hanson, and W. C. Cole. 2003. alpha-Tocopheryl succinate, the most effective form of vitamin E for adjuvant cancer treatment: A review. *J Am Coll Nutr* 22 (2), 108–117.
126. Pasbakhsh, P., N. Omidi, K. Mehrannia, A. G. Sobhani, I. Ragerdi Kashani, M. Abbasi, and A. Kord Valeshabad. 2008. The protective effect of vitamin E on locus coeruleus in early model of Parkinson's disease in rat: Immunoreactivity evidence. *Iran Biomed J* 12 (4), 217–222.
127. Roghani, M., and G. Behzadi. 2001. Neuroprotective effect of vitamin E on the early model of Parkinson's disease in rat: Behavioral and histochemical evidence. *Brain Res* 892 (1), 211–217.
128. Chaturvedi, R. K., S. Shukla, K. Seth, S. Chauhan, C. Sinha, Y. Shukla, and A. K. Agrawal. 2006. Neuroprotective and neurorescue effect of black tea extract in 6-hydroxydopamine–lesioned rat model of Parkinson's disease. *Neurobiol Dis* 22 (2), 421–434.
129. Khaldy, H., G. Escames, J. Leon, L. Bikjdaouene, and D. Acuna-Castroviejo. 2003. Synergistic effects of melatonin and deprenyl against MPTP-induced mitochondrial damage and DA depletion. *Neurobiol Aging* 24 (3), 491–500.
130. Silva-Adaya, D., V. Perez-De La Cruz, M. N. Herrera-Mundo, K. Mendoza-Macedo, J. Villeda-Hernandez, Z. Binienda, S. F. Ali, and A. Santamaria. 2008. Excitotoxic damage, disrupted energy metabolism, and oxidative stress in the rat brain: Antioxidant and neuroprotective effects of l-carnitine. *J Neurochem* 105 (3), 677–689.
131. Virmani, A., F. Gaetani, and Z. Binienda. 2005. Effects of metabolic modifiers such as carnitines, coenzyme Q10, and PUFAs against different forms of neurotoxic insults: Metabolic inhibitors, MPTP, and methamphetamine. *Ann NY Acad Sci* 1053, 183–191.
132. Choi, J. Y., C. S. Park, D. J. Kim, M. H. Cho, B. K. Jin, J. E. Pie, and W. G. Chung. 2002. Prevention of nitric oxide-mediated 1-methyl-4-phenyl-1,2,3,6-tetrahydropyridine-induced Parkinson's disease in mice by tea phenolic epigallocatechin 3-gallate. *Neurotoxicology* 23 (3), 367–374.
133. Jia, H., X. Li, H. Gao, Z. Feng, L. Zhao, X. Jia, H. Zhang, and J. Liu. 2008. High doses of nicotinamide prevent oxidative mitochondrial dysfunction in a cellular model and improve motor deficit in a Drosophila model of Parkinson's disease. *J Neurosci Res* 86 (9), 2083–2090.
134. Jia, H., Z. Liu, X. Li, Z. Feng, J. Hao, W. Shen, H. Zhang, and J. Liu. 2010. Synergistic anti-Parkinsonism activity of high doses of B vitamins in a chronic cellular model. *Neurobiol Aging* 31, 636–646.

135. Liu, D., M. Pitta, and M. P. Mattson. 2008. Preventing NAD(+) depletion protects neurons against excitotoxicity: Bioenergetic effects of mild mitochondrial uncoupling and caloric restriction. *Ann NY Acad Sci* 1147, 275–282.
136. Green, K. N., J. S. Steffan, H. Martinez-Coria, X. Sun, S. S. Schreiber, L. M. Thompson, and F. M. LaFerla. 2008. Nicotinamide restores cognition in Alzheimer's disease transgenic mice via a mechanism involving sirtuin inhibition and selective reduction of Thr231-phosphotau. *J Neurosci* 28 (45), 11500–11510.
137. Alcain, F. J., and J. M. Villalba. 2009. Sirtuin inhibitors. *Expert Opin Ther Pat* 19 (3), 283–294.
138. Guarente, L. 2007. Sirtuins in aging and disease. *Cold Spring Harb Symp Quant Biol* 72, 483–488.
139. Hallows, W. C., B. N. Albaugh, and J. M. Denu. 2008. Where in the cell is SIRT3?—Functional localization of an NAD$^+$-dependent protein deacetylase. *Biochem J* 411 (2), e11–e13.
140. Garske, A. L., B. C. Smith, and J. M. Denu. 2007. Linking SIRT2 to Parkinson's disease. *ACS Chem Biol* 2 (8), 529–532.
141. Shoulson, I. 1998. DATATOP: a decade of neuroprotective inquiry. Parkinson Study Group. Deprenyl and tocopherol antioxidative therapy of parkinsonism. *Ann Neurol* 44 (3 Suppl 1), S160–S166.
142. Group, T. P. S. 1993. Effects of tocopherol and deprenyl on the progression of disability in early Parkinson's disease. *N Engl J Med*, 176–183.
143. Prasad, K. N., C. Hernandez, J. Edwards-Prasad, J. Nelson, T. Borus, and W. A. Robinson. 1994. Modification of the effect of tamoxifen, cis-platin, DTIC, and interferon-alpha 2b on human melanoma cells in culture by a mixture of vitamins. *Nutr Cancer* 22 (3), 233–245.
144. Prasad, K. N., and R. Kumar. 1996. Effect of individual and multiple antioxidant vitamins on growth and morphology of human nontumorigenic and tumorigenic parotid acinar cells in culture. *Nutr Cancer* 26 (1), 11–19.
145. Fahn, S. 1992. A pilot trial of high-dose alpha-tocopherol and ascorbate in early Parkinson's disease. *Ann Neurol* 32 Suppl, S128–S132.
146. Shults, C. W., D. Oakes, K. Kieburtz, M. F. Beal, R. Haas, S. Plumb, J. L. Juncos, et al. 2002. Effects of coenzyme Q10 in early Parkinson disease: Evidence of slowing of the functional decline. *Arch Neurol* 59 (10), 1541–1550.
147. Weber, C. A., and M. E. Ernst. 2006. Antioxidants, supplements, and Parkinson's disease. *Ann Pharmacother* 40 (5), 935–938.
148. Storch, A., W. H. Jost, P. Vieregge, J. Spiegel, W. Greulich, J. Durner, T. Muller, et al. 2007. Randomized, double-blind, placebo-controlled trial on symptomatic effects of coenzyme Q(10) in Parkinson disease. *Arch Neurol* 64 (7), 938–944.
149. Lohr, J. B., and M. P. Caligiuri. 1996. A double-blind placebo-controlled study of vitamin E treatment of tardive dyskinesia. *J Clin Psychiatry* 57 (4), 167–173.
150. Birkmayer, J. G., C. Vrecko, D. Volc, and W. Birkmayer. 1993. Nicotinamide adenine dinucleotide (NADH)—A new therapeutic approach to Parkinson's disease. Comparison of oral and parenteral application. *Acta Neurol Scand Suppl* 146, 32–35.
151. Kuhn, W., T. Muller, R. Winkel, S. Danielczik, A. Gerstner, R. Hacker, C. Mattern, and H. Przuntek. 1996. Parenteral application of NADH in Parkinson's disease: Clinical improvement partially due to stimulation of endogenous levodopa biosynthesis. *J Neural Transm* 103 (10), 1187–1193.
152. Dizdar, N., B. Kagedal, and B. Lindvall. 1994. Treatment of Parkinson's disease with NADH. *Acta Neurol Scand* 90 (5), 345–347.
153. Swerdlow, R. H. 1998. Is NADH effective in the treatment of Parkinson's disease? *Drugs Aging* 13 (4), 263–268.
154. Zhang, S. M., M. A. Hernan, H. Chen, D. Spiegelman, W. C. Willett, and A. Ascherio. 2002. Intakes of vitamins E and C, carotenoids, vitamin supplements, and PD risk. *Neurology* 59 (8), 1161–1169.
155. Etminan, M., S. S. Gill, and A. Samii. 2005. Intake of vitamin E, vitamin C, and carotenoids and the risk of Parkinson's disease: A meta-analysis. *Lancet Neurol* 4 (6), 362–365.
156. Krinsky, N. I. 1989. Antioxidant functions of carotenoids. *Free Radic Biol Med* 7 (6), 617–635.
157. Hazuka, M. B., J. Edwards-Prasad, F. Newman, J. J. Kinzie, and K. N. Prasad. 1990. Beta-carotene induces morphological differentiation and decreases adenylate cyclase activity in melanoma cells in culture. *J Am Coll Nutr* 9 (2), 143–149.
158. Zhang, L. X., R. V. Cooney, and J. S. Bertram. 1992. Carotenoids up-regulate connexin43 gene expression independent of their provitamin A or antioxidant properties. *Cancer Res* 52 (20), 5707–5712.
159. Carter, C. A., M. Pogribny, A. Davidson, C. D. Jackson, L. J. McGarrity, and S. M. Morris. 1996. Effects of retinoic acid on cell differentiation and reversion toward normal in human endometrial adenocarcinoma (RL95-2) cells. *Anticancer Res* 16 (1), 17–24.

160. Meyskens, Jr., F. L. 1995. Role of vitamin A and its derivatives in the treatment of human cancer. In *Nutrients in Cancer Prevention and Treatment*, ed. K. N. Prasad, L. Santamaria, and R. M. Williams, 349–362. Totowa, NJ: Humana Press.
161. Vile, G. F., and C. C. Winterbourn. 1988. Inhibition of adriamycin-promoted microsomal lipid peroxidation by beta-carotene, alpha-tocopherol and retinol at high and low oxygen partial pressures. *FEBS Lett* 238 (2), 353–356.
162. McCay, P. B. 1985. Vitamin E: Interactions with free radicals and ascorbate. *Annu Rev Nutr* 5, 323–340.
163. Schwartz, J. L. 1995. Molecular and biochemical control of tumor growth following treatment with carotenoids or tocopherols. In *Nutrients in Cancer Prevention and Treatment*, ed. Prasad, K. N., Santamaria, L., and Williams, R. M., 287–316. Totwa, NJ: Humana Press.
164. Prasad, K. N., and J. Edwards-Prasad. 1992. Vitamin E and cancer prevention: Recent advances and future potentials. *J Am Coll Nutr* 11 (5), 487–500.
165. Vali, S., R. B. Mythri, B. Jagatha, J. Padiadpu, K. S. Ramanujan, J. K. Andersen, F. Gorin, and M. M. Bharath. 2007. Integrating glutathione metabolism and mitochondrial dysfunction with implications for Parkinson's disease: A dynamic model. *Neuroscience* 149 (4), 917–930.
166. Witschi, A., S. Reddy, B. Stofer, and B. H. Lauterburg. 1992. The systemic availability of oral glutathione. *Eur J Clin Pharmacol* 43 (6), 667–669.
167. Shen, W., K. Liu, C. Tian, L. Yang, X. Li, J. Ren, L. Packer, C. W. Cotman, and J. Liu. 2008. R-alpha-Lipoic acid and acetyl-L-carnitine complementarily promote mitochondrial biogenesis in murine 3T3-L1 adipocytes. *Diabetologia* 51 (1), 165–174.
168. Niki, E. 1997. Mechanisms and dynamics of antioxidant action of ubiquinol. *Mol Aspects Med* 18 Suppl, S63–S70.
169. Hiramatsu, M., R. D. Velasco, D. S. Wilson, and L. Packer. 1991. Ubiquinone protects against loss of tocopherol in rat liver microsomes and mitochondrial membranes. *Res Commun Chem Pathol Pharmacol* 72 (2), 231–241.
170. Chen, R. S., C. C. Huang, and N. S. Chu. 1997. Coenzyme Q10 treatment in mitochondrial encephalomyopathies. Short-term double-blind, crossover study. *Eur Neurol* 37 (4), 212–218.
171. Prasad, K. N., F. G. La Rosa, and J. E. Prasad. 1998. Prostaglandins act as neurotoxin for differentiated neuroblastoma cells in culture and increase levels of ubiquitin and beta-amyloid. *In Vitro Cell Dev Biol Anim* 34 (3), 265–274.
172. Shalit, F., B. Sredni, L. Stern, E. Kott, and M. Huberman. 1994. Elevated interleukin-6 secretion levels by mononuclear cells of Alzheimer's patients. *Neurosci Lett* 174 (2), 130–132.
173. Sharif, S. F., R. J. Hariri, V. A. Chang, P. S. Barie, R. S. Wang, and J. B. Ghajar. 1993. Human astrocyte production of tumour necrosis factor-alpha, interleukin-1 beta, and interleukin-6 following exposure to lipopolysaccharide endotoxin. *Neurol Res* 15 (2), 109–112.
174. Eikelenboom, P., J. M. Rozemuller, G. Kraal, F. C. Stam, P. A. McBride, M. E. Bruce, and H. Fraser. 1991. Cerebral amyloid plaques in Alzheimer's disease but not in scrapie-affected mice are closely associated with a local inflammatory process. *Virchows Arch B Cell Pathol Incl Mol Pathol* 60 (5), 329–336.
175. Eikelenboom, P., and F. C. Stam. 1982. Immunoglobulins and complement factors in senile plaques. An immunoperoxidase study. *Acta Neuropathol (Berl)* 57 (2–3), 239–242.
176. Rogers, J., N. R. Cooper, S. Webster, J. Schultz, P. L. McGeer, S. D. Styren, W. H. Civin, et al. 1992. Complement activation by beta-amyloid in Alzheimer disease. *Proc Natl Acad Sci U S A* 89 (21), 10016–10020.
177. Rogers, J., L.-F. Lue, L. Brachova, S. Webster, and J. Schultz. 1995. Inflammation as a response and a cause of Alzheimer's pathophysiology. *Dementia* 9, 133–138.
178. Webster, S., S. O'Barr, and J. Rogers. 1994. Enhanced aggregation and beta structure of amyloid beta peptide after coincubation with C1q. *J Neurosci Res* 39 (4), 448–456.
179. Frohman, E. M., T. C. Frohman, S. Gupta, A. de Fougerolles, and S. van den Noort. 1991. Expression of intercellular adhesion molecule 1 (ICAM-1) in Alzheimer's disease. *J Neurol Sci* 106 (1), 105–111.
180. Rozemuller, J. M., P. Eikelenboom, S. T. Pals, and F. C. Stam. 1989. Microglial cells around amyloid plaques in Alzheimer's disease express leucocyte adhesion molecules of the LFA-1 family. *Neurosci Lett* 101 (3), 288–292.
181. Verbeek, M. M., I. Otte-Holler, J. R. Westphal, P. Wesseling, D. J. Ruiter, and R. M. de Waal. 1994. Accumulation of intercellular adhesion molecule-1 in senile plaques in brain tissue of patients with Alzheimer's disease. *Am J Pathol* 144 (1), 104–116.
182. Anderton, B. 1994. Free radicals on the mind. Hydrogen peroxide mediates amyloid beta protein toxicity. *Hum Exp Toxicol* 13 (10), 719.
183. Harman, D. 1992. Free radical theory of aging. *Mutat Res* 275 (3–6), 257–266.

184. Smith, M. A., L. M. Sayre, V. M. Monnier, and G. Perry. 1995. Radical AGEing in Alzheimer's disease. *Trends Neurosci* 18 (4), 172–176.
185. Olanow, C. W., and G. W. Arendash. 1994. Metals and free radicals in neurodegeneration. *Curr Opin Neurol* 7 (6), 548–558.
186. Abate, A., G. Yang, P. A. Dennery, S. Oberle, and H. Schroder. 2000. Synergistic inhibition of cyclooxygenase-2 expression by vitamin E and aspirin. *Free Radic Biol Med* 29 (11), 1135–1142.
187. Melamed, E., D. Offen, A. Shirvan, R. Djaldetti, A. Barzilai, and I. Ziv. 1998. Levodopa toxicity and apoptosis. *Ann Neurol* 44 (3 Suppl 1), S149–S154.
188. Fahn, S., D. Oakes, I. Shoulson, K. Kieburtz, A. Rudolph, A. Lang, C. W. Olanow, C. Tanner, and K. Marek. 2004. Levodopa and the progression of Parkinson's disease. *N Engl J Med* 351 (24), 2498–2508.
189. Fahn, S. 2005. Does levodopa slow or hasten the rate of progression of Parkinson's disease? *J Neurol* 252 Suppl 4, IV37–IV42.
190. Abdin, A. A., and H. E. Hamouda. 2008. Mechanism of the neuroprotective role of coenzyme Q10 with or without l-dopa in rotenone-induced parkinsonism. *Neuropharmacology* 55 (8), 1340–1346.

11 Micronutrients in Prevention and Improvement of the Standard Therapy in Hearing Disorders

INTRODUCTION

The hearing disorders are a complex disease of the ear and include a partial or full loss of hearing, tinnitus, and Meniere's disease (MD) that are caused by diverse groups of biological, chemical, and environmental agents. There is no adequate strategy for prevention except avoiding the agents or conditions that can induce hearing disorders. Earplugs are used to reduce the intensity of noise that is known to induce hearing disorders. The effective treatment includes primarily hearing aids of various kinds. Anti-inflammatory drugs are used to reduce inflammation and improve hearing loss induced by certain agents. At present, there are no effective biological strategies for prevention or improved treatment of hearing disorders. In order to develop such strategies, it is essential to know some of the biochemical mechanisms that contribute to the damage of cells responsible for hearing. The analysis of published data on hearing disorders suggest that increased oxidative stress and products of inflammation, such as proinflammatory cytokines, play a central role in the initiation and progression of hearing loss induced by diverse groups of biological, chemical, and environmental agents. Since high-dose dietary and endogenous antioxidants neutralize free radicals and reduce inflammation, they should be useful in prevention and improved management of hearing disorders in combination with physical devices currently in use.

The main objective of this chapter is to describe briefly the incidence and cost, types, and causative agents of hearing disorders. The evidence for the involvement of oxidative stress and inflammation in the initiation and progression of hearing disorders are also discussed. In addition, this chapter presents scientific rationale and evidence for using multiple micronutrients including dietary and endogenous antioxidants in order to improve the efficacy of currently used physical devices in prevention and improved treatment of hearing disorders.

INCIDENCE AND COST

The number of Americans with hearing loss appears to have doubled during the past 30 years. The number of adult Americans with hearing loss was 13.2 million in 1971, 14.2 million in 1977, 20.3 million in 1991, 24.2 million in 1993, and 28.6 million in 2000.[1–3]

It has been estimated that about 14.9% of U.S. children have hearing disorders in one or both ears.[4] Early onset of deafness may be present in 4–11 cases per 10,000 children, and about 50% of them are attributed to genetic causes.[5] Among U.S. ethnic groups, 391,000 school-age children have unilateral hearing loss.[6] It has been estimated by the American Academy of Otolaryngology–Head and Neck Surgery that hearing loss, one of the most common birth defects, occurs in about three cases per 1000 babies born. About 60% of them are due to genetic defects. In the United States, about 1.4 million children under the age of 18 have a hearing loss (Better Hearing Institute, an advocacy group).

In sudden sensorineural hearing loss (SSHL), also referred to as sudden deafness, a rapid hearing loss occurs within a few hours or over a period of 3 days.[7] The incidence of SSHL is estimated to be 5–20 cases per 100,000 persons.[8]

It has been estimated that about one-third of adult Americans experience tinnitus at some time in their lives. About 10–15% of adults have prolonged tinnitus requiring medical attention.[9] The incidence of tinnitus vary markedly, from 7.9 million[10] to more than 37 million.[11] About 90% of patients with tinnitus have varying degrees of hearing loss.

It has been estimated that about 0.2% to 2% of the U.S. population suffer from MD. The majority of the people with MD are over 40 years of age. Men and women are equally affected by this disease.

The economics of lifetime cost, direct and indirect, of hearing loss could be 1 million per child, if no early treatment is provided. The loss of income for 24 million adult Americans with untreated hearing loss could be $122 billion a year due to underperformance on the job (Better Hearing Institute, an advocacy group).

TYPES OF HEARING DISORDERS

CONDUCTIVE HEARING LOSS

Conductive hearing loss may occur when sound is not transmitted properly through the outer or middle ear or both. This form of hearing loss is generally mild to moderate because sound still can be detected by the inner ear. However, otosclerosis can induce severe hearing loss. Conductive hearing loss occurs due to ear canal obstruction, damage to tympanic membrane, and ossicles of the middle ear, injury to inner ear, and otosclerosis.

SENSORINEURAL HEARING LOSS

Sensorineural hearing loss is due to insensitivity of the inner ear, the cochlea, or to impaired function of the auditory nervous system. This form of hearing loss could be moderate to severe and can lead to complete deafness. The sensorineural hearing loss is caused due to damage to hair cells of the cochlea. It also can be caused by the damage to the VIII cranial nerve and the vestibulocochlear nerve.

TINNITUS

Injury to the hair cells can cause hearing loss, tinnitus, or balance problems. When hair cells are damaged, glutamate, an excitatory neurotransmitter responsible for converting vibrational sound into electrical signal, is produced in excessive amounts. Excessive amounts of glutamate are very toxic to neurons. Damage to peripheral auditory and somatosensory systems causes imbalance between excitatory and inhibitory neurotransmitters in the midbrain auditory cortex and brain stem. This imbalance causes hyperactivity in the auditory cortex leading to the perception of phantom sounds (tinnitus).

MENIERE'S DISEASE (MD)

MD is a disorder of the inner ear that can cause episodes of vertigo (the abnormal sensation of movement), dizziness, ringing in the ears (tinnitus), fluctuating and progressive hearing loss, balance problems, and a feeling of fullness or pressure. In addition to hearing loss, sounds may appear distorted in some patients experiencing unusual sensitivity to noises (hyperacusis). These changes can occur in one or both ears. This disease is named after a French physician Prosper Meniere who first described this inner ear disorder in 1861.

MD usually starts in one ear, and over time (usually within 5 years), both ears are affected with the disease. In most cases, progressive hearing loss occurs in the affected ears. MD causes death of cochlear (hearing) hair cells, and it also gradually damages vestibular (motion-sensing) hair cells.

The fluid-filled hearing and balance membranous structures of the inner ear normally function independent of other fluid systems in the body, and the volume of the fluid (known as endolymph) remains constant. However, this changes with the injury or degeneration of the inner ear structures. One of the established pathological features includes fluctuating pressure of the fluid within the inner ear, referred to as endolymphatic hydrops or excess fluid in the inner ear. The membranous structure in the inner ear called labyrinth contains endolymph. This structure can become dilated like a balloon when pressure increases due to either blockage of the drainage system or entry of excess amounts of fluid. It is believed that endolymphatic fluid bursts from its normal channel in the ear and flows into other areas causing damage to the auditory and vestibular systems.

AGENTS OR CONDITIONS CAUSING HEARING DISORDERS

Prolonged exposure to intense noise is known to be a risk factor for hearing loss.[12] It is estimated that more than 30 million Americans are exposed to hazardous levels of sound intensity on a regular basis.[13] In addition, industrial workers and troops in training and in combat are exposed to high intensity noise and vibration. Additional agents that can cause hearing loss include cancer chemotherapeutic agents, such as cisplatin, antibiotics such as gentamicin, diseases such as ear infection (otitis media) and meningitis, MD, trauma, aging, and heredity. Cytomegalovirus (CMV) is the leading cause of infectious-related congenital sensorineural hearing loss worldwide. The CMV inflammatory genes play a significant role in causing hearing loss.[14] Age-related hearing loss, referred to as presbycusis, is caused by cochlear degeneration that is induced by increased oxidative stress and mutations in mitochondria. Hearing loss progresses very slowly as a function of aging. This condition is called presbycusis. Causes of tinnitus include blows to the head, large doses of certain drugs such as aspirin, anemia, hypertension, noise exposure, stress, earwax blockage, and certain types of tumor. Both dominant and recessive genes exist, which can cause mild to severe hearing loss.

MEASUREMENTS OF HEARING LOSS

The severity of hearing loss is measured by the degree of loudness, as measured in decibels (dB). The levels of dB range as function of severity of hearing loss are described below.

Mild hearing loss: between 25 and 40 dB
Moderate hearing loss: between 41 and 55 dB
Severe hearing loss: between 71 and 90 dB

CURRENT PREVENTION AND TREATMENT STRATEGIES

Although physical ear protection devices can reduce the impact of noise and vibration somewhat, the energy generated from high levels of noise intensity and vibration can penetrate the inner ear to cause damage to hair cells. Physical protection of the ear plays no role in chemical-induced or age-related hearing loss. Some individuals, such as troops in combat, musicians, or industrial workers do develop varying degrees of hearing loss in spite of physical ear protection. There is no biological protection strategy to reduce the risk of hearing loss. The development of such a strategy may compliment the physical ear protection devices in the prevention of hearing disorders.

Except for hearing aids of various types and cochlear transplant, there are no effective biological treatment strategies to improve the efficacy of physical ear devices. The hearing loss progresses in spite of hearing aids. Therefore, the development of a biological treatment strategy may compliment the ear devices in improving the management of hearing disorders.

Glucocorticoids are widely used to treat SSHL possibly because of involvement of inflammation. Treatment of mice with dexamethasone improves the synthesis of glutathione in the cochlear spiral ganglion by increasing the expression of gamma-glutamylcysteine synthetase, a rate-limiting enzyme in the biosynthesis of glutathione.[15] Thus, the mechanisms of protection by dexamethasone involve both reduction in inflammation and oxidative stress.

The current treatment of MD includes medication, surgery, and diet. Medications commonly used for acute episodes are Meclizine (Antivert), Lorazepam (Ativan), Phenergan, Compazine, Dexamethasone (Decadron), and calcium channel blockers. Medications used between attacks include diuretics, dyazide (Triamterine/HCTZ). Steroids and immune suppressants are rarely used. Surgical treatment is the last resort in severe cases of MD. Dietary recommendations include food and adequate fluid intake evenly throughout the day, reduced intake of salt and sugar, avoidance of caffeine and foods containing monosodium glutamate, and limited alcohol consumption. These treatment methodologies have been useful to manage the symptoms of the disease, but have failed to prevent the progressive damage to cochlear and vestibular hair cells. To address this problem, it is essential to understand the mechanisms that are involved in the death of these cells.

In order to develop an effective biological strategy for prevention or treatment of hearing disorders, it is important to identify some major biochemical events that contribute to the initiation and progression of hearing disorders. From the analysis of published data on laboratory and clinical studies, it appears that increased oxidative stress and chronic inflammation play a central role in the pathogenesis of hearing disorders.

INVOLVEMENT OF OXIDATIVE STRESS IN HEARING DISORDERS

Several studies have shown that increased oxidative stress due to production of excessive amounts of free radicals derived from oxygen and nitrogen, and acute and/or chronic inflammation produced by diverse groups of agents such as high intensity noise, vibration, cisplatin, gentamicin, aging, and MD are one of the major factors that play a central role in the initiating and progression of hearing disorders.

The data for the involvement of increased oxidative stress in hearing disorders comes from two sources, directly by measuring oxidative stress and indirectly by the use of antioxidants. An exposure to high-intensity noise causes a decrease in serum total antioxidant capacity and an increase in nitric oxide in guinea pigs.[16] Increased nitric oxide causes formation of peroxynitrite, which is very damaging to hair cells. Formation of free radicals following exposure to impulse noise has been reported in some animal studies.[17-23] The exposure to vibration also produces hearing disorders. In animal models (guinea pig), the older animals were twofold more sensitive to vibration-induced hearing loss than younger animals.[24]

Certain chemotherapeutic agents such as cisplatin and antibiotics such as aminoglycosides induced hearing loss by increasing oxidative stress, and this effect is reduced by antioxidants. Reactive oxygen species are involved in cisplatin-induced hearing loss.[25] Carboplatin depressed significantly the levels of antioxidant enzymes, superoxide dismutase (SOD), glutathione peroxidase, glutathione reductase, glutathione transferase and catalase, and elevated the levels of products of lipid peroxidation.[26] Carboplatin also depleted the level of glutathione.[19]

The levels of nitric oxide, peroxynitrite, oxidative stress, nuclear factor kappa-beta (NF-kappaB), glutamate receptor (N-methyl-D-aspartate) and calcium are elevated in tinnitus.[27,28] About 21% to 42% of tinnitus is induced by exposure to noise.[29] About 34% of tinnitus patients had posttraumatic stress disorder (PTSD), suggesting that there may be some linkage of neuronal mechanisms that cause both tinnitus and PTSD.[30] Evidence for increased oxidative stress and chronic inflammation has also been found in patients with PTSD.

The role of oxidative stress in MD is supported by the fact that free radical scavengers such as rebamipide, vitamin C, and glutathione, when administered orally for 8 weeks to 25 patients with poorly controlled MD, improved tinnitus, hearing loss, and disability[31].

Age-related cochlear structural alterations and degeneration of sensory and neural cells also occur.[32] Increased oxidative stress and chronic inflammation are also associated with aging.

INVOLVEMENT OF INFLAMMATION IN HEARING DISORDERS

In addition to increased oxidative stress, inflammation also appears to be a contributing factor in hearing loss induced by certain agents. For example, in a randomized double-blind, placebo controlled study, aspirin reduced the risk of gentamicin-induced hearing loss.[33] Anti-inflammatory drugs reduced inflammation and improved hearing loss.[34] Noise can damage cochlear function through inflammation in animal models. This is supported by the fact that the levels of intracellular adhesion molecules and migration of leukocytes increased after exposure to noise.[35] Intense noise can activate the nuclear transcription factor-kappaB (NF-kappaB) in the cochlea of mice.[36] This causes overexpression of inflammatory products in the inner ear including intracellular adhesion molecule-1 (ICAM-1), vascular cell adhesion molecule-1 (VCAM-1), and inducible nitric oxide synthase (iNOS) that contribute to hearing loss.[37]

Proinflammatory cytokines and activation of NF-kappaB play an important role in cisplatin-induced ototoxicity in mice and in cultures of immortalized cochlear cells.[38,39] Tumor necrosis factor-alpha (TNF-alpha) plays an important role in cochlear degeneration after bacterial meningitis. This is supported by the fact that administration of TNF-alpha antibody reduced post-meningitis hearing loss in Mongolian gerbils.[40] Furthermore, increase in the levels of TNF-alpha is associated with trauma-induced hearing loss,[41] and TNF-alpha–induced toxicity in the organ of Corti explant cultures was blocked by dexamethasone.[42] It has been reported that otosclerosis-induced sensorineural hearing loss is due to the chronic release of TNF-alpha from the foci of the otic capsule.[43] It has been proposed that repeated inflammatory reactions can produce sac dysfunction leading to MD.[44]

BENEFICIAL EFFECTS OF ANTIOXIDANTS IN HEARING DISORDERS

Antioxidants are known to reduce oxidative stress and inflammation; therefore, the supplementation with antioxidants appears to be one of the most rational approaches to prevent and improve hearing disorders in combination with standard therapy. Several animal and some human studies showed that supplementation with antioxidants has produced beneficial effects in improving hearing disorders.

Animal Studies

Vitamin E when administered intraperitoneally 3 days before and 3 days after noise exposure reduced noise-induced cochlear damage and hearing loss in guinea pigs.[45,46] Vitamin E protected against noise-induced damage to the inner ear in cyrinid fish.[47] Alpha lipoic acid protects against noise-induced hearing loss in guinea pigs.[16] An intraperitoneal injection of N-acetylcysteine (NAC) or glutathione significantly reduced hair cell loss in cochlear cells of rats and guinea pigs.[48,49] NAC attenuated noise-induced hearing disorders in guinea pigs.[50] Acetyl-L-carnitine and NAC administered twice a day for 2 days and 1 h before and 1 h after noise exposure for an additional 2 days provided protection against hearing loss in the chinchilla model.[51] The role of NAC in reducing noise-induced hearing loss has been recently reviewed.[52] Coenzyme Q_{10} helped in recovery from hypoxia-induced sudden deafness by protecting damage to auditory hair cells as well as preventing respiratory metabolic impairment of hair cells.[53] Idebenone, a synthetic analog of coenzyme Q_{10} with antioxidant properties, protected guinea pigs against noise-induced hearing loss.[54] The soluble form of coenzyme Q_{10} was effective in reducing noise-induced hearing loss by promoting the survival of hair cells in guinea pigs.[55] The combination of vitamin E and idebenone did not produce additive protective effect against noise-induced hearing loss, suggesting that these two antioxidants may be acting by similar mechanisms.[56] Vitamin C also protected against noise-induced hearing loss in albino guinea pigs.[57] D-Methionine, an antioxidant, attenuated noise-induced oxidative stress and functional loss of cochlea in mice.[58]

Vitamin E protected against cisplatin-induced damage to cochlear hair cells in rats.[59] Trolox, a water-soluble analog of vitamin E, when applied locally, reduced cisplatin-induced ototoxicity in guinea pigs.[60] Vitamin E reduced gentamicin-induced hearing loss and vestibular dysfunction.[61] Cisplatin-induced cochlear damage is reduced by vitamin E in an animal model.[62] An in vitro study suggested that NAC protected against cisplatin-induced damage to inner ear auditory sensory cells.[63] Antioxidants attenuate aminoglycoside-induced hearing loss and vestibular dysfunction in an animal model (chinchilla).[64] Alpha-lipoic acid protected against carboplatin-induced toxicity in hair cells in rats.[65]

In mice and dogs, a diet rich in antioxidants reduced age-related cochlear degeneration.[32] Age-related hearing loss is characterized by a progressive decline in sensitivity to sound; however, caloric restriction and treatment with individual antioxidants such as vitamin E, vitamin C, acetyl-L-carnitine, alpha-lipoic acid, and melatonin improved auditory sensitivity to sound and reduced mitochondrial DNA deletion and loss of hair cells in aging rats.[66–68] In a mice model of premature age-related hearing loss, treatment with N-acetyl-L-carnitine failed to protect against hearing loss.[69]

Human Studies

In a prospective, double-blind study design, supplementation with vitamin E alone provided better recovery than the standard therapy in patients with idiopathic sudden hearing loss.[45] In a prospective, double-blind study, vitamin E alone administered orally improved the efficacy of standard therapy.[46] In a prospective randomized study, intravenous administration of magnesium sulfate improved hearing recovery in patients with idiopathic SSHL.[70] Coenzyme Q_{10} delayed the progression of hearing loss in patients with a genetic defect, 7445A→G mitochondrial mutation.[71] The use of glutamate antagonists, steroids, and antioxidants may be useful in the management of hearing loss and tinnitus.[72] An oral supplementation with antioxidants [vitamin E, vitamin C, beta-carotene (BC), and phospholipids] reduced the subjective discomfort and tinnitus intensity in patients with idiopathic tinnitus.[73] NAC protected against aminoglycoside-induced ototoxicity in hemodialysis patients.[74] An antioxidant mixture containing reduced glutathione, alpha-lipoic acid, cysteine, and other antioxidants improved the symptoms of MD.[75]

RATIONALE FOR USING MULTIPLE MICRONUTRIENTS IN HEARING DISORDERS

Since increased oxidative stress and chronic inflammation are involved in hearing disorders, and since antioxidants reduce oxidative stress and chronic inflammation, supplementation with multiple micronutrients including dietary and endogenous antioxidants may improve the current prevention program with physical devices and improve the efficacy of standard therapy in patients with hearing disorders. Several studies with antioxidants and hearing disorders discussed above support this rationale. Although supplementation with a single antioxidant in these studies has produced some beneficial effects in improving hearing disorders, this is not recommended for an optimal improvement in hearing disorders.

Experimental designs of clinical studies with individual antioxidants may not be suitable for determining the efficacy of micronutrient strategy in reducing the risk of hearing disorders in individuals who are exposed daily to intense noise, vibration, and factors that are known to induce hearing disorders. Such a strategy is also not suitable for improving the efficacy of standard therapy in patients with hearing disorders. This is due to the fact that these individuals have a high internal oxidative environment, and it is known that individual antioxidants can act as pro-oxidants when oxidized. In addition, their mechanisms of action and distribution at cellular and organ levels differ, their internal cellular and organ environments (oxygenation, aqueous and lipid components) differ, and their affinity for various types of free radicals differ. For example, BC is more effective in quenching oxygen radicals than most other antioxidants.[76] BC can perform certain biological functions that cannot be produced by its metabolite vitamin A, and vice verss.[77,78] It has been reported that BC treatment enhances the expression of the connexin gene, which codes for a gap junction protein in mammalian fibroblasts in culture, whereas vitamin A treatment does not produce such an effect.[78] Vitamin A can induce differentiation in certain normal and cancer cells, whereas BC and other carotenoids do not.[79,80] Thus, BC and vitamin A have, in part, different biological functions. Therefore, the addition of both BC and vitamin A into a multiple micronutrient preparation is essential for improving the efficacy of micronutrients therapy.

The gradient of oxygen pressure varies within cells. Some antioxidants, such as vitamin E, are more effective as quenchers of free radicals in reduced oxygen pressure, whereas BC and vitamin A are more effective in higher atmospheric pressures.[81] Vitamin C is necessary to protect cellular components in aqueous environments, whereas carotenoids and vitamins A and E protect cellular components in lipid environments. In addition, vitamin C is necessary for the activity of tyrosine hydroxylase, which is the rate-limiting enzyme in the synthesis of catecholamines. Vitamin C also plays an important role in maintaining cellular levels of vitamin E by recycling vitamin E radical (oxidized) to the reduced (antioxidant) form.[82] Also, oxidative DNA damage produced by the high levels of vitamin C could be protected by vitamin E. Oxidized forms of vitamins C and E can also act as radicals; therefore, excessive amounts of any one of these forms, when used as a single agent, could be harmful over a long period.

The form of vitamin E used is also important in any clinical trial. It has been established that D-alpha-tocopheryl succinate (alpha-TS) is the most effective form of vitamin both in vitro and in vivo.[83,84] This form of vitamin E is more soluble than alpha-tocopherol and enters cells more readily. Therefore, it is expected to cross the blood–brain barrier in greater amounts than alpha-tocopherol. However, this has not yet been demonstrated in animals or humans. We have reported that an oral ingestion of alpha-TS (800 IU/day) in humans increased plasma levels of not only alpha-tocopherol, but also alpha-TS, suggesting that a portion of alpha-TS can be absorbed from the intestinal tract before hydrolysis.[85] This observation is important because the conventional assumption based on rodents has been that esterified forms of vitamin E, such as alpha-TS, alpha-tocopheryl nicotinate, and alpha-tocopheryl acetate, can be absorbed from the intestinal tract only after they are hydrolyzed to alpha-tocopherol. Our preliminary data showed that this assumption may not be true for the absorption of alpha-TS in humans. Therefore, the addition of both forms of vitamin E into a multiple micronutrient preparation is essential for improving the efficacy of micronutrients therapy.

Carboplatin, which is known to induce hearing loss, depleted the level of glutathione,[19] which may increase oxidative stress and eventually degeneration of hair cells. In hair cells and the auditory nervous system, mitochondria are very sensitive to oxidative stress, and impaired mitochondria can generate excessive amounts of reactive oxygen species. Thus, improving the function of impaired mitochondria or protecting mitochondria from oxidative damage becomes very necessary for prevention and better management of hearing disorders. Glutathione is effective in catabolizing H_2O_2 and anions. However, oral supplementation with glutathione failed to significantly increase plasma levels of glutathione in human subjects,[86] suggesting that this tripeptide is completely hydrolyzed in the GI tract. Therefore, I propose to utilize NAC and alpha-lipoic acid that increase the cellular levels of glutathione by different mechanisms in a multiple micronutrient preparation. In addition, R-alpha-lipoic acid and acetyl-L-carnitine together promoted mitochondrial biogenesis in murine adipocytes in culture; however, no effect was observed when these antioxidants were used individually.[87] This type of study further emphasized the value of using more than one antioxidant in any clinical or laboratory study.

Other endogenous antioxidants, coenzyme Q_{10}, may have some potential value in prevention and improved treatment of hearing disorders. Since mitochondrial dysfunction may be associated with hair cells and the auditory nervous system, and since coenzyme Q_{10} is needed for the generation of ATP by mitochondria, it is essential to add this antioxidant in multiple micronutrient preparation in order to improve the function of mitochondria. A study has shown that Ubiquinol (coenzyme Q_{10}) scavenges peroxy radicals faster than alpha-tocopherol[88] and, like vitamin C, can regenerate vitamin E in a redox cycle.[89] However, it is a weaker antioxidant than alpha-tocopherol.

Selenium is a cofactor of glutathione peroxidase, and Se-glutathione peroxidase also acts as an antioxidant by increasing the intracellular level of antioxidants. There may be some other mechanisms of selenium. Therefore, these agents should be added to a multiple micronutrient preparation for prevention and improved treatment of hearing disorders. Because of the biology of antioxidants discussed above, the use of single antioxidants in clinical trials cannot be considered rational for prevention or improving treatment outcomes in patients with hearing disorders.

In addition to dietary and endogenous antioxidants, B vitamins that are necessary for general health should be added to a multiple micronutrient preparation for reducing the incidence or improved treatment of hearing disorders.

In addition to physical protection, the multiple micronutrient preparation should be consumed daily prior to exposure to the agents or conditions that induce hearing disorders in order to reduce the risk of developing tinnitus, hearing loss, or a balancing problem. People suffering from hearing disorders should take antioxidants in combination with standard therapy. However, the selection of the appropriate type of antioxidant preparation and dose schedule is very critical for enhancing their effectiveness. I recommend supplementation with multiple micronutrients containing dietary and endogenous antioxidants for reducing the risk of hearing disorders and improving the efficacy of standard therapy to improve the management of hearing disorders.

Doses are very important because, at certain low doses, antioxidants may reduce free radicals but may not decrease chronic inflammation. At higher doses (totally safe in humans), they reduce oxidative stress as well as inflammation. These issues have been discussed in detail in a recent review paper.[90]

A multiple micronutrient preparation containing iron, copper, or manganese is not recommended because these trace minerals interact with vitamin C and generate excessive amounts of free radicals. In addition, these trace minerals in the presence of vitamin C are absorbed better than in its absence, and the nature has provided no significant mechanisms of excretion of iron or copper in men of all ages and women after menopause. Increased free iron or copper stores in the body increases the risk of many chronic diseases. The addition of heavy metals such as molybdenum, zirconium, and vanadium is also not recommended because there are no significant mechanisms of removal of these heavy metals from the body. An accumulation of these metals after long-term consumption could be toxic to nervous tissue including the brain. The inclusion of herbs or herbal antioxidants into a multiple dietary and endogenous antioxidant preparation is not recommended because they do not produce any unique beneficial effect that cannot be produced by standard antioxidants. In addition, certain herbs are known to interact with the prescription and non-prescription drugs in an adverse manner. These issues have been discussed in detail in two review papers.[90,91]

A dose schedule of twice a day (half in the morning and half in the evening) is equally important in increasing the effectiveness of the micronutrient preparation. Taking micronutrients once a day may create large fluctuations in the tissue levels of micronutrients because the biological half-lives of micronutrients markedly vary. We have observed that a twofold change in the level of vitamin E succinate markedly alters gene expression profiles in neuroblastoma cells (unpublished data). Thus, the genetic machinery of the cell constantly has to re-adjust to cope with the variations in the levels of micronutrients, and this could create cellular stress over a long period. These issues have been discussed in detail in a recent review paper.[91]

A commercial formulation of multiple micronutrients was tested in a clinical study in troops returning from Iraq with mild to moderate traumatic brain injury. Thirty-four patients with posttraumatic dizziness were admitted to the Naval Medical Center San Diego Clinic over a 2-month period and agreed to participate in the study under the supervision of Dr. Michael Hoffer and his colleagues. All patients had received their injury 3–20 weeks prior to admission, and they received identical treatment consisting of medical therapy (for any migraines), supportive care, steroids, and vestibular rehabilitation therapy. Fifteen of the 34 patients also received a dose of an antioxidant and micronutrient formula (two capsules by mouth twice a day). At the onset of therapy, all patients were evaluated in outcome measures, which included the Sensory Organization Test (SOT) by Computerized Dynamic Posturography (CDP), the Dynamic Gait Index (DGI), the Activities Balance Confidence (ABC) scale, the Dizziness Handicap Index (DHI), the Vestibular Disorders Activities of Daily Living (VADL) score, and the Balance Scoring System (BESS) test. The study was carried out for 12 weeks. The therapist who graded these outcomes and performed the testing was blinded as to whether the patient was receiving antioxidant therapy or not. The pretrial test scores did not differ significantly between the two groups on any of the tests.

The results showed that both groups of patients showed trends toward significant improvement on all tests after the 12 weeks of therapy, but the combination treatment trend was stronger than that of the standard therapy alone group. After only 4 weeks, the SOT score by CDP was 78 for the antioxidant group compared to 63 for the non-antioxidant group. This difference was statistically significant at the $P < 0.05$ level. The improvement noted by the antioxidant group on the other tests was also greater than the non-antioxidant group, although these differences did not reach statistical significance because of the short trial period and small sample size.[92]

PROPOSED MICRONUTRIENT RECOMMENDATION FOR PREVENTION AND IMPROVED TREATMENT OF HEARING DISORDERS

A formulation of multiple micronutrients may include vitamin A (retinyl palmitate), vitamin E (both D-alpha-tocopherol and D-TS), natural mixed carotenoids, vitamin C (calcium ascorbate), coenzyme Q_{10}, R-alpha-lipoic acid, NAC, L-carnitine, vitamin D, B vitamins, selenium, zinc, and chromium. No iron, copper, or manganese would be included because these trace minerals are known to interact with vitamin C to produce free radicals. These trace minerals are absorbed from the intestinal tract more in the presence of antioxidants than in their absence that could result in increased body stores of free forms of these minerals. Increased iron stores have been linked to increased risk of several chronic diseases. Previous multiple micronutrients tested in a clinical study with U.S. troops lacked natural BC; however, it is essential to add this dietary antioxidant because BC not only acts as a precursor of vitamin A, but it performs other biological functions that cannot be produced by vitamin A.

A randomized, double-blind, placebo-controlled trial using the proposed micronutrient preparation should be initiated in the individuals who are frequently exposed to agents that induce hearing disorders. A similar clinical trial in combination with standard therapy can be initiated in the individuals who suffer from hearing disorders. In the meanwhile, the proposed micronutrient recommendations can be adopted by the individuals who are exposed to agents or conditions that can induce hearing disorders or those who are suffering from this disease in consultation with their physicians or health professionals. It is expected that the proposed recommendations would reduce the risk of developing hearing disorders and retard the rate of progression of the disease in patients who suffer from this disease and, in combination with standard therapy, may improve the treatment outcomes more than that produced by standard therapy alone.

CONCLUSIONS

The hearing disorders are a complex disease of the ear and include a partial or full loss of hearing, tinnitus, and MD that are caused by diverse groups of biological, chemical, and environmental agents. There are no adequate strategies for prevention or treatment of hearing disorders. The analysis of published data on hearing disorders suggest that increased oxidative stress and products of inflammation such as reactive oxygen species, proinflammatory cytokines, prostaglandin E_2, compliment proteins, and adhesion molecules play a central role in the initiation and progression of hearing disorders. Since high-dose dietary and endogenous antioxidants neutralize free radicals and reduce inflammation, they should be useful in prevention and improved management of hearing disorders in combination with currently used physical devices. Indeed, several laboratory studies using cell culture and animal models showed that supplementation with individual dietary or endogenous antioxidants reduced noise- and chemical-induced hearing disorders to varying degrees. A few human studies also confirm the value of antioxidants in reducing the levels of induced hearing loss and tinnitus as well as improved the symptoms of MD. The scientific rationale and evidence in support of using multiple micronutrients including dietary and endogenous antioxidants for prevention and improved treatment of hearing disorders were discussed. The results of a pilot randomized clinical study with a commercial preparation of multiple micronutrients showed that daily oral supplementation with this micronutrient preparation for a period of 12 weeks improved the efficacy of standard therapy (supportive care, steroids, and vestibular rehabilitation therapy) in U.S. troops returning from Iraq with mild to moderate traumatic brain injury. Therefore, I propose a shift in a paradigm of experimental design of clinical studies from using a single micronutrient to multiple micronutrients for evaluating their efficacy in prevention and improved treatment of hearing disorders.

A randomized, double-blind, placebo-controlled trial using the proposed micronutrient preparation should be initiated in the individuals who are frequently exposed to agents that induce hearing disorders. A similar clinical trial in combination with standard therapy can be initiated in the individuals who suffer from hearing disorders. In the meanwhile, the proposed micronutrient recommendations can be adopted by the individuals who are exposed to agents or conditions that can induce hearing disorders or those who are suffering from this disease in consultation with their physicians or health professionals.

REFERENCES

1. Ries, P. W. 1994. Prevalence and characteristics of persons with hearing trouble: United States, 1990–1991. *Vital Health Stat* 188: 9–10.
2. Benson, V., and M. A. Marano. 1995. Current estimates from the National Health Interview Survey, 1993. National Center for Health Statistics. *Vital Health Stat* 10 (190).
3. Kochkin, S., and V. I. MarkeTrak. 2001. The VA and direct mail sales spark growth in hearing aid market. *The Hearing Review* 8: 16–24, 63–65.
4. Niskar, A. S., S. M. Kieszak, A. Holmes, E. Esteban, C. Rubin, and D. J. Brody. 1998. Prevalence of hearing loss among children 6 to 19 years of age: The Third National Health and Nutrition Examination Survey. *JAMA* 279 (14): 1071–1075.
5. Marazita, M. L., L. M. Ploughman, B. Rawlings, E. Remington, K. S. Arnos, and W. E. Nance. 1993. Genetic epidemiological studies of early-onset deafness in the U.S. school-age population. *Am J Med Genet* 46 (5): 486–491.
6. Lee, D. J., O. Gomez-Marin, and H. M. Lee. 1998. Prevalence of unilateral hearing loss in children: The National Health and Nutrition Examination Survey II and the Hispanic Health and Nutrition Examination Survey. *Ear Hear* 19 (4): 329–332.
7. National Institute on Deafness and Other Communication Disorders, 2003. Sudden deafness (NIH pub. No. 00-4757), Bethesda, MD.
8. Byl, F. M., Jr. 1984. Sudden hearing loss: Eight years' experience and suggested prognostic table. *Laryngoscope* 94 (5 Pt 1): 647–661.
9. Heller, A. J. 2003. Classification and epidemiology of tinnitus. *Otolaryngol Clinics N Am* 36, 239–248.
10. Adams, P. F. 1999. Current estimates from the National Health Interview Survey, 1996. National Center for Health Statistics. *Vital Health Stat*, 10 (200).
11. Noell, C. A., and W. L. Meyerhoff. 2003. Tinnitus. Diagnosis and treatment of this elusive symptom. *Geriatrics* 58 (2): 28–34.

12. Dalton, D. S., K. J. Cruickshanks, T. L. Wiley, B. E. Klein, R. Klein, and T. S. Tweed. 2001. Association of leisure-time noise exposure and hearing loss. *Audiology* 40 (1): 1–9.
13. National Institute on Deafness and Other Communication Disorders. 2002. Noise-induced hearing loss (NIH Pub. No. 97-4233, Bethesda, MD.
14. Schraff, S. A., D. K. Brown, M. R. Schleiss, J. Meinzen-Derr, J. H. Greinwald, and D. I. Choo. 2007. The role of CMV inflammatory genes in hearing loss. *Otol Neurotol* 28 (7), 964–969.
15. Nagashima, R., and K. Ogita. 2006. Enhanced biosynthesis of glutathione in the spiral ganglion of the cochlea after in vivo treatment with dexamethasone in mice. *Brain Res* 1117 (1): 101–108.
16. Diao, M. F., H. Y. Liu, Y. M. Zhang, and W. Y. Gao. 2003. Changes in antioxidant capacity of the guinea pig exposed to noise and the protective effect of alpha-lipoic acid against acoustic trauma. *Sheng Li Xue Bao* 55 (6): 672–676.
17. Clerici, W. J., D. L. DiMartino, and M. R. Prasad. 1995. Direct effects of reactive oxygen species on cochlear outer hair cell shape in vitro. *Hear Res* 84 (1–2): 30–40.
18. Henderson, D., E. C. Bielefeld, K. C. Harris, and B. H. Hu. 2006. The role of oxidative stress in noise-induced hearing loss. *Ear Hear* 27 (1): 1–19.
19. Henderson, D., S. L. McFadden, C. C. Liu, N. Hight, and X. Y. Zheng. 1999. The role of antioxidants in protection from impulse noise. *Ann N Y Acad Sci* 884: 368–380.
20. Ohlemiller, K. K., J. S. Wright, and L. L. Dugan. 1999. Early elevation of cochlear reactive oxygen species following noise exposure. *Audiol Neurootol* 4 (5): 229–236.
21. Van Campen, L. E., W. J. Murphy, J. R. Franks, P. I. Mathias, and M. A. Toraason. 2002. Oxidative DNA damage is associated with intense noise exposure in the rat. *Hear Res* 164 (1–2): 29–38.
22. Yamane, H., Y. Nakai, M. Takayama, K. Konishi, H. Iguchi, T. Nakagawa, S. Shibata, A. Kato, K. Sunami, and C. Kawakatsu. 1995. The emergence of free radicals after acoustic trauma and strial blood flow. *Acta Otolaryngol Suppl* 519: 87–92.
23. Yamashita, D., H. Y. Jiang, J. Schacht, and J. M. Miller. 2004. Delayed production of free radicals following noise exposure. *Brain Res* 1019 (1–2): 201–209.
24. Zou, J., P. Bretlau, I. Pyykko, J. Starck, and E. Toppila. 2001. Sensorineural hearing loss after vibration: An animal model for evaluating prevention and treatment of inner ear hearing loss. *Acta Otolaryngol* 121 (2): 143–148.
25. Minami, S. B., S. H. Sha, and J. Schacht. 2004. Antioxidant protection in a new animal model of cisplatin-induced ototoxicity. *Hear Res* 198 (1–2): 137–143.
26. Husain, K., R. B. Scott, C. Whitworth, S. M. Somani, and L. P. Rybak. 2001. Dose response of carboplatin-induced hearing loss in rats: Antioxidant defense system. *Hear Res* 151 (1–2): 71–78.
27. Neri, S., S. Signorelli, D. Pulvirenti, B. Mauceri, D. Cilio, F. Bordonaro, G. Abate, et al. 2006. Oxidative stress, nitric oxide, endothelial dysfunction and tinnitus. *Free Radic Res* 40 (6): 615–618.
28. Pall, M. L., and S. A. Bedient. 2007. The NO/ONOO- cycle as the etiological mechanism of tinnitus. *Int Tinnitus J* 13 (2): 99–104.
29. Kowalska, S., and W. Sulkowski. 2001. Tinnitus in noise-induced hearing impairment. *Med Pr* 52 (5): 305–313.
30. Fagelson, M. A. 2007. The association between tinnitus and posttraumatic stress disorder. *Am J Audiol* 16 (2): 107–117.
31. Takumida, M., M. Anniko, and M. Ohtani. 2003. Radical scavengers for Meniere's disease after failure of conventional therapy: A pilot study. *Acta Otolaryngol* 123 (6): 697–703.
32. Le, T., and E. M. Keithley. 2007. Effects of antioxidants on the aging inner ear. *Hear Res* 226 (1–2): 194–202.
33. Chen, Y., W. G. Huang, D. J. Zha, J. H. Qiu, J. L. Wang, S. H. Sha, and J. Schacht. 2007. Aspirin attenuates gentamicin ototoxicity: From the laboratory to the clinic. *Hear Res* 226 (1–2): 178–182.
34. Wang, X., T. Truong, P. B. Billings, J. P. Harris, and E. M. Keithley. 2003. Blockage of immune-mediated inner ear damage by etanercept. *Otol Neurotol* 24 (1): 52–57.
35. Shi, X., and A. L. Nuttall. 2007. Expression of adhesion molecular proteins in the cochlear lateral wall of normal and PARP-1 mutant mice. *Hear Res* 224 (1–2): 1–14.
36. Masuda, M., R. Nagashima, S. Kanzaki, M. Fujioka, K. Ogita, and K. Ogawa. 2006. Nuclear factor-kappa B nuclear translocation in the cochlea of mice following acoustic overstimulation. *Brain Res* 1068 (1): 237–247.
37. Yamamoto, H., I. Omelchenko, X. Shi, and A. L. Nuttall. 2009. The influence of NF-kappaB signal-transduction pathways on the murine inner ear by acoustic overstimulation. *J Neurosci Res* 87 (8): 1832–1840.

38. Kim, H. J., H. S. So, J. H. Lee, C. Park, J. B. Lee, M. J. Youn, S. J. Kim, et al. 2008. Role of proinflammatory cytokines in cisplatin-induced vestibular hair cell damage. *Head Neck* 30 (11): 1445–1456.
39. So, H., H. Kim, J. H. Lee, C. Park, Y. Kim, E. Kim, J. K. Kim, et al. 2007. Cisplatin cytotoxicity of auditory cells requires secretions of proinflammatory cytokines via activation of ERK and NF-kappaB. *J Assoc Res Otolaryngol* 8 (3): 338–355.
40. Aminpour, S., S. P. Tinling, and H. A. Brodie. 2005. Role of tumor necrosis factor-alpha in sensorineural hearing loss after bacterial meningitis. *Otol Neurotol* 26 (4): 602–609.
41. Haake, S. M., C. T. Dinh, S. Chen, A. A. Eshraghi, and T. R. Van De Water. 2009. Dexamethasone protects auditory hair cells against TNFalpha-initiated apoptosis via activation of PI3K/Akt and NFkappaB signaling. *Hear Res* 255 (1–2): 22–32.
42. Van De Water, T. R., C. T. Dinh, R. Vivero, G. Hoosien, A. A. Eshraghi, and T. J. Balkany. 2009. Mechanisms of hearing loss from trauma and inflammation: Otoprotective therapies from the laboratory to the clinic. *Acta Otolaryngol* 1–4.
43. Sziklai, I., T. J. Batta, and T. Karosi. 2009. Otosclerosis: An organ-specific inflammatory disease with sensorineural hearing loss. *Eur Arch Otorhinolaryngol* 266 (11): 1711–1718.
44. Derebery, M. J. 1996. Allergic and immunologic aspects of Meniere's disease. *Otolaryngol Head Neck Surg* 114 (3): 360–365.
45. Hou, F., S. Wang, S. Zhai, Y. Hu, W. Yang, and L. He. 2003. Effects of alpha-tocopherol on noise-induced hearing loss in guinea pigs. *Hear Res* 179 (1–2): 1–8.
46. Joachims, H. Z., J. Segal, A. Golz, A. Netzer, and D. Goldenberg. 2003. Antioxidants in treatment of idiopathic sudden hearing loss. *Otol Neurotol* 24 (4): 572–575.
47. Scholik, A. R., U. S. Lee, C. K. Chow, and H. Y. Yan. 2004. Dietary vitamin E protects the fathead minnow, *Pimephales promelas*, against noise exposure. *Comp Biochem Physiol C Toxicol Pharmacol* 137 (4): 313–323.
48. Duan, M., J. Qiu, G. Laurell, A. Olofsson, S. A. Counter, and E. Borg. 2004. Dose and time-dependent protection of the antioxidant *N*-l-acetylcysteine against impulse noise trauma. *Hear Res* 192 (1–2): 1–9.
49. Ohinata, Y., T. Yamasoba, J. Schacht, and J. M. Miller. 2000. Glutathione limits noise-induced hearing loss. *Hear Res* 146 (1–2): 28–34.
50. Ohinata, Y., J. M. Miller, and J. Schacht. 2003. Protection from noise-induced lipid peroxidation and hair cell loss in the cochlea. *Brain Res* 966 (2): 265–273.
51. Kopke, R., E. Bielefeld, J. Liu, J. Zheng, R. Jackson, D. Henderson, and J. K. Coleman. 2005. Prevention of impulse noise-induced hearing loss with antioxidants. *Acta Otolaryngol* 125 (3): 235–243.
52. Kopke, R. D., R. L. Jackson, J. K. Coleman, J. Liu, E. C. Bielefeld, and B. J. Balough. 2007. NAC for noise: From the bench top to the clinic. *Hear Res* 226 (1–2): 114–125.
53. Sato, K. 1988. Pharmacokinetics of coenzyme Q10 in recovery of acute sensorineural hearing loss due to hypoxia. *Acta Otolaryngol Suppl* 458: 95–102.
54. Sergi, B., A. R. Fetoni, G. Paludetti, A. Ferraresi, P. Navarra, A. Mordente, and D. Troiani. 2006. Protective properties of idebenone in noise-induced hearing loss in the guinea pig. *Neuroreport* 17 (9): 857–861.
55. Fetoni, A. R., R. Piacentini, A. Fiorita, G. Paludetti, and D. Troiani. 2009. Water-soluble Coenzyme Q10 formulation (Q-ter) promotes outer hair cell survival in a guinea pig model of noise induced hearing loss (NIHL). *Brain Res* 1257: 108–116.
56. Fetoni, A. R., A. Ferraresi, C. L. Greca, D. Rizzo, B. Sergi, G. Tringali, R. Piacentini, and D. Troiani. 2008. Antioxidant protection against acoustic trauma by coadministration of idebenone and vitamin E. *Neuroreport* 19 (3): 277–281.
57. McFadden, S. L., J. M. Woo, N. Michalak, and D. Ding. 2005. Dietary vitamin C supplementation reduces noise-induced hearing loss in guinea pigs. *Hear Res* 202 (1–2): 200–208.
58. Samson, J., A. Wiktorek-Smagur, P. Politanski, E. Rajkowska, M. Pawlaczyk-Luszczynska, A. Dudarewicz, S. H. Sha, J. Schacht, and M. Sliwinska-Kowalska. 2008. Noise-induced time-dependent changes in oxidative stress in the mouse cochlea and attenuation by D-methionine. *Neuroscience* 152 (1): 146–150.
59. Kalkanis, J. G., C. Whitworth, and L. P. Rybak. 2004. Vitamin E reduces cisplatin ototoxicity. *Laryngoscope* 114 (3): 538–542.
60. Teranishi, M. A., and T. Nakashima. 2003. Effects of Trolox, locally applied on round windows, on cisplatin-induced ototoxicity in guinea pigs. *Int J Pediatr Otorhinolaryngol* 67 (2): 133–139.
61. Sergi, B., A. R. Fetoni, A. Ferraresi, D. Troiani, G. B. Azzena, G. Paludetti, and M. Maurizi. 2004. The role of antioxidants in protection from ototoxic drugs. *Acta Otolaryngol Suppl* (552): 42–45.
62. Fetoni, A. R., B. Sergi, A. Ferraresi, G. Paludetti, and D. Troiani. 2004. alpha-Tocopherol protective effects on gentamicin ototoxicity: An experimental study. *Int J Audiol* 43 (3): 166–171.

63. Feghali, J. G., W. Liu, and T. R. Van De Water. 2001. l-*N*-Acetyl-cysteine protection against cisplatin-induced auditory neuronal and hair cell toxicity. *Laryngoscope* 111 (7): 1147–1155.
64. Schacht, J. 1999. Antioxidant therapy attenuates aminoglycoside-induced hearing loss. *Ann N Y Acad Sci* 884: 125–130.
65. Husain, K., C. Whitworth, S. M. Somani, and L. P. Rybak. 2005. Partial protection by lipoic acid against carboplantin-induced ototoxicity in rats. *Biomed Environ Sci* 18 (3): 198–206.
66. Seidman, M. D. 2000. Effects of dietary restriction and antioxidants on presbyacusis. *Laryngoscope* 110 (5 Pt 1): 727–738.
67. Seidman, M. D., N. Ahmad, D. Joshi, J. Seidman, S. Thawani, and W. S. Quirk. 2004. Age-related hearing loss and its association with reactive oxygen species and mitochondrial DNA damage. *Acta Otolaryngol Suppl* (552): 16–24.
68. Derin, A., B. Agirdir, N. Derin, O. Dinc, K. Guney, H. Ozcaglar, and S. Kilincarslan. 2004. The effects of L-carnitine on presbyacusis in the rat model. *Clin Otolaryngol Allied Sci* 29 (3): 238–241.
69. Davis, R. R., M. W. Kuo, S. G. Stanton, B. Canlon, E. Krieg, and K. N. Alagramam. 2007. *N*-Acetyl L-cysteine does not protect against premature age-related hearing loss in C57BL/6J mice: A pilot study. *Hear Res* 226 (1–2): 203–208.
70. Gordin, A., D. Goldenberg, A. Golz, A. Netzer, and H. Z. Joachims. 2002. Magnesium: A new therapy for idiopathic sudden sensorineural hearing loss. *Otol Neurotol* 23 (4): 447–451.
71. Angeli, S. I., X. Z. Liu, D. Yan, T. Balkany, and F. Telischi. 2005. Coenzyme Q-10 treatment of patients with a 7445A→G mitochondrial DNA mutation stops the progression of hearing loss. *Acta Otolaryngol* 125 (5): 510–512.
72. Seidman, M. D. 1998. Glutamate antagonists, steroids, and antioxidants as therapeutic options for hearing loss and tinnitus and the use of an inner ear drug delivery system. *Int Tinnitus J* 4 (2): 148–154.
73. Savastano, M., G. Brescia, and G. Marioni. 2007. Antioxidant therapy in idiopathic tinnitus: Preliminary outcomes. *Arch Med Res* 38 (4): 456–459.
74. Tepel, M. 2007. *N*-Acetylcysteine in the prevention of ototoxicity. *Kidney Int* 72 (3): 231–232.
75. Raponi, G., D. Alpini, S. Volonte, S. Capobianco, and A. Cesarani. 2003. The role of free radicals and plasmatic antioxidant in Meniere's syndrome. *Int Tinnitus J* 9 (2): 104–108.
76. Krinsky, N. I. 1989. Antioxidant functions of carotenoids. *Free Radic Biol Med* 7 (6): 617–635.
77. Hazuka, M. B., J. Edwards-Prasad, F. Newman, J. J. Kinzie, and K. N. Prasad. 1990. Beta-carotene induces morphological differentiation and decreases adenylate cyclase activity in melanoma cells in culture. *J Am Coll Nutr* 9 (2): 143–149.
78. Zhang, L. X., R. V. Cooney, and J. S. Bertram. 1992. Carotenoids up-regulate connexin43 gene expression independent of their provitamin A or antioxidant properties. *Cancer Res* 52 (20): 5707–5712.
79. Carter, C. A., M. Pogribny, A. Davidson, C. D. Jackson, L. J. McGarrity, and S. M. Morris. 1996. Effects of retinoic acid on cell differentiation and reversion toward normal in human endometrial adenocarcinoma (RL95-2) cells. *Anticancer Res* 16 (1): 17–24.
80. Meyskens, Jr., F. L. 1995. Role of vitamin a and its derivatives in the treatment of human cancer. In *Nutrients in Cancer Prevention and Treatment*, ed. K. N. Prasad, L. Santamaria, and R. M. Williams, 349–362. Totowa, NJ: Humana Press.
81. Vile, G. F., and C. C. Winterbourn. 1988. Inhibition of adriamycin-promoted microsomal lipid peroxidation by beta-carotene, alpha-tocopherol and retinol at high and low oxygen partial pressures. *FEBS Lett* 238 (2): 353–356.
82. McCay, P. B. 1985. Vitamin E: Interactions with free radicals and ascorbate. *Annu Rev Nutr* 5: 323–340.
83. Prasad, K. N., B. Kumar, X. D. Yan, A. J. Hanson, and W. C. Cole. 2003. Alpha-tocopheryl succinate, the most effective form of vitamin E for adjuvant cancer treatment: A review. *J Am Coll Nutr* 22 (2): 108–117.
84. Schwartz, J. L. 1995. Molecular and biochemical control of tumor growth following treatment with carotenoids or tocopherols. In *Nutrients in Cancer Prevention and Treatment*, ed. K. N. Prasad, L. Santamaria, and R. M. Williams, 287–316. Totowa, NJ: Humana Press.
85. Prasad, K. N., and J. Edwards-Prasad. 1992. Vitamin E and cancer prevention: Recent advances and future potentials. *J Am Coll Nutr* 11 (5): 487–500.
86. Witschi, A., S. Reddy, B. Stofer, and B. H. Lauterburg. 1992. The systemic availability of oral glutathione. *Eur J Clin Pharmacol* 43 (6): 667–669.
87. Shen, W., K. Liu, C. Tian, L. Yang, X. Li, J. Ren, L. Packer, C. W. Cotman, and J. Liu. 2008. *R*-alpha-Lipoic acid and acetyl-L-carnitine complementarily promote mitochondrial biogenesis in murine 3T3-L1 adipocytes. *Diabetologia* 51 (1): 165–174.

88. Niki, E. 1997. Mechanisms and dynamics of antioxidant action of ubiquinol. *Mol Aspects Med* 18 (Suppl): S63–S70.
89. Hiramatsu, M., R. D. Velasco, D. S. Wilson, and L. Packer. 1991. Ubiquinone protects against loss of tocopherol in rat liver microsomes and mitochondrial membranes. *Res Commun Chem Pathol Pharmacol* 72 (2): 231–241.
90. Prasad, K. N., W. C. Cole, and K. C. Prasad. 2002. Risk factors for Alzheimer's disease: Role of multiple antioxidants, non-steroidal anti-inflammatory and cholinergic agents alone or in combination in prevention and treatment. *J Am Coll Nutr* 21 (6): 506–522.
91. Prasad, K. N. 2003. Antioxidants in cancer care: When and how to use them as an adjunct to standard and experimental therapies. *Expert Rev Anticancer Ther* 3 (6): 903–915.
92. Gottshall, K., M. E. Hoffer, and B. J. 2006. Use of antioxidants micronutrient compounds in vestibular rehabilitation after operational head trauma or blast injury. In *Barany International Balance Meeting*, Stockholm, Sweden, June 2006.

12 Micronutrients in Improvement of the Standard Therapy in Posttraumatic Stress Disorder

INTRODUCTION

Posttraumatic stress disorder (PTSD) is a complex mental disorder often resulting from exposure to sudden or repeatedly extreme traumatic events such as war, terrorism, natural, or human-caused disaster, as well as violent personal assault such as rape, mugging, domestic violence, and accidents. There is also a strong direct relationship between mild traumatic brain injury (TBI) and PTSD.[1,2] The symptoms of PTSD often appear within 3 months of the exposure to traumatic stressors, and they include unwanted reexperiencing of the trauma in memory (flashbacks, nightmares, triggered emotional responses), passive and active avoidance (emotional numbing, avoidance of discussions about the traumatic event), and hyperarousal.[3] In addition, PTSD is usually accompanied by other psychiatric and medical comorbidities, including depression, substance abuse, cognitive dysfunction, and other problems of physical and mental health. These problems may lead to impairment of the ability to function in social or family life including occupational instability, marital stress, and family problems. Some of the symptoms of PTSD overlap with other diseases including chronic fatigue syndrome, fibromyalgia, and multiple chemical sensitivities.[4] The current gold standard management of PTSD involves antidepressant medications that rarely yield better than a 40% reduction in the Clinician Administered PTSD Scale (CAPS) scores, but most patients still exhibit PTSD symptoms at the end of any treatment trial.[5] Therefore, additional approaches that attenuate some biochemical events that contribute to the progression of PTSD must be developed. In this chapter, among various biochemical events, the role of increased oxidative stress and chronic inflammation in the initiation and progression of PTSD will be discussed. If these biochemical processes are involved in PTSD, the role of micronutrients including dietary and endogenous antioxidants alone or in combination with standard therapy will be discussed in order to reduce the progression of PTSD and to improve the efficacy of standard therapy. In addition, a rational formulation of micronutrient to attenuate oxidative stress and chronic inflammation will be presented for further evaluation.

INCIDENCE AND COST OF PTSD

PTSD affects about 7.7 million Americans over the ages of 18 or about 3.5% of people in this age group in a given year.[6] In a recent large-scale study of military personnel in the current combat theaters, it was demonstrated that U.S. Army and Marine Corps personnel returning from duty in Iraq and Afghanistan exhibited PTSD rates of 18% and 20%, respectively.[7] Before deployment, only 5% of soldiers showed PTSD symptoms, but after a full year of deployment, about 17% of soldiers exhibited PTSD symptoms. The rate of increase in PTSD was proportional to the length of their

TABLE 12.1
Incidence of Partial and Fully Established PTSD in U.S. Military Personnel after Deployment

Source	Incident (%)
Veterans from Iraq, 2006	18–20
Veterans from Vietnam	30.9 in men
	26.9 in women
	22.5 partial PTSD in men
	21.2 partial PTSD in women

Note: The incidence of PTSD in U.S. troops before deployment was 5%. The incidence of PTSD appears to increase with time as well as with repeated combat deployment.

stay in Iraq[8] (Table 12.1). The number of soldiers with PTSD may further increase due to repeated combat deployments.[9]

In 2007, the National Center for Posttraumatic Disorder estimated that the incidence of PTSD among American Vietnam veterans is about 30.9% for men and 26.9% for women. An additional 22.5% of men and 21.2% of women have had partial PTSD. This constitutes about 1.7 million Vietnam veterans who have experienced clinically significant combat-related stress disorder.

The estimated societal cost of PTSD and depression among returning troops for 2 years after deployment varies from about $6000 to more than $25,000 per case. The total cost including direct medical treatment and care, lost productivity, and suicide for 2 years ranges from $4 billion to $6.2 billion (Rand Corporation analysis, 2008).

SYMPTOMS OF PTSD

Symptoms of PTSD typically appear within 3 months of the traumatic stressor often resulting in a diminished quality of life and considerable emotional suffering. Disabling PTSD symptoms include reexperiencing of the trauma in memory (flashbacks, nightmares, triggered emotional responses), passive and active avoidance (emotional numbing, avoidance of discussions about the traumatic event), and hyperarousal.[4,10] In addition, PTSD is usually accompanied by other psychiatric and medical comorbidities, including depression, substance abuse, problems in learning, memory and cognition, and other issues of physical and mental health.[11,12] These problems often times lead to impairment of the ability to function in social or family life including occupational instability, marital, and family problems. Some of the symptoms of PTSD overlap with other diseases including chronic fatigue syndrome, fibromyalgia, and multiple chemical sensitivity.[13]

The gold standard antidepressant medications yield approximately a 40% reduction in CAPS scores, and most patients will still meet criteria for PTSD at the end of an adequate treatment trial.[5] In order to identify new agents that can improve the efficacy of current treatments, it would be important to know at least some of the biochemical events that are associated with PTSD. Some biochemical evidence is described below.

BIOCHEMICAL EVENTS IN PTSD

The fact that reduced hippocampal volume, as determined by magnetic resonance imaging (MRI), is found in patients with PTSD[14–15] suggests a significant loss of cholinergic neurons that could account for cognitive dysfunction. It has been reported that PTSD is associated with general learning and memory impairment.[17] The biochemical events responsible for initiation and progression of

PTSD are not fully understood; however, some that contribute to the progression of PTSD include increased oxidative stress and chronic inflammation, and release of glutamate. These biochemical events can provide a basis for developing an effective strategy for reducing the risk of PTSD and improving its current management (Table 12.2).

INCREASED OXIDATIVE STRESS IN PTSD

There is mounting evidence indicating that free radicals may be involved in the initiation and development of many different human diseases including psychiatric disorders and PTSD.[18] Stress evokes a sustained increase in nitric oxide synthase (NOS) activity that can generate excessive amounts of nitric oxide (NO).[19,20] Oxidation of NO produces peroxynitrite that is very toxic to nerve cells.[13] It has been proposed that deficiency of tetrahydrobioptrin causes NOS to produce superoxide[21] that can oxidize NO to produce peroxynitrite. Peroxynitrite can then damage vital molecules, thus repeating a vicious cycle of producing increased levels of peroxynitrite. The combination of high NOS activity and low levels of tetrahydrobioptrin can produce a sustained increase in peroxynitrite level. Indeed, elevated levels of peroxynitrite and its precursor NO have been observed in patients with PTSD.[22] Platelet monoamine oxidase, which generates excessive amounts of free radicals while degrading catecholamines, is also elevated in patients with PTSD.[23] This is further confirmed by the fact that depletion of catecholamines has been observed in patients with PTSD.[24] Peroxynitrite and other free radicals increase the level of oxidative damage in brain tissue of patients with PTSD causing cognitive and other brain dysfunction. Recently, the expression profiles of certain genes in the mitochondria of autopsied samples of dorsolateral prefrontal cortex of patients with PTSD are altered in comparison to healthy control.[25] This study is important because the activity of dorsolateral prefrontal cortex region of the brain that regulates working memory and fear responses is decreased in PTSD patients.[25] The DNA microarray analysis of postmortem samples of prefrontal cortex from patients with major depression revealed that the gene expression profiles of some specific genes are altered in comparison to those from normal control.[26] The alterations in expression profile of certain genes are very interesting observations, but they have not been confirmed by real-time PCR; therefore, additional studies would be needed to establish changes in the levels of specific genes that are associated with PTSD. Increased levels of oxidative stress may contribute to the cognitive dysfunctions commonly observed in patients with PTSD. It is interesting to point out that increase in oxidative stress, chronic inflammation, and mitochondrial dysfunction have been observed in other neurological diseases such as Alzheimer's disease.[27] Thus, attenuation of oxidative stress appears to be one of the rational choices for reducing the risk of onset and progression of PTSD.

CHRONIC INFLAMMATION IN PTSD

In addition to increased oxidative stress, increased chronic inflammation due to activation of microglia may be associated with PTSD. For example, serum levels of interleukin-6 (IL-6) are elevated

TABLE 12.2
Biochemical Events Responsible for Initiation and Progression of PTSD

Biochemical Events	Status
Markers of oxidative stress	Increases
Markers of chronic inflammation	Increases
Glutamate release	Increases
Certain gene expression profiles	Altered
Extinction of conditioned fear	Impaired

in patients with PTSD.[28] Increased levels of IL-6 and IL-6 receptors were found in patients with PTSD.[29] High levels of tumor necrosis factor-alpha (TNF-alpha) and IL-1beta were elevated in patients with PTSD in comparison to control subjects.[30] Psychological stress induces a chronic inflammatory process.[31] Chronic fear of terror in women, but not in men, is associated with elevated levels of C-reactive protein (CRP) that may contribute to increased risk of cardiovascular disease in PTSD patients.[32] The levels of CRP and receptor to IL-6 were elevated in patients with PTSD.[33] A study has reported that in men, but not in women, the episodes of depression are associated with increased levels of CRP[34]; however, other studies have reported no such association.[35] Increased levels of chronic inflammation may also contribute to the cognitive dysfunctions commonly observed in patients with PTSD. Increased chronic inflammation is also associated with certain neurological diseases such as Alzheimer's disease.[27] Thus, attenuation of chronic inflammation may be one of the rational strategies for reducing the risk of onset and progression of PTSD.

Release of Glutamate in PTSD

The glutamatergic systems appear to play an important role in the pathophysiology of PTSD.[36] Stress-induced glutamate release and glucocorticoids have been implicated to cause hippocampal atrophy in patients with PTSD. This observation is not unexpected because glutamate in high doses is known to be neurotoxic. Glutamate and NO released during stress play a central role in maintaining anxiety disorders.[19,36–38] Stress activates glutamate-NMDA (N-methyl-D-aspartate) receptors and decreases brain-derived neurotrophic factors, and excessive amounts of glutamate can cause death to cholinergic neurons that may account for the cognitive dysfunction associated with PTSD. Therefore, blocking the release of glutamate and reducing the toxicity of glutamate would be useful in reducing the risk and progression of PTSD symptoms. Indeed, antiglutamatergic agents such as lamotrigine improve some of the symptoms of PTSD (reexperiencing hyperarousal and avoidance).[36]

STANDARD THERAPY IN PTSD

Standard therapy includes drugs and psychological/psychiatric treatment. Some examples of drug therapy that has produced limited success are described below.

In a 6-week randomized, double-blind, placebo-controlled trial using 22 chronic PTSD outpatients, it was found that D-serine, an endogenous agonist of NMDA receptor at the site of glycine may improve some of the symptoms of PTSD.[39] Antiglutamatergic agents, such as lamotrigine, were effective in reducing some of the symptoms of PTSD.[36] Selective serotonin reuptake inhibitors also were useful in improving the symptoms of PTSD.[40] The efficacy of other drugs in the treatment of PTSD, such as antidepressants, antiadrenergic agents, anticonvulsants, benzodiazepines, and atypical antipsychotics yielding variable degrees of improvement has been reviewed.[41]

Extinction of conditioned fear appears to be defective in patients with PTSD. D-Cycloserine, a partial agonist of NMDA receptor, was useful in enhancing extinction of learned fear in rats.[42] This was achieved when D-cycloserine was administered shortly before or after extinction training of rats.[43]

Persistent retrieval and maintenance of traumatic memories is a biological process that keeps these memories vivid and thereby maintains the symptoms of PTSD. It has been demonstrated that elevated glucocorticoid levels inhibit memory retrieval processes in animals and humans.[44] In patients with PTSD, low-dose cortisol treatment for 1 month reduced symptoms of traumatic memories without causing adverse health effects, probably by preventing recall of traumatic memories.[44,45]

None of the drugs that are currently used in the treatment of PTSD addressed the issue of increased oxidative stress and chronic inflammation that are associated with the initiation and progression of PTSD. Therefore, we propose a novel antioxidant strategy that can reduce the risk of onset of PTSD and, in combination with drug therapies, can improve their efficacy.

RATIONALE FOR USING MICRONUTRIENTS IN PTSD

In spite of strong scientific rationale for using antioxidants that can reduce the risk of onset of PTSD, no efforts have been made to evaluate the efficacy of antioxidants in deployed troops who have been exposed to traumatic events and environmental stressors during deployment. It is possible that increased oxidative stress, chronic inflammation, and glutamate release occur in these troops who develop PTSD. Intervention with multiple micronutrients including dietary and endogenous antioxidants may help to reduce the risk of developing PTSD.

It is well established that antioxidants are scavengers of free radicals; however, their role in reducing inflammation has not drawn significant attention. There are substantial amounts of data that show that dietary and endogenous antioxidants and antioxidants derived from herbs, fruits, and vegetables inhibit chronic inflammation.[46–58] One of their mechanisms of action may involve suppression of genes induced by proinflammatory cytokines released by microglia[59] and inhibition of TNF-alpha–induced NF-kappa B activation through enhancement of mitogen-activated protein kinase (MAPK).[60]

In spite of strong scientific rationale for using antioxidants in combination with drug therapies, no efforts have been made to evaluate their efficacy in reducing the rate of progression in patients with established PTSD. Increased oxidative stress, chronic inflammation, and glutamate release have been demonstrated in patients with PTSD, and they play an important role in the progression of the disease. Therefore, intervention with multiple micronutrients including dietary and endogenous antioxidants in combination with drug therapies may be more effective in reducing the progression of the disease than the individual agents.

Fear and anxiety release excessive amounts of glutamate. In addition, animal studies have suggested that increased proinflammatory stimuli and oxidative stress cause microglia to release excessive amounts of glutamate, which not only maintain anxiety disorders through the NMDA receptor, but which also contributes to neurodegeneration.[61] Release of glutamate was blocked by vitamin E,[61] and this could help in improving anxiety disorders. Indeed, an inhibitor of the NMDA receptor reduces anxiety,[62] but is toxic. Both vitamin E[63] and coenzyme Q_{10}[64] also protect against glutamate-induced neurotoxicity in cell culture models. Therefore, antioxidants that are nontoxic appear to be one of the rational choices for reducing the glutamate release in patients with PTSD.

Since increased oxidative stress, proinflammatory products of chronic inflammation, and glutamate release are observed in patients with PTSD, antioxidants that neutralize free radicals, reduce inflammation, and prevent glutamate release may be one of the rational choices for reducing the risk of onset and improving the efficacy of current drug therapies in patients with PTSD. Although no studies have been performed to evaluate the role of micronutrients in the prevention or management of PTSD patients, data from the animal and cell culture models and from other human neurological diseases suggest that antioxidants may be useful in reducing the initiation and progression of PTSD as well as improving the efficacy of standard therapy when used adjunctively. For example, mitochondria are considered one of the most sensitive targets of oxidative damage in adult neurons,[65] and impaired mitochondria, commonly found in neurological diseases, generate excessive amounts of free radicals.[66] In addition, it has been reported that beta-amyloid fragments that are associated with neurodegeneration in Alzheimer's disease mediate their action by free radicals.[67] This is supported by the fact that vitamin E protects neuronal cells in culture against beta-amyloid–induced toxicity.[68] Vitamin E at a dose of 2000 IU/day produced some beneficial effects in patients with Alzheimer's disease.[69] Patients consuming antioxidants showed reduced risk of vascular dementia and slower decline of cognitive function in cases of dementia and Alzheimer's disease.[70] We have reported that prostaglandin E_2 (PGE2), a product of inflammatory reactions, is very toxic to mature neurons, and a mixture of antioxidants reduces this toxicity.[71] Glutathione deficiency has been consistently found in autopsied brain samples from patients with neurological diseases such as Alzheimer's disease[72] and Parkinson's disease.[73,74] Administration of coenzyme Q_{10} has been shown to improve clinical symptoms of mitochondrial encephalomyopathies,[75] but only modest improvement in Parkinson's disease.[76] Others have reported inconsistent results with coenzyme Q_{10}.[77] In the MPTP rat model of Parkinson's disease, an administration of a mixture of dietary and endogenous antioxidants before treatment with MPTP blocked MPTP-induced depletion of tyrosine hydroxylase (TH), a rate-limiting enzyme in the biosynthesis of TH, as well as enhanced the expression of TH.[78] Antioxidants also blocked MPTP-induced hypokinesia. In addition, intravenous injection of vitamin B_{12} improved cognitive function in Alzheimer's disease.[79]

PROBLEMS OF USING A SINGLE MICRONUTRIENT IN PTSD

Although no well-designed clinical studies have been performed with one or more antioxidants in PTSD patients, previous clinical studies with a single antioxidant in high-risk populations of other diseases such as cancer, heart disease, and certain neurological diseases have produced inconsistent results. It is well established that the internal oxidative environment of high-risk populations of these diseases is high. It is also known that an individual antioxidant, when oxidized, acts as a pro-oxidant. Therefore, administration of a single antioxidant under the above conditions may produce pro-oxidant effects rather than antioxidant effects. This effect of a single antioxidant may have contributed to the inconsistent results varying from beneficial effects, to no effect, or to harmful effects. I propose that high doses of multiple micronutrients including dietary and endogenous antioxidants, when administered as an adjunct to standard therapy, may increase the efficacy of therapy in reducing the progression of damage in PTSD patients. In addition, when they are administered during deployment, the initial levels of damage and rate of progression of damage may be reduced before intervention with standard therapy.

RATIONALE FOR RECOMMENDING MULTIPLE MICRONUTRIENTS INCLUDING DIETARY AND ENDOGENOUS ANTIOXIDANTS IN PTSD

Because of increased levels of oxidative stress and chronic inflammation, enhanced release of glutamate in PTSD, an oral supplementation with appropriate multiple micronutrients including dietary and endogenous antioxidants appears to be one of the rational choices for improving neurological dysfunction including cognitive impairment. In addition, such a micronutrient preparation in combination with standard therapy may improve its efficacy in the management of PTSD. Experimental designs of most previous clinical studies that have utilized only one or two antioxidants are not suitable for determining the efficacy of multiple micronutrients in improving the efficacy of standard therapy in the management of PTSD. This is due to the fact that their mechanisms of action and distribution at cellular and organ levels differ, their cellular and organ environments (oxygenation, aqueous and lipid components) differ, and their affinity for various types of free radicals differs. For example, beta-carotene (BC) is more effective in quenching oxygen radicals than most other antioxidants.[80] BC can perform certain biological functions that cannot be produced by its metabolite vitamin A, and vice versa.[81,82] It has been reported that BC treatment enhances the expression of the connexin gene, which codes for a gap junction protein in mammalian fibroblasts in culture, whereas vitamin A treatment does not produce such an effect.[82] Vitamin A can induce differentiation in certain normal and cancer cells, whereas BC and other carotenoids do not.[83,84] Thus, BC and vitamin A have, in part, different biological functions.

The gradient of oxygen pressure varies within cells. Some antioxidants, such as vitamin E, are more effective as quenchers of free radicals in reduced oxygen pressure, whereas BC and vitamin A are more effective in higher atmospheric pressures.[85] Vitamin C is necessary to protect cellular components in aqueous environments, whereas carotenoids and vitamins A and E protect cellular components in lipid environments. Vitamin C also plays an important role in maintaining cellular levels of vitamin E by recycling vitamin E radical (oxidized) to the reduced (antioxidant) form.[86] Also, oxidative DNA damage produced by high levels of vitamin C could be protected by vitamin

E. Oxidized forms of vitamins C and E can also act as radicals; therefore, excessive amounts of any one of these forms, when used as a single agent, could be harmful over a long period.

The form of vitamin E used is also important in any clinical trial. It has been established that D-alpha-tocopheryl succinate (alpha-TS) is the most effective form of vitamin E both in vitro and in vivo.[87,88] This form of vitamin E is more soluble than alpha-tocopherol and enters cells more readily. Therefore, it is expected to cross the blood–brain barrier in greater amounts than alpha-tocopherol. However, this has not yet been demonstrated in animals or humans. We have reported that an oral ingestion of alpha-TS (800 IU/day) in humans increased plasma levels of not only alpha-tocopherol, but also alpha-TS, suggesting that a portion of alpha-TS can be absorbed from the intestinal tract before hydrolysis.[89] This observation is important because the conventional assumption based on the rodent studies has been that esterified forms of vitamin E, such as alpha-TS, alpha-tocopheryl nicotinate, or alpha-tocopheryl acetate, can be absorbed from the intestinal tract only after they are hydrolyzed to alpha-tocopherol. Our preliminary data showed that this assumption may not be true for the absorption of alpha-TS in humans.

Glutathione is effective in catabolizing H_2O_2 and anions. However, oral supplementation with glutathione failed to significantly increase plasma levels of glutathione in human subjects,[90] suggesting that this tripeptide is completely hydrolyzed in the gastrointestinal tract. Therefore, I propose to utilize N-acetylcysteine and alpha-lipoic acid that increase the cellular levels of glutathione by different mechanisms in a multiple micronutrient preparation. In addition, R-alpha-lipoic acid and acetyl-L-carnitine together promoted mitochondrial biogenesis in murine adipocytes in culture; however, no effect was observed when these antioxidants were used individually.[91] These types of studies further emphasized the value of using more than one antioxidant in any clinical or laboratory studies involving PTSD.

Another endogenous antioxidant, coenzyme Q_{10}, may also have some potential value in reducing the risk of developing PTSD in high-risk populations and improving the efficacy of standard therapy in PTSD. Since mitochondrial dysfunction may occur in patients with PTSD, and since coenzyme Q_{10} is needed for the generation of ATP by mitochondria, it is essential to add this antioxidant in a multiple micronutrient preparation in order to improve the function of mitochondria. A study has shown that Ubiquinol (coenzyme Q_{10}) scavenges peroxy radicals faster than alpha-tocopherol[92] and, like vitamin C, can regenerate vitamin E in a redox cycle.[93] However, it is a weaker antioxidant than alpha-tocopherol. Coenzyme Q_{10} administration has been shown to improve clinical symptoms in patients with mitochondrial encephalomyopathies.[75]

Selenium is a cofactor of glutathione peroxidase, and Se-glutathione peroxidase increases the intracellular level of glutathione that is a powerful antioxidant. There may be some other mechanisms of action of selenium. Therefore, selenium and coenzyme Q_{10} should be added to a multiple micronutrient preparation.

The values of antioxidants in reducing the risk of cognitive dysfunction have been evaluated in other neurological diseases such as Alzheimer's disease and Parkinson's disease. It has been reported that beta-amyloid fragments that are associated with neurodegeneration in Alzheimer's disease mediate their action by free radicals.[67] This is supported by the fact that vitamin E protects neuronal cells in culture against beta-amyloid–induced toxicity.[68] Vitamin E at a dose of 2000 IU/day produced some beneficial effects in patients with Alzheimer's disease.[69] Patients consuming antioxidants showed reduced risk of vascular dementia and slower decline of cognitive function in cases of dementia and Alzheimer's disease.[70] We have reported that PGE2, a product of inflammatory reactions, is very toxic to mature neurons, and a mixture of antioxidants reduces this toxicity.[71] Glutathione deficiency has been consistently found in autopsied brain samples from patients with neurological diseases such as Alzheimer's disease[72] and Parkinson's disease.[73,74] Administration of coenzyme Q_{10} has been shown to improve clinical symptoms of mitochondrial encephalomyopathies[75] and only modest improvement in Parkinson's disease.[76] Others have reported inconsistent results with coenzyme Q_{10}.[77] These studies suggest that antioxidant micronutrients have neuroprotective value and provide a scientific rationale for testing the efficacy of multiple micronutrients including dietary and endogenous antioxidants in combination with standard therapy in patients with PTSD for reducing the progression of damage. In addition to dietary and endogenous antioxidants, all B vitamins that are necessary for general health should be added to a multiple micronutrient preparation.

A commercial formulation of multiple micronutrients was tested in a clinical study in troops returning from Iraq with mild to moderate TBI. Thirty-four patients with posttraumatic dizziness were admitted to the Naval Medical Center San Diego Clinic over a 2-month period and agreed to participate in the study under the supervision of Dr. Michael Hoffer and his colleagues.[94] All patients had received their injury 3–20 weeks before admission, and they received identical treatment consisting of medical therapy (for any migraines), supportive care, steroids, and vestibular rehabilitation therapy. Fifteen of the 34 patients also received a dose of an antioxidant and micronutrient formula (two capsules by mouth twice a day). At the onset of therapy, all patients were evaluated in outcome measures, which included the Sensory Organization Test (SOT) by Computerized Dynamic Posturography (CDP), the Dynamic Gait Index (DGI), the Activities Balance Confidence (ABC) scale, the Dizziness Handicap Index (DHI), the Vestibular Disorders Activities of Daily Living (VADL) score, and the Balance Scoring System (BESS) test. The study was carried out for 12 weeks. The therapist who graded these outcomes and performed the testing was blinded as to whether the patient was receiving antioxidant therapy or not. The pretrial test scores did not differ significantly between the two groups on any of the tests.

Both groups of patients showed trends toward significant improvement on all tests after the 12 weeks of therapy, but the combination treatment trend was stronger than that of the standard therapy alone group. After only 4 weeks, the SOT score by CDP was 78 for the antioxidant group compared to 63 for the non-antioxidant group. This difference was statistically significant at the $P < 0.05$ level. The improvement noted by the antioxidant group on the other tests was also greater than the non-antioxidant group, although these differences did not reach statistical significance because of the short trial period and small sample size. This study should be expanded using a randomized, double-blind, and placebo-controlled clinical study design in which the efficacy of the proposed multiple micronutrients preparation should be tested in soldiers returning from combat theaters exhibiting mild to moderate TBI or any sign of mental disorders such as anxiety, fear, and depression.

RECOMMENDED MICRONUTRIENTS FOR REDUCING THE RISK OF PTSD IN HIGH-RISK POPULATIONS

High-risk populations for developing PTSD include troops who are in combat theater or those who are returning from combat after one or multiple deployments, family exposed to sudden death in the family, individuals exposed to natural disasters such as earthquake and flood in which a lot of fatalities occur, victims of rape, car accidents, or terrorist attack. These individuals are at high risk for developing PTSD-associated symptoms such as cognitive dysfunction and other neurological abnormalities several years later. They provide an excellent opportunity to study the efficacy of a multiple micronutrients preparation in reducing the risk of developing PTSD in these populations.

A preparation of multiple micronutrients may include vitamin A (retinyl palmitate), vitamin E (both D-alpha-tocopherol and D-alpha-TS), natural mixed carotenoids, vitamin C (calcium ascorbate), coenzyme Q_{10}, R-alpha-lipoic acid, N-acetylcysteine, L-carnitine, vitamin D, all B vitamins, selenium, zinc, chromium, and omega-3 fatty acids. No iron, copper, or manganese would be included because these trace minerals are known to interact with vitamin C to produce free radicals. These trace minerals are absorbed from the intestinal tract more in the presence of antioxidants than in their absence that could result in increased body stores of free forms of these minerals. Increased iron stores have been linked to increased risk of several chronic diseases.[95] Antioxidants from herbs, fruits, and vegetables were not included because they do not produce any unique biological effects that cannot be produced by antioxidants present in the micronutrient preparation.

The recommended micronutrient supplements should be taken orally and divided into two doses, half in the morning and the other half in the evening with meal. This is because the biological half-lives of micronutrients are highly variable which can create high levels of fluctuations in the tissue levels of micronutrients. A twofold difference in the levels of certain micronutrients such as alpha-TS can cause a marked difference in the expression of gene profiles (our unpublished data). To maintain relatively consistent levels of micronutrients in the brain, the proposed micronutrients should be taken twice a day.

The efficacy of the proposed micronutrient formulation in high-risk populations should be tested in well-designed clinical studies. In the meanwhile, the proposed micronutrient recommendations may be adopted by the individuals who are in combat theater or who have suffered from concussive injury during deployment in consultation with their physicians or health professionals. It is expected that the proposed recommendations would reduce risk of developing PTSD.

RECOMMENDED MICRONUTRIENTS IN COMBINATION WITH STANDARD THERAPY IN PTSD

Increased oxidative stress and acute inflammation, and glutamate release have been found in PTSD. The current standard therapies are not considered sufficient in the management of PTSD. The addition of a preparation of multiple micronutrients such as that described in the previous paragraph with high-risk populations of PTSD may improve the efficacy of standard therapy in the management of PTSD. Therefore, the efficacy of this preparation in combination with standard therapy should be tested in patients with PTSD by well-designed clinical studies. In the meanwhile, the proposed micronutrient recommendations may be adopted by the individuals who are suffering from PTSD in consultation with their physicians or health professionals. It is expected that the proposed recommendations would enhance the efficacy of standard therapy in the management of PTSD.

DIET AND LIFESTYLE RECOMMENDATIONS FOR PTSD

In addition to supplementation with multiple micronutrients, a balanced diet low in fat and high in fiber and rich in fruits and vegetables is very necessary for reducing the risk of developing PTSD, as well as for improving the efficacy of standard therapy in the management of PTSD. Lifestyle recommendations include daily moderate exercise, reduced stress, no tobacco smoking, and reduced intake of caffeine and alcoholic beverages.

CONCLUSIONS

In summary, PTSD is a complex mental disorder resulting from exposure to sudden or repeated extreme traumatic events and possibly other stressful environmental stressors. The current standard management of PTSD that includes drug therapies and psychological counseling is considered unsatisfactory. The major biochemical events that contribute to the initiation and progression of PTSD include increased oxidative stress, chronic inflammation, and release of glutamate. Standard therapies do not influence these biochemical events. Since antioxidants neutralize free radicals, reduce inflammation, and inhibit the release and toxicity of glutamate, they may be useful in reducing the risk of onset of PTSD when administered orally before or soon after exposure to traumatic events. In addition, they can improve the efficacy of standard therapies when administered orally in patients with PTSD. A well-designed clinical study to test the efficacy of the proposed multiple micronutrient preparation in reducing the risk of PTSD and improving the efficacy of standard therapy in PTSD should be initiated.

REFERENCES

1. Hoge, C. W., D. McGurk, J. L. Thomas, A. L. Cox, C. C. Engel, and C. A. Castro. 2008. Mild traumatic brain injury in U.S. soldiers returning from Iraq. *N Engl J Med* 358 (5): 453–463.
2. Schneiderman, A. I., E. R. Braver, and H. K. Kang. 2008. Understanding sequelae of injury mechanisms and mild traumatic brain injury incurred during the conflicts in Iraq and Afghanistan: Persistent postconcussive symptoms and posttraumatic stress disorder. *Am J Epidemiol* 167 (12): 1446–1452.
3. King, D., L. King, G. A. Leskin, and F. W. Weathers. 1998. Confirmatory factor analysis of the clinician-administered PTSD scale: Evidence for the dimensionality of posttraumatic stress disorder. *Psychological Assessment* 10: 90–96.
4. Stander, V. A., L. L. Merrill, C. J. Thomsen, and J. S. Milner. 2007. Posttraumatic stress symptoms in Navy personnel: Prevalence rates among recruits in basic training. *J Anxiety Disord* 21 (6): 860–870.
5. Hamner, M. B., S. Robert, and B. C. Frueh. 2004. Treatment-resistant posttraumatic stress disorder: Strategies for intervention. *CNS Spectr* 9 (10): 740–752.
6. Kessler, R. C., W. T. Chiu, O. Demler, K. R. Merikangas, and E. E. Walters. 2005. Prevalence, severity, and comorbidity of 12-month DSM-IV disorders in the National Comorbidity Survey Replication. *Arch Gen Psychiatry* 62 (6): 617–627.
7. Hoge, C. W., C. A. Castro, S. C. Messer, D. McGurk, D. I. Cotting, and R. L. Koffman. 2004. Combat duty in Iraq and Afghanistan, mental health problems, and barriers to care. *N Engl J Med* 351 (1): 13–22.
8. Castro, C., and C. W. Hoge. 2005. Building psychological resiliency and mitigating the risks of combat and deployment stressors faced by soldiers. Presented at NATO Human Factors and Medicine Panel Symposium, Prague, Czech Republic, October 3–5, 2005.
9. Friedman, M. J. 2005. Veterans' mental health in the wake of war. *N Engl J Med* 352 (13): 1287–1290.
10. Leskin, G. A., D. G. Kaloupek, and T. M. Keane. 1998. Treatment for traumatic memories: Review and recommendations. *Clin Psychol Rev* 18 (8): 983–1001.
11. Brewin, C. R. 2001. A cognitive neuroscience account of posttraumatic stress disorder and its treatment. *Behav Res Ther* 39: 373–393.
12. King, L. A., D. W. King, J. A. Fairbank, T. M. Keane, and G. A. Adams. 1998. Resilience-recovery factors in post-traumatic stress disorder among female and male Vietnam veterans: Hardiness, postwar social support, and additional stressful life events. *J Pers Soc Psychol* 74 (2): 420–434.
13. Pall, M. L., and J. D. Satterlee. 2001. Elevated nitric oxide/peroxynitrite mechanism for the common etiology of multiple chemical sensitivity, chronic fatigue syndrome, and posttraumatic stress disorder. *Ann N Y Acad Sci* 933: 323–329.
14. Bremner, J. D., T. M. Scott, R. C. Delaney, S. M. Southwick, J. W. Mason, D. R. Johnson, R. B. Innis, G. McCarthy, and D. S. Charney. 1993. Deficits in short-term memory in posttraumatic stress disorder. *Am J Psychiatry* 150 (7): 1015–1019.
15. Tischler, L., S. R. Brand, K. Stavitsky, E. Labinsky, R. Newmark, R. Grossman, M. S. Buchsbaum, and R. Yehuda. 2006. The relationship between hippocampal volume and declarative memory in a population of combat veterans with and without PTSD. *Ann NY Acad Sci* 1071: 405–409.
16. Villarreal, G., D. A. Hamilton, H. Petropoulos, I. Driscoll, L. M. Rowland, J. A. Griego, P. W. Kodituwakku, B. L. Hart, R. Escalona, and W. M. Brooks. 2002. Reduced hippocampal volume and total white matter volume in posttraumatic stress disorder. *Biol Psychiatry* 52 (2): 119–125.
17. Burriss, L., E. Ayers, J. Ginsberg, and D. A. Powell. 2008. Learning and memory impairment in PTSD: Relationship to depression. *Depress Anxiety* 25 (2): 149–157.
18. Bremner, J. D. 2006. Stress and brain atrophy. *CNS Neurol Disord Drug Targets* 5 (5): 503–512.
19. Harvey, B. H., T. Bothma, A. Nel, G. Wegener, and D. J. Stein. 2005. Involvement of the NMDA receptor, NO-cyclic GMP and nuclear factor K-beta in an animal model of repeated trauma. *Hum Psychopharmacol* 20 (5): 367–373.
20. Harvey, B. H., F. Oosthuizen, L. Brand, G. Wegener, and D. J. Stein 2004. Stress–restress evokes sustained iNOS activity and altered GABA levels and NMDA receptors in rat hippocampus. *Psychopharmacology (Berl)* 175 (4): 494–502.
21. Pall, M. L. 2007. Nitric oxide synthase partial uncoupling as a key switching mechanism for the NO/ONOO-cycle. *Med Hypotheses* 69 (4): 821–825.
22. Tezcan, E., M. Atmaca, M. Kuloglu, and B. Ustundag. 2003. Free radicals in patients with post-traumatic stress disorder. *Eur Arch Psychiatry Clin Neurosci* 253 (2): 89–91.
23. Richardson, J. S. 1993. On the functions of monoamine oxidase, the emotions, and adaptation to stress. *Int J Neurosci* 70 (1–2): 75–84.

24. Pivac, N., J. Knezevic, D. Kozaric-Kovacic, M. Dezeljin, M. Mustapic, D. Rak, T. Matijevic, J. Pavelic, and D. Muck-Seler. 2007. Monoamine oxidase (MAO) intron 13 polymorphism and platelet MAO-B activity in combat-related posttraumatic stress disorder. *J Affect Disord* 103 (1–3): 131–138.
25. Su, Y. A., J. Wu, L. Zhang, Q. Zhang, D. M. Su, P. He, B. D. Wang, et al. 2008. Dysregulated mitochondrial genes and networks with drug targets in postmortem brain of patients with posttraumatic stress disorder (PTSD) revealed by human mitochondria-focused cDNA microarrays. *Int J Biol Sci* 4 (4): 223–235.
26. Tochigi, M., K. Iwamoto, M. Bundo, T. Sasaki, N. Kato, and T. Kato. 2008. Gene expression profiling of major depression and suicide in the prefrontal cortex of postmortem brains. *Neurosci Res* 60 (2): 184–191.
27. Prasad, K. N., W. C. Cole, and K. C. Prasad. 2002. Risk factors for Alzheimer's disease: Role of multiple antioxidants, non-steroidal anti-inflammatory and cholinergic agents alone or in combination in prevention and treatment. *J Am Coll Nutr* 21 (6): 506–522.
28. Yehuda, R. 2001. Biology of posttraumatic stress disorder. *J Clin Psychiatry* 62 (Suppl 17): 41–46.
29. Maes, M., A. H. Lin, L. Delmeire, A. Van Gastel, G. Kenis, R. De Jongh, and E. Bosmans. 1999. Elevated serum interleukin-6 (IL-6) and IL-6 receptor concentrations in posttraumatic stress disorder following accidental man-made traumatic events. *Biol Psychiatry* 45 (7): 833–839.
30. von Kanel, R., U. Hepp, B. Kraemer, R. Traber, M. Keel, L. Mica, and U. Schnyder. 2007. Evidence for low-grade systemic proinflammatory activity in patients with posttraumatic stress disorder. *J Psychiatr Res* 41 (9): 744–752.
31. Sutherland, A. G., D. A. Alexander, and J. D. Hutchison. 2003. Disturbance of pro-inflammatory cytokines in post-traumatic psychopathology. *Cytokine* 24 (5): 219–225.
32. Melamed, S., A. Shirom, S. Toker, S. Berliner, and I. Shapira. 2004. Association of fear of terror with low-grade inflammation among apparently healthy employed adults. *Psychosom Med* 66 (4): 484–491.
33. Miller, R. J., A. G. Sutherland, J. D. Hutchison, and D. A. Alexander. 2001. C-reactive protein and interleukin 6 receptor in post-traumatic stress disorder: A pilot study. *Cytokine* 13 (4): 253–255.
34. Danner, M., S. V. Kasl, J. L. Abramson, and V. Vaccarino. 2003. Association between depression and elevated C-reactive protein. *Psychosom Med* 65 (3): 347–356.
35. Douglas, K. M., A. J. Taylor, and P. G. O'Malley. 2004. Relationship between depression and C-reactive protein in a screening population. *Psychosom Med* 66 (5): 679–683.
36. Nair, J., and S. Singh Ajit. 2008. The role of the glutamatergic system in posttraumatic stress disorder. *CNS Spectr* 13 (7): 585–591.
37. Joca, S. R., F. R. Ferreira, and F. S. Guimaraes. 2007. Modulation of stress consequences by hippocampal monoaminergic, glutamatergic and nitrergic neurotransmitter systems. *Stress* 10 (3): 227–249.
38. Trist, D. G. 2000. Excitatory amino acid agonists and antagonists: Pharmacology and therapeutic applications. *Pharm Acta Helv* 74 (2–3): 221–229.
39. Heresco-Levy, U., A. Vass, B. Bloch, H. Wolosker, E. Dumin, L. Balan, L. Deutsch, and I. Kremer. 2009. Pilot controlled trial of D-serine for the treatment of post-traumatic stress disorder. *Int J Neuropsychopharmacol* 12: 1275–1282.
40. Ipser, J., S. Seedat, and D. J. Stein. 2006. Pharmacotherapy for post-traumatic stress disorder—A systematic review and meta-analysis. *S Afr Med J* 96 (10): 1088–1096.
41. Ravindran, L. N., and M. B. Stein. 2009. Pharmacotherapy of PTSD: Premises, principles, and priorities. *Brain Res* 1293: 24–39.
42. Richardson, R., L. Ledgerwood, and J. Cranney. 2004. Facilitation of fear extinction by D-cycloserine: Theoretical and clinical implications. *Learn Mem* 11 (5): 510–516.
43. Vervliet, B. 2008. Learning and memory in conditioned fear extinction: Effects of D-cycloserine. *Acta Psychol (Amst)* 127 (3): 601–613.
44. de Quervain, D. J., and J. Margraf. 2008. Glucocorticoids for the treatment of post-traumatic stress disorder and phobias: A novel therapeutic approach. *Eur J Pharmacol* 583 (2–3): 365–371.
45. Schelling, G. 2002. Effects of stress hormones on traumatic memory formation and the development of posttraumatic stress disorder in critically ill patients. *Neurobiol Learn Mem* 78 (3): 596–609.
46. Abate, A., G. Yang, P. A. Dennery, S. Oberle, and H. Schroder. 2000. Synergistic inhibition of cyclooxygenase-2 expression by vitamin E and aspirin. *Free Radic Biol Med* 29 (11): 1135–1142.
47. Devaraj, S., R. Tang, B. Adams-Huet, A. Harris, T. Seenivasan, J. A. de Lemos, and I. Jialal. 2007. Effect of high-dose alpha-tocopherol supplementation on biomarkers of oxidative stress and inflammation and carotid atherosclerosis in patients with coronary artery disease. *Am J Clin Nutr* 86 (5): 1392–1398.
48. Fu, Y., S. Zheng, J. Lin, J. Ryerse, and A. Chen. 2008. Curcumin protects the rat liver from CCl4-caused injury and fibrogenesis by attenuating oxidative stress and suppressing inflammation. *Mol Pharmacol* 73 (2): 399–409.

49. Hori, K., D. Hatfield, F. Maldarelli, B. J. Lee, and K. A. Clouse. 1997. Selenium supplementation suppresses tumor necrosis factor alpha-induced human immunodeficiency virus type 1 replication in vitro. *AIDS Res Hum Retroviruses* 13 (15): 1325–1332.
50. Jesudason, E. P., J. G. Masilamoni, B. S. Ashok, B. Baben, V. Arul, K. S. Jesudoss, W. C. Jebaraj, S. Dhandayuthapani, S. Vignesh, and R. Jayakumar. 2008. Inhibitory effects of short-term administration of DL-alpha-lipoic acid on oxidative vulnerability induced by Abeta amyloid fibrils (25–35) in mice. *Mol Cell Biochem* 311 (1–2): 145–156.
51. Kuhlmann, M. K., and N. W. Levin. 2008. Potential interplay between nutrition and inflammation in dialysis patients. *Contrib Nephrol* 161: 76–82.
52. Lee, H. S., K. K. Jung, J. Y. Cho, M. H. Rhee, S. Hong, M. Kwon, S. H. Kim, and S. Y. Kang. 2007. Neuroprotective effect of curcumin is mainly mediated by blockade of microglial cell activation. *Pharmazie* 62 (12): 937–942.
53. Li, Y., L. Liu, S. W. Barger, R. E. Mrak, and W. S. Griffin. 2001. Vitamin E suppression of microglial activation is neuroprotective. *J Neurosci Res* 66 (2): 163–170.
54. Peairs, A. T., and J. W. Rankin. 2008. Inflammatory response to a high-fat, low-carbohydrate weight loss diet: Effect of antioxidants. *Obesity (Silver Spring)* 16 (7): 1573–1578.
55. Rahman, S., K. Bhatia, A. Q. Khan, M. Kaur, F. Ahmad, H. Rashid, M. Athar, F. Islam, and S. Raisuddin. 2008. Topically applied vitamin E prevents massive cutaneous inflammatory and oxidative stress responses induced by double application of 12-*O*-tetradecanoylphorbol-13-acetate (TPA) in mice. *Chem Biol Interact* 172 (3): 195–205.
56. Suzuki, Y. J., B. B. Aggarwal, and L. Packer. 1992. Alpha-lipoic acid is a potent inhibitor of NF-kappa B activation in human T cells. *Biochem Biophys Res Commun* 189 (3): 1709–1715.
57. Wood, L. G., M. L. Garg, H. Powell, and P. G. Gibson. 2008. Lycopene-rich treatments modify noneosinophilic airway inflammation in asthma: Proof of concept. *Free Radic Res* 42 (1): 94–102.
58. Zhu, J., W. Yong, X. Wu, Y. Yu, J. Lv, C. Liu, X. Mao, et al. 2008. Anti-inflammatory effect of resveratrol on TNF-alpha-induced MCP-1 expression in adipocytes. *Biochem Biophys Res Commun* 369 (2): 471–477.
59. Wang, J. Y., L. L. Wen, Y. N. Huang, Y. T. Chen, and M. C. Ku. 2006. Dual effects of antioxidants in neurodegeneration: Direct neuroprotection against oxidative stress and indirect protection via suppression of glia-mediated inflammation. *Curr Pharm Des* 12 (27): 3521–3533.
60. Lee, C. K., E. Y. Lee, Y. G. Kim, S. H. Mun, H. B. Moon, and B. Yoo. 2008. Alpha-lipoic acid inhibits TNF-alpha induced NF-kappa B activation through blocking of MEKK1-MKK4-IKK signaling cascades. *Int Immunopharmacol* 8 (2): 362–370.
61. Barger, S. W., M. E. Goodwin, M. M. Porter, and M. L. Beggs. 2007. Glutamate release from activated microglia requires the oxidative burst and lipid peroxidation. *J Neurochem* 101 (5): 1205–1213.
62. Davis, M., K. Ressler, B. O. Rothbaum, and R. Richardson. 2006. Effects of D-cycloserine on extinction: Translation from preclinical to clinical work. *Biol Psychiatry* 60 (4): 369–375.
63. Schubert, D., H. Kimura, and P. Maher. 1992. Growth factors and vitamin E modify neuronal glutamate toxicity. *Proc Natl Acad Sci U S A* 89 (17): 8264–8267.
64. Sandhu, J. K., S. Pandey, M. Ribecco-Lutkiewicz, R. Monette, H. Borowy-Borowski, P. R. Walker, and M. Sikorska. 2003. Molecular mechanisms of glutamate neurotoxicity in mixed cultures of NT2-derived neurons and astrocytes: Protective effects of coenzyme Q10. *J Neurosci Res* 72 (6): 691–703.
65. Wallace, D. C. 1992. Mitochondrial genetics: A paradigm for aging and degenerative diseases? *Science* 256 (5057): 628–632.
66. Mutisya, E. M., A. C. Bowling, and M. F. Beal. 1994. Cortical cytochrome oxidase activity is reduced in Alzheimer's disease. *J Neurochem* 63 (6): 2179–2184.
67. Schubert, D., C. Behl, R. Lesley, A. Brack, R. Dargusch, Y. Sagara, and H. Kimura. 1995. Amyloid peptides are toxic via a common oxidative mechanism. *Proc Natl Acad Sci U S A* 92 (6): 1989–1993.
68. Behl, C., J. Davis, G. M. Cole, and D. Schubert. 1992. Vitamin E protects nerve cells from amyloid beta protein toxicity. *Biochem Biophys Res Commun* 186 (2): 944–950.
69. Sano, M., C. Ernesto, R. G. Thomas, M. R. Klauber, K. Schafer, M. Grundman, P. Woodbury, et al. 1997. A controlled trial of selegiline, alpha-tocopherol, or both as treatment for Alzheimer's disease. The Alzheimer's Disease Cooperative Study. *N Engl J Med* 336 (17): 1216–1222.
70. Maxwell, C. J., M. S. Hicks, D. B. Hogan, J. Basran, and E. M. Ebly. 2005. Supplemental use of antioxidant vitamins and subsequent risk of cognitive decline and dementia. *Dement Geriatr Cogn Disord* 20 (1): 45–51.
71. Yan, X. D., B. Kumar, P. Nahreini, A. J. Hanson, J. E. Prasad, and K. N. Prasad. 2005. Prostaglandin-induced neurodegeneration is associated with increased levels of oxidative markers and reduced by a mixture of antioxidants. *J Neurosci Res* 81 (1): 85–90.

72. Liu, H., H. Wang, S. Shenvi, T. M. Hagen, and R. M. Liu. 2004. Glutathione metabolism during aging and in Alzheimer disease. *Ann NY Acad Sci* 1019: 346–349.
73. Chinta, S. J., M. J. Kumar, M. Hsu, S. Rajagopalan, D. Kaur, A. Rane, D. G. Nicholls, J. Choi, and J. K. Andersen. 2007. Inducible alterations of glutathione levels in adult dopaminergic midbrain neurons result in nigrostriatal degeneration. *J Neurosci* 27 (51), 13997–14006.
74. Hsu, M., B. Srinivas, J. Kumar, R. Subramanian, and J. Andersen. 2005. Glutathione depletion resulting in selective mitochondrial complex I inhibition in dopaminergic cells is via an NO-mediated pathway not involving peroxynitrite: Implications for Parkinson's disease. *J Neurochem* 92 (5): 1091–1103.
75. Chen, R. S., C. C. Huang, and N. S. Chu. 1997. Coenzyme Q10 treatment in mitochondrial encephalomyopathies. Short-term double-blind, crossover study. *Eur Neurol* 37 (4): 212–218.
76. Muller, T., T. Buttner, A. F. Gholipour, and W. Kuhn. 2003. Coenzyme Q10 supplementation provides mild symptomatic benefit in patients with Parkinson's disease. *Neurosci Lett* 341 (3): 201–204.
77. The NINDS NET-PD Investigators. 2007. A randomized clinical trial of coenzyme Q10 and GPI-1485 in early Parkinson disease. *Neurology* 68: 20–28.
78. King, J., V. Mackey, K. Prasad and C. Charlton. 2008. Blockage of the proposed precipitating stage for Parkinson's disease by antioxidants: A potential preventive measure for PD. *FASEB J* 22: 715.2a.
79. Ikeda, T., K. Yamamoto, K. Takahashi, Y. Kaku, M. Uchiyama, K. Sugiyama, and M. Yamada. 1992. Treatment of Alzheimer-type dementia with intravenous mecobalamin. *Clin Ther* 14 (3): 426–437.
80. Krinsky, N. I. 1989. Antioxidant functions of carotenoids. *Free Radic Biol Med* 7 (6): 617–635.
81. Hazuka, M. B., J. Edwards-Prasad, F. Newman, J. J. Kinzie, and K. N. Prasad. 1990. Beta-carotene induces morphological differentiation and decreases adenylate cyclase activity in melanoma cells in culture. *J Am Coll Nutr* 9 (2): 143–149.
82. Zhang, L. X., R. V. Cooney, and J. S. Bertram. 1992. Carotenoids up-regulate connexin43 gene expression independent of their provitamin A or antioxidant properties. *Cancer Res* 52 (20): 5707–5712.
83. Carter, C. A., M. Pogribny, A. Davidson, C. D. Jackson, L. J. McGarrity, and S. M. Morris. 1996. Effects of retinoic acid on cell differentiation and reversion toward normal in human endometrial adenocarcinoma (RL95-2) cells. *Anticancer Res* 16 (1): 17–24.
84. Meyskens, Jr., F. L. 1995. Role of vitamin A and its derivatives in the treatment of human cancer. In *Nutrients in Cancer Prevention and Treatment*, ed. K. N. Prasad, L. Santamaria, and R. M. Williams, 349–362. Totowa, NJ: Humana Press.
85. Vile, G. F., and C. C. Winterbourn. 1988. Inhibition of adriamycin-promoted microsomal lipid peroxidation by beta-carotene, alpha-tocopherol and retinol at high and low oxygen partial pressures. *FEBS Lett* 238 (2): 353–356.
86. McCay, P. B. 1985. Vitamin E: Interactions with free radicals and ascorbate. *Annu Rev Nutr* 5: 323–340.
87. Prasad, K. N., B. Kumar, X. D. Yan, A. J. Hanson, and W. C. Cole. 2003. Alpha-tocopheryl succinate, the most effective form of vitamin E for adjuvant cancer treatment: A review. *J Am Coll Nutr* 22 (2): 108–117.
88. Schwartz, J. L. 1995. Molecular and biochemical control of tumor growth following treatment with carotenoids or tocopherols. In *Nutrients in Cancer Prevention and Treatment*, ed. K. N. Prasad, L. Santamaria, and R. M. Williams, 287–316. Totowa, NJ: Humana Press.
89. Prasad, K. N., and J. Edwards-Prasad. 1992. Vitamin E and cancer prevention: Recent advances and future potentials. *J Am Coll Nutr* 11 (5): 487–500.
90. Witschi, A., S. Reddy, B. Stofer, and B. H. Lauterburg. 1992. The systemic availability of oral glutathione. *Eur J Clin Pharmacol* 43 (6): 667–669.
91. Shen, W., K. Liu, C. Tian, L. Yang, X. Li, J. Ren, L. Packer, C. W. Cotman, and J. Liu. 2008. R-alpha-Lipoic acid and acetyl-L-carnitine complementarily promote mitochondrial biogenesis in murine 3T3-L1 adipocytes. *Diabetologia* 51 (1): 165–174.
92. Niki, E. 1997. Mechanisms and dynamics of antioxidant action of ubiquinol. *Mol Aspects Med* 18 (Suppl): S63–S70.
93. Hiramatsu, M., R. D. Velasco, D. S. Wilson, and L. Packer. 1991. Ubiquinone protects against loss of tocopherol in rat liver microsomes and mitochondrial membranes. *Res Commun Chem Pathol Pharmacol* 72 (2): 231–241.
94. Gottshall, K., M. E. Hoffer, and B. J. Balough. 2006. Use of antioxidants micronutrient compounds in vestibular rehabilitation after operational head trauma or blast injury. *Barany International Balance Meeting*, Stockholm, Sweden, June 2006.
95. Olanow, C. W., and G. W. Arendash. 1994. Metals and free radicals in neurodegeneration. *Curr Opin Neurol* 7 (6): 548–558.

13 Micronutrients in Improvement of the Standard Therapy in Traumatic Brain Injury

INTRODUCTION

Traumatic brain injury (TBI), also called head injury, occurs when a sudden trauma causes damage to the brain. TBI can occur with or without penetrating head injury. TBI without penetrating head injury is also called concussive injury that may express as a mild, moderate, or severe form. A concussion occurs when the brain is violently rocked back and forth within the skull following a blow to the head or neck such as that observed in contact sports like football or when in close proximity to a concussive blast pressure wave. Most TBIs occur as a mild form. TBI with penetrating head injury could also be mild, moderate, or severe and occur when an object penetrates the skull and damages the brain. This form of TBI is often associated with vehicle crashes, improvised explosive devices (IEDs), and combat-related injuries. TBI with penetrating head injury is easily recognizable, but concussive injury is difficult to identify after injury.

Despite measures such as standardized treatment guidelines, several clinical studies aimed at identifying therapeutic agents, and improved understanding of the mechanisms of cellular damage, treatment strategies for patients with TBI remain unsatisfactory. In addition, there is no effective strategy to reduce the risk of dementia and other forms of mental disorders associated with TBI. In order to develop a rational strategy for reducing the progression of TBI, it would be important to identify major biological events that play a crucial role in the progression of this type of injury.

A few studies suggested that increased levels of oxidative stress, inflammation, and release of glutamate are involved in the progression of damage following acute TBI or concussive injury. Since antioxidants neutralize free radicals and reduce inflammation, and can prevent the release and toxicity of glutamate, they appear to be one of the rational choices for improving the current management of TBI and concussive injury as adjunctive therapy. The clinical studies to evaluate the efficacy of antioxidants in these injuries have not been performed in a satisfactory manner. Most studies with a single antioxidant have been performed in animal models or cell culture models. The results of these studies have consistently shown beneficial effects in TBI.

This chapter describes briefly the causes, incidence and cost, symptoms, and major biochemicals contributing to the progression of TBI. In addition, this chapter presents scientific rationale and evidence in support of a hypothesis that daily supplementation with multiple micronutrients, including dietary and endogenous antioxidants, may improve the efficacy of standard therapy in acute and long-term management of TBI.

CAUSES OF TBI

Among U.S. soldiers deployed to the wars in Iraq and Afghanistan, blasts including IEDs, vehicle crashes, and other combat-related injuries are the main causes of the increased incidence of TBI with penetrating head injury. The exposure to blast pressure waves can induce varying degrees of concussive injury in combat troops. Most troops in combat theater suffer from this form of TBI.

Among civilians, transportation accidents involving automobiles, motorcycles, bicycles, and pedestrians are the major causes of TBI with penetrating head injury. Sports, especially contact sports such as football, soccer, and hockey, can cause concussive injury.

INCIDENCE AND COST OF TBI

U.S. TROOPS

There is no precise estimate of TBI in injured soldiers returning from Iraq and Afghanistan. About 65% of soldiers are injured by explosive devices. Because of an excellent trauma care in the battlefield, the number of survivors has increased, resulting in a higher number of soldiers with TBI. In the Editorial section of *The Lancet* (a British clinical medical journal), December, 6, 2007, it was mentioned that the proportion of injured soldiers with TBI increased from 14% to 20% in the previous U.S. wars to 60% in the current wars in Iraq and Afghanistan. Others estimate that about 30% of all soldiers with combat-related injuries seen at Walter Reed Army Medical Center from 2003 to 2005 sustained a TBI. At present, about 320,000 soldiers who served in Iraq and Afghanistan have a mild TBI. About 90% of TBI are of the mild type.

U.S. CIVILIANS

In the U.S. civilian population, about 1.4 million people suffer from a TBI every year, about 235,000 are hospitalized, and about 1.1 million are treated and released from an emergency department, and about 50,000 people die.[1] Among children ages 0 to 14 years 2685 deaths, 37,000 hospitalizations, and 435,000 visits annually occur due to a TBI. The CDC Injury Center has estimated that about 3.8 million sports- and recreation-related concussions occur in the United States each year. The CDC has estimated that at least 5.3 million Americans who suffered from TBI have a long-term or lifelong need for help to perform activities of daily living.

The cost per year per person with mild TBI is about $32,000; with moderate to severe TBI is $268,000 to more than $408,000. Thus, the economic cost of TBI is enormous; the emotional cost of the individuals with TBI and their families cannot be measured. In 2000, the direct medical costs and indirect costs, such as lost productivity because of TBI, are estimated to be $60 billion in the United States.[2]

SYMPTOMS AND CONSEQUENCES OF TBI

Symptoms of TBI can be mild, moderate, or severe, depending upon the extent of damage to the brain. Most TBI's are of the mild type. Individuals with a mild TBI may remain conscious or may become unconscious for a few seconds or minutes. Other symptoms of a mild TBI include headache, confusion, light-headedness, dizziness, blurred vision, tinnitus (ringing in the ears), fatigue, alterations in sleeping patterns, mood changes, trouble with memory, concentration, and thinking. Individuals with a moderate or severe TBI may exhibit additional symptoms. They include a headache that gets worse or remains persistent, repeated vomiting or nausea, convulsions or seizures, an inability to awaken from sleep, dilation of one or both pupils of the eyes, slurred speech, weakness or numbness in the extremities, loss of coordination, and increased confusion, restlessness, or agitation. The long-term quality of life remains very poor in individuals with TBI with or without penetrating head injury.

SYMPTOMS AND CONSEQUENCES OF CONCUSSIVE INJURY

Despite evolutionary changes in protective equipment, concussive injuries remain a major health risk for professional football players.[3,4] Cerebral concussion is a type of TBI that is normally produced by acceleration and deceleration of the head. It can also happen during the rapid displacement and rotation of the cranium after peak head acceleration and momentum transfer by helmet impacts.[5] It is characterized by a sudden brief impairment of consciousness, paralysis of reflex activity, and loss of memory. Sports-related concussions have been classified into simple and complex concussions (recommendation of the Second International Conference on Concussion in Sport, 2005). Athletes who are slow to recover (i.e., more than 10 days) are classified as having complex concussions. Brain deformation may occur after the primary head acceleration.[5] Damage to the midbrain correlated with memory and cognitive problems after concussion. The major depression commonly observed after concussion contributes to impairment of memory, processing speed, verbal memory, and executive function.[6-8] An early onset of dementia may be initiated by repetitive cerebral concussions in professional football players.[9,10] Balance disorders are also considered one of the major health problems associated with the TBI.[10,11]

RISK OF POSTTRAUMATIC DISORDER ASSOCIATED WITH TBI

Extensive studies on TBI and its relationship with posttraumatic stress disorder (PTSD) and concussive injuries have been discussed in two recent epidemiologic studies in U.S. soldiers returning from Iraq and Afghanistan.[12,13] In one study, among 2525 soldiers, 4.9% reported injury with loss of consciousness, 10.3% reported injuries with altered mental status, and 17.2% reported other injuries during deployment. Among those who reported loss of consciousness, the incidence of PTSD was about 43.9%; among those reporting altered mental status, it was 27.3%; and those reporting other injuries, it was 16.2%. In contrast, those soldiers reporting no injury in combat, the incidence of PTSD was only 9.1%. It was proposed that the strong association between mild TBI and PTSD may be due to life-threatening combat experiences; in some cases, it could reflect neurological deficits as well as traumatic stress. Female soldiers had a higher incidence of PTSD than male soldiers.

BIOCHEMICAL EVENTS THAT CONTRIBUTE TO THE PROGRESSION OF DAMAGE FOLLOWING TBI

Both animal and human studies show that TBI causes a significant loss of cortical tissue at the site of injury (primary damage) that is followed by a secondary damage involving increased oxidative damage, mitochondrial dysfunction, release of predominantly proinflammatory cytokines and glutamate leading to neurological dysfunction. The major biochemical events that contribute to the progression of acute and chronic damage following TBI include increased oxidative stress and chronic inflammation, and mitochondrial dysfunction and release of excessive amounts of glutamate. Therefore, attenuation of these biochemical events in TBI patients may help to reduce the progression of damage when combined with standard therapy, and reduced the risk of neurological abnormalities including cognitive impairment.

EVIDENCE FOR INCREASED OXIDATIVE STRESS IN TBI

Increased oxidative stress due to production of excessive amounts of free radicals derived from oxygen and nitrogen occur after TBI.[14-17] Increased production of superoxide radicals has been demonstrated in mice.[18] The extent of oxidative damage appeared to be directly proportional to the severity of TBI in a rat model of TBI.[19] The levels of antioxidant enzymes Mn-SOD (manganese-dependent superoxide dismutase) and glutathione reductase decreased more in older rats than the younger ones following TBI, whereas the levels of markers of oxidative damage such as products of lipid peroxidation (acrolein and 4-hydroxynonenal) increased more in the older rats than the younger rats.[17] In rats, there appears to be a close relationship between degree of oxidative stress and severity of brain damage following TBI as evidenced by the highest values of malondialdehyde

(MDA) and lowest value of ascorbate.[20] The total antioxidant reserves of brain homogenates and water-soluble antioxidants reserves as well as tissue concentration of ascorbate, glutathione, sulfhydryl proteins were reduced after TBI in rats.[21] TBI induced peroxynitrite-mediated oxidative damage to mitochondrial function that precedes neuronal loss in the brain. The oxidation of nitric oxide (NO) forms peroxynitrite. Animal studies have revealed that TBI increased NO production that impairs mitochondrial function by inhibiting cytochrome oxidase.[22] Cytochrome oxidase is a key enzyme needed to generate energy. Thus, the energy level in tissue decreased after TBI that may interfere with repair process. TBI also increased inducible nitric oxide synthase (iNOS) activity that contributes to neurological deficits but not to cerebral edema by generating excessive amounts of NO.[23] In a rat model of traumatic injury (unilateral moderate cortical contusion), increased oxidative damage occurs as early as 3 h following TBI that adversely affects synaptic function and plasticity of hippocampal neurons and, thereby, enhances cognitive dysfunction.[24] In another model of TBI (fluid percussion brain injury in rat), it was observed that protein carbonylation and thiobarbituric acid-reactive substances (TBARS) levels increased in parietal cortex 1 and 3 months after injury. These changes in markers of oxidative damage were associated with the progressive decrease in the activity of Na^+,K^+-ATPase.[25] These results suggest that increase in oxidative stress associated with decrease in Na^+,K^+-ATPase activity may account for cognitive dysfunction observed following TBI.

A few human studies also confirm the role of oxidative stress in the progression of TBI. F_2-isoprostane is a marker of lipid peroxidation, whereas neuron-specific enolase (NSE) is considered a marker of neuronal damage. The levels of F_2-isoprostane and NSE increased in the cerebrospinal fluid (CSF) samples following TBI in children and infants.[26] Both the levels of ascorbate and glutathione decreased in the CSF of children and infants following TBI.[27] In a recent study, the level of 3-nitrotyrosine increased in the CSF of the patients with TBI.[28] It has been reported that the levels of beta-amyloid fragment (A beta-42) increased in CSF of patients after severe TBI.[29] This peptide has been implicated in causing neuronal damage in patients with Alzheimer's disease, and one of the mechanisms of injury induced by amyloid beta fragments (A beta-42) generated from splicing of amyloid precursor protein (APP) involves increased oxidative stress.[30–33]

MITOCHONDRIAL DYSFUNCTION IN TBI

Animal studies. Increased oxidative stress contributes to the mitochondrial dysfunction that plays a central role in causing cognitive impairment and eventually cell death following TBI.[34,35] Experimental TBI causes a significant loss of cortical tissue at the site of injury (primary damage) that is followed by a secondary injury involving mitochondria that enhances the primary injury leading to neurological dysfunction. In a rat model of TBI, several mitochondrial proteins involved in bioenergetics were oxidized following injury causing mitochondrial dysfunction that eventually leads to cell death.[36] In a rat model of TBI, it was found that the activity of mitochondrial enzyme pyruvate dehydrogenase (PDH) decreased, acid–base balance disrupted, and levels of oxidative stress increased in blood following injury. The decrease in blood levels of PDH was associated with increased gliosis and loss of subunit PDHE1-infinity of PDH in brain tissue, and these effects can be prevented by pyruvate treatment.[37] These changes contribute to the severity of brain injury. Cytochrome *c* oxidase is important for oxidative phosphorylation in the mitochondria. The expression of cytochrome *c* oxidase I, II, and III mRNA in injured cortex was reduced following TBI in rats, whereas the expression of these mRNAs was slightly elevated in contralateral cortex.[38] Generally, oxidative stress–induced mitochondrial dysfunction in rat model of TBI is observed 1–3 h after TBI, suggesting the importance of an early intervention to reduce the oxidative stress.[39] In a mice model of TBI, it was observed that cortical mitochondrial damage includes swelling, a disruption of cristae and rupture of outer membranes, a decrease in calcium-buffering capacity, and an increase in oxidation of protein and lipids. The levels of cortical 3-nitrotyrosine were elevated as early as 30 min after injury.[40]

Human studies. There is a direct link between energy metabolism and N-acetylaspartate. In a clinical study involving 14 patients (6 patients with diffuse brain injury and 8 with focal brain lesions), it was observed that reduction in the brain levels of N-acetylaspartate in the absence of ischemic insult reflected mitochondrial dysfunction.[41] It has been proposed that extracellular levels of N-acetylaspartate can be used as a potential marker for mitochondrial function in humans after TBI.[42] The role of mitochondrial dysfunction in the progression of damage following TBI is further supported by the fact that treatment with mitochondrial uncouplers, 2-4-dinitrophenol (2,4-DNP) and 2,4-dinitrophenol-p-trifluoromethoxyphenylhydrazene (FCCP), significantly reduced loss of cortical damage and improved behavioral deficits following TBI in rats.[43]

EVIDENCE FOR INCREASED LEVELS OF MARKERS OF INFLAMMATION IN TBI

Human studies. Following TBI, resident cells in the brain such as microglia generate excessive amounts of proinflammatory cytokines, prostaglandins, reactive oxygen species, compliment proteins, and adhesion molecules that are highly toxic to neurons.[44-48] The evidence of inflammation is also found by the infiltration and accumulation of polymorphonuclear leukocytes. Proinflammatory cytokines increased the expression of iNOS, which can produce excessive amounts of NO that may, in turn, become oxidized to form peroxynitrite that contribute to the pathogenesis of TBI.[49-59] An inhibitor of iNOS provided neuroprotection against damage produced by peroxynitrite.[52] The proinflammatory cytokine interleukin-6 (IL-6) is elevated in patients with acute TBI, and a significant relationship exists between the severity of TBI and the transcranial IL-6 gradient at admission.[53] In addition, activation of nuclear factor-kappa B (NF-kappaB) occurs after TBI in both animals and humans.[54,55] Treatment with beta-Aescin inhibited activation of NF-kappaB and expression of tumor necrosis factor-alpha (TNF-alpha).[54] The levels of IL-10 in 46 adult patients with TBI ($N = 18$), nontraumatic intracranial hemorrhage ($N = 11$), and polytrauma with concomitant brain injury ($N = 17$) were detectable independent of types of lesion,[56] whereas it was barely detectable in control subjects.[57] The significance of this rise in the levels of IL-10 remains uncertain; however, it was associated with increased rate of infection and mild to moderate to severe damage to blood–brain barrier (BBB). In a clinical study involving 75 patients with moderate to severe TBI, the role of cytokines and lipids in patient outcomes on the criteria of 30-day mortality was evaluated. The results showed that the levels of cytokines (IL-6 and IL-8) increased, and lipid decreased in all patients compared to healthy control. In addition, the levels of two cytokines were higher, and the levels of LDL were lower in nonsurvivors than in survivors. These results suggested that the level of LDL alone or in combination with IL-6 and IL-8 could be a prognostic value for a 30-day survival outcome.[58] Severe TBI in infants and children ($N = 36$) increased the levels of proinflammatory cytokines (IL-1beta, IL-6, and IL-12p70) and anti-inflammatory cytokines (IL-10) and chemokines (IL-8 and MIP-1alpha) compared to controls. Moderate hypothermia did not decrease the levels of cytokines in children with TBI.[59]

Animal studies. The levels of inflammation markers such as iNOS and cyclooxygenase 2 (COX-2) activity, and markers of oxidative stress (loss of glutathione and oxidized/reduced glutathione ratio, 3-nitrotyrosine, and 4-hydroxynonenal) increased after TBI in an animal model, and treatment with fenofibrate reduced the levels of these markers.[60] The levels of proinflammatory cytokines, TNF-alpha increased after TBI in rats. The delayed elevation of soluble tumor necrosis factor receptors p75 and p55 was observed in CSF and plasma after TBI.[61] The levels of TNF-alpha and Fas are elevated after TBI. Using TNF-alpha- and Fas-deficient transgenic mice (TNFalpha/Fas$^{-/-}$), it was demonstrated that the motor performance and spatial memory acquisition were improved in transgenic animals compared to wild-type mice after subjecting them with a controlled cortical impact (a model of TBI). The results suggested that TNF-alpha and FAS play an important role in TBI-induced neurological dysfunction. This was further confirmed by the fact that in immature normal mice subjected to controlled cortical impact, genetic inhibition of TNF-alpha and Fas conferred beneficial effects on histology and spatial memory acquisition in adulthood.[62] In a rat model of TBI, an animal received impact-acceleration head injury as a sustained mild head injury or a severe head injury. The levels of NO metabolites decreased in the cortex, cerebellum, hippocampus, and brain stem in both groups after 5 min. The extent of decrease in NO levels depended upon the extent of injury, being lowest in the brain regions where the direct trauma was most severe.[63] Nuclear factor erythroid-2-related factor 2 (Nrf2) is an important transcriptional factor that provides protection against toxic products of inflammation. Using transgenic mice deficient in Nrf2$^{-/-}$, it was demonstrated that upon activation of NF-kappaB, the levels of proinflammatory cytokines, TNF-alpha, IL-1beta and IL-6, and expression of intracellular adhesion molecule 1 (ICAN-1) were higher in the brain compared to the wild-type Nrf2$^{+/+}$ mice following TBI (moderate to severe weight-drop impact head injury).[64,65]

The role of proinflammatory cytokines in the progression of damage followed by TBI is further supported by the fact that inhibitors of these cytokines improved neuronal loss and cognitive dysfunction in animal models of TBI. For example, IL-1 beta neutralizing antibody (IgG2a/k),[66] an inhibitor of TNF-alpha at a posttranscriptional stage, dexanabinol (HU-211)[67] and antioxidants,[68] inhibitor of glial activation and proinflammatory cytokines, Minozac (Mzc),[69] and a synthetic analogue of tripeptide Glypromate (NNZ-2566),[70] an inhibitor of activation of astrocytes (simvastatin)[71] provide neuroprotection by reducing neuronal loss and neurological deficits.

EVIDENCE FOR INCREASED RELEASE OF GLUTAMATE IN TBI

Human studies. The excitatory amino acids play a significant role in the progression of injury following TBI. The levels of extracellular glutamate and aspartate increased in the brain regions following TBI in animals.[72] Excessive amounts of glutamate in the extracellular space may lead to an uncontrolled shift of sodium, potassium, and calcium that may cause swelling, edema, and eventually cell death. In addition, increased synaptic release of glutamate also occurs at the site of injury.[73,74] In a clinical study involving 80 patients with severe head injury, it was observed that the levels of excitatory amino acids increased that may enhance neuronal damage in these patients.[75] In patients with focal and diffuse brain injury, the levels of glutamate were elevated in both CSF and extracellular space following TBI.[76] In another clinical study, it was found that patients who died of their head injury had higher levels of dialysate glutamate and aspartame compared to those who recovered. The highest levels were present in patients with gunshot wounds, followed by those who had mass lesions. Patients with diffuse brain injury had the lowest levels of glutamate and aspartame.[72] Excessive amounts of glutamate and aspartame are released in 85 severely head-injured patients, and the patients with contusions had the highest level of glutamate and aspartate.[77] In a clinical study involving 28 severely brain-injured patients, the levels of glutamate and taurine in ventricular CSF were elevated in patients with subdural or epidural hematomas, contusions, and generalized brain edema. The simultaneous release of taurine, which has inhibitory and anti-excitotoxic functions with glutamate, suggests that the injured brain is attempting to counteract the action of glutamate.[78] Similar results were obtained in a rat model of TBI.[79] In a clinical study involving 27 children with severe TBI and 21 children without TBI or meningitis, it was observed that the levels of adenosine and glutamate were elevated in the ventricular CSF following TBI. The release of adenosine following TBI may reflect an attempt by adenosine to provide neuroprotection against glutamate-induced toxicity.[80]

Animal studies. In a rat model of TBI, it was shown that the levels of two high-affinity sodium-dependent glial transporters, glutamate transporter 1 (GLT-1), and glutamate-aspartame transporter (GLAST) decreased following TBI.[74,81] This suggested that decreased glial transporter function may contribute to the increased levels of extracellular glutamate. Treatment with hypothermia reduces the neuronal damage in remote cortical and subcortical regions following TBI. In a rat model of TBI, hypothermia treatment reduced the levels of hydroxyl radicals and glutamate release.[82] The involvement of glutamate in the progression of damage following TBI is further suggested by the fact that administration of N-methyl-D-aspartame, an (NMDA) antagonist, significantly reduced glutamate release,[83,84] and improved motor function and cognitive dysfunction following TBI in animal models. Activation of presynaptic group II metabotropic glutamate (mGlu II) receptor reduces synaptic glutamate release. Indeed, (−)-2-oxa-4-aminobicyclo(3.1.0)hexane-4,6-dicarboxylate (LY379268), a selective agonist of mGlu II, significantly reduced cell death following TBI in mice.[85] In another animal model of TBI (lateral fluid percussion-induced brain injury), administration of mGlu II agonist protected improved behavior deficits compared to control following injury.[86]

ROLE OF MATRIX METALLOPROTEINASES IN TBI

Experimental data in animal models of TBI suggest that the levels of matrix metalloproteinases (MMPs) increased following TBI; therefore, it has been suggested that they may enhance posttraumatic edema by increasing BBB permeability. In a clinical study involving 20 patients with a mild head injury and normal CT scan, 15 patients with moderate polytrauma without TBI, and 20 healthy volunteers, it was observed that the levels of MMP-2 and MMP-9 increased in the plasma and microdialysis samples of patients compared to control volunteers; this was followed by a significant decrease in the levels of both MMP-2 and MMP-9.[87]

TREATMENTS OF TBI

TBI is extremely difficult to treat because of the inherent complexity of the brain structures and functions as well as extreme variation in the pattern of injury. Approximately half of severely brain-injured patients will need surgery to remove or repair hematomas (rupture of blood vessels) or contusions (bruised brain tissue) (National Institute of Neurological Disorders and Stroke, 2009). Initial treatment focuses on preventing secondary injury following TBI. This includes proper oxygen supply to the brain and the rest of the body, maintaining adequate blood flow, and controlling blood pressure. Patients with moderate to severe TBI receive rehabilitation therapy that includes individually tailored treatment program in the area of physical therapy, occupational therapy, speech/language therapy, medications, psychology/psychiatry therapy, and social support. Recently, hypothermia (32–33°C) has been used in the management of TBI. In a clinical study, it was demonstrated that hypothermia attenuated the levels of markers of oxidative stress in infants and children after severe TBI.[88]

Based on the studies on animal models of TBI, several potential therapeutic agents have been identified. They include erythropoietin,[89,90] antibodies of serotonin receptors,[91] histone deacetylase inhibitor,[92] protease inhibitors,[93] fenofibrate, a peroxisome proliferator-activated receptor alpha agonist,[60] meloxicam, a COX-2 inhibitor,[94] and interferon-gamms.[95]

Treatments of Sports-Related Concussive Injury

Current efforts on reducing the impact of concussion have focused on the development of physical protection. Indeed, the introduction of newer football helmets appears to lower the risk of concussion by about 10–20%.[11] Even among protected groups, the long-term consequences of undetectable concussion have not been evaluated. There is no effective preventive strategy to reduce the risk of neurological disorders in athletes who have suffered concussive injury. Therefore, a novel biological protection strategy that can reduce the acute and long-term impacts of concussion should be developed. Since increased oxidative stress, chronic inflammation, and glutamate release are involved in the development and progression of neurological deficits, and since antioxidants are known to reduce oxidative stress, inflammation, and glutamate release, daily supplementation with appropriate types of multiple micronutrients including dietary and endogenous antioxidants appears to be one of the rational choices for reducing the risk of neurological dysfunction.

Treatments of TBI with Antioxidants

Despite great potential of antioxidants in the management of TBI, very little attention has been paid to test the efficacy of these micronutrients alone or in combination with standard therapy in animals or humans. A few studies are described below. Resveratrol, a phenolic antioxidant, administered immediately after TBI, reduced oxidative damage and lesion volume in rats.[96,97] Edaravone, a FDA-approved drug, reduced oxidative damage by neutralizing free radicals after TBI in humans.[98] Superoxide dismutase improved TBI-induced mitochondrial dysfunction in transgenic mice overexpressing CuZn SOD or Mn SOD.[99] In transgenic mice overexpressing glutathione peroxidase (GPxTg), it was observed that markers of oxidative stress including nitrotyrosine were reduced and spatial memory improved compared to wild-type animals following TBI.[100] Treatment with alpha-lipoic acid reduced markers of proinflammatory cytokines and oxidative stress, and improved histological changes in the brain, and preserved BBB permeability and reduced edema following TBI in animals.[101] Administration of N-acetylcysteine (NAC) provided neuroprotection (reduction in brain edema and BBB permeability) in animal models following TB by reducing markers of proinflammatory cytokines and adhesion molecules.[102] The early rise in complex I and complex II proteins of mitochondria that regulate excitatory neurotransmitter release following TBI was blocked by NAC.[73] In addition, TBI-induced elevation of heme oxygenase-1 (HO-1) levels in glial cells as well as neurons and loss of tissue volume was markedly reduced by NAC treatment in an animal model of TBI (lateral fluid percussion injury).[103] Melatonin, a pineal hormone exhibiting antioxidant activity, protected against TBI-induced damage by attenuating the activation of NF-kappaB and AP-1.[104]

In a rat model of TBI (mild fluid percussion injury), increased oxidation of proteins and reduced levels of SOD and Sir2 (silent information regulator), and poor performance associated with a decline in the levels of brain-derived neurotrophic factor (BDNF) and its downstream effectors on synaptic plasticity, synapsin I and cAMP-response element-binding protein (CREB), were observed following injury. Dietary supplementation with vitamin E or Curcumin protected the brain against mild TBI-induced damage by reducing the above biochemical changes involved in synaptic plasticity and cognitive function.[105,106] Repetitive concussive injury increased brain lipid peroxidation, and accelerated beta-amyloid fragments (Abeta) formation and deposition, as well as cognitive impairment in Tg2526 mice. Dietary supplementation with vitamin E prevented TBI-induced biochemical changes and cognitive function.[107] Vitamin E and Curcumin have been shown to block the toxic effects of A-beta-42.[108–110] Vitamin E also inhibited the release and toxicity of glutamate.[111,112] TBI decreased alpha7 neuronal nicotinic cholinergic receptor (nAChR) expression. Supplementation with dietary choline, a selective agonist of nAChR, improved spatial memory, reduced loss of cortical tissue and brain inflammation, and normalized nAChR expression following TBI in a rat model of TBI (cortical contusion injury).[113]

It has been reported that dietary supplementation of omega-3 fatty acids in animal model of TBI (mild fluid percussion injury) protected against TBI-induced reduced synaptic plasticity and cognitive impairment.[114] In contrast, supplementation with saturated fat diet[115] or caffeine[116] aggravated TBI-induced injury in animals.

It is well established that antioxidants are scavengers of free radicals; however, their role in reducing inflammation has not drawn significant attention. There are substantial amounts of data that show that dietary and endogenous antioxidants and antioxidants derived from herbs and fruits and vegetables inhibit inflammation.[117–129] The role of antioxidants in reducing inflammation following TBI has been discussed in the above paragraph.

Antioxidants Reduce Glutamate Release

Glutamate is released following TBI. It has been reported that increased proinflammatory stimuli and oxidative stress cause microglia to release excessive amounts of glutamate, which contributes to loss of neurons.[130] Release of glutamate was blocked by vitamin E.[130] Both vitamin E[112] and coenzyme Q_{10}[111] also protect against glutamate-induced neurotoxicity in cell culture models.

PROBLEMS OF USING A SINGLE AGENT IN TBI

Laboratory studies with animal models of TBI consistently showed that supplementation with a single micronutrient such as an antioxidant may protect the brain against TBI-induced biochemical and structural damage. Although no well-designed clinical studies have been performed with one or more antioxidants following TBI, previous clinical studies with a single antioxidant in high-risk populations of other diseases such as cancer, heart disease, and certain neurological diseases have produced inconsistent results. It is well established that the internal oxidative environment of high-risk populations of these diseases are high. It is also known that an individual antioxidant when oxidized acts as a pro-oxidant. Therefore, administration of a single antioxidant under the above conditions may produce pro-oxidant effects rather than antioxidant effects. This effect of a single antioxidant may have contributed to the inconsistent results varying from beneficial effects, no effect, to harmful effects. I propose that high doses of multiple micronutrients including dietary and endogenous antioxidants, when administered as an adjunct to standard therapy, may increase the efficacy of therapy in reducing the progression of damage following TBI. In addition, when they are administered before the TBI, the initial levels of damage and rate of progression of damage may be reduced before intervention with standard therapy.

RATIONALE FOR USING MULTIPLE MICRONUTRIENTS IN TBI

Because of increased levels of oxidative stress and chronic inflammation, enhanced release of glutamate following TBI with a closed head injury (concussive injury during contact sports or due to an exposure to blast wave pressure), an oral supplementation with appropriate multiple micronutrients including dietary and endogenous antioxidants appears to be one of the rational choices for reducing the risk of late adverse effects on brain function including cognitive impairment. In addition, such a micronutrient preparation, in combination with standard therapy, may improve its efficacy in the management of TBI with penetrating head injury. Experimental designs of most previous clinical studies that have utilized only one or two antioxidants are not suitable for determining the efficacy of multiple micronutrients in reducing the late adverse effects or improving the efficacy of standard therapy in the management of TBI. This is due to the fact that their mechanisms of action and distribution at cellular and organ levels differ, their cellular and organ environments (oxygenation, aqueous, and lipid components) differ, and their affinity for various types of free radicals differs. For example, beta-carotene (BC) is more effective in quenching oxygen radicals than most other antioxidants.[131] BC can perform certain biological functions that cannot be produced by its metabolite vitamin A, and vice versa.[132,133] It has been reported that BC treatment enhances the expression of the connexin gene, which codes for a gap junction protein in mammalian fibroblasts in culture, whereas vitamin A treatment does not produce such an effect.[133] Vitamin A can induce differentiation in certain normal and cancer cells, whereas BC and other carotenoids do not.[134,135] Thus, BC and vitamin A have, in part, different biological functions.

The gradient of oxygen pressure varies within cells. Some antioxidants, such as vitamin E, are more effective as quenchers of free radicals in reduced oxygen pressure, whereas BC and vitamin A are more effective in higher atmospheric pressures.[136] Vitamin C is necessary to protect cellular components in aqueous environments, whereas carotenoids and vitamins A and E protect cellular components in lipid environments. Vitamin C also plays an important role in maintaining cellular levels of vitamin E by recycling vitamin E radical (oxidized) to the reduced (antioxidant) form.[137] Also, oxidative DNA damage produced by high levels of vitamin C could be protected by vitamin E. Oxidized forms of vitamins C and E can also act as radicals; therefore, excessive amounts of any one of these forms, when used as a single agent, could be harmful over a long period of time.

The form of vitamin E used is also important in any clinical trial. It has been established that D-alpha-tocopheryl succinate (alpha-TS) is the most effective form of vitamin E both in vitro and in vivo.[138,139] This form of vitamin E is more soluble than alpha-tocopherol and enters cells more readily. Therefore, it is expected to cross the BBB in greater amounts than alpha-tocopherol. However, this has not yet been demonstrated in animals or humans. We have reported that an oral ingestion of alpha-TS (800 IU/day) in humans increased plasma levels of not only alpha-tocopherol, but also alpha-TS, suggesting that a portion of alpha-TS can be absorbed from the intestinal tract before hydrolysis.[140] This observation is important because the conventional assumption based on the rodent studies has been that esterified forms of vitamin E, such as alpha-TS, alpha-tocopheryl nicotinate, or alpha-tocopheryl acetate, can be absorbed from the intestinal tract only after they are hydrolyzed to alpha-tocopherol. Our preliminary data showed that this assumption may not be true for the absorption of alpha-TS in humans.

Glutathione is effective in catabolizing H_2O_2 and anions. However, oral supplementation with glutathione failed to significantly increase plasma levels of glutathione in human subjects,[141] suggesting that this tripeptide is completely hydrolyzed in the gastrointestinal tract. Therefore, I propose to utilize NAC and alpha-lipoic acid that increase the cellular levels of glutathione by different mechanisms in a multiple micronutrient preparation. In addition, R-alpha-lipoic acid and acetyl-L-carnitine together promoted mitochondrial biogenesis in murine adipocytes in culture; however, no effect was observed when these antioxidants were used individually.[142] These types of studies further emphasized the value of using more than one antioxidant in any clinical or laboratory studies involving TBI.

Other endogenous antioxidants, coenzyme Q_{10}, may also have some potential value in prevention and improved treatment of diabetes. Since mitochondrial dysfunction occurs in patients with diabetes, and since coenzyme Q_{10} is needed for the generation of ATP by mitochondria, it is essential to add this antioxidant in multiple micronutrient preparation in order to improve the function of mitochondria. A study has shown that Ubiquinol (coenzyme Q_{10}) scavenges peroxy radicals faster than alpha-tocopherol,[143] and like vitamin C, can regenerate vitamin E in a redox cycle.[144] However, it is a weaker antioxidant than alpha-tocopherol. Coenzyme Q_{10} administration has been shown to improve clinical symptoms in patients with mitochondrial encephalomyopathies.[145]

Selenium is a cofactor of glutathione peroxidase, and Se-glutathione peroxidase increases the intracellular level of glutathione that is a powerful antioxidant. There may be some other mechanisms of action of selenium. Therefore, selenium and coenzyme Q_{10} should be added to a multiple micronutrient preparation for prevention and improved treatment of diabetes.

The values of antioxidants in reducing the risk of neurological dysfunction have been evaluated in other neurological diseases such as Alzheimer's disease and Parkinson's disease in humans. It has been reported that beta-amyloid fragments that are associated with neurodegeneration in Alzheimer's disease mediate their action by free radicals.[146] This is supported by the fact that vitamin E protects neuronal cells in culture against beta-amyloid–induced toxicity.[147] Vitamin E at a dose of 2000 IU/day produced some beneficial effects in patients with Alzheimer's disease.[148] Patients consuming antioxidants showed reduced risk of vascular dementia and slower decline of cognitive function in cases of dementia and Alzheimer's disease.[149] We have reported that PGE2, a product of inflammatory reactions, is very toxic to mature neurons, and a mixture of antioxidants reduces this toxicity.[150] Glutathione deficiency has been consistently found in autopsied brain samples from patients with neurological diseases such as Alzheimer's disease[151] and Parkinson's disease.[152,153] Administration of coenzyme Q_{10} has been shown to improve clinical symptoms of mitochondrial encephalomyopathies[145] and only modest improvement in Parkinson's disease.[154] Others have reported inconsistent results with coenzyme Q_{10}.[155] These studies suggest that antioxidant micronutrients have neuroprotective value and provide a scientific rationale for testing the efficacy of multiple micronutrients including dietary and endogenous antioxidants in combination with standard therapy in patients with TBI for reducing the progression of damage.

In addition to dietary and endogenous antioxidants, all B vitamins that are necessary for general health should be added to a multiple micronutrient preparation for reducing the risk of neurological disorders following TBI or improving the treatment of TBI in combination with the standard therapy.

A commercial formulation of multiple micronutrients was tested in a clinical study in troops returning from Iraq with mild to moderate TBI. Thirty-four patients with posttraumatic dizziness were admitted to the Naval Medical Center San Diego Clinic over a 2-mo period of time and agreed to participate in the study under the supervision of Dr. Michael Hoffer and his colleagues.[156] All patients had received their injury 3–20 weeks before admission, and they received identical treatment consisting of medical therapy (for any migraine), supportive care, steroids, and vestibular rehabilitation therapy. Fifteen of the 34 patients also received a dose of an antioxidant and micronutrient formula (two capsules by mouth twice a day). At the onset of therapy, all patients were evaluated in outcome measures, which included the Sensory Organization Test (SOT) by Computerized Dynamic Posturography (CDP), the Dynamic Gait Index (DGI), the Activities Balance Confidence (ABC) scale, the Dizziness Handicap Index (DHI), the Vestibular Disorders Activities of Daily Living (VADL) score, and the Balance Scoring System (BESS) test. The study was carried out for 12 weeks. The therapist who graded these outcomes and performed the testing was blinded as to whether the patient was receiving antioxidant therapy or not. The pretrial test scores did not differ significantly between the two groups on any of the tests.

Both groups of patients showed trends toward significant improvement on all tests after the 12 weeks of therapy, but the combination treatment trend was stronger than that of the standard therapy alone group. After only 4 weeks, the SOT score by CDP was 78 for the antioxidant group compared to 63 for the non-antioxidant group. This difference was statistically significant at the $P < 0.05$ level. The improvement noted by the antioxidant group on the other tests was also greater than the non-antioxidant group, although these differences did not reach statistical significance because of the short trial period and small sample size.

RECOMMENDED MICRONUTRIENTS FOR REDUCING THE LATE ADVERSE EFFECTS IN HIGH-RISK POPULATIONS

The high-risk populations include persons who have suffered repeated concussive injury (TBI with closed head injury) such as that observed during contact sports or due to an exposure to blast wave pressure. These individuals are at high risk for developing cognitive dysfunction and other neurological abnormalities several years later. They provide an excellent opportunity to study the efficacy of multiple micronutrients in reducing the risk of abnormal brain function.

A preparation of multiple micronutrients may include vitamin A (retinyl palmitate), vitamin E (both D-alpha-tocopherol and D-TS), natural mixed carotenoids, vitamin C (calcium ascorbate), coenzyme Q_{10}, R-alpha-lipoic acid, NAC, L-carnitine, vitamin D, all B vitamins, selenium, zinc, chromium, and omega-3 fatty acids. No iron, copper, or manganese would be included because these trace minerals are known to interact with vitamin C to produce free radicals. These trace minerals are absorbed from the intestinal tract more in the presence of antioxidants than in their absence that could result in increased body stores of free forms of these minerals. Increased iron stores have been linked to increased risk of several chronic diseases.[157] Antioxidants from herbs, fruits, and vegetables were not included because they do not produce any unique biological effects that cannot be produced by antioxidants present in the micronutrient preparation.

The recommended micronutrient supplements should be taken orally and divided into two doses, half in the morning and the other half in the evening with meal. This is because the biological half-lives of micronutrients are highly variable, which can create high levels of fluctuations in the tissue levels of micronutrients. A twofold difference in the levels of certain micronutrients such as alpha-TS can cause a marked difference in the expression of gene profiles (our unpublished data). In order to maintain relatively consistent levels of micronutrients in the brain, the proposed micronutrients should be taken twice a day.

The efficacy of proposed micronutrient formulation in high-risk populations should be tested by well-designed clinical studies. In the meanwhile, the proposed micronutrient recommendations may be adopted by the individuals who are being exposed to or who have been exposed to concussive injury in consultation with their physicians or health professionals. It is expected that the proposed recommendations would reduce the risk of late adverse effects on brain function in these populations.

RECOMMENDED MICRONUTRIENT SUPPLEMENT IN COMBINATION WITH STANDARD THERAPY IN TBI PATIENTS WITH PENETRATING HEAD INJURY

Increased oxidative stress, acute inflammation, and glutamate release have been found in TBI patients with penetrating head injury. The current medications are not considered sufficient either in the management of acute injury or long-term adverse effects on brain function in survivors of these injuries. The addition of a formulation of multiple micronutrients such as that described in the previous paragraph with high-risk populations of TBI may improve the efficacy of standard therapy in the acute and long-term management of TBI. The efficacy of this formulation in combination with standard therapy should be tested by well-designed clinical studies. In the meanwhile, the proposed micronutrient recommendations may be adopted by the individuals who have survived TBI with penetrating head injury and who are receiving standard therapy in consultation with their physicians or health professionals. It is expected that the proposed recommendations would enhance the efficacy of standard therapy in the management of TBI.

DIET AND LIFESTYLE RECOMMENDATIONS FOR TBI

A balanced diet is very necessary, in addition to supplementation with multiple micronutrients, for reducing the risk of long-term adverse effects on brain functions, as well as improving the efficacy of standard therapy in the management of acute and long-term management of TBI with penetrating head injury. I recommend a balanced diet containing low-fat and plenty of fruits and vegetables. Lifestyle recommendations include daily moderate exercise, reduced stress, no tobacco smoking, and reduced intake of caffeine. High saturated fat diet[115] and caffeine[116] appear to increase the progression of damage following TBI in animal models.

CONCLUSIONS

TBI occurs when a sudden trauma causes damage to the brain. TBI that results when the head suddenly and violently hits a solid object is called closed head injury or concussive injury that is commonly observed in contact sports, such as football, soccer, and hockey. A concussion occurs when the brain is violently rocked back and forth within the skull following a blow to the head or neck, or when in close proximity to a concussive blast pressure wave. TBI can also result when an object penetrates the skull and damages the brain. Penetrating type of head injuries are easily recognizable, but closed head injuries are difficult to identify after injury. TBI may increase the risk of PTSD and dementia. Despite progress that includes standardized treatment guidelines, several clinical studies aimed at identifying therapeutic agents and improved understanding of the mechanisms of cellular damage, treatment strategies for patients with acute TBI remain unsatisfactory. In addition, there are no therapeutic agents that can reduce the risk of dementia and other mental disorders appearing as a late effect of TBI. Based on the mechanistic data on TBI that include increased oxidative stress, and release of proinflammatory cytokines and glutamate, I have proposed to evaluate the efficacy of a proposed multiple micronutrient preparation including dietary and endogenous antioxidants, and modifications in the diet and lifestyle, in combination with standard therapy, for improving its efficacy in the management of acute injury, as well as in reducing the risk of late adverse effects on brain functions including dementia and PTSD. This is due to the fact that antioxidants reduce oxidative stress, inflammation, and glutamate release. In the meanwhile, the proposed micronutrient recommendations may be adopted by the individuals who have survived TBI and who are receiving standard therapy in consultation with their physicians or health professionals. It is expected that the proposed recommendations would enhance the efficacy of standard therapy in the management of TBI.

REFERENCES

1. Langlois, J. A., W. Rutland-Brown, and K. E. Thomas. 2004. Traumatic brain injury in the United States: Emergency department visits, hospitalizations, and death. Centers for Disease Control and Prevention, National Center for Injury Prevention and Control, Atlanta, GA.
2. Finkelstein, E. A., P. S. Corso, and T. R. Miller. 2006. *The Incidence and Economic Burden of Injuries in the United States*. New York, NY: Oxford University Press.
3. Guskiewicz, K. M., N. L. Weaver, D. A. Padua, and W. E. Garrett Jr. 2000. Epidemiology of concussion in collegiate and high school football players. *Am J Sports Med* 28 (5): 643–650.
4. Levy, M. L., B. M. Ozgur, C. Berry, H. E. Aryan, and M. L. Apuzzo. 2004. Analysis and evolution of head injury in football. *Neurosurgery* 55 (3): 649–655.
5. Viano, D. C., I. R. Casson, E. J. Pellman, C. A. Bir, L. Zhang, D. C. Sherman, and M. A. Boitano. 2005. Concussion in professional football: Comparison with boxing head impacts—Part 10. *Neurosurgery* 57 (6): 1154–1172; discussion 1154–1172.
6. Rapoport, M. J., S. McCullagh, P. Shammi, and A. Feinstein. 2005. Cognitive impairment associated with major depression following mild and moderate traumatic brain injury. *J Neuropsychiatry Clin Neurosci* 17 (1): 61–65.
7. van Donkelaar, P., J. Langan, E. Rodriguez, A. Drew, C. Halterman, L. R. Osternig, and L. S. Chou. 2005. Attentional deficits in concussion. *Brain Inj* 19 (12): 1031–1039.
8. Halterman, C. I., J. Langan, A. Drew, E. Rodriguez, L. R. Osternig, L. S. Chou, and P. van Donkelaar. 2006. Tracking the recovery of visuospatial attention deficits in mild traumatic brain injury. *Brain* 129 (Pt 3): 747–753.
9. Guskiewicz, K. M., S. W. Marshall, J. Bailes, M. McCrea, R. C. Cantu, C. Randolph, and B. D. Jordan. 2005. Association between recurrent concussion and late-life cognitive impairment in retired professional football players. *Neurosurgery* 57 (4): 719–726; discussion 719–726.
10. Gottshall, K., A. Drake, N. Gray, E. McDonald, and M. E. Hoffer. 2003. Objective vestibular tests as outcome measures in head injury patients. *Laryngoscope* 113 (10): 1746–1750.
11. Viano, D. C., E. J. Pellman, C. Withnall, and N. Shewchenko. 2006. Concussion in professional football: Performance of newer helmets in reconstructed game impacts—Part 13. *Neurosurgery* 59 (3): 591–606; discussion 591–606.
12. Hoge, C. W., D. McGurk, J. L. Thomas, A. L. Cox, C. C. Engel, and C. A. Castro. 2008. Mild traumatic brain injury in U.S. soldiers returning from Iraq. *N Engl J Med* 358 (5): 453–463.
13. Schneiderman, A. I., E. R. Braver, and H. K. Kang. 2008. Understanding sequelae of injury mechanisms and mild traumatic brain injury incurred during the conflicts in Iraq and Afghanistan: Persistent postconcussive symptoms and posttraumatic stress disorder. *Am J Epidemiol* 167 (12): 1446–1452.
14. Graham, D. I., T. K. McIntosh, W. L. Maxwell, and J. A. Nicoll. 2000. Recent advances in neurotrauma. *J Neuropathol Exp Neurol* 59 (8): 641–651.
15. Bayir, H., P. M. Kochanek, and V. E. Kagan. 2006. Oxidative stress in immature brain after traumatic brain injury. *Dev Neurosci* 28 (4–5): 420–431.
16. Rael, L. T., R. Bar-Or, C. W. Mains, D. S. Slone, A. S. Levy, and D. Bar-Or. 2009. Plasma oxidation–reduction potential and protein oxidation in traumatic brain injury. *J Neurotrauma*.
17. Shao, C., K. N. Roberts, W. R. Markesbery, S. W. Scheff, and M. A. Lovell. 2006. Oxidative stress in head trauma in aging. *Free Radic Biol Med* 41 (1): 77–85.
18. Mikawa, S., H. Kinouchi, H. Kamii, G. T. Gobbel, S. F. Chen, E. Carlson, C. J. Epstein, and P. H. Chan. 1996. Attenuation of acute and chronic damage following traumatic brain injury in copper, zinc-superoxide dismutase transgenic mice. *J Neurosurg* 85 (5): 885–891.

19. Petronilho, F., G. Feier, B. de Souza, C. Guglielmi, L. S. Constantino, R. Walz, J. Quevedo, and F. Dal-Pizzol. 2009. Oxidative stress in brain according to traumatic brain injury intensity. *J Surg Res* in press.
20. Tavazzi, B., S. Signoretti, G. Lazzarino, A. M. Amorini, R. Delfini, M. Cimatti, A. Marmarou, and R. Vagnozzi. 2005. Cerebral oxidative stress and depression of energy metabolism correlate with severity of diffuse brain injury in rats. *Neurosurgery* 56 (3): 582–589; discussion 582–589.
21. Singh, I. N., P. G. Sullivan, and E. D. Hall. 2007. Peroxynitrite-mediated oxidative damage to brain mitochondria: Protective effects of peroxynitrite scavengers. *J Neurosci Res* 85 (10): 2216–2223.
22. Huttemann, M., I. Lee, C. W. Kreipke, and T. Petrov. 2008. Suppression of the inducible form of nitric oxide synthase prior to traumatic brain injury improves cytochrome c oxidase activity and normalizes cellular energy levels. *Neuroscience* 151 (1): 148–154.
23. Louin, G., C. Marchand-Verrecchia, B. Palmier, M. Plotkine, and M. Jafarian-Tehrani. 2006. Selective inhibition of inducible nitric oxide synthase reduces neurological deficit but not cerebral edema following traumatic brain injury. *Neuropharmacology* 50 (2): 182–190.
24. Ansari, M. A., K. N. Roberts, and S. W. Scheff. 2008. Oxidative stress and modification of synaptic proteins in hippocampus after traumatic brain injury. *Free Radic Biol Med* 45 (4): 443–452.
25. Lima, F. D., M. A. Souza, A. F. Furian, L. M. Rambo, L. R. Ribeiro, F. V. Martignoni, M. S. Hoffmann, et al. 2008. Na^+,K^+-ATPase activity impairment after experimental traumatic brain injury: Relationship to spatial learning deficits and oxidative stress. *Behav Brain Res* 193 (2): 306–310.
26. Varma, S., K. L. Janesko, S. R. Wisniewski, H. Bayir, P. D. Adelson, N. J. Thomas, and P. M. Kochanek. 2003. F_2-isoprostane and neuron-specific enolase in cerebrospinal fluid after severe traumatic brain injury in infants and children. *J Neurotrauma* 20 (8): 781–786.
27. Bayir, H., V. E. Kagan, Y. Y. Tyurina, V. Tyurin, R. A. Ruppel, P. D. Adelson, S. H. Graham, K. Janesko, R. S. Clark, and P. M. Kochanek. 2002. Assessment of antioxidant reserves and oxidative stress in cerebrospinal fluid after severe traumatic brain injury in infants and children. *Pediatr Res* 51 (5): 571–578.
28. Darwish, R. S., N. Amiridze, and B. Aarabi. 2007. Nitrotyrosine as an oxidative stress marker: Evidence for involvement in neurologic outcome in human traumatic brain injury. *J Trauma* 63 (2): 439–442.
29. Emmerling, M. R., M. C. Morganti-Kossmann, T. Kossmann, P. F. Stahel, M. D. Watson, L. M. Evans, P. D. Mehta, et al. 2000. Traumatic brain injury elevates the Alzheimer's amyloid peptide A beta 42 in human CSF. A possible role for nerve cell injury. *Ann N Y Acad Sci* 903, 118–122.
30. Pappolla, M. A., Y. J. Chyan, R. A. Omar, K. Hsiao, G. Perry, M. A. Smith, and P. Bozner. 1998. Evidence of oxidative stress and in vivo neurotoxicity of beta-amyloid in a transgenic mouse model of Alzheimer's disease: A chronic oxidative paradigm for testing antioxidant therapies in vivo. *Am J Pathol* 152 (4): 871–877.
31. Butterfield, D. A. 2002. Amyloid beta-peptide (1–42)–induced oxidative stress and neurotoxicity: Implications for neurodegeneration in Alzheimer's disease brain. A review. *Free Radic Res* 36 (12): 1307–1313.
32. Butterfield, D. A., A. Castegna, C. M. Lauderback, and J. Drake. 2002. Evidence that amyloid beta-peptide–induced lipid peroxidation and its sequelae in Alzheimer's disease brain contribute to neuronal death. *Neurobiol Aging* 23 (5): 655–664.
33. Qi, X. L., J. Xiu, K. R. Shan, Y. Xiao, R. Gu, R. Y. Liu, and Z. Z. Guan. 2005. Oxidative stress induced by beta-amyloid peptide(1–42) is involved in the altered composition of cellular membrane lipids and the decreased expression of nicotinic receptors in human SH-SY5Y neuroblastoma cells. *Neurochem Int* 46 (8): 613–621.
34. Robertson, C. L., S. Scafidi, M. C. McKenna, and G. Fiskum. 2009. Mitochondrial mechanisms of cell death and neuroprotection in pediatric ischemic and traumatic brain injury. *Exp Neurol* 218 (2): 371–380.
35. Mazzeo, A. T., A. Beat, A. Singh, and M. R. Bullock. 2009. The role of mitochondrial transition pore, and its modulation, in traumatic brain injury and delayed neurodegeneration after TBI. *Exp Neurol* 218 (2): 363–370.
36. Opii, W. O., V. N. Nukala, R. Sultana, J. D. Pandya, K. M. Day, M. L. Merchant, J. B. Klein, P. G. Sullivan, and D. A. Butterfield. 2007. Proteomic identification of oxidized mitochondrial proteins following experimental traumatic brain injury. *J Neurotrauma* 24 (5): 772–789.
37. Sharma, P., B. Benford, Z. Z. Li, and G. S. Ling. 2009. Role of pyruvate dehydrogenase complex in traumatic brain injury and Measurement of pyruvate dehydrogenase enzyme by dipstick test. *J Emerg Trauma Shock* 2 (2): 67–72.
38. Dai, W., H. L. Cheng, R. Q. Huang, Z. Zhuang, and J. X. Shi. 2009. Quantitative detection of the expression of mitochondrial cytochrome c oxidase subunits mRNA in the cerebral cortex after experimental traumatic brain injury. *Brain Res* 1251: 287–295.

39. Gilmer, L. K., K. N. Roberts, K. Joy, P. G. Sullivan, and S. W. Scheff. 2009. Early mitochondrial dysfunction after cortical contusion injury. *J Neurotrauma* 26 (8): 1271–1280.
40. Singh, I. N., P. G. Sullivan, Y. Deng, L. H. Mbye, and E. D. Hall. 2006. Time course of post-traumatic mitochondrial oxidative damage and dysfunction in a mouse model of focal traumatic brain injury: Implications for neuroprotective therapy. *J Cereb Blood Flow Metab* 26 (11): 1407–1418.
41. Aygok, G. A., A. Marmarou, P. Fatouros, B. Kettenmann, and R. M. Bullock. 2008. Assessment of mitochondrial impairment and cerebral blood flow in severe brain injured patients. *Acta Neurochir Suppl* 102, 57–61.
42. Belli, A., J. Sen, A. Petzold, S. Russo, N. Kitchen, M. Smith, B. Tavazzi, R. Vagnozzi, et al. 2006. Extracellular *N*-acetylaspartate depletion in traumatic brain injury. *J Neurochem* 96 (3): 861–869.
43. Pandya, J. D., J. R. Pauly, V. N. Nukala, A. H. Sebastian, K. M. Day, A. S. Korde, W. F. Maragos, E. D. Hall, and P. G. Sullivan. 2007. Post-injury administration of mitochondrial uncouplers increases tissue sparing and improves behavioral outcome following traumatic brain injury in rodents. *J Neurotrauma* 24 (5): 798–811.
44. Lucas, S. M., N. J. Rothwell, and R. M. Gibson. 2006. The role of inflammation in CNS injury and disease. *Br J Pharmacol* 147 (Suppl 1): S232–S240.
45. Goodman, J. C., M. Van, S. P. Gopinath, and C. S. Robertson. 2008. Pro-inflammatory and pro-apoptotic elements of the neuroinflammatory response are activated in traumatic brain injury. *Acta Neurochir Suppl* 102: 437–439.
46. Hutchinson, P. J., M. T. O'Connell, N. J. Rothwell, S. J. Hopkins, J. Nortje, K. L. Carpenter, I. Timofeev, P. G. Al-Rawi, D. K. Menon, and J. D. Pickard. 2007. Inflammation in human brain injury: Intracerebral concentrations of IL-1alpha, IL-1beta, and their endogenous inhibitor IL-1ra. *J Neurotrauma* 24 (10): 1545–1557.
47. You, Z., J. Yang, K. Takahashi, P. H. Yager, H. H. Kim, T. Qin, G. L. Stahl, R. A. Ezekowitz, M. C. Carroll, and M. J. Whalen. 2007. Reduced tissue damage and improved recovery of motor function after traumatic brain injury in mice deficient in complement component C4. *J Cereb Blood Flow Metab* 27 (12): 1954–1964.
48. Hein, A. M., and M. K. O'Banion. 2009. Neuroinflammation and memory: The role of prostaglandins. *Mol Neurobiol* 40 (1): 15–32.
49. Dietrich, W. D., K. Chatzipanteli, E. Vitarbo, K. Wada, and K. Kinoshita. 2004. The role of inflammatory processes in the pathophysiology and treatment of brain and spinal cord trauma. *Acta Neurochir Suppl* 89: 69–74.
50. Potts, M. B., S. E. Koh, W. D. Whetstone, B. A. Walker, T. Yoneyama, C. P. Claus, H. M. Manvelyan, and L. J. Noble-Haeusslein. 2006. Traumatic injury to the immature brain: Inflammation, oxidative injury, and iron-mediated damage as potential therapeutic targets. *NeuroRx* 3 (2): 143–153.
51. Hall, E. D., M. R. Detloff, K. Johnson, and N. C. Kupina. 2004. Peroxynitrite-mediated protein nitration and lipid peroxidation in a mouse model of traumatic brain injury. *J Neurotrauma* 21 (1): 9–20.
52. Gahm, C., S. Holmin, P. N. Wiklund, L. Brundin, and T. Mathiesen. 2006. Neuroprotection by selective inhibition of inducible nitric oxide synthase after experimental brain contusion. *J Neurotrauma* 23 (9): 1343–1354.
53. Minambres, E., A. Cemborain, P. Sanchez-Velasco, et al. 2003. Correlation between transcranial interleukin-6 gradient and outcome in patients with acute brain injury. *Crit Care Med* 31: 33–38.
54. Xiao, G. M., and J. Wei. 2005. Effects of beta-Aescin on the expression of nuclear factor-kappaB and tumor necrosis factor-alpha after traumatic brain injury in rats. *J Zhejiang Univ Sci B* 6 (1): 28–32.
55. Hang, C. H., G. Chen, J. X. Shi, X. Zhang, and J. S. Li. 2006. Cortical expression of nuclear factor kappaB after human brain contusion. *Brain Res* 1109 (1): 14–21.
56. Dziurdzik, P., L. Krawczyk, P. Jalowiecki, Z. Kondera-Anasz, and L. Menon. 2004. Serum interleukin-10 in ICU patients with severe acute central nervous system injuries. *Inflamm Res* 53 (8): 338–343.
57. Kirchhoff, C., S. Buhmann, V. Bogner, J. Stegmaier, B. A. Leidel, V. Braunstein, W. Mutschler, and P. Biberthaler. 2008. Cerebrospinal IL-10 concentration is elevated in non-survivors as compared to survivors after severe traumatic brain injury. *Eur J Med Res* 13 (10): 464–468.
58. Venetsanou, K., K. Vlachos, A. Moles, G. Fragakis, G. Fildissis, and G. Baltopoulos. 2007. Hypolipoproteinemia and hyperinflammatory cytokines in serum of severe and moderate traumatic brain injury (TBI) patients. *Eur Cytokine Netw* 18 (4): 206–209.
59. Buttram, S. D., S. R. Wisniewski, E. K. Jackson, P. D. Adelson, K. Feldman, H. Bayir, R. P. Berger, R. S. Clark, and P. M. Kochanek. 2007. Multiplex assessment of cytokine and chemokine levels in cerebrospinal fluid following severe pediatric traumatic brain injury: Effects of moderate hypothermia. *J Neurotrauma* 24 (11): 1707–1717.

60. Chen, X. R., V. C. Besson, B. Palmier, Y. Garcia, M. Plotkine, and C. Marchand-Leroux. 2007. Neurological recovery-promoting, anti-inflammatory, and anti-oxidative effects afforded by fenofibrate, a PPAR alpha agonist, in traumatic brain injury. *J Neurotrauma* 24 (7): 1119–1131.
61. Maier, B., M. Lehnert, H. L. Laurer, A. E. Mautes, W. I. Steudel, and I. Marzi. 2006. Delayed elevation of soluble tumor necrosis factor receptors p75 and p55 in cerebrospinal fluid and plasma after traumatic brain injury. *Shock* 26 (2): 122–127.
62. Bermpohl, D., Z. You, E. H. Lo, H. H. Kim, and M. J. Whalen. 2007. TNF alpha and Fas mediate tissue damage and functional outcome after traumatic brain injury in mice. *J Cereb Blood Flow Metab* 27 (11): 1806–1818.
63. Tuzgen, S., N. Tanriover, M. Uzan, E. Tureci, T. Tanriverdi, K. Gumustas, and C. Kuday. 2003. Nitric oxide levels in rat cortex, hippocampus, cerebellum, and brainstem after impact acceleration head injury. *Neurol Res* 25 (1): 31–34.
64. Jin, W., H. Wang, W. Yan, L. Xu, X. Wang, X. Zhao, X. Yang, G. Chen, and Y. Ji. 2008. Disruption of Nrf2 enhances upregulation of nuclear factor-kappaB activity, proinflammatory cytokines, and intercellular adhesion molecule-1 in the brain after traumatic brain injury. *Mediators Inflamm* 2008, 725174.
65. Jin, W., H. Wang, W. Yan, L. Zhu, Z. Hu, Y. Ding, and K. Tang. 2009. Role of Nrf2 in protection against traumatic brain injury in mice. *J Neurotrauma* 26 (1): 131–139.
66. Clausen, F., A. Hanell, M. Bjork, L. Hillered, A. K. Mir, H. Gram, and N. Marklund. 2009. Neutralization of interleukin-1beta modifies the inflammatory response and improves histological and cognitive outcome following traumatic brain injury in mice. *Eur J Neurosci* 30 (3): 385–396.
67. Shohami, E., R. Gallily, R. Mechoulam, R. Bass, and T. Ben-Hur. 1997. Cytokine production in the brain following closed head injury: Dexanabinol (HU-211) is a novel TNF-alpha inhibitor and an effective neuroprotectant. *J Neuroimmunol* 72 (2): 169–177.
68. Trembovler, V., E. Beit-Yannai, F. Younis, R. Gallily, M. Horowitz, and E. Shohami. 1999. Antioxidants attenuate acute toxicity of tumor necrosis factor-alpha induced by brain injury in rat. *J Interferon Cytokine Res* 19 (7): 791–795.
69. Lloyd, E., K. Somera-Molina, L. J. Van Eldik, D. M. Watterson, and M. S. Wainwright. 2008. Suppression of acute proinflammatory cytokine and chemokine upregulation by post-injury administration of a novel small molecule improves long-term neurologic outcome in a mouse model of traumatic brain injury. *J Neuroinflammation* 5: 28.
70. Wei, H. H., X. C. Lu, D. A. Shear, A. Waghray, C. Yao, F. C. Tortella, and J. R. Dave. 2009. NNZ-2566 treatment inhibits neuroinflammation and pro-inflammatory cytokine expression induced by experimental penetrating ballistic-like brain injury in rats. *J Neuroinflammation* 6, 19.
71. Wu, H., A. Mahmood, D. Lu, H. Jiang, Y. Xiong, D. Zhou, and M. Chopp. 2009. Attenuation of astrogliosis and modulation of endothelial growth factor receptor in lipid rafts by simvastatin after traumatic brain injury. *J Neurosurg* in press
72. Gopinath, S. P., A. B. Valadka, J. C. Goodman, and C. S. Robertson. 2000. Extracellular glutamate and aspartate in head injured patients. *Acta Neurochir Suppl* 76: 437–438.
73. Yi, J. H., R. Hoover, T. K. McIntosh, and A. S. Hazell. 2006. Early, transient increase in complexin I and complexin II in the cerebral cortex following traumatic brain injury is attenuated by *N*-acetylcysteine. *J Neurotrauma* 23 (1): 86–96.
74. Yi, J. H., and A. S. Hazell. 2006. Excitotoxic mechanisms and the role of astrocytic glutamate transporters in traumatic brain injury. *Neurochem Int* 48 (5): 394–403.
75. Bullock, R., A. Zauner, J. J. Woodward, J. Myseros, S. C. Choi, J. D. Ward, A. Marmarou, and H. F. Young. 1998. Factors affecting excitatory amino acid release following severe human head injury. *J Neurosurg* 89 (4): 507–518.
76. Yamamoto, T., S. Rossi, M. Stiefel, E. Doppenberg, A. Zauner, R. Bullock, and A. Marmarou. 1999. CSF and ECF glutamate concentrations in head injured patients. *Acta Neurochir Suppl* 75: 17–19.
77. Koura, S. S., E. M. Doppenberg, A. Marmarou, S. Choi, H. F. Young, and R. Bullock. 1998. Relationship between excitatory amino acid release and outcome after severe human head injury. *Acta Neurochir Suppl* 71: 244–246.
78. Stover, J. F., M. C. Morganti-Kosmann, P. M. Lenzlinger, R. Stocker, O. S. Kempski, and T. Kossmann. 1999. Glutamate and taurine are increased in ventricular cerebrospinal fluid of severely brain-injured patients. *J Neurotrauma* 16 (2): 135–142.
79. Stover, J. F., and A. W. Unterberg. 2000. Increased cerebrospinal fluid glutamate and taurine concentrations are associated with traumatic brain edema formation in rats. *Brain Res* 875 (1–2): 51–55.

80. Robertson, C. L., M. J. Bell, P. M. Kochanek, P. D. Adelson, R. A. Ruppel, J. A. Carcillo, S. R. Wisniewski, et al. 2001. Increased adenosine in cerebrospinal fluid after severe traumatic brain injury in infants and children: Association with severity of injury and excitotoxicity. *Crit Care Med* 29 (12): 2287–2293.
81. Rao, V. L., M. K. Baskaya, A. Dogan, J. D. Rothstein, and R. J. Dempsey. 1998. Traumatic brain injury down-regulates glial glutamate transporter (GLT-1 and GLAST) proteins in rat brain. *J Neurochem* 70 (5): 2020–2027.
82. Globus, M. Y., O. Alonso, W. D. Dietrich, R. Busto, and M. D. Ginsberg. 1995. Glutamate release and free radical production following brain injury: Effects of posttraumatic hypothermia. *J Neurochem* 65 (4): 1704–1711.
83. Panter, S. S., and A. I. Faden. 1992. Pretreatment with NMDA antagonists limits release of excitatory amino acids following traumatic brain injury. *Neurosci Lett* 136 (2): 165–168.
84. Obrenovitch, T. P., and J. Urenjak. 1997. Is high extracellular glutamate the key to excitotoxicity in traumatic brain injury? *J Neurotrauma* 14 (10): 677–698.
85. Movsesyan, V. A., and A. I. Faden. 2006. Neuroprotective effects of selective group II mGluR activation in brain trauma and traumatic neuronal injury. *J Neurotrauma* 23 (2): 117–127.
86. Allen, J. W., S. A. Ivanova, L. Fan, M. G. Espey, A. S. Basile, and A. I. Faden. 1999. Group II metabotropic glutamate receptor activation attenuates traumatic neuronal injury and improves neurological recovery after traumatic brain injury. *J Pharmacol Exp Ther* 290 (1): 112–120.
87. Vilalta, A., J. Sahuquillo, A. Rosell, M. A. Poca, M. Riveiro, and J. Montaner. 2008. Moderate and severe traumatic brain injury induce early overexpression of systemic and brain gelatinases. *Intensive Care Med* 34 (8): 1384–1392.
88. Bayir, H., P. D. Adelson, S. R. Wisniewski, P. Shore, Y. Lai, D. Brown, K. L. Janesko-Feldman, V. E. Kagan, and P. M. Kochanek. 2009. Therapeutic hypothermia preserves antioxidant defenses after severe traumatic brain injury in infants and children. *Crit Care Med* 37 (2): 689–695.
89. Grasso, G., A. Sfacteria, F. Meli, V. Fodale, M. Buemi, and D. G. Iacopino. 2007. Neuroprotection by erythropoietin administration after experimental traumatic brain injury. *Brain Res* 1182, 99–105.
90. Xiong, Y., M. Chopp, and C. P. Lee. 2009. Erythropoietin improves brain mitochondrial function in rats after traumatic brain injury. *Neurol Res* 31 (5): 496–502.
91. Sharma, H. S., R. Patnaik, S. Patnaik, S. Mohanty, A. Sharma, and P. Vannemreddy. 2007. Antibodies to serotonin attenuate closed head injury induced blood brain barrier disruption and brain pathology. *Ann N Y Acad Sci* 1122: 295–312.
92. Zhang, B., E. J. West, K. C. Van, G. G. Gurkoff, J. Zhou, X. M. Zhang, A. P. Kozikowski, and B. G. Lyeth. 2008. HDAC inhibitor increases histone H3 acetylation and reduces microglia inflammatory response following traumatic brain injury in rats. *Brain Res* 1226: 181–191.
93. Foley, K., R. E. Kast, and E. L. Altschuler. 2009. Ritonavir and disulfiram have potential to inhibit caspase-1 mediated inflammation and reduce neurological sequelae after minor blast exposure. *Med Hypotheses* 72 (2): 150–152.
94. Hakan, T., H. Z. Toklu, N. Biber, H. Ozevren, S. Solakoglu, P. Demirturk, and F. V. Aker. 2009. Effect of COX-2 inhibitor meloxicam against traumatic brain injury-induced biochemical, histopathological changes and blood–brain barrier permeability. *Neurol Res*.
95. Chen, X., I. Y. Choi, T. S. Chang, Y. H. Noh, C. Y. Shin, C. F. Wu, K. H. Ko, and W. K. Kim. 2009. Pretreatment with interferon-gamma protects microglia from oxidative stress via up-regulation of Mn-SOD. *Free Radic Biol Med* 46 (8): 1204–1210,
96. Ates, O., S. Cayli, E. Altinoz, I. Gurses, N. Yucel, M. Sener, A. Kocak, and S. Yologlu. 2007. Neuroprotection by resveratrol against traumatic brain injury in rats. *Mol Cell Biochem* 294 (1–2): 137–144.
97. Sonmez, U., A. Sonmez, G. Erbil, I. Tekmen, and B. Baykara. 2007. Neuroprotective effects of resveratrol against traumatic brain injury in immature rats.*Neurosci Lett* 420 (2): 133–137.
98. Dohi, K., K. Satoh, Y. Mihara, S. Nakamura, Y. Miyake, H. Ohtaki, T. Nakamachi, T. Yoshikawa, S. Shioda, and T. Aruga. 2006. Alkoxyl radical-scavenging activity of edaravone in patients with traumatic brain injury. *J Neurotrauma* 23 (11): 1591–1599.
99. Xiong, Y., F. S. Shie, J. Zhang, C. P. Lee, and Y. S. Ho. 2005. Prevention of mitochondrial dysfunction in post-traumatic mouse brain by superoxide dismutase. *J Neurochem* 95 (3): 732–744.
100. Tsuru-Aoyagi, K., M. B. Potts, A. Trivedi, T. Pfankuch, J. Raber, M. Wendland, C. P. Claus, S. E. Koh, D. Ferriero, and L. J. Noble-Haeusslein. 2009. Glutathione peroxidase activity modulates recovery in the injured immature brain. *Ann Neurol* 65 (5): 540–549.

101. Toklu, H. Z., T. Hakan, N. Biber, S. Solakoglu, A. V. Ogunc, and G. Sener. 2009. The protective effect of alpha lipoic acid against traumatic brain injury in rats. *Free Radic Res* 43 (7): 658–667.
102. Chen, G., J. Shi, Z. Hu, and C. Hang. 2008. Inhibitory effect on cerebral inflammatory response following traumatic brain injury in rats: A potential neuroprotective mechanism of N-acetylcysteine. *Mediators Inflamm* 2008: 716458.
103. Yi, J. H., and A. S. Hazell. 2005. N-Acetylcysteine attenuates early induction of heme oxygenase-1 following traumatic brain injury. *Brain Res* 1033 (1): 13–19.
104. Beni, S. M., R. Kohen, R. J. Reiter, D. X. Tan, and E. Shohami. 2004. Melatonin-induced neuroprotection after closed head injury is associated with increased brain antioxidants and attenuated late-phase activation of NF-kappaB and AP-1. *FASEB J* 18 (1): 149–151.
105. Wu, A., Z. Ying, and F. Gomez-Pinilla. 2009. Vitamin E protects against oxidative damage and learning disability after mild traumatic brain injury in rats. *Neurorehabil Neural Repair* 24 (3): 290–298.
106. Wu, A., Z. Ying, and F. Gomez-Pinilla. 2006. Dietary curcumin counteracts the outcome of traumatic brain injury on oxidative stress, synaptic plasticity, and cognition. *Exp Neurol* 197 (2): 309–317.
107. Conte, V., K. Uryu, S. Fujimoto, Y. Yao, J. Rokach, L. Longhi, J. Q. Trojanowski, V. M. Lee, T. K. McIntosh, and D. Pratico. 2004. Vitamin E reduces amyloidosis and improves cognitive function in Tg2576 mice following repetitive concussive brain injury. *J Neurochem* 90 (3): 758–764.
108. Butterfield, D. A., T. Koppal, R. Subramaniam, and S. Yatin. 1999. Vitamin E as an antioxidant/free radical scavenger against amyloid beta-peptide-induced oxidative stress in neocortical synaptosomal membranes and hippocampal neurons in culture: Insights into Alzheimer's disease. *Rev Neurosci* 10 (2): 141–149.
109. Montiel, T., R. Quiroz-Baez, L. Massieu, and C. Arias. 2006. Role of oxidative stress on beta-amyloid neurotoxicity elicited during impairment of energy metabolism in the hippocampus: Protection by antioxidants. *Exp Neurol* 200 (2): 496–508.
110. Ono, K., K. Hasegawa, H. Naiki, and M. Yamada. 2004. Curcumin has potent anti-amyloidogenic effects for Alzheimer's beta-amyloid fibrils in vitro. *J Neurosci Res* 75 (6): 742–750.
111. Sandhu, J. K., S. Pandey, M. Ribecco-Lutkiewicz, R. Monette, H. Borowy-Borowski, P. R. Walker, and M. Sikorska. 2003. Molecular mechanisms of glutamate neurotoxicity in mixed cultures of NT2-derived neurons and astrocytes: Protective effects of coenzyme Q10. *J Neurosci Res* 72 (6): 691–703.
112. Schubert, D., H. Kimura, and P. Maher. 1992. Growth factors and vitamin E modify neuronal glutamate toxicity. *Proc Natl Acad Sci U S A* 89 (17): 8264–8267.
113. Guseva, M. V., D. M. Hopkins, S. W. Scheff, and J. R. Pauly. 2008. Dietary choline supplementation improves behavioral, histological, and neurochemical outcomes in a rat model of traumatic brain injury. *J Neurotrauma* 25 (8): 975–983.
114. Wu, A., Z. Ying, and F. Gomez-Pinilla. 2004. Dietary omega-3 fatty acids normalize BDNF levels, reduce oxidative damage, and counteract learning disability after traumatic brain injury in rats. *J Neurotrauma* 21 (10): 1457–1467.
115. Wu, A., R. Molteni, Z. Ying, and F. Gomez-Pinilla. 2003. A saturated-fat diet aggravates the outcome of traumatic brain injury on hippocampal plasticity and cognitive function by reducing brain-derived neurotrophic factor. *Neuroscience* 119 (2): 365–375.
116. Al Moutaery, K., S. Al Deeb, H. Ahmad Khan, and M. Tariq. 2003. Caffeine impairs short-term neurological outcome after concussive head injury in rats. *Neurosurgery* 53 (3): 704–711; discussion 711–712.
117. Abate, A., G. Yang, P. A. Dennery, S. Oberle, and H. Schroder. 2000. Synergistic inhibition of cyclooxygenase-2 expression by vitamin E and aspirin, *Free Radic Biol Med* 29 (11): 1135–1142.
118. Devaraj, S., R. Tang, B. Adams-Huet, A. Harris, T. Seenivasan, J. A. de Lemos, and I. Jialal. 2007. Effect of high-dose alpha-tocopherol supplementation on biomarkers of oxidative stress and inflammation and carotid atherosclerosis in patients with coronary artery disease. *Am J Clin Nutr* 86 (5): 1392–1398.
119. Fu, Y., S. Zheng, J. Lin, J. Ryerse, and A. Chen. 2008. Curcumin protects the rat liver from CCl4-caused injury and fibrogenesis by attenuating oxidative stress and suppressing inflammation. *Mol Pharmacol* 73 (2): 399–409.
120. Hori, K., D. Hatfield, F. Maldarelli, B. J. Lee, and K. A. Clouse. 1997. Selenium supplementation suppresses tumor necrosis factor alpha-induced human immunodeficiency virus type 1 replication in vitro. *AIDS Res Hum Retroviruses* 13 (15): 1325–1332.
121. Jesudason, E. P., J. G. Masilamoni, B. S. Ashok, B. Baben, V. Arul, K. S. Jesudoss, W. C. Jebaraj, S. Dhandayuthapani, S. Vignesh, and R. Jayakumar. 2008. Inhibitory effects of short-term administration of dl-alpha-lipoic acid on oxidative vulnerability induced by Abeta amyloid fibrils (25–35) in mice. *Mol Cell Biochem* 311 (1–2): 145–156.
122. Kuhlmann, M. K., and N. W. Levin. 2008. Potential interplay between nutrition and inflammation in dialysis patients. *Contrib Nephrol* 161: 76–82.

123. Lee, H. S., K. K. Jung, J. Y. Cho, M. H. Rhee, S. Hong, M. Kwon, S. H. Kim, and S. Y. Kang. 2007. Neuroprotective effect of curcumin is mainly mediated by blockade of microglial cell activation. *Pharmazie* 62 (12): 937–942.
124. Masliah, E., E. Rockenstein, I. Veinbergs, Y. Sagara, M. Mallory, M. Hashimoto, and L. Mucke. 2001. Beta-amyloid peptides enhance alpha-synuclein accumulation and neuronal deficits in a transgenic mouse model linking Alzheimer's disease and Parkinson's disease. *Proc Natl Acad Sci U S A* 98 (21): 12245–12250.
125. Peairs, A. T., and J. W. Rankin. 2008. Inflammatory response to a high-fat, low-carbohydrate weight loss diet: Effect of antioxidants, *Obesity (Silver Spring)* 16 (7): 1573–1578.
126. Rahman, S., K. Bhatia, A. Q. Khan, M. Kaur, F. Ahmad, H. Rashid, M. Athar, F. Islam, and S. Raisuddin. 2008. Topically applied vitamin E prevents massive cutaneous inflammatory and oxidative stress responses induced by double application of 12-O-tetradecanoylphorbol-13-acetate (TPA) in mice. *Chem Biol Interact* 172 (3): 195–205.
127. Suzuki, Y. J., B. B. Aggarwal, and L. Packer. 1992. Alpha-lipoic acid is a potent inhibitor of NF-kappa B activation in human T cells. *Biochem Biophys Res Commun* 189 (3): 1709–1715.
128. Wood, L. G., M. L. Garg, H. Powell, and P. G. Gibson. 2008. Lycopene-rich treatments modify noneosinophilic airway inflammation in asthma: Proof of concept. *Free Radic Res* 42 (1): 94–102.
129. Zhu, J., W. Yong, X. Wu, Y. Yu, J. Lv, C. Liu, X. Mao, et al. 2008. Anti-inflammatory effect of resveratrol on TNF-alpha-induced MCP-1 expression in adipocytes. *Biochem Biophys Res Commun* 369 (2): 471–477.
130. Barger, S. W., M. E. Goodwin, M. M. Porter, and M. L. Beggs. 2007. Glutamate release from activated microglia requires the oxidative burst and lipid peroxidation. *J Neurochem* 101 (5): 1205–1213.
131. Krinsky, N. I. 1989. Antioxidant functions of carotenoids. *Free Radic Biol Med* 7 (6): 617–635.
132. Hazuka, M. B., J. Edwards-Prasad, F. Newman, J. J. Kinzie, and K. N. Prasad. 1990. Beta-carotene induces morphological differentiation and decreases adenylate cyclase activity in melanoma cells in culture. *J Am Coll Nutr* 9 (2): 143–149.
133. Zhang, L. X., R. V. Cooney, and J. S. Bertram. 1992. Carotenoids up-regulate connexin43 gene expression independent of their provitamin A or antioxidant properties. *Cancer Res* 52 (20): 5707–5712.
134. Carter, C. A., M. Pogribny, A. Davidson, C. D. Jackson, L. J. McGarrity, and S. M. Morris. 1996. Effects of retinoic acid on cell differentiation and reversion toward normal in human endometrial adenocarcinoma (RL95-2) cells. *Anticancer Res* 16 (1): 17–24.
135. Meyskens, Jr., F. L. 1995. Role of vitamin A and its derivatives in the treatment of human cancer. In *Nutrients in Cancer Prevention and Treatment*, ed. K. N. Prasad, L. Santamaria, and R. M. Williams, 349–362. Totowa, NJ: Humana Press.
136. Vile, G. F., and C. C. Winterbourn. 1988. Inhibition of adriamycin-promoted microsomal lipid peroxidation by beta-carotene, alpha-tocopherol and retinol at high and low oxygen partial pressures. *FEBS Lett* 238 (2): 353–356.
137. McCay, P. B. 1985. Vitamin E: Interactions with free radicals and ascorbate. *Annu Rev Nutr* 5: 323–340.
138. Prasad, K. N., B. Kumar, X. D. Yan, A. J. Hanson, and W. C. Cole. 2003. Alpha-tocopheryl succinate, the most effective form of vitamin E for adjuvant cancer treatment: A review. *J Am Coll Nutr* 22 (2): 108–117.
139. Schwartz, J. L. 1995. Molecular and biochemical control of tumor growth following treatment with carotenoids or tocopherols. In *Nutrients in Cancer Prevention and Treatment*, ed. K. N. Prasad, L. Santamaria, and R. M. Williams, 287–316. Totowa, NJ: Humana Press.
140. Prasad, K. N., and J. Edwards-Prasad. 1992. Vitamin E and cancer prevention: Recent advances and future potentials. *J Am Coll Nutr* 11 (5): 487–500.
141. Witschi, A., S. Reddy, B. Stofer, and B. H. Lauterburg. 1992. The systemic availability of oral glutathione. *Eur J Clin Pharmacol* 43 (6): 667–669.
142. Shen, W., K. Liu, C. Tian, L. Yang, X. Li, J. Ren, L. Packer, C. W. Cotman, and J. Liu. 2008. R-alpha-Lipoic acid and acetyl-L-carnitine complementarily promote mitochondrial biogenesis in murine 3T3-L1 adipocytes. *Diabetologia* 51 (1): 165–174.
143. Niki, E. 1997. Mechanisms and dynamics of antioxidant action of ubiquinol. *Mol Aspects Med* 18 (Suppl): S63–S70.
144. Hiramatsu, M., R. D. Velasco, D. S. Wilson, and L. Packer. 1991. Ubiquinone protects against loss of tocopherol in rat liver microsomes and mitochondrial membranes. *Res Commun Chem Pathol Pharmacol* 72 (2): 231–241.
145. Chen, R. S., C. C. Huang, and N. S. Chu. 1997. Coenzyme Q10 treatment in mitochondrial encephalomyopathies. Short-term double-blind, crossover study. *Eur Neurol* 37 (4): 212–218.

146. Schubert, D., C. Behl, R. Lesley, A. Brack, R. Dargusch, Y. Sagara, and H. Kimura. 1995. Amyloid peptides are toxic via a common oxidative mechanism. *Proc Natl Acad Sci U S A* 92 (6): 1989–1993.
147. Behl, C., J. Davis, G. M. Cole, and D. Schubert. 1992. Vitamin E protects nerve cells from amyloid beta protein toxicity. *Biochem Biophys Res Commun* 186 (2): 944–950.
148. Sano, M., C. Ernesto, R. G. Thomas, M. R. Klauber, K. Schafer, M. Grundman, P. Woodbury, et al. 1997. A controlled trial of selegiline, alpha-tocopherol, or both as treatment for Alzheimer's disease. The Alzheimer's Disease Cooperative Study. *N Engl J Med* 336 (17): 1216–1222.
149. Maxwell, C. J., M. S. Hicks, D. B. Hogan, J. Basran, and E. M. Ebly. 2005. Supplemental use of antioxidant vitamins and subsequent risk of cognitive decline and dementia. *Dement Geriatr Cogn Disord* 20 (1): 45–51.
150. Yan, X. D., B. Kumar, P. Nahreini, A. J. Hanson, J. E. Prasad, and K. N. Prasad. 2005. Prostaglandin-induced neurodegeneration is associated with increased levels of oxidative markers and reduced by a mixture of antioxidants. *J Neurosci Res* 81 (1): 85–90.
151. Liu, H., H. Wang, S. Shenvi, T. M. Hagen, and R. M. Liu. 2004. Glutathione metabolism during aging and in Alzheimer disease. *Ann N Y Acad Sci* 1019, 346–349.
152. Chinta, S. J., M. J. Kumar, M. Hsu, S. Rajagopalan, D. Kaur, A. Rane, D. G. Nicholls, J. Choi, and J. K. Andersen. 2007. Inducible alterations of glutathione levels in adult dopaminergic midbrain neurons result in nigrostriatal degeneration. *J Neurosci* 27 (51): 13997–14006.
153. Hsu, M., B. Srinivas, J. Kumar, R. Subramanian, and J. Andersen. 2005. Glutathione depletion resulting in selective mitochondrial complex I inhibition in dopaminergic cells is via an NO-mediated pathway not involving peroxynitrite: Implications for Parkinson's disease. *J Neurochem* 92 (5): 1091–1103.
154. Muller, T., T. Buttner, A. F. Gholipour, and W. Kuhn. 2003. Coenzyme Q10 supplementation provides mild symptomatic benefit in patients with Parkinson's disease. *Neurosci Lett* 341 (3): 201–204.
155. The NINDS NET-PD Investigators. 2007. A randomized clinical trial of coenzyme Q10 and GPI-1485 in early Parkinson disease. *Neurology* 68: 20–28.
156. Gottshall, K., M. E. Hoffer, and B. J. Balough. 2006. Use of antioxidants micronutrient compounds in vestibular rehabilitation after operational head trauma or blast injury. Barany International Balance Meeting, Stockholm, Sweden, June 2006.
157. Olanow, C. W., and G. W. Arendash. 1994. Metals and free radicals in neurodegeneration. *Curr Opin Neurol* 7 (6): 548–558.

14 Micronutrients in Prevention and Improvement of the Standard Therapy in HIV/AIDS

INTRODUCTION

The emergence of pathogenic human immunodeficiency virus (HIV) has markedly alarmed public and health professionals alike throughout the world. Similar viruses have been found in monkeys. These viruses may have coexisted with their respective hosts throughout the entire evolutionary processes and maintained their species specificity. The presence of genetic variants of viruses within the host suggests that these viruses can be mutated. Mutations may occur spontaneously or may be induced by increased oxidative stress in the host due to adverse environmental and dietary conditions that generate excessive amounts of free radicals. Some mutated forms of virus may acquire aggressive traits and kill the host, whereas other mutated forms may infect different species and may become pathogenic in the new host.

Although most HIV-infected persons progress to acquired immunodeficiency syndrome (AIDS), some do not. This implies that the immune system of some individuals is competent enough to mount a defensive response against HIV infection. The role of the immune system in HIV infection is further supported by the fact that micronutrient deficiency and illicit drugs that are known to impair immune function increase the risk of HIV infection. This may be due to the fact that micronutrient deficiency increased the levels of oxidative stress that can induce inflammation in the individuals. Increased oxidative stress and inflammation are also associated with the progression of HIV infection. The current prevention strategy has emphasized safe sex by using condoms and the use of clean needles for intravenous (IV) drug users. Micronutrients such as dietary and endogenous antioxidants that reduce oxidative stress and inflammation and play a prominent role in stimulating host's immune function have not drawn adequate attention for reducing the risk of HIV infection or slowing down the rate of progression of HIV to AIDS.

The introduction of highly active antiretroviral therapy (HAART) has improved the survival time of patients with AIDS, but it has failed to affect the risk of developing dementia, and it is very toxic. Low-dose HAART is also used in reducing the risk of transmission of virus from the infected to uninfected persons with limited success. Antiviral therapy also increases oxidative stress; therefore, the use of antioxidants in combination with HAART appears to be one of the rational choices for improving the efficacy of HAART in patients with AIDS. Unfortunately, most previous studies utilized a single antioxidant in combination with HAART, and they produced inconsistent results with respect to producing clinical outcomes better than HAART alone. In rare cases where more than one antioxidant was used in combination with HAART, only dietary antioxidants were used. For optimal effects, it would be essential to utilize multiple micronutrients including both dietary and endogenous antioxidants.

This chapter discusses the incidence and cost of HIV infection, and the role of immune function, oxidative stress, and inflammation in HIV infection and progression to AIDS. This chapter also provides a scientific rationale for using a comprehensive micronutrient preparation containing multiple dietary and endogenous antioxidants for reducing the risk of infection and transmission, and as an adjunct to HAART for improving the treatment outcomes in HIV/AIDS patient.

HISTORY, INCIDENCE, AND COST OF HIV/AIDS

The first case of unusual defects in the immune system was detected among gay men in the United States in 1981. In 1982, AIDS was defined, and HIV was isolated in 1983. The main types of HIV are HIV-1 and HIV-2, HIV-2 being less transmissible and less pathogenic. There are several subtypes of HIV-1, and genetic recombination of subtypes results in the generation of mosaic and recombinant viruses. Certain recombinant strains of HIV are present in the circulating blood. The prevalence of a specific subtype of HIV or their recombinants varies depending upon the region of the world. It has been shown that HIV primarily kills cells of the immune system (CD4 lymphocytes and macrophages playing a key defensive role in viral infection). HIV infection thus results in the progressive decline in the function of the immune system. This then makes the host more susceptible to additional infections such as esophageal candidiasis; HIV infection eventually progresses to AIDS.

At the end of 2004, about 1 million adults and children were living with HIV infection, about 44,000 new cases of HIV infection were detected, and about 16,000 died of AIDS in the United States.[40] During the same period in the world, about 39.4 million adults and children were living with HIV infection, about 4.9 million new cases were identified, and about 3.1 million died of AIDS. Sub-Saharan Africa has about 10% of the world's population, but about 65% of them are infected with HIV.[40] The exact reasons for the difference in the HIV infection rate between the United States and the sub-Saharan populations are unknown; however, the higher prevalence of micronutrient deficiency that can adversely affect the immune function may, in part, account for the increased rates of HIV infection in Sub-Saharan populations.

Based on the study published in 2008,[1] the Center for Disease Control and Prevention (CDC) estimated that in 2006, 56,300 new cases of HIV infection occurred in the United States, and about 50% of them were found in gay and bisexual men. The incidence of this infection among blacks/African Americans was 7 times higher than that found among whites. This increase in incidence of HIV infection was primarily due to improved detection techniques rather than new infections. The annual incidence of about 40,000 remained stable since 1992. In 2007, new cases of HIV were estimated to be 35,934 (26,355 males and 9579 females). The difference in incidence between male and female appears to be about threefold. Estimated number of deaths due to HIV/AIDS was 14,105 in adults and 5 in children under the age of 13 years. These studies suggest that the incidence rate of HIV infection did not increase in the United States as predicted earlier by some experts in the field.

Average annual costs of treating HIV/AIDS patients is about $1200/month per person in the United States, whereas it is about $50/month in the developing countries. In 2001, the annual estimated economic loss (including productive losses) among the U.S. population was about $18.2 billion, of which direct medical cost alone was estimated to be about $9.2 billion.

ROLE OF IMMUNE FUNCTION IN HIV INFECTION

The immune status of the host is one of the most important determining factors in HIV infection. This is evidenced by the fact that HIV infection does not progress to AIDS in some infected individuals. The primary cellular target of HIV is immune cells. In addition, micronutrient deficiency and illicit drugs that are known to impair immune function also increase the risk of HIV infection and the rate of progression of the HIV infection to AIDS.

MICRONUTRIENT DEFICIENCY IMPAIRS IMMUNE FUNCTION

Micronutrient deficiency can increase oxidative stress and inflammation that could damage the immune system, and thereby, makes the individuals more susceptible to HIV infection. It can also increase the toxicity of antiviral drugs, mortality, disease progression, and the risk of maternal–fetal transmission of HIV. Indeed, the deficiency of antioxidants and other micronutrients is a common feature of adults and children with HIV/AIDS. The deficiency of micronutrients includes selenium, vitamin E, vitamin A, beta-carotene (BC), lycopene, glutathione, coenzyme Q_{10}, vitamin C, vitamin B_6, vitamin B_{12}, and Zn.[2-7] Micronutrient deficiency that includes selenium, lycopene, BC, retinol, vitamin A, and vitamin E has also been reported in children with HIV infection.[8-9] Low plasma levels of antioxidants in pregnant women were associated with increased risks of fetal death and HIV transmission through the intrapartum route.[10]

Other than the poor diet, the mechanisms of nutritional deficiency associated with HIV infection and/or AIDS are not fully understood. One study showed that individuals infected with HIV or patients with AIDS exhibit increased excretion of vitamin A and vitamin E.[11] The malabsorption may account for deficiency in some nutrients such as selenium and BC.[12] Furthermore, HIV-1 encodes for one of the human glutathione peroxidase, and therefore, its replication may cause deficiency in glutathione, selenium, cysteine, glutamine, and tryptophan.[13] Increased oxidative stress in HIV-infected individuals can also deplete antioxidant levels in the body. Therefore, a preventive strategy to protect immune function by improving micronutrient deficiency may be one of the rational choices for reducing the rate of HIV infection.

The consequences of these nutritional deficiencies have been also investigated. For example, low serum levels of selenium in HIV-infected population is associated with loss of $CD4^+$ cells, increased levels of markers of cytokines (interleukin-8), and soluble tumor necrosis factor receptors (sTNFR).[14] Selenium deficiency causes an adverse effect on immune function and thereby makes the individuals more susceptible to HIV infection.[15] Malnutrition and selenium deficiency increase the risk of mycobacterial infection in illicit drug abusers as well as in HIV-infected individuals.[16] Low serum levels of vitamin B_{12} are associated with increased neurological abnormalities and more rapid progression of HIV infection to AIDS and an increase in AZT-induced bone marrow toxicity.[17] Vitamin A deficiency is associated with increased mortality and more rapid disease progression and increased maternal–fetal transmission.[17] Thus, micronutrient deficiency plays a central role in enhancing the rate of progression of HIV infection to AIDS, the risk of AIDS-related neurological deficits, mortality, and maternal–fetal transmission, as well as AZT-induced toxicity to bone marrow.

ILLICIT DRUGS IMPAIR IMMUNE FUNCTION

According to the CDC, about 70% of HIV infection occurs among drug users, suggesting that these illicit drugs may play an important role in increasing the risk of HIV infection. Illicit drugs, such as Ecstasy, are one of the agents that suppress immune function.[18-22] They also enhance the progression of HIV infection to AIDS.[22] The illicit drugs may also increase the activation of microglia in the brain that may contribute to dementia in some HIV-infected individuals.[23] The use of IV drugs may impair short- and long-term CD4 cell recovery in HIV-positive patients during active antiviral therapy.[24] Several clinical observations, neuroimaging, and neuropathological studies suggested that the use of illicit drugs enhanced the adverse effects of HIV infection on the central nervous system. The investigations on cell culture models support this conclusion. Furthermore, the IV injection of illicit drugs is also a risk factor for acquiring HIV infection, the incidence of which continues to rise in IV drug users even in countries with access to antiviral therapy.[25] Thus, a preventive strategy that is based on protecting the immune system and brain against the adverse effects of illicit drugs may be one of the rational choices for reducing the rate of HIV infection and dementia.

INCREASED OXIDATIVE STRESS AND INFLAMMATION ENHANCE THE RISK AND PROGRESSION OF HIV INFECTION

Many conditions can induce increased oxidative stress in the body. They include micronutrient deficiency,[2-6,8,9] and illicit drugs.[18-23] HIV infection also increased oxidative stress in humans and animal models. For example, evidence for high oxidative stress has been found in patients with AIDS.[3,26–30] Additionally, increased oxidative stress in human erythrocytes was observed in asymptomatic patients infected with HIV and patients with AIDS.[31] These studies suggest that increased oxidative stress is one of the major initiators of HIV infection, probably by impairing the immune function. In the autopsied brain samples from AIDS patients with dementia, the levels of 3-nitrotyrosine, a marker of oxidative damage, was elevated in comparison to those observed in the autopsied brain samples from the uninfected nondemented persons.[32] This result suggests that simultaneous production of nitric oxide and superoxide anion increases the levels of peroxynitrite that may contribute to the neuropathology of HIV-1 infection. In cats, feline immunodeficiency virus increased the levels of oxidative stress during the acute phase of viral infection.[33] These studies suggest that increased oxidative stress occurs during HIV infection and its progression.

Proinflammatory cytokines released during inflammatory reactions are also associated with the HIV infection.[14] Increased oxidative stress and proinflammatory cytokines can further impair immune function and thereby increase the susceptibility of the individuals to HIV infection. Both free radicals and TNF-alpha activate NF-kappa-B that is required for HIV proliferation.[34,35] Therefore, both increased oxidative stress and inflammatory reactions play an important role in determining the rate of the progression of the disease. They also play an important role in the development of complications associated with AIDS including cognitive dysfunction and the increased rate of myocardial infarction in patients with AIDS.[36–39] Therefore, attenuating the production and action of free radicals and proinflammatory cytokines by antioxidants should be considered as one of the crucial strategies for reducing the risk and progression of HIV/AIDS.

CURRENT AND PROPOSED PREVENTION STRATEGIES FOR HIV INFECTION

The HIV prevention strategies are discussed under two categories, primary prevention and secondary prevention. Primary prevention refers to a strategy that would reduce the risk of HIV infection in normal unexposed populations. Secondary prevention refers to a strategy that would prevent the transmission of HIV from the infected to the uninfected persons.

Primary Prevention

Although the primary prevention strategy appears to be the most rational for reducing the risk of HIV infection, adequate attention has not been paid to this approach. At present, there are no specific recommendations for the primary prevention. Since the immune system is considered one of the primary determining factors in HIV infection, the use of nontoxic agents such as multiple micronutrients including dietary and endogenous antioxidants that are known to neutralize free radicals and stimulate immune function appears to be one of the rational choices for reducing the risk of HIV infection. In addition, avoiding the consumption of illicit drugs that impairs immune function may also help in reducing the risk of HIV infection throughout the world. This strategy is cheap and nontoxic and could markedly reduce the risk of HIV infection in individuals, especially those who are malnourished and those who regularly consume illicit drugs. Vaccines against HIV infection that are currently in the development phase could be of great help in the primary prevention strategy. Until then, daily supplementation with multiple micronutrient preparations including dietary and endogenous antioxidants at doses that are higher than those for RDA, and are totally safe, may be very useful in reducing the risk of HIV infection. The recommended micronutrients include vitamin A, natural mixed-carotenoids, vitamin C, vitamin E (D-alpha-tocopherol acetate and D-alpha-tocopheryl succinate), alpha-lipoic acid, N-acetylcysteine (NAC), (a glutathione-elevating agent), coenzyme Q_{10}, L-carnitine, vitamin D, all B-vitamins, selenium, and zinc, but no iron, copper, or manganese.

Secondary Prevention

The recommendations for the secondary prevention in adults include safe sex, use of clean needles for illicit drug users, testing for HIV infection, and administration of low-dose antiviral drugs to those individuals who are tested positive for HIV. Low-dose antiviral drugs are also used in secondary prevention and reported to produce benefits in some cases. Daily supplementation with multiple micronutrients such as that proposed in the section on Primary Prevention may also be useful in reducing the risk of HIV transmission from the infected adults to the uninfected adults.

HIV transmission from mother to child during pregnancy, delivery, or breastfeeding is referred to as prenatal transmission. This mode of transmission is the most common route of HIV infection in children in the United States. Most the children with AIDS are from the minority ethnic groups.[40] Antiviral therapy administered to HIV-positive mothers during pregnancy, labor, and delivery, as well as during an elective cesarean and then to the newborn, can reduce the rate of prenatal HIV transmission to 2% or less.[41] If antiviral therapy to HIV-positive mothers is started during labor and delivery, the rate of HIV transmission to newborn can be decreased to less than 10%.[42] Although the rate of HIV infection was markedly decreased in newborns by antiviral therapy to their mothers during pregnancy, labor, and delivery, the subsequent health status of these children has not been evaluated. In view of the fact that antiviral therapy even at low doses has a potential to produce some late adverse health effects in children, this therapy is known to increase oxidative stress. Antioxidants that are known to reduce oxidative stress in combination with antiviral therapy could be useful in reducing the potential harmful effects of this therapy in children. The multiple micronutrients such as those proposed in the section of Primary Prevention at lower doses may be useful in reducing the risk of prenatal transmission. Indeed, certain micronutrients may also reduce the rate of prenatal transmission of HIV. A well-designed clinical study in which only one micronutrient (vitamin A containing 30 mg BC and 5000 IU preformed vitamin A) or multiple micronutrients containing two dietary antioxidants (500 mg vitamins C and 30 mg E), B-vitamins (20 mg B_1, 20 mg B_2, 25 mg B_6, 100 mg niacin, 50 μg vitamin B_{12}), and 0.8 mg folic acid were administered orally to immunologically and nutritionally compromised Tanzanian breastfeeding mothers. Some beneficial effects included reduced vertical transmission of HIV through breastfeeding to children and child mortality were observed.[43,44] Micronutrient treatment during pregnancy that improved the body weight of fetuses and immune function, and lowered viral load and hypertension, was observed.[45]

EVIDENCE FOR MICRONUTRIENTS REDUCING PROGRESSION OF HIV INFECTION

Micronutrient deficiency including antioxidants often exists in adult and child patients with HIV/AIDS[2–6,8,9,12]; therefore, supplementation with micronutrients including antioxidants should reduce the rate of progression of the disease. Indeed, some studies have reported that supplementation with one or two antioxidants improved health outcomes (enhanced immune function, reduced the rate of progression of the disease, oxidative damage, and inflammation in the HIV/AIDS patients).[35,46,47] For example, vitamin E and selenium also produce some beneficial effects in a mouse model of AIDS.[48] Selenium supplementation decreased progression of HIV infection by reducing viral load and improving CD4 counts.[49] Selenium supplementation also inhibited abnormally high levels of proinflammatory cytokines (TNF-alpha and IL-8) in HIV/AIDS disease, which is often associated with neurological abnormalities, Kaposi's sarcoma, wasting syndromes, and increased viral replication.[2] In addition, antioxidants and their derivatives such as alpha-lipoic acid, NAC, selenium, and alpha-tocopheryl succinate inhibited HIV replication by reducing activation of NF-kappa B that is required for HIV replication.[35,46,47,50] In Botswana, supplementation with glutathione and amino acids (cysteine, tryptophan, and glutamine) reversed AIDS in 99% of the patients. Vitamin E supplementation protected T lymphocytes of HIV-infected patients from apoptosis by suppressing the expression of CD95L (a physiological ligand that stimulates CD95, a death receptor) that is involved in this mechanism of cell death.[51] Low concentration of BC is a common observation in patients with HIV/AIDS, and it can predict mortality rate. Supplementation with micronutrients and natural mixed carotenoids may improve the survival rates by correcting the deficiency.[52] A short-term supplementation with BC may increase CD4+ cell count in a patient with AIDS.[53] In addition, BC (60 mg/day) supplementation showed objective and subjective improvements in patients with AIDS, but it did not affect lymphadenopathy.[54] Higher doses of BC in combination with hyperthermia were effective even in patients with advanced AIDS.[55] Alpha-tocopheryl succinate inhibited HIV replication and reduced the toxicity of AZT in lymphocytes in vitro.[55] Supplementation with vitamin A, vitamin C, vitamin E, BC, vitamin B_6, and vitamin B_{12} retarded the development of immune dysfunction.[4] Supplementation with BC and selenium improved immunological function and decreased lipid peroxidation.[12] Supplementation with BC (5450 IU of vitamin A), vitamin C (250 mg), vitamin E (100 IU), selenium (100 μg), and coenzyme Q_{10} (50 mg) improved some parameters of oxidative stress, but did not decrease the viral load.[56] On the other hand, supplementation with high doses of NAC and vitamin C for 60 days in HIV patients with advanced immunodeficiency can reduce viral load and improve immunological function.[57]

Supplementation with multiple vitamins to HIV-infected women during pregnancy and lactation resulted in better health of their children than those not taking vitamins.[58] Anemia is a frequent complication among HIV-infected individuals and is associated with faster disease progression and mortality. Supplementation with multiple vitamins in women during pregnancy and in the postpartum period provided a significant improvement in hematological status among HIV-infected women and their children.[59] It is interesting to note that certain antioxidants inhibit viral replication, the mechanism of which is different from that of antiviral drugs. Antioxidants inhibit viral replication by reducing activation of NF-kappa B, whereas antiviral drugs decreased it by inhibiting reverse transcriptase activity. Therefore, the combination of the two should reduce viral load more than that produced by the individual agents.

CURRENT TREATMENTS OF HIV/AIDS

The evolution of antiviral therapy for the treatments of HIV/AIDS has led to the development of HAART that includes a combination of three or more classes of antiviral drugs. They represent nucleoside and nucleotide reverse transcriptase inhibitors (nNRTI), non-nucleoside nucleotide reverse transcriptase inhibitors (NNRTI), protease inhibitors, integrase inhibitors, and entry inhibitors. nNRTI inhibits reverse transcriptase by incorporating themselves into the newly synthesized viral DNA preventing its function; NNRTI inhibits reverse transcriptase directly by binding to the enzyme and prevents further transcription of viruses; protease inhibitors stop the viral replication by inhibiting activity of protease, which is needed to complete the final assembly of HIV; the integrase inhibitor inhibits enzyme integrase, which is responsible for integration of viral DNA into the DNA of infected cells, and thus stops virus production, and entry inhibitors help to prevent the virus from entering and infecting cells.

HAART has been useful in increasing the survival time of HIV/AIDS patients and slowing the rate of disease progression; but it has largely failed to produce any beneficial effect on HIV-related dementia.[60] At present, there is no effective treatment for HIV dementia. It has been reported that patients with apolipoprotein E (ApoE) 4 allele are more susceptible to oxidative damage-induced dementia.[60] The introduction of HAART has decreased HIV-associated oral lesions, but the incidence of oral warts and HIV-associated salivary gland disease increased in Brazil.[61] In addition, HAART increased oxidative stress that caused toxicities including metabolic bone diseases such as osteopenia and osteoporosis,[62] distal sensory polyneuropathy, cataracts, retinitis, cystoids macular edema,[63] and hyperlipidemia.[64] Some patients are forced to discontinue antiviral drugs because of toxicity. In addition, some HIV-infected individuals cannot tolerate antiviral drugs; some of them cannot afford these drugs financially. The introduction of HAART into HIV-infected people of

Nicaragua has increased the death rate.[65] This could have been, in part, due to a nutritional deficiency that is common in developing countries. Therefore, additional approaches to improve the efficacy and reduce the toxicity of HAART are needed.

ROLE OF MICRONUTRIENTS IN COMBINATION WITH ANTIVIRAL DRUGS

Since most antiviral drugs can increase oxidative stress and are very toxic, supplementation with multiple micronutrients including antioxidants in combination with antiviral drugs appears to be one of the rational choices for improving the efficacy of the antiviral therapy in patients with HIV/AIDS. Indeed, alpha-tocopheryl succinate reduced the toxicity of AZT in lymphocyte culture.[50] Vitamin C and vitamin E supplementation reduced AZT-induced cardiac damage in mice.[66] The coadministration of antioxidants and AZT increases the therapeutic potential of AZT.[67]

In contrast to laboratory studies, clinical trials with one or two antioxidants, in combination with antiviral therapy, have produced inconsistent results varying from no effects to beneficial effects. In a randomized-placebo-controlled trial in which 49 HIV-positive patients participated, supplementation with DL-alpha-tocopheryl acetate (800 IU/day) and vitamin C (1000 mg/day) was administered orally for a period of 3 months. The results showed that supplementation reduced oxidative stress compared to placebo control. In addition, a trend toward a reduction in viral load was observed in a supplemented group.[68] A review on the efficacy of micronutrient supplementation in HIV-positive patients taking HAART has concluded that supplementation did not improve the efficacy of HAART.[69] Supplementation with NAC, a glutathione-elevating agent, inhibited inflammatory responses and reduced HIV replication.[70] In a randomized, 8-week double-blind, placebo-controlled trial, an oral supplementation with NAC increased the levels of glutathione in red blood cells and T cell lymphocytes.[71] In a pilot study with 8 HIV-positive patients, supplementation with NAC and vitamin C for 6 days had no effect on viral load or CD4+ lymphocyte counts; however, in some patients with most advanced immunodeficiency, supplementation reduced viral load.[57] In a randomized, double-blind, placebo-controlled trial with HIV-positive patients receiving antiviral therapy, supplementation with NAC alone for 180 days did not improve the efficacy of antiviral therapy.[72] In a prospective, double-blind, placebo-controlled trial, 40 HIV-positive patients taking HAART were randomized to receive micronutrients or placebo twice daily for 12 weeks. The results showed that micronutrients supplementation significantly improved CD4+ lymphocyte counts in patients taking HAART.[73]

RATIONALE FOR USING MULTIPLE MICRONUTRIENTS IN PRIMARY AND SECONDARY PREVENTION OF HIV INFECTION

High-risk populations include malnourished individuals, illicit drug users, and uninfected partners of HIV-infected people. Because of the increased levels of oxidative stress and chronic inflammation associated with the impaired immune function of individuals of these populations, oral supplementation with appropriate multiple micronutrients that reduce oxidative stress and chronic inflammation, and improve immune function, appears to be one of the rational choices for the prevention of HIV infection in high-risk populations. The use of one or two antioxidants may provide some short-term beneficial effects depending upon the dose, type of antioxidants, and observation period; however, it is well established that an individual antioxidant, when oxidized, acts as a pro-oxidant. As a matter of fact, all human studies with a single antioxidant in a population with high internal oxidative environment (e.g., heavy tobacco smokers) have produced adverse effects.[74–77] On the other hand, a study on the same single antioxidant in a population with a normal oxidative environment (physicians and nurses) showed no adverse effects on cancer or heart disease risk.[78] Therefore, I recommend taking multiple micronutrients including dietary and endogenous antioxidants for the prevention of HIV infection.

Humans have multiple antioxidants, most of which are derived from the diet, while others are made endogenously. Different types of free radicals derived from oxygen and nitrogen are produced. Free radicals can be quenched by both dietary antioxidants such as vitamins A, C, and E, carotenoids, lutein, lycopene, bioflavanoids, and a variety of phenolic compounds, and endogenous antioxidants such as glutathione, alpha-lipoic acid, coenzyme Q_{10}, and antioxidant enzymes such as catalase, glutathione peroxidase, and mitochondrial Mn-superoxide dismutase-1 (Mn-SOD-1) and cytosolic Cu/Zn-SOD-2. In addition, their mechanisms of action and distribution at the cellular and organ levels differ, their internal cellular and organ environments (oxygenation, aqueous and lipid components) differ, and their affinity for various types of free radicals differ. For example, BC is more effective in quenching oxygen radicals than most other antioxidants.[79] BC can perform certain biological functions that cannot be produced by its metabolite vitamin A, and vice versa.[80,81] It has been reported that BC treatment enhances the expression of the connexin gene, which codes for a gap junction protein in mammalian fibroblasts in culture, whereas vitamin A treatment does not produce such an effect.[81] Vitamin A can induce differentiation in certain normal and cancer cells, whereas BC and other carotenoids do not.[82,83] Thus, BC and vitamin A have, in part, different biological functions. Therefore, addition of both BC and vitamins in a multiple micronutrient is essential in order to increase its efficacy.

The gradient of oxygen pressure varies within cells. Some antioxidants, such as vitamin E, are more effective as quenchers of free radicals in reduced oxygen pressure, whereas BC and vitamin A are more effective in higher atmospheric pressures.[84] Vitamin C is necessary to protect cellular components in aqueous environments, whereas carotenoids and vitamins A and E protect cellular components in lipid environments. Vitamin C also plays an important role in maintaining cellular levels of vitamin E by recycling vitamin E radical (oxidized) to the reduced (antioxidant) form.[85] Also, oxidative DNA damage produced by high levels of vitamin C could be protected by vitamin E. Oxidized forms of vitamin C and vitamin E can also act as radicals; therefore, excessive amounts of any one of these forms, when used as a single agent, could be harmful over a long period of time.

The form of vitamin E used is also important in any clinical trial. It has been established that D-alpha-tocopheryl succinate (alpha-TS) is the most effective form of vitamin E both in vitro and in vivo.[86,87] This form of vitamin E is more soluble than alpha-tocopherol and enters cells more readily. Therefore, it is expected to cross the blood–brain barrier in greater amounts than alpha-tocopherol. However, this has not yet been demonstrated in animals or humans. We have reported that an oral ingestion of alpha-TS (800 IU/day) in humans increased plasma levels of not only alpha-tocopherol, but also alpha-TS, suggesting that a portion of alpha-TS can be absorbed from the intestinal tract before hydrolysis.[88] This observation is important because the conventional assumption based on the rodent studies has been that esterified forms of vitamin E such as alpha-TS, alpha-tocopheryl nicotinate, or alpha-tocopheryl acetate, can be absorbed from the intestinal tract only after they are hydrolyzed to alpha-tocopherol. Our preliminary data showed that this assumption may not be true for the absorption of alpha-TS in humans.

Glutathione is effective in catabolizing H_2O_2 and anions. However, oral supplementation with glutathione failed to significantly increase plasma levels of glutathione in human subjects,[90] suggesting that this tripeptide is completely hydrolyzed in the gastrointestinal tract. Therefore, I propose to utilize NAC and alpha-lipoic acid that increase the cellular levels of glutathione by different mechanisms in a multiple micronutrient preparation. In addition, R-alpha-lipoic acid and acetyl-L-carnitine together promoted mitochondrial biogenesis in murine adipocytes in culture; however, no effect was observed when these antioxidants were used individually.[91] These types of studies further emphasized the value of using more than one antioxidant in any clinical or laboratory studies for reducing the risk of HIV infection in high-risk populations.

Other endogenous antioxidants, coenzyme Q_{10}, may be needed for reducing the risk of HIV infection. Since increased oxidative stress can cause mitochondrial dysfunction and since coenzyme Q_{10} is needed for the generation of ATP by mitochondria, it is essential to add this antioxidant in multiple micronutrient preparation in order to improve the function of mitochondria. A study has shown that Ubiquinol (coenzyme Q_{10}) scavenges peroxy radicals faster than alpha–tocopherol[92] and, like vitamin C, can regenerate vitamin E in a redox cycle.[93] However, it is a weaker antioxidant than alpha-tocopherol.

Selenium is a cofactor of glutathione peroxidase, and Se-glutathione peroxidase increases the intracellular level of glutathione that is a powerful antioxidant. There may be some other mechanisms of action of selenium. Therefore, selenium and coenzyme Q_{10} should be added to a multiple micronutrient preparation for reducing the risk of HIV infection.

In addition to dietary and endogenous antioxidants, B vitamins that are necessary for general health should be added to a multiple micronutrient preparation for reducing the risk of HIV infection.

RECOMMENDED MICRONUTRIENTS FOR PRIMARY AND SECONDARY PREVENTION OF HIV INFECTION

A formulation of multiple micronutrients may include vitamin A (retinyl palmitate), vitamin E (both D-alpha-tocopherol and D-alpha-TS), natural mixed carotenoids, vitamin C (calcium ascorbate), coenzyme Q_{10}, R-alpha-lipoic acid, NAC, L-carnitine, vitamin D, all B vitamins, selenium, zinc, and chromium. No iron, copper, or manganese would be included in this micronutrient preparation because these trace minerals are known to interact with vitamin C to produce free radicals. These trace minerals are absorbed from the intestinal tract more in the presence of antioxidants than in their absence that could result in increased body stores of these minerals. Increased iron or copper stores have been linked to increased risk of several chronic diseases.[94] The efficacy of the proposed micronutrient formulation in high-risk populations susceptible to HIV infection remains to be tested; however, all proposed micronutrients have been used by consumers for several decades without any reported toxicity. In the meanwhile, the proposed micronutrient recommendations may be adopted by the individuals among high-risk populations in consultation with their physicians or health professionals. It is expected that the proposed recommendations would reduce the risk of HIV infection in high-risk populations.

The recommended micronutrient supplements should be taken orally and divided into two doses: half in the morning and the other half in the evening with meal. This is because the biological half-lives of micronutrients are highly variable, which can create high levels of fluctuations in the tissue levels of micronutrients. A twofold difference in the levels of certain micronutrients such as alpha-TS can cause a marked difference in the expression of gene profiles (our unpublished data). To maintain relatively consistent levels of micronutrients in the brain, the proposed micronutrients should be taken twice a day.

RECOMMENDED MICRONUTRIENTS FOR IMPROVING THE EFFICACY OF ANTIVIRAL THERAPY

Most of the previous clinical studies with antioxidants alone or in combination with antiviral therapy have primarily utilized either one or two antioxidants alone or in combination with antiviral therapy. This has produced inconsistent results with respect to the progression of the disease or the efficacy of HAART in the management of HIV/AIDS. I propose the use of multiple micronutrients at doses higher than those recommended for prevention of HIV infection. The rationale for recommending multiple micronutrients rather than one or two antioxidants is discussed in the section of prevention of HIV infection. Unfortunately, none of the clinical trials with antioxidants alone or in combination with antiviral therapy have considered these important scientific rationales, while designing studies with antioxidants in HIV-positive patients with or without HAART. The efficacy of proposed micronutrient formulation in combination with HAART remains to be tested; however, all proposed micronutrients have been used by the consumers for several decades without reported toxicity. In the meanwhile, the proposed micronutrient recommendations may be adopted by the

HIV/AIDS patients receiving HAART in consultation with their physicians or health professionals. It is expected that the proposed recommendations would enhance the efficacy of HAART in reducing viral load as well as the toxicity of antiviral therapy.

DIET AND LIFESTYLE RECOMMENDATIONS

In addition to micronutrient supplementation, I recommend a low-fat and high-fiber diet with plenty of fruits and vegetables for maximal effects on reducing the risk of HIV infection in high-risk populations, and improving the efficacy of antiviral therapy in patients with HIV/AIDS. Lifestyle recommendations include daily moderate exercise, reduced stress, and no tobacco smoking or illicit drug consumption.

CONCLUSIONS

Emergence pathogenic HIV has greatly alarmed health professionals throughout the world. Although most HIV-infected persons progress to AIDS, some do not. This implies that the immune system of some individuals is competent enough to mount a defensive response against HIV. The role of immune systems in HIV infection is further supported by the fact that micronutrient deficiency and illicit drugs that are known to impair immune function increase the risk of HIV infection. However, the current primary prevention strategy has not emphasized the importance of stimulating immune systems for reducing the risk of HIV infection. The introduction of HAART has improved the survival time of patients with AIDS, but it has failed to affect the risk of developing dementia, and it is very toxic. Low-dose HAART is also used in secondary prevention (transmission of virus from the infected to uninfected persons) with limited success. The increased oxidative stress and chronic inflammation appear to increase the risk of HIV infection as well as enhance the progression of the disease. Antioxidants that are known to reduce oxidative stress and chronic inflammation produced some beneficial effects in AIDS patients. Free radicals and proinflammatory cytokines such as tumor necrosis factor-alpha activate NF kappa-beta that is required for HIV replication. Some antioxidants such as alpha-lipoic acid and vitamin E reduce the activation of NF kappa beta, and thereby reduce the rate of viral replication. Clinical studies with antioxidants alone or in combination with antiviral therapy in HIV-positive patients have utilized one or two antioxidants resulting in inconsistent results with respect to reducing viral load or toxicity of antiviral drugs. The possible reasons for these inconsistent results have been discussed in this chapter. I have proposed that a preparation of multiple micronutrients containing dietary and endogenous antioxidants, all B vitamins, vitamin D, and certain minerals such as zinc and selenium, but no iron, copper, or manganese is expected to reduce the risk of HIV infection in uninfected persons by stimulating immune function. It can also reduce the transmission of HIV from the infected person to uninfected persons, possibly by decreasing the viral load in the infected persons and by stimulating the immune function in the uninfected person. In addition, a similar preparation of multiple micronutrients may also improve the efficacy of antiviral therapy by decreasing the viral load by a mechanism that is different from those of antiviral drugs and by decreasing the toxicity of the drugs. A clinical study with the proposed preparations of multiple micronutrients in high-risk populations and in HIV-positive patients should be initiated in order to evaluate their efficacy in reducing the risk of HIV infection and improving the efficacy of antiviral drugs. In the meanwhile, those individuals who are at high risk for HIV infection and those patients with HIV infection with or without antiviral drugs may like to adopt the proposed micronutrient preparations in consultation with their doctors.

REFERENCES

1. Hall, H. I., R. Song, P. Rhodes, J. Prejean, Q. An, L. M. Lee, J. Karon, et al. 2008. Estimation of HIV incidence in the United States. *JAMA* 300 (5): 520–529.

2. Baum, M. K., M. J. Miguez-Burbano, A. Campa, and G. Shor-Posner. 2000. Selenium and interleukins in persons infected with human immunodeficiency virus type 1. *J Infect Dis* 182 (Suppl 1): S69–S73.
3. Favier, A., C. Sappey, P. Leclerc, P. Faure, and M. Micoud. 1994. Antioxidant status and lipid peroxidation in patients infected with HIV. *Chem Biol Interact* 91 (2–3): 165–180.
4. Liang, B., S. Chung, M. Araghiniknam, L. C. Lane, and R. R. Watson. 1996. Vitamins and immunomodulation in AIDS. *Nutrition* 12 (1): 1–7.
5. Patrick, L. 2000. Nutrients and HIV: Part two—Vitamins A and E, zinc, B-vitamins, and magnesium. *Altern Med Rev* 5 (1): 39–51.
6. Ullrich, R., T. Schneider, W. Heise, W. Schmidt, R. Averdunk, E. O. Riecken, and M. Zeitz. 1994. Serum carotene deficiency in HIV-infected patients. Berlin Diarrhoea/Wasting Syndrome Study Group. *Aids* 8 (5): 661–665.
7. Dworkin, B. M. 1994. Selenium deficiency in HIV infection and the acquired immunodeficiency syndrome (AIDS). *Chem Biol Interact* 91 (2–3): 181–186.
8. Omene, J. A., C. R. Easington, R. H. Glew, M. Prosper, and S. Ledlie. 1996. Serum beta-carotene deficiency in HIV-infected children. *J Natl Med Assoc* 88 (12): 789–793.
9. Periquet, B. A., N. M. Jammes, W. E. Lambert, J. Tricoire, M. M. Moussa, J. Garcia, J. Ghisolfi, and J. Thouvenot. 1995. Micronutrient levels in HIV-1-infected children. *Aids* 9 (8): 887–893.
10. Kupka, R., M. Garland, G. Msamanga, D. Spiegelman, D. Hunter, and W. Fawzi. 2005. Selenium status, pregnancy outcomes, and mother-to-child transmission of HIV-1. *J Acquir Immune Defic Syndr* 39 (2): 203–210.
11. Jordao Junior, A. A., S. Silveira, J. F. Figueiredo, and H. Vannucchi. 1998. Urinary excretion and plasma vitamin E levels in patients with AIDS. *Nutrition* 14 (5): 423–426.
12. Patrick, L. 1999. Nutrients and HIV: Part one—Beta carotene and selenium. *Altern Med Rev* 4 (6): 403–413.
13. Foster, H. D. 2004. How HIV-1 causes AIDS: Implications for prevention and treatment. *Med Hypotheses* 62 (4): 549–553.
14. Look, M. P., J. K. Rockstroh, G. S. Rao, K. A. Kreuzer, U. Spengler, and T. Sauerbruch. 1997. Serum selenium versus lymphocyte subsets and markers of disease progression and inflammatory response in human immunodeficiency virus-1 infection. *Biol Trace Elem Res* 56 (1): 31–41.
15. Rayman, M. P., and M. P. Rayman. 2002. The argument for increasing selenium intake. *Proc Nutr Soc* 61 (2): 203–215.
16. Shor-Posner, G., M. J. Miguez, L. M. Pineda, A. Rodriguez, P. Ruiz, G. Castillo, X. Burbano, R. Lecusay, and M. Baum. 2002. Impact of selenium status on the pathogenesis of mycobacterial disease in HIV-1-infected drug users during the era of highly active antiretroviral therapy. *J Acquir Immune Defic Syndr* 29 (2): 169–173.
17. Tang, A. M., and E. Smit. 1998. Selected vitamins in HIV infection: A review. *AIDS Patient Care STDS* 12 (4): 263–273.
18. Friedman, H., C. Newton, and T. W. Klein. 2003. Microbial infections, immunomodulation, and drugs of abuse. *Clin Microbiol Rev* 16 (2): 209–219.
19. Connor, T. J. 2004. Methylenedioxymethamphetamine (MDMA, 'Ecstasy'): A stressor on the immune system. *Immunology* 111 (4): 357–367.
20. Lugoboni, F., G. Quaglio, B. Pajusco, P. Civitelli, L. Romano, C. Bossi, I. Spilimbergo, and P. Mezzelani. 2004. Immunogenicity, reactogenicity and adherence to a combined hepatitis A and B vaccine in illicit drug users. *Addiction* 99 (12): 1560–1564.
21. Nair, M. P., S. Mahajan, R. Hewitt, Z. R. Whitney, and S. A. Schwartz. 2004. Association of drug abuse with inhibition of HIV-1 immune responses: Studies with long-term of HIV-1 non-progressors. *J Neuroimmunol* 147 (1–2): 21–25.
22. Nair, M. P., S. A. Schwartz, S. D. Mahajan, C. Tsiao, R. P. Chawda, R. Whitney, B. B. Don Sykes, and R. Hewitt. 2004. Drug abuse and neuropathogenesis of HIV infection: Role of DC-SIGN and IDO. *J Neuroimmunol* 157 (1–2): 56–60.
23. Arango, J. C., P. Simmonds, R. P. Brettle, and J. E. Bell. 2004. Does drug abuse influence the microglial response in AIDS and HIV encephalitis? *Aids* 18 (Suppl 1): S69–S74.
24. Dronda, F., J. Zamora, S. Moreno, A. Moreno, J. L. Casado, A. Muriel, M. J. Perez-Elias, A. Antela, L. Moreno, and C. Quereda. 2004. CD4 cell recovery during successful antiretroviral therapy in naive HIV-infected patients: The role of intravenous drug use. *Aids* 18 (16): 2210–2212.
25. Anthony, I. C., J. C. Arango, B. Stephens, P. Simmonds, and J. E. Bell. 2008. The effects of illicit drugs on the HIV infected brain. *Front Biosci* 13: 1294–1307.

26. Greenspan, H. C. 1993. The role of reactive oxygen species, antioxidants and phytopharmaceuticals in human immunodeficiency virus activity. *Med Hypotheses* 40 (2): 85–92.
27. Jarstrand, C., and B. Akerlund. 1994. Oxygen radical release by neutrophils of HIV-infected patients. *Chem Biol Interact* 91 (2–3): 141–146.
28. Ogunro, P. S., T. O. Ogungbamigbe, M. O. Ajala, and B. E. Egbewale. 2005. Total antioxidant status and lipid peroxidation in HIV-1 infected patients in a rural area of south western Nigeria. *Afr J Med Med Sci* 34 (3): 221–225.
29. Gil, L., G. Martinez, I. Gonzalez, A. Tarinas, A. Alvarez, A. Giuliani, R. Molina, R. Tapanes, J. Perez, and O. S. Leon. 2003. Contribution to characterization of oxidative stress in HIV/AIDS patients. *Pharmacol Res* 47 (3): 217–224.
30. Suttajit, M. 2007. Advances in nutrition support for quality of life in HIV/AIDS. *Asia Pac J Clin Nutr* 16 (Suppl 1): 318–322.
31. Repetto, M., C. Reides, M. L. Gomez Carretero, M. Costa, G. Griemberg, and S. Llesuy. 1996. Oxidative stress in blood of HIV infected patients. *Clin Chim Acta* 255 (2): 107–117.
32. Boven, L. A., L. Gomes, C. Hery, F, Gray, J. Verhoef, P. Portegies, M. Tardieu, and H. S. Nottet. 1999. Increased peroxynitrite activity in AIDS dementia complex: Implications for the neuropathogenesis of HIV-1 infection. *J Immunol* 162 (7): 4319–4327.
33. Webb, C., T. Lehman, K. McCord, P. Avery, and S. Dow. 2008. Oxidative stress during acute FIV infection in cats. *Vet Immunol Immunopathol* 122 (1–2): 16–24.
34. Suzuki, Y. J., B. B. Aggarwal, and L. Packer. 1992. Alpha-lipoic acid is a potent inhibitor of NF-kappa B activation in human T cells. *Biochem Biophys Res Commun* 189 (3): 1709–1715.
35. Suzuki, Y. J., and L. Packer. 1993. Inhibition of NF-kappa B activation by vitamin E derivatives. *Biochem Biophys Res Commun* 193 (1): 277–283.
36. Mollace, V., H. S. Nottet, P. Clayette, M. C. Turco, C. Muscoli, D. Salvemini, and C. F. Perno. 2001. Oxidative stress and neuroAIDS: Triggers, modulators and novel antioxidants. *Trends Neurosci* 24 (7): 411–416.
37. Shor-Posner, G. 2000. Cognitive function in HIV-1–infected drug users. *J Acquir Immune Defic Syndr* 25 (Suppl 1): S70–S73.
38. Shor-Posner, G., R. Lecusay, G. Morales, A. Campa, and M. J. Miguez-Burbano. 2002. Neuroprotection in HIV-positive drug users: Implications for antioxidant therapy. *J Acquir Immune Defic Syndr* 31 (Suppl 2): S84–S88.
39. Turchan, J., C. B. Pocernich, C. Gairola, A. Chauhan, G. Schifitto, D. A. Butterfield, S. Buch, et al. 2003. Oxidative stress in HIV demented patients and protection ex vivo with novel antioxidants. *Neurology* 60 (2): 307–314.
40. CDC, HIV/AIDS Surveillance Report, 2005, vol. 17 ed. US Department of Health and Human Services Atlanta, 2007.
41. Cooper, E. R., M. Charurat, L. Mofenson, I. C. Hanson, J. Pitt, C. Diaz, K. Hayani, et al. 2002. Combination antiretroviral strategies for the treatment of pregnant HIV-1-infected women and prevention of perinatal HIV-1 transmission. *J Acquir Immune Defic Syndr* 29 (5): 484–494.
42. Wade, N. A., G. S. Birkhead, B. L. Warren, T. T. Charbonneau, P. T. French, L. Wang, J. B. Baum, J. M. Tesoriero, and R. Savicki. 1998. Abbreviated regimens of zidovudine prophylaxis and perinatal transmission of the human immunodeficiency virus. *N Engl J Med* 339 (20): 1409–1414.
43. Fawzi, W. W., G. I. Msamanga, D. Hunter, B. Renjifo, G. Antelman, H. Bang, K. Manji, et al. 2002. Randomized trial of vitamin supplements in relation to transmission of HIV-1 through breastfeeding and early child mortality. *Aids* 16 (14): 1935–1944.
44. Fawzi, W. W., G. I. Msamanga, D. Spiegelman, R. Wei, S. Kapiga, E. Villamor, D. Mwakagile, et al. 2004. A randomized trial of multivitamin supplements and HIV disease progression and mortality. *N Engl J Med* 351 (1): 23–32.
45. Merchant, A. T., G. Msamanga, E. Villamor, E. Saathoff, M. O'Brien, E. Hertzmark, D. J. Hunter, and W. W. Fawzi. 2005. Multivitamin supplementation of HIV-positive women during pregnancy reduces hypertension. *J Nutr* 135 (7): 1776–1781.
46. Harakeh, S., R. J. Jariwalla, and L. Pauling. 1990. Suppression of human immunodeficiency virus replication by ascorbate in chronically and acutely infected cells. *Proc Natl Acad Sci U S A* 87 (18): 7245–7249.
47. Hori, K., D. Hatfield, F. Maldarelli, B. J. Lee, and K. A. Clouse. 1997. Selenium supplementation suppresses tumor necrosis factor alpha-induced human immunodeficiency virus type 1 replication in vitro. *AIDS Res Hum Retroviruses* 13 (15): 1325–1332.
48. Wang, Y., and R. R. Watson. 1994. Vitamin E supplementation at various levels alters cytokine production by thymocytes during retrovirus infection causing murine AIDS. *Thymus* 22 (3): 153–165.

49. Hurwitz, B. E., J. R. Klaus, M. M. Llabre, A. Gonzalez, P. J. Lawrence, K. J. Maher, J. M. Greeson, et al. 2007. Suppression of human immunodeficiency virus type 1 viral load with selenium supplementation: A randomized controlled trial. *Arch Intern Med* 167 (2): 148–154.
50. Gogu, S. R., J. J. Lertora, W. J. George, N. E. Hyslop, and K. C. Agrawal. 1991. Protection of zidovudine-induced toxicity against murine erythroid progenitor cells by vitamin E. *Exp Hematol* 19 (7): 649–652.
51. Li-Weber, M., M. A. Weigand, M. Giaisi, D. Suss, M. K. Treiber, S. Baumann, E. Ritsou, R. Breitkreutz, and P. H. Krammer. 2002. Vitamin E inhibits CD95 ligand expression and protects T cells from activation-induced cell death. *J Clin Invest* 110 (5): 681–690.
52. Austin, J., N. Singhal, R. Voigt, F. Smaill, M. J. Gill, S. Walmsley, I. Salit, et al. 2006. A community randomized controlled clinical trial of mixed carotenoids and micronutrient supplementation of patients with acquired immunodeficiency syndrome. *Eur J Clin Nutr* 60 (11): 1266–1276.
53. Fryburg, D. A., R. J. Mark, B. P. Griffith, P. W. Askenase, and T. F. Patterson. 1995. The effect of supplemental beta-carotene on immunologic indices in patients with AIDS: A pilot study. *Yale J Biol Med* 68 (1–2): 19–23.
54. Santamaria, L., A. Bianchi-Santamaria, and M. dell'Orti. 1996. Carotenoids in cancer, mastalgia, and AIDS: Prevention and treatment—An overview. *J Environ Pathol Toxicol Oncol* 15 (2–4): 89–95.
55. Pontiggia, P., A. Bianchi Santamaria, K. Alonso, and L. Santamaria. 1995. Whole body hyperthermia associated with beta-carotene supplementation in patients with AIDS, *Biomed Pharmacother* 49 (5): 263–265.
56. Batterham, M., J. Gold, D. Naidoo, O. Lux, S. Sadler, S. Bridle, M. Ewing, and C. Oliver. 2001. A preliminary open label dose comparison using an antioxidant regimen to determine the effect on viral load and oxidative stress in men with HIV/AIDS. *Eur J Clin Nutr* 55 (2): 107–114.
57. Muller, F., A. M. Svardal, I. Nordoy, R. K. Berge, P. Aukrust, and S. S. Froland. 2000. Virological and immunological effects of antioxidant treatment in patients with HIV infection. *Eur J Clin Invest* 30 (10): 905–914.
58. Fawzi, W. W., G. I. Msamanga, R. Wei, D. Spiegelman, G. Antelman, E. Villamor, K. Manji, and D. Hunter. 2003. Effect of providing vitamin supplements to human immunodeficiency virus-infected, lactating mothers on the child's morbidity and CD4+ cell counts. *Clin Infect Dis* 36 (8): 1053–1062.
59. Fawzi, W. W., G. I. Msamanga, R. Kupka, D. Spiegelman, E. Villamor, F. Mugusi, R. Wei, and D. Hunter. 2007. Multivitamin supplementation improves hematologic status in HIV-infected women and their children in Tanzania. *Am J Clin Nutr* 85 (5): 1335–1343.
60. Steiner, J., N. Haughey, W. Li, A. Venkatesan, C. Anderson, R. Reid, T. Malpica, C. Pocernich, D. A. Butterfield, and A. Nath. 2006. Oxidative stress and therapeutic approaches in HIV dementia. *Antioxid Redox Signal* 8 (11–12): 2089–2100.
61. Ferreira, S., C. Noce, A. S. Junior, L. Goncalves, S. Torres, V. Meeks, R. Luiz, and E. Dias. 2007. Prevalence of oral manifestations of HIV infection in Rio De Janeiro, Brazil from 1988 to 2004. *AIDS Patient Care STDS* 21 (10): 724–731.
62. Pan, G., Z. Yang, S. W. Ballinger, and J. M. McDonald. 2006. Pathogenesis of osteopenia/osteoporosis induced by highly active anti-retroviral therapy for AIDS. *Ann N Y Acad Sci* 1068, 297–308.
63. Thorne, J. E., D. A. Jabs, J. H. Kempen, J. T. Holbrook, C. Nichols, and C. L. Meinert. 2006. Causes of visual acuity loss among patients with AIDS and cytomegalovirus retinitis in the era of highly active antiretroviral therapy. *Ophthalmology* 113 (8): 1441–1445.
64. Benesic, A., M. Zilly, F. Kluge, B. Weissbrich, R. Winzer, H. Klinker, and P. Langmann. 2004. Lipid lowering therapy with fluvastatin and pravastatin in patients with HIV infection and antiretroviral therapy: Comparison of efficacy and interaction with indinavir. *Infection* 32 (4): 229–233.
65. Matute, A. J., E. Delgado, J. J. Amador, and A. I. Hoepelman. 2008. The epidemiology of clinically apparent HIV infection in Nicaragua. *Eur J Clin Microbiol Infect Dis* 27 (2): 105–108.
66. de la Asuncion, J. G., M. L. Del Olmo, L. G. Gomez-Cambronero, J. Sastre, F. V. Pallardo, and J. Vina. 2004. AZT induces oxidative damage to cardiac mitochondria: Protective effect of vitamins C and E. *Life Sci* 76 (1): 47–56.
67. Romero-Alvira, D., and E. Roche. 1998. The keys of oxidative stress in acquired immune deficiency syndrome apoptosis. *Med Hypotheses* 51 (2): 169–173.
68. Allard, J. P., E. Aghdassi, J. Chau, C. Tam, C. M. Kovacs, I. E. Salit, and S. L. Walmsley. 1998. Effects of vitamin E and C supplementation on oxidative stress and viral load in HIV-infected subjects. *Aids* 12 (13): 1653–1659.
69. Drain, P. K., R. Kupka, F. Mugusi, and W. W. Fawzi. 2007. Micronutrients in HIV-positive persons receiving highly active antiretroviral therapy. *Am J Clin Nutr* 85 (2): 333–345.

70. Roederer, M., F. J. Staal, S. W. Ela, and L. A. Herzenberg. 1993. *N*-Acetylcysteine: Potential for AIDS therapy. *Pharmacology* 46 (3): 121–129.
71. De Rosa, S. C., M. D. Zaretsky, J. G. Dubs, M. Roederer, M. Anderson, A. Green, D. Mitra, et al. 2000. *N*-Acetylcysteine replenishes glutathione in HIV infection. *Eur J Clin Invest* 30 (10): 915–929.
72. Treitinger, A., C. Spada, I. Y. Masokawa, J. C. Verdi, M. Van Der Sander Silveira, M. C. Luis, M. Reis, S. I. Ferreira, and D. S. Abdalla. 2004. Effect of *N*-acetyl-L-cysteine on lymphocyte apoptosis, lymphocyte viability, TNF-alpha and IL-8 in HIV-infected patients undergoing anti-retroviral treatment. *Braz J Infect Dis* 8 (5): 363–371.
73. Kaiser, J. D., A. M. Campa, J. P. Ondercin, G. S. Leoung, R. F. Pless, and M. K. Baum. 2006. Micronutrient supplementation increases CD4 count in HIV-infected individuals on highly active antiretroviral therapy: A prospective, double-blinded, placebo-controlled trial. *J Acquir Immune Defic Syndr* 42 (5): 523–528.
74. Fariss, M. W., M. B. Fortuna, C. K. Everett, J. D. Smith, D. F. Trent, and Z. Djuric. 1994. The selective antiproliferative effects of alpha-tocopheryl hemisuccinate and cholesteryl hemisuccinate on murine leukemia cells result from the action of the intact compounds. *Cancer Res* 54 (13): 3346–3351.
75. Albanes, D., O. P. Heinonen, J. K. Huttunen, P. R. Taylor, J. Virtamo, B. K. Edwards, J. Haapakoski, et al. 1995. Effects of alpha-tocopherol and beta-carotene supplements on cancer incidence in the Alpha-Tocopherol Beta-Carotene Cancer Prevention Study. *Am J Clin Nutr* 62 (6 Suppl): 1427S–1430S.
76. Bairati, I., F. Meyer, M. Gelinas, A. Fortin, A. Nabid, F. Brochet, J. P. Mercier, et al. 2005. Randomized trial of antioxidant vitamins to prevent acute adverse effects of radiation therapy in head and neck cancer patients. *J Clin Oncol* 23 (24): 5805–5813.
77. Bowen, D. J., M. Thornquist, K. Anderson, M. Barnett, C. Powell, G. Goodman, and G. Omenn. 2003. Stopping the active intervention: CARET. *Control Clin Trials* 24 (1): 39–50.
78. Hennekens, C. H., J. E. Buring, J. E. Manson, M. Stampfer, B. Rosner, N. R. Cook, C. Belanger, et al. 1996. Lack of effect of long-term supplementation with beta carotene on the incidence of malignant neoplasms and cardiovascular disease. *N Engl J Med* 334 (18): 1145–1149.
79. Krinsky, N. I. 1989. Antioxidant functions of carotenoids. *Free Radic Biol Med* 7 (6): 617–635.
80. Hazuka, M. B., J. Edwards-Prasad, F. Newman, J. J. Kinzie, and K. N. Prasad. 1990. Beta-carotene induces morphological differentiation and decreases adenylate cyclase activity in melanoma cells in culture. *J Am Coll Nutr* 9 (2): 143–149.
81. Zhang, L. X., R. V. Cooney, and J. S. Bertram. 1992. Carotenoids up-regulate connexin43 gene expression independent of their provitamin A or antioxidant properties. *Cancer Res* 52 (20): 5707–5712.
82. Carter, C. A., M. Pogribny, A. Davidson, C. D. Jackson, L. J. McGarrity, and S. M. Morris. 1996. Effects of retinoic acid on cell differentiation and reversion toward normal in human endometrial adenocarcinoma (RL95-2) cells. *Anticancer Res* 16 (1): 17–24.
83. Meyskens, F. L., Jr. 1995. Role of vitamin A and its derivatives in the treatment of human cancer. In *Nutrients in Cancer Prevention and Treatment*, ed. K. N. Prasad, L. Santamaria, and R. M. Williams, 349–362. Totowa, NJ: Humana Press.
84. Vile, G. F., and C. C. Winterbourn. 1988. Inhibition of adriamycin-promoted microsomal lipid peroxidation by beta-carotene, alpha-tocopherol and retinol at high and low oxygen partial pressures. *FEBS Lett* 238 (2): 353–356.
85. McCay, P. B. 1985. Vitamin E: Interactions with free radicals and ascorbate. *Annu Rev Nutr* 5, 323–340.
86. Prasad, K. N., B. Kumar, X. D. Yan, A. J. Hanson, and W. C. Cole. 2003. Alpha-tocopheryl succinate, the most effective form of vitamin E for adjuvant cancer treatment: A review. *J Am Coll Nutr* 22 (2): 108–117.
87. Schwartz, J. L. 1995. Molecular and biochemical control of tumor growth following treatment with carotenoids or tocopherols. In *Nutrients in Cancer Prevention and Treatment*, ed. K. N. Prasad, L. Santamaria, and R. M. Williams, 287–316. Totowa, NJ: Humana Press.
88. Prasad, K. N., and J. Edwards-Prasad. 1992. Vitamin E and cancer prevention: Recent advances and future potentials. *J Am Coll Nutr* 11 (5): 487–500.
89. Vali, S., R. B. Mythri, B. Jagatha, J. Padiadpu, K. S. Ramanujan, J. K. Andersen, F. Gorin, and M. M. Bharath. 2007. Integrating glutathione metabolism and mitochondrial dysfunction with implications for Parkinson's disease: A dynamic model. *Neuroscience* 149 (4): 917–930.
90. Witschi, A., S. Reddy, B. Stofer, and B. H. Lauterburg. 1992. The systemic availability of oral glutathione. *Eur J Clin Pharmacol* 43 (6): 667–669.
91. Shen, W., K. Liu, C. Tian, L. Yang, X. Li, J. Ren, L. Packer, C. W. Cotman, and J. Liu. 2008. *R*-alpha-Lipoic acid and acetyl-L-carnitine complementarily promote mitochondrial biogenesis in murine 3T3-L1 adipocytes. *Diabetologia* 51 (1): 165–174.

92. Niki, E. 1997. Mechanisms and dynamics of antioxidant action of ubiquinol, *Mol Aspects Med* 18 (Suppl): S63–S70.
93. Hiramatsu, M., R. D. Velasco, D. S. Wilson, and L. Packer. 1991. Ubiquinone protects against loss of tocopherol in rat liver microsomes and mitochondrial membranes. *Res Commun Chem Pathol Pharmacol* 72 (2): 231–241.
94. Olanow, C. W., and G. W. Arendash. 1994. Metals and free radicals in neurodegeneration. *Curr Opin Neurol* 7 (6): 548–558.

15 Micronutrients in Protecting Against Late Adverse Health Effects of Diagnostic Radiation Doses

INTRODUCTION

It is established that ionizing radiation is a potent mutagen and carcinogen that can induce somatic and heritable mutations, and neoplastic and certain non-neoplastic diseases; however, it is also used in the diagnosis and treatment of certain human diseases. Children are more sensitive to ionizing radiation on all criteria of radiation damage, including cancer, than adults. Also, the time interval between radiation exposure and death in children is longer than adults, which would increase the risk of expression of deleterious effects in children more than in adults.[1,2] Growing use of x-ray–based devices in the early diagnosis of human diseases has raised concerns about potential hazards of such procedures in increasing the risk of cancer, and somatic and heritable mutations in individuals receiving diagnostic doses of radiation. These risks also exist in radiation workers who are exposed to higher doses of ionizing radiation per year than non-radiation workers. The number of radiation workers has increased proportionally with increased diagnostic radiation procedures. In 2008, it was estimated that over 60 million computed tomography (CT) scans were performed in the United States.[3] This estimate did not include other diagnostic procedures such as chest x-rays, dental x-rays, fluoroscopic imaging, positron emission tomography (PET), and other nuclear medicine scans. Therefore, it is likely that many more patients were exposed to diagnostic doses of radiation than the current estimates. Because of the potential health hazards of low doses of radiation, developing an effective radioprotective strategy that involves both physical and biological protection methods against potential damage from low doses of radiation has become an urgent issue for the present and future generations.

Efforts to develop protection against radiation damage began soon after the discovery of x-rays in 1895 by Dr. Roentgen, a German scientist. However, the observation by Dr. Muller of Columbia University, in 1927, that x-ray causes gene mutations in *Drosophila melanogaster* (common fruit fly) provided new impetus to develop an effective physical and biological protection against radiation damage. The initial physical concept of radiation protection involved three principles that can reduce dose levels: (1) lead-shielding of unexposed areas, especially radiosensitive organs such as bone marrow, intestine, gonads, and thyroid, if possible; (2) increased distance between the radiation source and radiation workers or patients; and (3) reduction of radiation exposure time. Each of these physical principles has been very useful in reducing dose levels during diagnostic procedures, but they have limitations. For example, during fluoroscopy, it may not be possible to protect the gastrointestinal tract (one of the most radiosensitive organs) against radiation damage by lead shielding alone. Increasing the distance between the radiation source and individuals to be exposed may not be practical for many radiation workers, patients, civilian, or military personnel. Reducing radiation exposure time may also not be pertinent to all populations, except those that are involved in taking care of patients who have received gamma-emitting radioisotopes for medical purposes or who are responsible for radioactive decontamination as a result of nuclear accidents or attack. To address the growing concerns of radiation-induced damage, the concept of ALARA (as low as reasonably achievable) with respect to dose was recommended by national and international radiation protection agencies for radiation workers and individuals receiving diagnostic doses of radiation.[4] At present, all radiologists and radiobiologists follow the principles of ALARA in order to reduce radiation doses to patients. Additional recommendations are being made to reduce the number of diagnostic procedures in patients, whenever possible, in order to reduce the doses as much as possible.[5-7] These recommendations represent physical principles of radiation protection, and they have been very useful in reducing the diagnostic radiation doses to patients; however, they do not provide any suggestions on how to provide biological protection in those patients who justifiably receive low-dose radiation during diagnostic procedures. They also do not provide any recommendation for biological protection in radiation workers who are exposed daily to radiation doses higher than those in non-radiation workers.

This chapter discusses the probable biochemical and genetic events involved in radiation-induced carcinogenesis, interaction of radiation with chemical and biological carcinogens and tumor promoters; risk estimates of radiation-induced cancer, current recommendations for radiation protection. In addition, this chapter proposes a novel concept of biological protection against low doses of radiation referred to as PAMARA (protection as much as reasonably achievable) that would compliment the existing physical radiation protection concept of ALARA that refers to dose reduction.

PROBABLE BIOCHEMICAL AND GENETIC STEPS INVOLVED IN RADIATION-INDUCED CARCINOGENESIS

Radiation-induced carcinogenesis is no different from that which occurs spontaneously or caused by other carcinogens/tumor promoters. It involves a gradual accumulation of multiple mutations over a long period. Radiation-induced human cancers have long latent periods; 10 years for leukemia and 30 years or more for solid tumors.[8] This implies that radiation-induced mutations (due to genetic mutations and/or chromosomal damage) that can be detected within 24 h of radiation exposure are not directly responsible for the development of carcinogenesis in normal human cells because such cells continue to divide and proliferate like unirradiated normal cells for a long time. However, radiation-induced mutations cause genetic instability in normal cells that can make these cells more sensitive to mutagenic changes caused by increased oxidative stress that continues to occur as a function of time. Such genetically unstable cells may continue to proliferate and differentiate like nonirradiated cells in spite of carrying genetic abnormalities until the expression of genes that regulate differentiation is altered. This defect in expression of differentiation genes prevents cells from going through differentiation and death and, thus, continue to divide. These cells are referred to as immortal cells, and they represent the first step in carcinogenesis. Immortalized cells can continue to proliferate and can form adenomas such as polyps in the colon or cysts in the breast. When some key cellular genes, oncogenes or antioncogenes, are altered by continued exposure to increased oxidative stress caused by mutagens, carcinogens, and/or tumor promoters, these cells then become fully transformed and can induce cancer when tested in the appropriate host.[9,10] The existence of a long-latent period for radiation-induced cancer provides an opportunity to intervene at any time after radiation exposure with appropriate radioprotective agents in order to reduce the risk of late adverse effects of radiation. Radiation-induced immediate damage to DNA is caused primarily by free radicals, and very little by direct ionization, and free radicals are also involved in subsequent mutations in the irradiated cells. Therefore, it appears rational to suggest that supplementation with antioxidants that are known to neutralize free radicals before radiation exposure or any time after irradiation, may reduce potential risk of developing cancer and other adverse effects of radiation after diagnostic doses of radiation.

INTERACTIONS BETWEEN RADIATION AND CHEMICAL AND BIOLOGICAL CARCINOGENS AND TUMOR PROMOTERS

It is established that ionizing radiation interacts with chemical and biological carcinogens, and tumor promoters resulting in increased cancer induction. Some examples are given below. X-radiation enhances chemical carcinogen-induced transformation in normal mammalian cells by about 9-fold[11] and UV-induced transformation by about 12-fold.[12] X-irradiation also enhances the level of ozone-[13] and viral-induced[14] transformation in cell culture. Radiation doses that alone do not transform normal fibroblasts do so when combined with a tumor promoter.[15] Ionizing radiation in combination with tobacco smoking increases the risk of lung cancer by about 50%.[8] A low dose of radiation (20 mSv) does not produce detectable levels of mutations as measured by chromosomal damage; however, in the presence of caffeine (which inhibits repair of DNA damage), mutations become detectable.[15] Low doses of radiation (20 and 50 mSv) can act as a mitogen,[16] and lower doses (about 1 mSv) do not activate double-strand DNA break repair mechanisms.[17] This lack of repair after exposure to low doses of radiation can lead to accumulation of mutations that can increase the risk of cancer. This issue of interaction of radiation with other carcinogens and tumor promoters is often ignored when estimating the risk of cancer in children or adults.

RISK ESTIMATES OF RADIATION-INDUCED CANCER

Two models of risk estimate for radiation-induced cancer have been proposed. The first model proposes that cancer risk in humans following exposure to low doses of radiation (100 mSv or less) may be best estimated by a linear no-threshold relationship, since any dose has the potential to induce cancer. The most recent Biological Effects of Ionizing Radiation (BEIR) report supports this model.[18] This model of risk estimation for radiation-induced cancer can also be applied to children.[19] The second model suggests that there is a threshold dose below which radiation may not induce cancer in humans.[20,21] The second model has relied primarily on mathematical modeling. Mathematical modeling may assume certain constant physical factors such as body weight[21] that may not reflect the inherent biological variations associated with radiation-induced carcinogenesis. These include differences in radiosensitivity with respect to age, organs, body mass, and differences in the efficacy of repair mechanisms.

Recently, a few excellent reviews have been published in support of the model of linear no-threshold model for radiation-induced cancer.[18,19] The typical radiation doses for an adult from a chest CT scan can range between 6 and 10 mSv.[22] The average annual dose from background radiation in the United States is approximately 3 mSv. Several radiation dose estimates for imaging studies in adults and children have been published.[22,23] A dose from a CT scan may increase the risk of cancer in children by 1 in 1000 exposed individuals[5,24,25]; however, another study has reported that the lifetime cancer mortality risks for a 1-year-old child exposed to a radiation dose from a CT scan are 0.18% (abdominal CT scan) and 0.07% (head CT scan). This risk estimate is an order of magnitude higher than for adults. It was further estimated that in 2001, approximately 600,000 abdominal and head CT scans were performed in children under the age of 15 years and that 500 of the exposed children might die from cancer attributed to the CT scan.[26] A Canadian study reported that an abdominal CT study in a 5-year-old child, may increase lifetime risk of radiation-induced cancer by approximately 26.1 per 100,000 in female and 20.4 per 100,000 in male patients.[27] Another study performed in Israel estimated an increase of about 0.29% over the total number of patients who are eventually expected to die from cancer.[7] If one considers the fact that patients receiving diagnostic doses of radiation and radiation workers may also be exposed to chemical and biological carcinogens, as well as tumor promoters that enhance radiation-induced cancer risk during their lifetime, the above estimates of cancer mortality risk could be higher.

Recently, dose estimates and cancer risk from cardiovascular imaging have been published.[28] It has been estimated that about 5 billion imaging examinations are performed worldwide each year,

TABLE 15.1
Summary of Estimated Effective Dose from Average Diagnostic Radiation Procedures

Type of Examination	Effective Dose (mSv)
Standard radiography	0.01–10.0
Computed tomography	2.0–20.0
Nuclear medicine	0.3–20.0
Interventional procedure	5.0–70.0

Source: Adapted from Mettler, F.A., Jr., W. Huda, T.T. Yoshizumi, and M. Mahesh, *Radiology* 248 (1), 254–263, 2008.

and 2 out of 3 involve ionizing radiation.[29] In 2006, the estimated medical radiation exposure dose in the United States has reached 3.2 mSv,[28] which is more than 6-fold higher than that estimated in 2004.[30] The analysis of the risk of cancer on the basis of the annual number of diagnostic x-rays taken in the United Kingdom and 14 other developing countries revealed the cumulative risk varied from 0.6% to 1.8%, whereas in Japan, which used the highest number of annual diagnostic x-rays, it was more than 3%.[30] Cardiologists prescribe and/or directly perform greater than 50% of radiation imaging examinations that contribute to about two-thirds of the total effective dose to patients.[31] It has been estimated that about 20 million nuclear medicine examinations were performed in 2006, and cardiac examinations accounted for about 57% of all nuclear medicine procedures and 85% of the radiation dose.[32] The BEIR VII report has estimated that a dose of 15 mSv may increase cancer risk by 1/750 cases. Others have estimated that coronary MSCT that delivers patients about 20 mSv may increase the risk of cancer by 1/500; coronary stent by 1/400 for 25 mSv.[33]

TABLE 15.2
Estimated Doses of Ionizing Radiation Delivered during Specific Diagnostic Procedures

Procedure Type	Effective Dose (mSv)
Chest or dental x-ray	0.01
Electron beam CT (cardiac)	10.0–1.3
Electron beam CT coronary angiography	1.5–2.0
Catheter coronary angiography	2.1–2.5
Electron beam CT whole body	5.2
CT (head)	2.0
CT (abdomen)	10.0
Barium enema	7.0
Upper GI exam	3.0
IV urogram	2.5
Lumbar spine	1.3
Mammogram	7.0
Passenger from Athens to New York	0.06
Occupational annual dose limit	50.0
General public annual dose limit	1.0
Background annual dose at sea level	1.0

Source: Adapted from Prasad, K.N., *Br J Radiol* 78 (930), 485–492, 2005.
Note: Occupational and general public dose limit does not include background radiation.

TABLE 15.3
Estimated Doses of Radiation from Selected Radioactive Nuclides Administered Once during Nuclear Medicine Procedures

Procedure Type	Effective Dose (mSv)
18F-Fluorodeoxyglucose, 10 mCi	4.8
99mTc-MAA lung scan, 5 mCi	0.60
99mTc-HDP bone scan, 20 mCi	4.0
201Tl thallium scan, 3 mCi	0.60

Source: Adapted from Prasad, K.N., *Br J Radiol* 78 (930), 485–492, 2005.

If one considers the fact that children may be exposed to chemical and biological carcinogens, as well as tumor promoters that enhance radiation-induced cancer risk, these estimates of cancer mortality risk could be higher for children. The effective radiation dose estimates from diagnostic procedures are presented in Table 15.1.[34] Other estimated doses and cancer risks are presented in Tables 15.2–15.4.

Military and civilian pilots and flight attendants are exposed to cosmic ionizing radiation, potential chemical carcinogens (fuel and jet engine exhaust), and electromagnetic fields from cockpit instruments, and disrupted sleep patterns. Several epidemiologic studies have evaluated the risk of cancer in these populations. Most studies suggest that there is an increased risk of prostate, melanoma, and other skin cancer, and acute myeloid leukemia in male pilots[35,36] and breast cancer, melanoma,[37,38] and breast cancer and bone cancer[39] in female flight attendants.

RISK OF LOW-DOSE RADIATION-INDUCED NON-NEOPLASTIC DISEASES

The incidence of non-neoplastic diseases and intermediate health risks measured by certain specific biochemical markers were studied in children living in radiation-contaminated areas near the Chernobyl nuclear accident site. The incidence of thyroid gland enlargement and vision disorders, mostly dry eye syndrome, was closely related to the levels of contamination.[40] Increased levels of oxidized conjugated dienes, products of lipid peroxidation, were found among these children. In another report, increased levels of spontaneous chemiluminescence, an indicator of enhanced oxygen radical activity, in leukocytes of children living in contaminated areas were observed.[41] The accuracy of these intermediate markers for predicting health risks after radiation exposure remains uncertain. Radiation exposure during interventional cardiovascular procedures can induce damage to DNA and can cause chromosomal aberrations.[42] The micronucleus assay in exfoliated buccal

TABLE 15.4
Estimated Increases in Cancer Risk from Exposure to One Computed Tomography (CT) Scan

Source and Dose of Radiation	Increase in Cancer Risk in Exposed Individuals
One CT scan	1 per 1000[5,24,25]
	1 per 1200[26]
	2.9 per 1000[7]
	0.26 per 1000 females[27]
	0.2 per 1000 males[27]
15 mSv	1 per 750[33]
20 mSv	1 per 500[33]
25 mSv	1 per 400[33]

cells is considered a useful and minimally invasive assay method for monitoring genetic damage in humans.[43] Dental x-ray can induce formation of micronuclei in buccal cells in both adults and children.[44,45]

CURRENT RECOMMENDATIONS FOR RADIATION PROTECTION

The concepts of physical protection and ALARA continue to be propagated and supported by radiobiologists and radiologists for reducing the doses from diagnostic radiation procedures in patients. Additionally, suggestions are being made to reduce overuse of diagnostic radiation procedures.[5–7,26] These are good practical suggestions to reduce the level of radiation doses in patients during diagnostic procedures. There is no doubt that these recommendations would reduce the dose levels and thereby reduce biological damage somewhat, but it is not adequate. The issue of biological protection against the damage produced by low doses of radiation has not drawn adequate attention from radiobiologists or radiologists. At present, there is no biological protection strategy available for patients receiving diagnostic doses of radiation or for those working in radiation environments (radiation workers).

EVIDENCE FOR A MICRONUTRIENT STRATEGY FOR BIOLOGICAL PROTECTION AGAINST RADIATION DAMAGE

Although the recommendation of ALARA can help to reduce the level of radiation doses to patients, this does not help to reduce the level of damage to those patients receiving diagnostic doses of radiation or to workers who are exposed daily to radiation doses higher than nonradiation workers. To provide biological protection against radiation damage, it would be important to identify nontoxic chemical or biological agents which, when administered orally before radiation exposure, could protect all normal tissues against radiation injury. Since antioxidants are known to neutralize free radicals and have shown to be of radioprotective value, they may represent one of the best strategies to provide biological protection against low doses of radiation. Such antioxidant protective strategy would help to extend the concept of ALARA from dose to biological protection.[46] This novel concept is referred to as PAMARA, which was initially referred to as DALARA.[46,47]

The search for nontoxic radioprotective agents, which can protect normal tissue against radiation damage, began soon after World War II. Extensive radiobiological studies identified numerous radioprotective agents. Unfortunately, most of them were toxic to humans; however, commonly used dietary and endogenous antioxidants that are nontoxic to humans exhibited radioprotective properties in cell culture and in animals, as well as in limited human studies. These studies with individual antioxidants are briefly described below.

RADIOPROTECTIVE STUDIES WITH ANTIOXIDANTS IN CELL CULTURE

It has been shown that vitamin E and selenium reduced radiation-induced transformation in cell culture; the combination was more effective than the individual agents.[48,49] Natural beta-carotene protected against radiation-induced neoplastic transformation in cell culture.[50] Vitamins E and C, beta-carotene reduced radiation-induced mutations and chromosomal damage in mammalian cells in culture.[51–59] These studies suggest that free radicals generated during irradiation can induce genetic damage that can be attenuated by antioxidants.

RADIOPROTECTIVE STUDIES WITH ANTIOXIDANTS IN ANIMALS

Alpha-lipoic acid, a glutathione-elevating agent, increases the LD_{50} (a dose producing 50% mortality within 30 days) in mice with a dose reduction factor of 1.26.[60] Vitamin E, Vitamin C, and beta-carotene protected rodents against the acute effects of irradiation.[56,58,59,61–68] Vitamin A and beta-carotene protected normal tissue during radiation therapy of cancer in an animal model.[69] A combination of vitamins A, C, and E protected against radiation-induced myelosuppression during radiation therapy of cancer in an animal model.[61] Supplementation with L-selenomethionine and several different types of antioxidants (vitamin C, vitamin E, glutathione, N-acetylcysteine (NAC), alpha-lipoic acid, and coenzyme Q_{10}, and soybean-derived Bowman–Birk inhibitor) protected human cells in culture and rats in vivo against oxidative stress produced by protons and 1 GeV iron ions.[70–72]

All previous animal studies with individual antioxidants have utilized primarily intraperitoneal route of administration before irradiation. The oral administration of antioxidants before irradiation was ineffective in these studies. Therefore, we developed a formulation of multiple antioxidants that include dietary antioxidants (vitamins A, C, and E, beta-carotene and mineral selenium) and endogenous antioxidants (alpha-lipoic acid, NAC, and coenzyme Q_{10}) to test its efficacy in reducing radiation damage in animal models. In a pilot study, we observed that this formulation of multiple antioxidants when administered orally before irradiation increased the survival of lethally irradiated mice (bone marrow syndrome dose) from 0% to 40% (unpublished results). The same formulation of antioxidants when administered orally before and after irradiation increased the survival time of irradiated sheep exposed to gastrointestinal (GI) syndrome dose from 7 to 38 days and reduced damage to the lung tissue in irradiated rabbits dying of central nervous system (CNS) syndrome within 4 h (Prasad and Jones, unpublished results).

The same antioxidant formulation also blocked proton radiation-induced cancer in female *D. melanogaster* carrying a dominant HOP (TUM-1) mutation that induces leukemia-like tumor (unpublished observation in collaboration with Dr. Bhattacharya et al. of NASA, Moffat Field, CA). This particular observation on fruit flies is of particular interest because, to my knowledge, this is a first demonstration in which a genetic basis of the disease can be prevented by antioxidants. Although the studies discussed above were performed with high radiation doses, free radicals are generated irrespective of dose levels, and the amounts of free radicals increase with the dose. These studies suggested that the biological protection against radiation damage can be obtained after oral administration of multiple antioxidants in animal models.

RADIOPROTECTIVE STUDIES WITH ANTIOXIDANTS IN HUMANS

Vitamin A and NAC may be effective against radiation-induced carcinogenesis.[73] An oral supplementation with alpha-lipoic acid for 28 days lowered the levels of lipid peroxidation among children chronically exposed to low doses of radiation in the area contaminated by the Chernobyl nuclear accident.[41] In another study, beta-carotene supplementation reduced cellular damage in the above population of children.[40] A combination of vitamin E and alpha-lipoic acid was more effective than the individual agents.[41] These studies in humans are very exciting because they demonstrate that very low doses of radiation can increase oxidative stress and induce cellular damage that can be protected by antioxidants. An oral supplementation with beta-carotene also protected against radiation-induced mucositis during radiation therapy of cancer of the head and neck.[65]

RECOMMENDED MICRONUTRIENT PREPARATIONS FOR BIOLOGICAL PROTECTION AGAINST LOW DOSES OF RADIATION

Based on the scientific results discussed above involving 12 cell culture studies, 15 animal studies, and 5 human studies, it should be possible to develop and implement antioxidant biological protection strategy that is safe and cost effective in order to reduce radiation damage in patients receiving radiation during diagnostic procedures or radiation workers receiving doses of radiation higher than nonradiation workers. This strategy requires separate oral preparation of micronutrients in capsules for patients receiving diagnostic radiation procedures and frequent flyers; and for radiation workers (individuals working with x-rays equipment and at the nuclear power plants, and pilots and crews of military and civilian aircrafts).

Individuals Receiving Diagnostic Radiation Procedures and Frequent Flyers

The micronutrient preparation in one capsule should contain vitamin C, D-alpha-tocopheryl succinate, natural mixed carotenoids, glutathione-elevating agents (NAC and alpha-lipoic acid), and mineral selenium. The antioxidant doses in each capsule for children under the age of 12 years would be lower than for adults. The patients receiving diagnostic doses of radiation will receive one capsule 30 to 60 min before and one capsule 6–8 h after a diagnostic radiation procedure. Those patients receiving a radionuclide may receive one capsule once before and twice a day for 3–5 days after administration of a radionuclide, depending upon the half-life of the radionuclide. The frequent flyers may take one capsule before boarding the flight and one capsule a few hours after arrival. This product is available commercially.

Radiation Workers, and Pilots and Flight Attendants

The micronutrient preparation in two capsules should contain vitamin A, natural mixed carotenoids, vitamin C, D-alpha-tocopherol, D-alpha-tocopheryl succinate, vitamin D, alpha-lipoic acid, NAC, coenzyme Q_{10}, L-carnitine, all B vitamins, mineral selenium, zinc, and chromium, but no iron, copper, or manganese. The radiation workers, and pilots and attendants of civilian and military aircrafts, may need consumption of these micronutrients twice (one capsule in the morning and one in the evening) daily throughout their lifetime in order to reduce potential risk of radiation damage. This product is available commercially.

Several in vitro and animal investigations and limited human studies on the radioprotective effects of antioxidants support the use of proposed micronutrient preparation that may reduce radiation damage in patients receiving diagnostic doses of radiation and frequent flyers as well as radiation workers, including pilots and crews of civilian and military aircrafts, no matter how small that damage might be. The implementation of PAMARA by micronutrient preparation will compliment the physical radiation protection concept of ALARA. In addition, implementation of the proposed PAMARA concept may also provide unique populations of individuals who have received antioxidants during diagnostic radiation procedures and those (radiation workers) who have received antioxidants daily during the period of employment, for further studies. In an epidemiologic experimental design, one can compare the risk of cancer in the population receiving a micronutrient preparation before radiation exposure with those receiving only radiation in order to establish an association between antioxidant consumption and risk of cancer in irradiated population.

The efficacy of proposed micronutrient preparation for biological radiation protection has not been tested by a randomized, double-blind, placebo-controlled clinical trial because of several inherent difficulties. For example, only the end point for which quantitative data after diagnostic examinations are available is cancer. The estimated increase in cancer incidence from exposure to one CT scan is about 1–2 per 1000 exposed individuals. This suggests that a sample size of thousands of individuals will be needed to detect any significant differences between irradiated control and experimental (irradiated individuals receiving micronutrients) groups. In addition, the latent period for the cancer can vary from 10 to more than 30 years; therefore, the completion of study may require 30 years or more. Such a clinical study will involve participation of a multicenter at the cost of multimillions of dollars. At this time, it is not practical to conduct such a study. Until such study is initiated and completed, the proposed micronutrient biological radiation protection strategy appears to be one of the most rational choices to reduce the potential damage caused by low doses of radiation.

It has been estimated that about two-thirds of radiation-induced damage are caused by free radicals. It is well established that antioxidants neutralize free radicals. If two-thirds of radiation damage during a CT procedure can be reduced by antioxidant supplementation, this is expected to reduce the current increase in cancer incidence of 1–2 per 1000 exposed individuals. At present, there is no strategy to provide biological protection against diagnostic doses of radiation. The proposed micronutrient preparation provides science- and evidenced-based strategy for biological radiation protection against damage, no matter how small that damage might be.

TOXICITY OF ANTIOXIDANTS

Dietary antioxidants (vitamins A, C, and E, beta-carotene, and selenium) and endogenous antioxidants glutathione-elevating agents (NAC), alpha-lipoic acid, coenzyme Q_{10}, and L-carnitine have been consumed by humans for decades without any reported toxicity. The ingredients in the proposed micronutrient preparation do not have any toxicity. The potential toxicity of a certain micronutrient at very high doses have been discussed in a review.[74]

CONCLUSIONS

The growing use of x-ray–based equipment in the early diagnosis of human diseases has raised concerns about potential hazards of such procedures in increasing the risk of cancer, and somatic and heritable mutations in patients. These risks also exist in radiation workers who are also exposed to higher doses of radiation per year than nonradiation workers. The number of radiation workers has increased proportionally with the increased use of diagnostic radiation procedures. The initial physical concept of radiation protection involved three principles: (a) lead-shielding; (b) increased distance between the radiation source and radiation workers or patients; and (c) reduction of radiation exposure time. In addition, the concept of ALARA continues to be propagated and supported by radiobiologists and radiologists for reducing the doses from diagnostic radiation procedures in patients. Additionally, suggestions are being made to reduce overuse of diagnostic radiation procedures. These recommendations would reduce the dose levels and, thereby, reduce some biological damage. However, these recommendations do not provide biological protection at the irradiated tissues. At present, there is no biological radiation protection strategy available for patients receiving diagnostic doses or radiation workers. Since radiation exposure generated excessive amounts of free radicals, and since antioxidants neutralize free radicals, the use of proposed micronutrient preparation may be one of the best strategies to provide biological radiation protection against low doses of radiation. The implementation of micronutrient biological radiation protection strategy would help to extend the concept of ALARA from radiation dose to biological protection that is referred to as PAMARA. The proposed micronutrient preparation that is applicable to patients receiving diagnostic doses of radiation should also be applicable to frequent flyers, and the micronutrient preparation for radiation workers should also be applicable to pilots and attendants of civilian and military aircrafts. The efficacy of proposed micronutrient preparation for biological radiation protection has not been tested by a randomized, double-blind, placebo-controlled clinical trial because of several inherent difficulties. Until such study is initiated and completed, the proposed micronutrient biological radiation protection strategy appears to be one of the most rational choices to reduce the potential damage caused by diagnostic doses of radiation.

REFERENCES

1. Kleinerman, R. A. 2006. Cancer risks following diagnostic and therapeutic radiation exposure in children. *Pediatr Radiol* 36 (Suppl 14): 121–125.
2. Prasad, K. N. 1995. *Handbook of Radiobiology*, 2nd ed. Boca Raton, FL, CRC Press.

3. Shah, N. B., and S. L. Platt. 2008. ALARA: Is there a cause for alarm? Reducing radiation risks from computed tomography scanning in children. *Curr Opin Pediatr* 20 (3): 243–247.
4. ICRP. 1991. 1990 Recommendations of the International Commission on Radiological Protection. Annals of the ICRP, 1–3.
5. Hall, E. J. 2009. Radiation biology for pediatric radiologists. *Pediatr Radiol* 39 (Suppl 1): S57–S64.
6. Brody, A. S., D. P. Frush, W. Huda, and R. L. Brent. 2007. Radiation risk to children from computed tomography. *Pediatrics* 120 (3): 677–682.
7. Chodick, G., C. M. Ronckers, V. Shalev, and E. Ron. 2007. Excess lifetime cancer mortality risk attributable to radiation exposure from computed tomography examinations in children. *Isr Med Assoc J* 9 (8): 584–587.
8. Committee on the Biological Effects of Ionizing Radiation. 1990. *Biological Effects of Ionizing Radiation (VRIE V)*. Washington, DC: National Academy Press.
9. Prasad, K. N., W. C. Cole, X. D. Yan, P. Nahreini, B. Kumar, A. Hanson, and J. E. Prasad. 2003. Defects in cAMP-pathway may initiate carcinogenesis in dividing nerve cells: A review. *Apoptosis* 8 (6): 579–586.
10. Prasad, K. N., A. R. Hovland, P. Nahreini, W. C. Cole, P. Hovland, B. Kumar, and K. C. Prasad. 2001. Differentiation genes: Are they primary targets for human carcinogenesis? *Exp Biol Med (Maywood)* 226 (9): 805–813.
11. DiPaolo, J. A., and P. J. Donovan. 1976. In vitro morphologic transformation of Syrian hamster cells by U.V.-irradiation is enhanced by x-irradiation and unaffected by chemical carcinogens. *Int J Radiat Biol Relat Stud Phys Chem Med* 30 (1): 41–53.
12. Borek, C., M. Zaider, A. Ong, H. Mason, and G. Witz. 1986. Ozone acts alone and synergistically with ionizing radiation to induce in vitro neoplastic transformation. *Carcinogenesis* 7 (9): 1611–1613.
13. Pollock, E. J., and G. J. Todaro. 1968. Radiation enhancement of SV40 transformation in 3T3 and human cells. *Nature* 219 (5153): 520–511.
14. Little, J. B. 1981. Influence of noncarcinogenic secondary factors on radiation carcinogenesis. *Radiat Res* 87 (2): 240–250.
15. Puck, T. T., H. Morse, R. Johnson, and C. A. Waldren. 1993. Caffeine enhanced measurement of mutagenesis by low levels of gamma-irradiation in human lymphocytes. *Somat Cell Mol Genet* 19 (5): 423–429.
16. Suzuki, K., S. Kodama, and M. Watanabe. 2001. Extremely low-dose ionizing radiation causes activation of mitogen-activated protein kinase pathway and enhances proliferation of normal human diploid cells. *Cancer Res* 61 (14): 5396–5401.
17. Rothkamm, K., and M. Lobrich. 2003. Evidence for a lack of DNA double-strand break repair in human cells exposed to very low x-ray doses. *Proc Natl Acad Sci U S A* 100 (9): 5057–5062.
18. BEIR, Phase 2, 2006. National Council of the National Academies Committee to Assess Health Risks from Exposure to Low Levels of Ionizing Radiation, Washington D.C.: The National Academies Press.
19. Brenner, D. J., and R. K. Sachs. 2006. Estimating radiation-induced cancer risks at very low doses: Rationale for using a linear no-threshold approach. *Radiat Environ Biophys* 44 (4): 253–256.
20. Cohen, B. L. 2002. Cancer risk from low-level radiation. *AJR Am J Roentgenol* 179 (5): 1137–1143.
21. Bond, V. P., V. Benary, and C. A. Sondhaus. 1991. A different perception of the linear, nonthreshold hypothesis for low-dose irradiation. *Proc Natl Acad Sci U S A* 88 (19): 8666–8670.
22. Robbins, E. 2008. Radiation risks from imaging studies in children with cancer. *Pediatr Blood Cancer* 51 (4): 453–457.
23. Hall, E., and A. J. Garcia. 2006. *Radiobiology for Radiologists*. Philadelphia, PA: Lippincott Williams & Wilkins.
24. Rice, H. E., D. P. Frush, D. Farmer, and J. H. Waldhausen. 2007. Review of radiation risks from computed tomography: Essentials for the pediatric surgeon. *J Pediatr Surg* 42 (4): 603–607.
25. Hall, E. J. 2002. Lessons we have learned from our children: Cancer risks from diagnostic radiology. *Pediatr Radiol* 32 (10): 700–706.
26. Brenner, D., C. Elliston, E. Hall, and W. Berdon. 2001. Estimated risks of radiation-induced fatal cancer from pediatric CT. *AJR Am J Roentgenol* 176 (2): 289–296.
27. Wan, M. J., M. Krahn, W. J. Ungar, E. Caku, L. Sung, L. S. Medina, and A. S. Doria. 2008. Acute appendicitis in young children: Cost-effectiveness of US versus CT in diagnosis—A Markov decision analytic model. *Radiology* 250 (2): 378–386.
28. Picano, E., E. Vano, R. Semelka, and D. Regulla. 2007. The American College of Radiology white paper on radiation dose in medicine: Deep impact on the practice of cardiovascular imaging. *Cardiovasc Ultrasound* 5, 37.
29. Picano, E. 2004. Sustainability of medical imaging. *BMJ* 328 (7439): 578–580.

30. Berrington de Gonzalez, A., and S. Darby. 2004. Risk of cancer from diagnostic x-rays: Estimates for the UK and 14 other countries. *Lancet* 363 (9406): 345–351.
31. Bedetti, G., N. Botto, M. G. Andreassi, C. Traino, E. Vano, and E. Picano. 2008. Cumulative patient effective dose in cardiology. *Br J Radiol* 81 (969): 699–705.
32. Amis, Jr., E. S., P. F. Butler, K. E. Applegate, S. B. Birnbaum, L. F. Brateman, J. M. Hevezi, F. A. Mettler, et al. 2007. American College of Radiology white paper on radiation dose in medicine. *J Am Coll Radiol* 4 (5): 272–284.
33. BEIR VII Report. 2006. Health risks from exposure to low levels of ionizing radiation, Washington, D.C.: The National Academies Press.
34. Mettler, Jr., F. A., W. Huda., T. T. Yoshizumi, and M. Mahesh. 2008. Effective doses in radiology and diagnostic nuclear medicine: A catalog. *Radiology* 248 (1): 254–263.
35. Buja, A., J. H. Lange, E. Perissinotto, G. Rausa, F. Grigoletto, C. Canova, and G. Mastrangelo. 2005. Cancer incidence among male military and civil pilots and flight attendants: An analysis on published data. *Toxicol Ind Health* 21 (10): 273–282.
36. Band, P. R., N. D. Le, R. Fang, M. Deschamps, A. J. Coldman, R. P. Gallagher, and J. Moody. 1996. Cohort study of Air Canada pilots: Mortality, cancer incidence, and leukemia risk. *Am J Epidemiol* 143 (2): 137–143.
37. Sigurdson, A. J., and E. Ron. 2004. Cosmic radiation exposure and cancer risk among flight crew. *Cancer Invest* 22 (5): 743–761.
38. Rafnsson, V., H. Tulinius, J. G. Jonasson, and J. Hrafnkelsson. 2001. Risk of breast cancer in female flight attendants: A population-based study (Iceland). *Cancer Causes Control* 12 (2): 95–101.
39. Pukkala, E., A. Auvinen, and G. Wahlberg. 1995. Incidence of cancer among Finnish airline cabin attendants, 1967–92. *BMJ* 311 (7006): 649–652.
40. Ben-Amotz, A., S. Yatziv, M. Sela, S. Greenberg, B. Rachmilevich, M. Shwarzman, and Z. Weshler. 1998. Effect of natural beta-carotene supplementation in children exposed to radiation from the Chernobyl accident. *Radiat Environ Biophys* 37 (3): 187–193.
41. Korkina, L. G., I. B. Afanas'ef, and A. T. Diplock. 1993. Antioxidant therapy in children affected by irradiation from the Chernobyl nuclear accident. *Biochem Soc Trans* 21 (Pt 3) (3): 314S.
42. Andreassi, M. G., A. Cioppa, S. Manfredi, C. Palmieri, N. Botto, and E. Picano. 2007. Acute chromosomal DNA damage in human lymphocytes after radiation exposure in invasive cardiovascular procedures. *Eur Heart J* 28 (18): 2195–2199.
43. Holland, N., C. Bolognesi, M. Kirsch-Volders, S. Bonassi, E. Zeiger, S. Knasmueller, and M. Fenech. 2008. The micronucleus assay in human buccal cells as a tool for biomonitoring DNA damage: The HUMN project perspective on current status and knowledge gaps. *Mutat Res* 659 (1–2): 93–108.
44. Angelieri, F., G. R. de Oliveira, E. K. Sannomiya, and D. A. Ribeiro. 2007. DNA damage and cellular death in oral mucosa cells of children who have undergone panoramic dental radiography. *Pediatr Radiol* 37 (6): 561–565.
45. Ribeiro, D. A., and F. Angelieri. 2008. Cytogenetic biomonitoring of oral mucosa cells from adults exposed to dental x-rays. *Radiat Med* 26 (6): 325–330.
46. Prasad, K. N., W. C. Cole, and G. M. Haase. 2004. Radiation protection in humans: Extending the concept of as low as reasonably achievable (ALARA) from dose to biological damage. *Br J Radiol* 77 (914): 97–99.
47. Prasad, K. N. 2005. Rationale for using multiple antioxidants in protecting humans against low doses of ionizing radiation. *Br J Radiol* 78 (930): 485–492.
48. Borek, C., A. Ong, H. Mason, L. Donahue, and J. E. Biaglow. 1986. Selenium and vitamin E inhibit radiogenic and chemically induced transformation in vitro via different mechanisms. *Proc Natl Acad Sci U S A* 83 (5): 1490–1494.
49. Radner, B. S., and A. R. Kennedy. 1986. Suppression of x-ray induced transformation by vitamin E in mouse C3H/10T1/2 cells. *Cancer Lett* 32 (1): 25–32.
50. Kennedy, A. R., and N. I. Krinsky. 1994. Effects of retinoids, beta-carotene, and canthaxanthin on UV- and X-ray-induced transformation of C3H10T1/2 cells in vitro. *Nutr Cancer* 22 (3): 219–232.
51. Gaziev, A. I., A. Podlutsky, B. M. Panfilov, and R. Bradbury. 1995. Dietary supplements of antioxidants reduce hprt mutant frequency in splenocytes of aging mice. *Mutat Res* 338 (1–6): 77–86.
52. Konopacka, M., M. Widel, and J. Rzeszowska-Wolny. 1998. Modifying effect of vitamins C, E and beta-carotene against gamma-ray-induced DNA damage in mouse cells. *Mutat Res* 417 (2–3): 85–94.
53. Kumar, B., M. N. Jha, W. C. Cole, J. S. Bedford, and K. N. Prasad. 2002. D-alpha-Tocopheryl succinate (vitamin E) enhances radiation-induced chromosomal damage levels in human cancer cells, but reduces it in normal cells. *J Am Coll Nutr* 21 (4): 339–343.

54. Ni, Q. G., and Y. Pei. 1997. Effect of beta-carotene on 60Co-gamma–induced mutation at T-lymphocyte hypoxanthine-guanine phosphoribosyl transferase locus in rats. *Zhongguo Yao Li Xue Bao* 18 (6): 535–536.
55. O'Connor, M. K., J. F. Malone, M. Moriarty, and S. Mulgrew. 1977. A radioprotective effect of vitamin C observed in Chinese hamster ovary cells. *Br J Radiol* 50 (596): 587–591.
56. Okunieff, P., S. Swarts, P. Keng, W. Sun, W. Wang, J. Kim, S. Yang, et al. 2008. Antioxidants reduce consequences of radiation exposure. *Adv Exp Med Biol* 614: 165–178.
57. Ushakova, T., H. Melkonyan, L. Nikonova, V. Afanasyev, A. I. Gaziev, N. Mudrik, R. Bradbury, and V. Gogvadze. 1999. Modification of gene expression by dietary antioxidants in radiation-induced apoptosis of mice splenocytes. *Free Radic Biol Med* 26 (7–8): 887–891.
58. Weiss, J. F., and M. R. Landauer. 2000. Radioprotection by antioxidants. *Ann N Y Acad Sci* 899, 44–60.
59. Weiss, J. F., and M. R. Landauer. 2003. Protection against ionizing radiation by antioxidant nutrients and phytochemicals. *Toxicology* 189 (1–2): 1–20.
60. Ramakrishnan, N., W. W. Wolfe, and G. N. Catravas. 1992. Radioprotection of hematopoietic tissues in mice by lipoic acid. *Radiat Res* 130 (3): 360–365.
61. Blumenthal, R. D., W. Lew, A. Reising, D. Soyne, L. Osorio, Z. Ying, and D. M. Goldenberg. 2000. Antioxidant vitamins reduce normal tissue toxicity induced by radio-immunotherapy. *Int J Cancer* 86 (2): 276–280.
62. El-Habit, O. H., H. N. Saada, K. S. Azab, M. Abdel-Rahman, and D. F. El-Malah. 2000. The modifying effect of beta-carotene on gamma radiation-induced elevation of oxidative reactions and genotoxicity in male rats. *Mutat Res* 466 (2): 179–186.
63. Ershoff, B. H., and C. W. Steers Jr. 1960. Antioxidants and survival time of mice exposed to multiple sublethal doses of x-irradiation. *Proc Soc Exp Biol Med* 104: 274–276.
64. Harapanhalli, R. S., V. Yaghmai, D. Giuliani, R. W. Howell, and D. V. Rao. 1996. Antioxidant effects of vitamin C in mice following x-irradiation. *Res Commun Mol Pathol Pharmacol* 94 (3): 271–287.
65. Mills, E. E. 1988. The modifying effect of beta-carotene on radiation and chemotherapy induced oral mucositis. *Br J Cancer* 57 (4): 416–417.
66. Mutlu-Turkoglu, U., Y. Erbil, S. Oztezcan, V. Olgac, G. Toker, and M. Uysal. 2000. The effect of selenium and/or vitamin E treatments on radiation-induced intestinal injury in rats. *Life Sci* 66 (20): 1905–1913.
67. Narra, V. R., R. S. Harapanhalli, R. W. Howell, K. S. Sastry, and D. V. Rao. 1994. Vitamins as radioprotectors in vivo. I. Protection by vitamin C against internal radionuclides in mouse testes: Implications to the mechanism of damage caused by the Auger effect. *Radiat Res* 137 (3): 394–399.
68. Umegaki, K., H. Uramoto, J. Suzuki, and T. Esashi. 1997. Feeding mice palm carotene prevents DNA damage in bone marrow and reduction of peripheral leukocyte counts, and enhances survival following x-ray irradiation. *Carcinogenesis* 18 (10): 1943–197.
69. Seifter, E., A. Rettura, J. Padawar, and S. M. Levenson. 1984. Vitamin A and beta-carotene as adjunctive therapy to tumor excision, radiation therapy and chemotherapy. In *Vitamins, Nutrition and Cancer*, ed. K. Prasad, 1–19. Basel: Karger.
70. Guan, J., X. S. Wan, Z. Zhou, J. Ware, J. J. Donahue, J. E. Biaglow, and A. R. Kennedy. 2004. Effects of dietary supplements on space radiation-induced oxidative stress in Sprague–Dawley rats. *Radiat Res* 162 (5): 572–579.
71. Kennedy, A. R., Z. Zhou, J. J. Donahue, and J. H. Ware. 2006. Protection against adverse biological effects induced by space radiation by the Bowman–Birk inhibitor and antioxidants. *Radiat Res* 166 (2): 327–332.
72. Wan, X. S., J. H. Ware, Z. Zhou, J. J. Donahue, J. Guan, and A. R. Kennedy. 2006. Protection against radiation-induced oxidative stress in cultured human epithelial cells by treatment with antioxidant agents. *Int J Radiat Oncol Biol Phys* 64 (5): 1475–1481.
73. Sminia, P., A. H. van der Kracht, W. M. Frederiks, and W. Jansen. 1996. Hyperthermia, radiation carcinogenesis and the protective potential of vitamin A and N-acetylcysteine. *J Cancer Res Clin Oncol* 122 (6): 343–350.
74. Prasad, K. N., W. C. Cole, and K. C. Prasad. 2002. Risk factors for Alzheimer's disease: Role of multiple antioxidants, non-steroidal anti-inflammatory and cholinergic agents alone or in combination in prevention and treatment. *J Am Coll Nutr* 21 (6): 506–522.

16 Micronutrients in Protecting Against Lethal Doses of Ionizing Radiation

INTRODUCTION

Ionizing radiation refers to photon energy that can knock out a negatively charged electron from the orbit of an atom leaving it positively charged and, thus, creating an ion pair after every such interaction. The process of creating an ion pair is referred to as ionization. Ionizing radiation has been divided into two categories, low linear energy transfer (LET) radiation and high LET radiation. The low LET radiation includes x-rays, gamma-rays, and beta-rays that cause cellular damage primarily (about two-thirds of damage) by generating free radicals during radiation exposure. The high LET radiation includes proton radiation, neutron radiation, alpha-particle radiation, and other heavy particle radiation that cause initial cellular damage primarily by ionization, while free radicals play a minor role. High LET radiation is generally 5–20 times more effective than the low LET radiation in causing damage, depending upon the type of radiation and criteria of radiation injury. The current unit used for low LET radiation dose is Gy (named after a famous radiobiologist, Dr. Gray), whereas the unit used for radiation protection recommendation is Sv (named after a famous health physicist, Dr. Sievert). The unit Sv accommodates any difference in relative biological efficiency (RBE) between low and high LET radiation. RBE is a ratio of a dose to produce an effect by low LET radiation and a dose to produce the same effect by high LET radiation. The above basic radiobiology concepts have been described in detail in several books including the one referred to here.[1]

Doses of radiation 0.25 Gy or more are referred to as high-dose radiation. At doses between 0.25 and 1.5 Gy delivered in a single dose to the whole body, no death is likely to occur, at a dose of 2 Gy a few deaths may occur, at a dose of 3 Gy, 50% may die, and at a dose of 6 Gy all will die. The survivors of high doses of radiation have increased risk of developing cancer and some non-neoplastic diseases. The risk of exposure to high doses of radiation exists in the event of a nuclear accident such as the Chernobyl nuclear accident in Russia, attack by terrorists using nuclear devices, or in case of unintentional nuclear conflicts. Furthermore, astronauts may receive high doses of proton radiation during exploration of the lunar surface from the solar flare-up.

Since the levels of free radicals can be modified by pharmacological agents, but the levels of ionization cannot, the earlier radiobiological concept was that the damage produced by low LET radiation can be protected by chemical agents that can neutralize free radicals during radiation exposure. Recent studies suggest that the damage caused by high LET radiation can also be protected by free radical scavengers.[2] According to an earlier radiobiological concept, it was thought that the free radicals formed during radiation exposure are only responsible for the damage caused by low LET radiation; therefore, in all earlier radiation protection studies, radioprotective agents were administered intraperitoneally (IP) only before irradiation. These radioprotective agents when administered shortly after irradiation were found to be ineffective.[1] Later, it was demonstrated that long-lived free radicals existed after irradiation for several hours,[3,4] and elevated levels of proinflammatory cytokines[5–8] were present after irradiation. Thus, in addition to short-lived free radicals generated during radiation exposure, the long-lived free radicals and products of inflammation (proinflammatory cytokines, prostaglandin E_2, adhesion molecules, and compliment proteins) contribute to the progression of postirradiation injury. These issues have not been considered in any experimental designs of the previous radiation protection studies with antioxidants. Therefore, the efficacy of radioprotective agents was determined when administered before irradiation.

This chapter discusses briefly the damage produced by high doses of ionizing radiation, a brief history and description of radiation protection studies, radiation protection studies primarily with antioxidants, currently available radiation therapeutic agents or procedures, rationale for using multiple micronutrients including dietary and endogenous antioxidants, and proposed multiple-micronutrient preparation in prevention and treatment of radiation injury.

RADIATION DAMAGE CAUSED BY HIGH DOSES OF IONIZING RADIATION

Most studies with high doses of radiation were performed in rodents (mice and rats) as well as in cell culture models of normal and cancer cells derived from both rodents and humans. The sources of radiation have been primarily x-rays from x-ray machines of varying energy, delivering radiation doses at varying dose rates, and gamma-radiation from radioactive isotopes such as ^{60}Co and ^{137}Cs of varying energy, delivering radiation doses at varying dose rates. Occasionally, a linear accelerator has been used to deliver radiation at a very high dose rate.

The extent of damage depends upon the dose, dose rate, mode of delivery (single vs. fractionated dose), surface area irradiated (whole body vs. partial body), and radiosensitivity of target organs. The most radiosensitive organs on the criterion of cell death include bone marrow, small intestine, hair follicles, and gonads. The responses to high-dose radiation differ among mammals and are generally measured in terms of mortality rate and survival time after irradiation. The mortality rate can be measured as LD_{50} (a dose that produces 50% lethality) or LD_{100} (a dose that produces 100% lethality). The efficacy of radiation protection is generally expressed as a dose reduction factor (DRF) that is the ratio of a dose that produces an effect in the presence of a radioprotective agent and a dose that produces the same effect in the absence of the same radioprotective agent.

The DRF should not be considered as the only way to express the relative efficacy of radioprotective agents. Other ways to express the efficacy can include an increase in survival rates and survival times compared to irradiated control groups.

High doses of radiation up to 1.5 Gy do not cause lethality, but they can increase the risk of some late adverse effects including cancer. They can induce chromosomal damage and gene mutations (somatic and heritable). High doses of radiation can cause lethality and produce organ-specific syndrome. The signs and symptoms produced by delivering high doses of radiation in a single dose to whole body are referred to as radiation syndrome. Radiation syndromes have been divided into three major categories: (1) bone marrow syndrome, (2) gastrointestinal (GI) syndrome, and (3) central nervous system (CNS) syndrome. Each radiation syndrome is characterized by specific doses, survival, survival time, and signs and symptoms. High doses of radiation can also cause acute or chronic damage to organ systems without causing lethality. The Handbook of Radiobiology has discussed radiation syndromes in great detail.[1]

BONE MARROW SYNDROME

The LD_{50} dose requirement to produce the bone marrow syndrome varies from one species to another (Table 16.1). The LD_{50} dose for rodents is about 3-fold higher than for humans. The bone marrow syndrome is often expressed in terms of $^{30}LD_{50}$ (50% lethality within 30 days). The deaths occur within 30 days in most species; however, in humans, most death occurs after 30 days, and 50% will die within 60 days of exposure. Therefore, for humans, the dose of bone marrow syndrome is expressed as $^{60}LD_{50}$. The bone marrow syndrome is primarily caused by extensive damage to bone marrow and the lymphatic system and is characterized by nausea, vomiting, and fatigue. Infection and bleeding are prominent. The major cause of death is infection. The persons exposed to

TABLE 16.1
Variations in Bone Marrow Syndrome Doses in Various Species

Species	LD_{50} Value (Gy)
Human	2.7–3.0
Monkey	3.98
Rodents (rat and mice)	8.5–9.0
Desert mice	11.0–12.0
Hamster	9.0
Rabbit	8.4
Dog	2.35
Sheep	1.55
Swine	1.94

Source: Prasad, K., *Handbook of Radiobiology*, 2nd ed. CRC Press, Boca Rotan, FL, 1995; Bond, V. P., Radiation mortality in different species, in *Comparative Cellular and Species Radiosensitivity*, Bond, V. P., and Sagahara, T. (eds.), Igaku Shoin, Tokyo, 1969.

doses that produce bone marrow syndrome should be treated like any other hematologic disorders. Although treatment with replacement therapy (blood transfusion and antibiotics when indicated) can save all 50% of exposed individuals who otherwise will die,[9,10] this treatment may not protect survivors from late adverse health effects. In addition, the requirements of antibiotic and blood transfusion per individual are so great that only a few individuals can be treated in any one medical institution. Therefore, additional approaches should be developed that not only can improve the efficacy of current radiation protection approaches, but can also reduce the late adverse health effects of ionizing radiation in survivors.

GI Syndrome

The dose requirement to produce the GI syndrome varies between rodents and humans. In rodents, it is 12–40.0 Gy, and in humans, it is 5–40 Gy. The doses that produce GI syndrome cause 100% mortality in 3.5 days (rodents) and 14 days (humans). The common signs and symptoms include loss of appetite, gastric complaint, nausea, vomiting, diarrhea (may be bloody in some cases), electrolyte imbalance, dehydration, hemoconcentration, and circulatory collapse, leading to death. The major cause of death is the denudation of villi of the small intestine; however, other factors such as infection, hemorrhage, and electrolyte imbalance contribute to the rate of progression of injury. The replacement therapy that includes administration of antibiotics, transfusion of blood, and electrolytes when indicated can increase the survival time of irradiated individuals by about 2-fold, from 14 to 28 days in humans. Only a bone marrow transplant can save the irradiated individuals dying from the GI syndrome, but all die later because of host versus graft reactions. Therefore, additional approaches that can increase the survival rate or survival time of individuals exposed to GI syndrome doses should be developed.

CNS Syndrome

The doses of 50 Gy or more can produce CNS syndrome in both humans and rodents. This syndrome is characterized by period of agitation, marked apathy, followed by disorientation, balance problems, ataxia, diarrhea, vomiting, opisthotonus, convulsion, coma, and death within 24 h. The major causes of death are increased inflammatory reactions damaging the blood vessels, neurons, and enhanced intracranial pressure. Death occurs so soon that no treatment is possible.

HIGH-DOSE RADIATION-INDUCED DAMAGE TO ORGANS

The radiation responses of skin are referred to as radiation dermatitis and can be induced by doses between 2 and 40 Gy. The sequences of acute responses include initial erythema, dry desquamation, and erythema proper and moist desquamation. The chronic responses may include development of necrosis that may occur following infection or high radiation doses that can damage blood vessels and connective tissues. Radiation-induced necrotic ulcer is difficult to heal because of damage to the blood vessels and connective tissues that interfere with the regeneration of epithelial cells. The hair follicles are very sensitive to radiation. During radiation therapy involving the head region, loss of hair frequently occurs.

Radiation responses of the mucous membrane are referred to as radiation mucositis. The sequences of changes are similar to the skin, except that the changes are seen earlier than those observed in the skin.

Radiation responses of non-dividing organs such as lung (radiation pneumonitis), liver (radiation hepatitis), brain, bone, and muscle are characterized by acute inflammatory reactions that are followed by fibrosis (lung and liver) and necrosis (brain, muscle, and bone). Radiation-induced necrosis is difficult to heal.

LATE EFFECTS OF HIGH DOSES OF RADIATION ON CANCER INCIDENCE

Most data for the adverse effects of high doses of radiation come primarily from populations exposed to radiation following the explosion of the atomic bomb in Hiroshima and Nagasaki, and cancer survivors who received radiation therapy and/or chemotherapy. The late adverse health effects of high doses of radiation include both neoplastic and non-neoplastic disease. High doses of radiation can induce cancer in all organs that have dividing cells or that have non-dividing cells with a capacity to proliferate following an appropriate stimulus. The increase in leukemia incidence following radiation exposure can be seen within 10 years; however, the risk of solid tumor persists for 30 years or more after irradiation. Thyroid cancer, breast cancer, and hematopoietic cancer are most frequent after irradiation. Thyroid cancer occurs generally in children; however, a 10-fold increase in incidence of this cancer was observed in children living in Belarus, Russia, and Ukraine who were exposed to radioactive fallout following the Chernobyl nuclear accident after 10 years of exposure.[11] Among children surviving the treatment of leukemia and brain tumor with standard therapy, the risk of developing secondary primary CNS tumors is high. Radiation exposure was associated with the increased risk of glioma and meningioma. Glioma occurred after a median of 9 years and meningioma after 17 years from initial cancer treatment.[12] The higher risk of secondary primary glioma in children survivors who were irradiated at an early age may suggest greater susceptibility of the developing brain to radiation. In addition to tumors of the CNS, children survivors of cancer treatment appear to have more than a 9-fold increase in the risk of secondary sarcomas compared to the general population.[13] An epidemiologic study reported that the survivors of childhood cancer treatment had increased risk for the second primary cancer, including non-melanoma skin cancer.[14] It has been reported that two patients who were treated for malignant disease by surgery and gamma-radiation (36–40 Gy fractionated doses) developed melanoma in tattoo sites used for marking the radiation field.[15] At present, there are no preventive strategies to reduce the risk of second primary tumors in survivors of cancer treatment.

LATE EFFECTS OF HIGH DOSES OF RADIATION ON THE RISK OF NON-NEOPLASTIC DISEASES

In survivors of childhood cancer, ovarian and testicular failure has been reported after treatment with tumor therapeutic agents.[16,17] Patients who received radiation doses 10 to 40 Gy fractionated doses for the treatment of other malignant diseases developed hypothyroidism a few months to several years after radiation therapy.[18] Other non-neoplastic diseases include cataract and delayed necrosis in the brain, muscle, auditory ossicles, and bone.[1] At present, there are no preventive strategies to reduce the risk of non-neoplastic diseases in survivors of childhood or adult cancer treatment.

BRIEF HISTORY AND DESCRIPTION OF RADIATION PROTECTION STUDIES

Efforts to protect normal tissue were started soon after the discovery of x-ray by Dr. Roentgen in 1995. However, it was not until World War II when the search for radioprotective agents began in earnest. Extensive radiobiological research identified numerous agents which, when administered IP shortly before irradiation, protected animals (primarily rodents) against radiation-induced mortality.[1,19,20] Some of these agents, when added before irradiation, were also effective in reducing chromosomal aberrations, gene mutations, and DNA damage. Most of these agents were ineffective when administered IP after irradiation.

Agents that reduce radiation damage have been divided into two groups: radioprotective agents and radiation therapeutic agents. Initially, agents which provided radiation protection only when administered before irradiation were called radioprotective agents. They were ineffective when administered after irradiation. Agents which provided radiation protection only when administered after irradiation were called radiation therapeutic agents. This strict differentiation between radioprotective radiation therapeutic agents may not be applicable now. This is due to long-lived free radicals, and toxic products of inflammation contribute to the rate of progression of damage after irradiation. Therefore, in order to maximize the efficacy of any radioprotective agents, administration of these agents before and after irradiation may be necessary.

Most widely studied radioprotective agents include (SH) compounds like cysteamine, cystamine, and aminoethylisothiourea (AET) and a cysteamine analogue, amifostine. These were powerful radioprotective agents against radiation doses that produce bone marrow syndrome in rodents without producing any adverse effects; however, all were considered toxic in humans even at doses 1/10 or less.[1,19,21–24] The primary mechanisms of protection against radiation injury by these agents include scavenging of free radicals and production of hypoxia. The effects of radioprotective agents on inflammation were never investigated, until recently.

RADIATION PROTECTION STUDIES WITH ANTIOXIDANTS IN CELL CULTURE MODELS

Several studies revealed that dietary antioxidants such as vitamin A, vitamin E [alpha tocopheryl acetate and alpha-tocopheryl succinate (alpha-TS)], vitamin C, selenium, and endogenous antioxidants such as alpha-lipoic acid, N-acetylcysteine (NAC), and L-carnitine that are non-toxic to humans produced varying degrees of radiation protection. It has been shown that alpha-TS and selenium, but not alpha-tocopheryl acetate reduced radiation-induced transformation in mammalian cells in culture; the combination of alpha-TS and selenium was more effective than the individual agents.[25,26] Natural beta-carotene (BC) was more effective than the synthetic one in reducing radiation-induced transformation in mammalian cells in culture.[27] Vitamin E (alpha tocopherol and alpha-TS), vitamin C, and BC inhibited radiation-induced mutations, chromosomal damage, and lethality in mammalian cells in culture.[28–34] In addition, endogenous antioxidants such as NAC, a glutathione-elevating agent, attenuated radiation-induced toxicity in mammalian cells in culture.[35] Calcitriol, the hormonally active vitamin D metabolite, protected keratinocytes against radiation-induced caspase-dependent and -independent programmed cell death in mammalian cells in culture.[36]

It was thought earlier that the radiation damage produced by high LET radiation cannot be modified by any pharmacological agents because most of the damage is produced by direct ionization. However, recent studies with antioxidant and space radiation (proton radiation and HZE particles radiation) revealed that antioxidants can protect against space radiation-induced injury. For example, space radiation induced cytotoxicity in human breast epithelial cells in culture and transformation in human thyroid cells in culture. Pretreatment of these cells with a mixture of soy-derived Bowman–Birk inhibitor (BBI), ascorbic acid, coenzyme Q_{10}, selenomethionine, and alpha-TS protected against space radiation-induced cytotoxicity and transformation in mammalian cells in culture.[37] It has been reported that the treatment of culture of human thyroid epithelial cells with selenomethionine alone also protected against space radiation-induced increase in oxidative stress, cytotoxicity, and cell transformation possibly by enhancing DNA repair machinery in irradiated cells.[38] These studies suggest that the early radiobiology concept that the effect of high LET radiation cannot be modified is not valid.

RADIATION PROTECTION STUDIES WITH ANTIOXIDANTS IN ANIMAL MODELS

Using animal models, several studies revealed that single IP or subcutaneous (SC) administrations of individual dietary or endogenous antioxidants shortly before whole-body gamma-irradiation with high doses enhanced the survival rate in varying degrees in rodents.[31,39–50] IP administration of vitamin E and L-carnitine individually before irradiation markedly reduced radiation-induced cataract formation in rats.[51,52] Preirradiation treatment of rats with vitamin E or L-carnitine alone significantly reduced severity of brain and retinal damage in rats; however, the combination of the two did not provide an additive protective effect.[53] It has been reported that IP administration of L-carnitine reduced gamma-radiation–induced cochlear damage in guinea pigs.[54] Vitamin E administered IP before irradiation reduced radiation-induced damage to salivary glands.[55] Pre- or postirradiation treatment of mice with NAC reduced radiation-induced liver injury.[56]

Melatonin, the chief secretory product of the pineal gland, exhibited strong radioprotective effects both in cell culture and in animal models.[57] Melatonin and vitamin E administered IP before irradiation reduced radiation-induced damage in brain.[58] Melatonin significantly reduced radiation-induced edema, necrosis, and neuronal degeneration, whereas vitamin E reduced only necrosis. The reasons for these differential effects of melatonin and vitamin E are unknown.

The radiation protection studies with antioxidants and high LET radiation performed in mammalian cells in culture were confirmed in animal models. For example, space radiation-induced increase in oxidative stress in mice was reduced by dietary supplementation with Bowman–Birk inhibitor concentrate (BBIC), L-selenomethionine, or a combination of NAC, sodium ascorbate, coenzyme Q_{10}, alpha-lipoic acid, L-selenomethionine, and alpha-TS.[59] Alpha-lipoic acid administered IP before whole-body irradiation significantly attenuated high LET radiation (^{56}Fe beams)–induced impairment in the reference memory, apoptotic damage in cerebellum, and increase in DNA and markers of oxidative damage.[65]

In addition to standard dietary and endogenous antioxidants, herbal antioxidants when administered IP shortly before high doses of radiation also protected irradiated animals against radiation damage.[61–65]

A few studies have shown that a mixture of dietary antioxidants administered IP before and during radiation exposure reduced radiation-induced myelosuppression and oxidative stress in rodents.[59,66] They were ineffective when injected after irradiation. An oral administration of antioxidants before or after whole–body x-irradiation was ineffective. It was thought that only free radicals generated during radiation exposure contribute to radiation injury; therefore, antioxidants were used only before irradiation.

Administration of manganese superoxide dismutase-plasmid liposome (MnSOD-PL) provided local radiation protection to the lung, esophagus, oral cavity, urinary bladder, and intestine when administered before gamma-irradiation.[67] It is not known whether MnSOD-PL can reduce the risk of late adverse effects of high doses of radiation. The relevance of this observation in humans remains uncertain.

Additional approaches for radiation protection are being developed including vaccine,[68] anti-apoptotic peptides,[69] and hormone derivative.[70] These approaches will require FDA approval before use in humans because of their potential toxicity.

RADIATION PROTECTION STUDIES WITH ANTIOXIDANTS IN HUMANS

Direct radiation protection studies with antioxidants cannot be performed in humans for obvious reasons. The limited data on this issue primarily come from experiences of patients and radiation oncologists during radiation therapy of cancer or individuals exposed to high doses of radiation following an accident in nuclear plants. Administration of BC orally reduced the severity of radiation-induced mucositis during radiation therapy of the head and neck cancer.[71] A combination of dietary antioxidants was more effective in protecting normal tissue during radiation therapy than the individual agents.[72,73] Vitamin A and NAC may be effective against radiation-induced cancer.[74] Alpha-lipoic acid treatment alone for 28 days lowered lipid peroxidation among children chronically exposed to low doses of radiation daily in the area contaminated by the Chernobyl nuclear accident.[75] In another study, supplementation with BC alone reduced cellular damage in the above population of children.[76] A combination of vitamin E and alpha lipoic acid was more effective than the individual agents.[75] These studies strongly suggest that dietary and endogenous antioxidants can be of radioprotective value in humans.

SCIENTIFIC RATIONALE FOR USING MULTIPLE ANTIOXIDANTS IN RADIATION PROTECTION

Individual antioxidants when administered orally only once before or after irradiation failed to provide any significant degree of protection. It was thought that a mixture of dietary and endogenous antioxidants when administered orally shortly before irradiation may be able to provide protection. In addition, their mechanisms of action and distribution at cellular and organ levels differ, their internal cellular and organ environments (oxygenation, aqueous and lipid components) differ, and their affinity for various types of free radicals differ. For example, BC is more effective in quenching oxygen radicals than most other antioxidants.[77] BC can perform certain biological functions that cannot be produced by its metabolite vitamin A, and vice versa.[78,79] It has been reported that BC treatment enhances the expression of the connexin gene, which codes for a gap junction protein in mammalian fibroblasts in culture, whereas vitamin A treatment does not produce such an effect.[79] Vitamin A can induce differentiation in certain normal and cancer cells, whereas BC and other carotenoids do not.[80,81] Thus, BC and vitamin A have, in part, different biological functions.

The gradient of oxygen pressure varies within cells. Some antioxidants, such as vitamin E, are more effective as quenchers of free radicals in reduced oxygen pressure, whereas BC and vitamin A are more effective in higher atmospheric pressures.[82] Vitamin C is necessary to protect cellular components in aqueous environments, whereas carotenoids and vitamins A and E protect cellular components in lipid environments. Vitamin C also plays an important role in maintaining cellular levels of vitamin E by recycling vitamin E radical (oxidized) to the reduced (antioxidant) form.[83] Also, oxidative DNA damage produced by high levels of vitamin C could be protected by vitamin E. Oxidized forms of vitamins C and E can also act as radicals; therefore, excessive amounts of any one of these forms, when used as a single agent, could be harmful over a long period.

The form of vitamin E used is also important in any clinical trial. It has been established that D-alpha-TS is the most effective form of vitamin E both in vitro and in vivo.[84,85] This form of vitamin E is more soluble than alpha-tocopherol and enters cells more readily. Therefore, it is expected to cross the blood–brain barrier in greater amounts than alpha-tocopherol. However, this has not yet been demonstrated in animals or humans. We have reported that an oral ingestion of alpha-TS (800 IU/day) in humans increased plasma levels of not only alpha-tocopherol, but also alpha-TS, suggesting that a portion of alpha-TS can be absorbed from the intestinal tract before hydrolysis.[86] This observation is important because the conventional assumption based on the rodent studies has been that esterified forms of vitamin E such as alpha-TS, alpha-tocopheryl nicotinate, or alpha-tocopheryl acetate can be absorbed from the intestinal tract only after they are hydrolyzed to alpha-tocopherol. Our preliminary data showed that this assumption may not be true for the absorption of alpha-TS in humans.

Glutathione is effective in catabolizing H_2O_2 and anions. However, an oral supplementation with glutathione failed to significantly increase plasma levels of glutathione in human subjects,[87] suggesting that this tripeptide is completely hydrolyzed in the GI tract. Therefore, I propose to utilize NAC and alpha-lipoic acid that increase the cellular levels of glutathione by different mechanisms in a multiple-micronutrient preparation.

Other endogenous antioxidants, coenzyme Q_{10}, may also have some potential value in radiation protection. Since mitochondrial dysfunction may be associated with acute and late effects of radiation, and since coenzyme Q_{10} is needed for the generation of ATP by mitochondria, it is essential to add this antioxidant in multiple-micronutrient preparation in order to improve the function of the mitochondria. A study has shown that Ubiquinol (coenzyme Q_{10}) scavenges peroxy radicals faster than alpha-tocopherol[88] and, like vitamin C, can regenerate vitamin E in a redox cycle.[89] However, it is a weaker antioxidant than alpha-tocopherol.

Selenium is a cofactor of glutathione peroxidase, and Se-glutathione peroxidase increases the intracellular level of glutathione that is a powerful antioxidant. There may be some other mechanisms of action of selenium. Therefore, selenium and coenzyme Q_{10} should be added to a multiple-micronutrient preparation for an optimal radiation protection.

SCIENTIFIC BASIS FOR USING ANTIOXIDANTS ORALLY BEFORE AND AFTER IRRADIATION FOR AN OPTIMAL RADIOPROTECTIVE EFFICACY

Individual antioxidants when administered orally only once before or after irradiation failed to provide any significant degree of protection. This could be due to the fact that absorption of a single antioxidant through the intestine was not sufficient to increase the tissue level of antioxidants high enough to provide any significant radiation protection. In addition, a single antioxidant could not quench different types of free radicals that are produced during irradiation. Therefore, it is possible that a preparation of multiple micronutrients, containing dietary and endogenous antioxidants administered orally once shortly before irradiation, may be effective in reducing the radiation damage.

Short-lived free radicals are generated during irradiation, and long-lived free radicals exist after irradiation. In addition, reactive oxygen species (ROS) are released from inflammatory reactions that occur after irradiation. The inflammatory reactions also release toxic chemicals such as proinflammatory cytokines, adhesion molecules, and compliment proteins all of which are toxic to cells. In addition to free radicals that are generated during irradiation, these postirradiation biological events should be attenuated in order to maximize the efficacy of potential radioprotective agents. Therefore, pre- and postirradiation treatment with a radioprotective agent is essential. Antioxidants not only neutralize free radicals, but also reduce inflammatory reactions[5,90]; therefore, both pre- and postirradiation treatments with antioxidants become essential in order to maximize their effectiveness in reducing radiation damage. Preirradiation treatment periods may include 3–7 days in order to increase the tissue levels of antioxidants optimally, and postirradiation treatment may continue for the entire observation period. No such studies have been performed as yet. In spite of the fact that antioxidants are fairly non-toxic in humans and that they exhibit radioprotective potential that has a mechanistic basis, no research was conducted to explore the capacity of antioxidants in radiation protection, using a proposed multiple-micronutrient preparation including dietary and endogenous antioxidants and dose schedule.

RADIATION PROTECTION STUDY WITH A MIXTURE OF MULTIPLE ANTIOXIDANTS ADMINISTERED ORALLY BEFORE AND AFTER IRRADIATION IN SHEEP

The GI syndrome in sheep appears to be more sensitive than in rodents or humans. A pilot study was performed to evaluate the effects of a mixture of multiple dietary [vitamins A, C, E (D-alpha-TS and D-alpha tocopheryl acetate)] and selenomethionine, and endogenous antioxidants (NAC, R-alpha-lipoic acid, coenzyme Q_{10}) in sheep, in collaboration with Dr. Jones (NASA, Houston, TX).

The results showed that a dose of 4.41 Gy produced GI syndrome associated with a mild CNS syndrome in sheep, causing 100% lethality in 7 days, compared to a dose of 7–8 Gy in rodents, and about 6 Gy in humans. An oral administration of the antioxidant mixture daily for 7 days before and daily for 7 days after irradiation increased the survival time of irradiated sheep from 7 to 38 days. To our knowledge, this is a first demonstration in which antioxidant treatment before and after irradiation increased the survival time of irradiated animals exhibiting GI syndrome by about 5-fold. It should be noted that these animals received no supportive care such as antibiotic, fluid replacement, or blood transfusion. The exact mechanisms of this high level of radiation protection in irradiated sheep exhibiting GI syndrome remain unknown. However, I suggest that in addition to scavenging free radicals during radiation exposure, the antioxidant mixture administered after irradiation also neutralized radiation-induced long-lived free radicals and reduced inflammation. It remains uncertain whether the continuation of antioxidant treatment after irradiation for a period longer than 7 days would have provided a better radiation protection. It also remains unknown whether the concentration of antioxidants used in this study represented an optimal dose. It is possible that the use of other treatment modalities such as restoration of electrolyte imbalance, blood transfusions, and antibiotic treatment in combination with multiple antioxidants may have increased the survival rate in irradiated sheep. At present, except for bone marrow transplant, no other strategy is available and approved for treating irradiated individuals exhibiting GI syndromes, but nearly all survivors of bone marrow transplants eventually die of host versus graft rejection.

RADIATION PROTECTION STUDY WITH A MIXTURE OF MULTIPLE ANTIOXIDANTS ADMINISTERED ORALLY BEFORE AND AFTER IRRADIATION IN RABBITS

A pilot study was performed to evaluate the effects of a mixture of multiple antioxidants (same as used in sheep) in collaboration with Dr. Jones.

The GI syndrome in rabbits appears to be more sensitive than in sheep. The results showed that a dose of 9.011 Gy produced GI syndrome associated with a CNS syndrome. About 25% of irradiated rabbits died of CNS syndrome within 4 h, the remaining died within 7 days.

An oral administration of the mixture of antioxidants did not prolong the survival time of irradiated rabbits. This was expected because the dose used to produce GI syndrome was closer to a dose that produced CNS syndrome in a significant number of irradiated animals. However, the necropsy of those irradiated rabbits dying of CNS syndrome showed that damage to the lungs was markedly reduced in the antioxidant-treated group in comparison to that observed in the placebo-treated group (Figure 16.1).

RADIATION PROTECTION STUDY WITH A MIXTURE OF MULTIPLE ANTIOXIDANTS ADMINISTERED ORALLY BEFORE IRRADIATION IN MICE

A pilot study was performed at the Armed Forces of Radiobiology Research Institute (AFRRI) to evaluate the effects of a mixture of multiple antioxidants (same as used in sheep) in mice. The results showed that a dose of 8.5 Gy produced bone marrow syndrome with a 100% lethality in 30 days. An oral administration of the antioxidant mixture daily for 7 days or 24 h before whole-body gamma-irradiation increased the survival rate of irradiated animals from 0% to 40% (Table 16.2). Placebo treatment of irradiated mice was ineffective. To our knowledge, this level of protection has not been achieved by an oral administration of a single antioxidant or its derivatives before whole-body gamma-irradiation with a dose that produced bone marrow syndrome with a 100% mortality.

The results also revealed that placebo-containing cellulose and dextrose administered orally exhibited radioprotective effect in mice at lower doses of radiation that is similar to that produced by the antioxidant mixture (data not shown). Thus, our initial assumption that the placebo used in

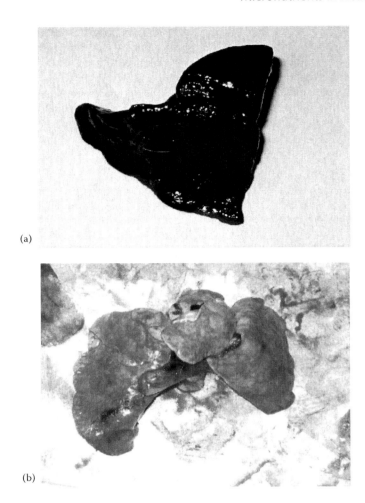

FIGURE 16.1 Protection of lung in rabbits exposed to CNS syndrome (dose, 9.011 Gy), by mixture of dietary and endogenous antioxidants. Autopsy of irradiated rabbits receiving placebo (and died in 4 h exhibiting CNS syndromes) revealed that (a) the lung was necrotic and without a lobular architecture, whereas (b) antioxidant-treated irradiated rabbits showed minimal pulmonary hemorrhage while maintaining the lobular architecture of the lung. This level of protection has never been achieved by any pharmacological or biological agents (unpublished observation, in collaboration with Dr. Jones of NASA, Houston, TX).

this study was inert was found to be incorrect. It is interesting to point out that certain polysaccharides when administered IP shortly before whole-body irradiation have been reported to be of some radioprotective value in irradiated mice.[91–93] Therefore, it is not surprising that a mixture of cellulose and dextrose provided some degree of protection at lower doses; however, the protective effect of the placebo was not observed at higher radiation doses in mice. In contrast to the observation made in mice, placebo treatment was totally ineffective in irradiated sheep and rabbits.

Additional approaches for radiation protection are being developed including vaccine,[68] antiapoptotic peptides,[69] and hormone derivative.[70] These approaches will require FDA approval before use in humans because of their potential toxicity. Until then, the use of multiple dietary and endogenous antioxidants remains one of the best choices for protection against radiation injury in humans.

Based on the results of our present study and those published by others, and based on the fact that antioxidants neutralize free radicals and reduce inflammation that contribute to the progression of radiation damage, it is possible to develop formulations of micronutrients containing both dietary

TABLE 16.2
Effect of Antioxidant Mixture or Placebo Administered Orally at a Dose of 222.5 mg/kg of Body Weight 7 Days before Various Doses of Whole-Body Gamma-Irradiation on Survival in Mice

Agents	Dose (Gy)	Survival (%)
Placebo	7.5	90
Antioxidant mixture	7.5	80
Placebo	8.0	30
Antioxidant mixture	8.0	60
Placebo	8.5	0
Antioxidant mixture	8.5	40
Placebo	9.0	0
Antioxidant mixture	9.0	0
Placebo	9.25	0
Antioxidant mixture	9.25	0

Note: Antioxidant mixture contained neither microcrystalline cellulose nor dextrose, but it contained about 11% silica by weight. Doses administered orally to animals 7 days before irradiation were corrected for the presence of 11% silica. Each group contained 10 animals.

and endogenous antioxidants for reducing radiation damage produced by high doses of ionizing radiation in humans. Such formulations would be considered safe in humans.

RADIATION PROTECTION STUDY WITH A MIXTURE OF MULTIPLE ANTIOXIDANTS ADMINISTERED ORALLY BEFORE AND AFTER IRRADIATION IN *DROSOPHILA MELANOGASTER*

A pilot study was performed to evaluate the effects of a mixture of multiple antioxidants (same as used in sheep) in collaboration with Dr. Sharmila Bhattacharya of NASA, Moffat Field, CA, on proton radiation–induced cancer in *D. melanogaster* (fruit fly).

The female flies carrying mutant HOP (TUM-1) become very sensitive to developing leukemia-like cancer. Dietary supplementation with the antioxidant mixture 7 days daily before and for the entire observation period after irradiation prevented proton radiation-induced cancer in female fruit flies carrying mutant HOP (TUM-1). It is impossible to extrapolate data obtained from fruit flies to humans. However, the possibility exists that daily supplementation with a mixture of antioxidants may reduce the risk of cancer among survivors of high doses of radiation. A clinical study with a multiple-micronutrient preparation containing dietary and endogenous antioxidants should be initiated among survivors of radiation exposure (radiation therapy and survivors of accidental radiation exposure).

STUDIES WITH RADIATION THERAPEUTIC AGENTS OR PROCEDURES

In the events of a terrorist attack by nuclear devices, unintended nuclear conflicts, or accidents in a nuclear plant, physicians, physicists, radiation biologists, nurses, and other health care professionals, and their private or public hospitals, will assume responsibility of treating individuals exposed to high doses of radiation. Under the above scenarios, radiation exposures may result in a few to mass casualties. In order to provide a guideline for the management of a large number of radiation-exposed individuals, the Strategic National Stockpile Radiation Working Group developed a consensus document.[94,95] This document recommends that individual radiation dose is estimated by determining the time of onset and severity of nausea, vomiting, decline in peripheral lymphocyte counts over several hours or days after irradiation, and appearance of chromosomal aberrations (including dicentrics and ring forms) in peripheral blood lymphocytes. In addition, documentation of clinical signs and symptoms characteristic of bone marrow syndrome, GI syndrome, and CNS syndrome or skin responses over time is essential in order to provide a rational basis for the selection of therapeutic agents and expected prognosis of the exposed individuals. The potential therapeutic agents may include replacement therapy (antibiotics, and transfusion of blood and electrolytes when indicated), which is most suitable for treating individuals exposed to doses that produce bone marrow syndrome. However, for those individuals who are exposed to doses that produce GI syndrome, additional agents such as certain cytokines, bone marrow, or stem cells transplant should be administered. In the explosion of nuclear devices containing radioactive iodine, immediate supplementation with potassium iodide may be necessary. The administration of potassium iodide will not be effective if taken several hours after exposure to radioactive iodine. It is also not affective against other radioactive isotopes.

The radiation therapeutic agents can be grouped into two broad categories: (1) chemical agents and (2) biological agents.

Chemical Agents

Antibiotics, blood, and electrolytes. The effectiveness of antibiotics in protecting against high doses of radiation that produce bone marrow syndrome is observed only when infection is present after irradiation. This is due to the fact that infection is the major cause of death in irradiated animals dying of bone marrow syndrome. In addition, loss of electrolytes and depletion of platelets and leukocytes occur after irradiation; therefore, transfusion with electrolytes and blood when indicated becomes necessary to prevent the irradiated animals from dying of bone marrow syndrome. These treatments can safely be applied to humans. They are ineffective in reducing mortality in irradiated animals or humans exposed to doses that cause GI syndrome.

Erythropoietin. The survival of mice irradiated whole body with a dose of 10 Gy increased from 0% to 40% when administered after irradiation.[96] The DRF value of erythropoietin dose (10 U) injected 1 h after whole-body irradiation with a dose of 6.51 Gy is 1.12.[97] The efficacy of erythropoietin in an irradiated individual has not been evaluated, but it is an FDA-approved drug that is used in certain human diseases to boost hemoglobin levels; therefore, it can be used as a radiation therapeutic agent.

Nucleic acid derivatives. Postirradiation treatment with DNA or RNA (3–6 h after irradiation) increased the survival of irradiated mice from 50% to 85%, an increase of 35%.[19,98] Guanosine or inosine administered IP 15 min after whole-body irradiation with a dose of 7 Gy delivered in a single dose produced a DRF value of 1.23 for guanosine and 1.15 for inosine. This effect is mediated by preventing oxidative damage and reducing the generation of ROS.[99,100] Thus, these two compounds act as an antioxidant and promoted complete and rapid repair of DNA in mouse leukocytes in vitro.[100] The relevance of these observations in treating radiation-exposed individuals remains unknown.

Statins. Statins are commonly used to lower cholesterol levels in humans. They exhibit both antioxidant and anti-inflammatory activities; therefore, it is expected that they will be of some radioprotective value. Indeed, pravastatin administered through drinking water daily 3 days before and 14 days after irradiation of surgically exteriorized small intestine with a dose of 19 Gy protected intestinal injury, but it did not protect tumor cells in culture against radiation injury.[101] Pravastatin also reduced radiation-induced skin lesions in mice when administered daily for 28 days.[102] The efficacy of statins in treating radiation-exposed individuals remains uncertain. It is very interesting to note that they mimic the effects of antioxidants in reducing radiation injury. These statins are FDA-approved drugs, and therefore, can be used in the short-term management of radiation injury in humans.

Cytokines and growth factors. Interleukin-4 (IL-4) injected once or for 5 consecutive days 2 h after whole-body irradiation of mice with doses of 7–10 Gy increased the survival of irradiated animals in the presence of poor recovery of hematopoietic systems.[103] The cytokines IL-4 and IL-13 appear to have pleiotropic effects affecting both pathological changes and tissue remodeling. Comparing the effects of IL-13Ralpha2 (IL-13 receptor alpha2) in irradiated wild-type mice and IL-4 receptor alpha gene-deficient mice revealed that IL-13Ralpha2 plays a major role in regeneration of epithelial cells after irradiation.[104]

Pre- or postirradiation of mice treated with recombinant murine (rM) colony-stimulating factor granulocyte-macrophage (CSF-gm) or recombinant human (rh) CSF-granulocyte reduced radiation damage. These growth factors were injected 20 h before irradiation or soon after irradiation.[105] The efficacy of recombinant human interleukin-3 (rhIL-3) and granulocyte-macrophage colony-stimulating factor (GM-CSF) on the peripheral lymphocytes of a rhesus monkey after whole-body irradiation with a dose of 3 Gy gamma-radiation was evaluated. The results showed that GM-CSF alone or GM-CSF + rhIL-3 reduced radiation-induced apoptosis in peripheral lymphocytes. The combination was more effective than the individual agents.[106] Acidic or basic fibroblast factor (FGF-1 or FGF-2) injected intravenously 24 h before or 1 h after whole-body irradiation with a dose of 7–18 Gy reduced radiation-induced apoptosis in crypt stem cells of intestines of mice.[107] These growth factors can be used in the management of radiation injury associated with GI syndrome in humans.

Imidazole. IP administration of Imidazole immediately after whole-body irradiation increased the survival of irradiated mice from 14% to 42%.[97] It increased the survival of irradiated mice from 14% to 80% when administered IP 5 min before whole-body irradiation.[108] The toxicity of this drug is unknown, therefore, not recommended in the management of radiation injury in humans.

Lipid. Olive oil injected IP 30 min after irradiation increased the survival of irradiated mice from 50% to 87.5%. Larger radiation doses or longer time intervals after irradiation had no therapeutic value.[19] The relevance of this observation to humans remains uncertain.

BIOLOGICAL AGENTS

Bone marrow and newborn liver cell transplant. Bone marrow transplant is often administered intravenously to irradiated individuals exposed to doses of radiation that produce GI syndrome because replacement therapy is not effective in increasing the survival of irradiated individuals. On the other hand, bone marrow transplantation can save many irradiated individuals dying from GI syndrome; however, these individuals die within a few years because of host versus graft rejection events.

A recent study has revealed that transplantation of newborn liver cells (as a source of hematopoietic stem cells) plus newborn thymus markedly improved the survival rate of mice irradiated with a dose that produced GI syndrome.[109] The relevance of this observation in the treatment of irradiated individuals remains uncertain.

The Chernobyl experience in treating irradiated individuals. On April 26, 1986, the world's most serious nuclear accident occurred at the Chernobyl nuclear power station in the former Soviet Union, releasing excessive amounts of radioactive substances into the atmosphere.[110] The care and treatment of individuals receiving high doses of radiation has been discussed in a book.[111] The medical response to this emergency involved five phases: assessment and containment, reduction of radiation exposure, estimation of dose to individuals, and treatment of irradiated individuals.

Assessments were made on important parameters such as amount and type of radioactive substance released. Measures to contain the spread of radioactivity were carried out. To limit the radiation exposure to individuals located near the reactor, massive evacuations were conducted. Within 36 h of the accident, 45,000 persons were evacuated, and 2 weeks later, 90,000 additional individuals were evacuated.

In order to reduce the dose to an exposed individual, exposed persons are thoroughly washed. In the event of exposure to radioactive ^{131}Iodine (^{131}I), a dose of potassium iodide is recommended as soon as possible in order to block the uptake of ^{131}I by the thyroid gland. An oral administration of potassium iodide 2 h after exposure to ^{131}I will reduce the uptake by the gland by 80%, and 6 h after, by about 30%.[112]

After ingestion of ^3H_2O (radioactive water), most of the radioactivity can be removed from the body in a few days by excessive drinking of cold water; however, if ^3H is present as ^3H-thymidine that incorporated into DNA, the above treatment would be useless. Chelating agents can remove certain radioactive metals by binding with them, but they could be toxic in humans if not properly monitored.

Physical dosimeter, such as the use of individual radiation meters or film badges, was of limited value at Chernobyl because the monitoring devices were either unrecoverable or destroyed by the high radiation doses. Biological dosimeter proved more effective at providing information on exposure levels, but demanded enormous amounts of medical and technical expertise and resources. Furthermore, there were limitations to the accuracy of the doses because of thermal and chemical injuries that have an impact on biological damage.[113]

About 200 people were exposed to large doses of whole-body radiation. One hundred and five received about 1–2 Gy or more, 33 received less than 6 Gy, and 10 received 6 Gy or more. Thirteen persons who received doses of 5.6–13.4 Gy, exhibited GI syndrome, and received bone marrow transplants.[113] Two transplanted patients who received an estimated dose of 5.6 and 8.7 Gy survived 3 years after the accident. Six irradiated patients received fetal liver transplant. Most died in about 3 months, and two patients who survived after 3 years also died primarily due to host versus graft rejection events.

The studies discussed above suggest that the current treatment of irradiated patients exposed to doses that produce GI syndrome is not effective; therefore, additional approaches should be developed.

RECOMMENDED MULTIPLE MICRONUTRIENTS FOR RADIATION PROTECTION IN HUMANS

A preparation of multiple micronutrients include vitamin A (retinyl palmitate), vitamin E (both D-alpha-tocopherol and D-alpha-TS), natural mixed carotenoids, vitamin C (calcium ascorbate), coenzyme Q_{10}, R-alpha-lipoic acid, NAC, L-carnitine, vitamin D, B vitamins, selenium, zinc, and chromium. No iron, copper, or manganese would be included because these trace minerals are known to interact with vitamin C to produce free radicals. These trace minerals are absorbed from the intestinal tract more in the presence of antioxidants than in their absence that could result in increased body stores of these minerals. Increased free iron stores have been linked to increased risk of several chronic diseases.

There would be two different preparations of micronutrients, one for treating individuals exposed to doses that can produce lethality, and the other for treating individuals who are exposed to doses of radiation that does not cause lethality and those who survive lethal doses of radiation. The ingredients of a micronutrient preparation for reducing acute effects of high doses of radiation will have higher levels of dietary and endogenous antioxidants than that for reducing the risk of late health adverse effects of radiation.

The micronutrient for reducing acute effects of high doses of radiation should be administered orally twice a day (morning and evening with meal, if possible) as soon as possible after radiation exposure and continued throughout the observation period of at least 60 days, and then switched to micronutrient formulation for reducing the late adverse effects for the entire lifespan. These products are commercially available.

COMBINATION OF A MULTIPLE-MICRONUTRIENT PREPARATION WITH REPLACEMENT THERAPY

Replacement therapy (antibiotics, and blood and electrolyte transfusion) should be provided whenever indicated to all individuals exposed to lethal doses of radiation. The micronutrient preparation should be started as soon as possible after radiation exposure, and then the schedule followed as described in the above paragraph. The study using the proposed micronutrient preparation in combination with replacement therapy should be initiated in animal models to determine the efficacy of this strategy on the criteria of survival rate and survival time in irradiated animals with doses that produce bone marrow syndrome and GI syndrome.

It is possible that the combination of a micronutrient mixture, administered before and after irradiation, and replacement therapy (when indicated after irradiation) may prevent irradiated animals or humans dying from GI syndrome or bone marrow syndrome caused by higher doses of radiation. Advantage of combining a micronutrient preparation with the replacement therapy is that continued treatment with micronutrients may also reduce the risk of later adverse health effects (neoplastic and non-neoplastic diseases) in survivors of radiation exposure. In the meanwhile, those individuals who are at risk of receiving low or high doses of radiation and those who are already exposed to these doses of radiation may like to adopt the proposed recommendation of micronutrients in consultation with their physicians.

CONCLUSIONS

High doses of ionizing radiation can cause extensive damage to organ systems including lethality, depending upon the total dose, dose rate, modes of delivery (single dose vs. fractionated dose), and surface area irradiated (whole body vs. partial body). High LET radiation (proton, neutron, alpha particles, and other heavy particles radiation) is 5–20 times more effective than the low LET radiation (x-ray and gamma-rays). In humans, the $^{60}LD_{50}$ (dose producing 50% mortality in 60 days) is about 3 Gy or more that produces bone marrow syndrome, the $^{7}LD_{100}$ (dose producing 100% mortality in 7 days) is 6 Gy or more that produces GI syndrome, and CNS syndrome is produced by dose 50 Gy or more that causes 100% mortality within 24 h.

Numerous radioprotective agents have been identified utilizing cell culture, both animal and human models, but except for antioxidants, all are found to be toxic in humans. The previous radiation protection studies with individual antioxidants in animal models have utilized primarily IP route of administration and, occasionally, SC route. These routes of administration are not relevant to humans. Oral administration of individual antioxidants before irradiation was ineffective in reducing radiation-induced mortality. In most previous radiation protection studies, an individual antioxidant was administered only before irradiation. In view of the fact that radiation-induced long-lived free radicals and inflammation that release ROS, and other toxic products, and in view of the fact that antioxidants neutralize free radicals and reduce inflammation, treatment with antioxidants before and after irradiation becomes necessary in order to optimize the radiation protection efficacy of these agents. Using a mixture of micronutrient formulation containing dietary and endogenous antioxidants, we have demonstrated that oral administration of antioxidants increased the survival time of gamma-irradiated sheep exposed to a dose that produces GI syndrome from 7 to 38 days without any other therapeutic intervention. The same mixture of antioxidants administered orally 7 days before irradiation protected lungs of irradiated rabbits that died of CNS syndrome within 4 h. The same mixture of antioxidants administered orally 7 days before irradiation increased the survival of irradiated rats exposed to doses that produce bone marrow syndrome from 0% to 40% without any other therapeutic intervention.

Except for replacement therapy (antibiotics, transfusion of blood and electrolytes when indicated), most others are not effective in increasing the survival rate of animals irradiated with high doses of radiation that can produce bone marrow syndrome. Transplantations with bone marrow or hematopoietic stem cells are effective in improving the survival rate of individuals exposed to doses of radiation that produce GI syndrome, but all later died because of host versus graft rejection events. I have proposed that the combination of micronutrient therapy with the replacement therapy may improve their effectiveness in increasing the survival rates of irradiated animals after exposure to doses that produce GI syndrome.

The survivors of high doses of radiation (accidentally exposed individuals or survivors of cancer treatment) have an increased risk of developing neoplastic and non-neoplastic diseases. At present, there are no effective strategies to reduce the late adverse effects of radiation in survivors of radiation exposure. Continuation of micronutrient therapy for the entire life span may reduce the adverse effects of radiation therapy/chemotherapy in radiation survivors.

Two different preparations of micronutrients have been proposed: one for testing in irradiated animals exposed to high doses of x-rays or gamma-rays that produce bone marrow syndrome or GI syndrome, the other to be tested in radiation survivors. In the meanwhile, I have proposed that radiation survivors may like to use the proposed strategy in consultation with their physicians.

REFERENCES

1. Prasad, K. 1995. *Handbook of Radiobiology*, 2nd ed. Boca Rotan, FL: CRC Press.
2. Guan, J., X. S. Wan, Z. Zhou, J. Ware, J. J. Donahue, J. E. Biaglow, and A. R. Kennedy. 2004. Effects of dietary supplements on space radiation-induced oxidative stress in Sprague–Dawley rats. *Radiat Res* 162 (5): 572–579.
3. Kumagai, J., K. Masui, Y. Itagaki, M. Shiotani, S. Kodama, M. Watanabe, and T. Miyazaki. 2003. Long-lived mutagenic radicals induced in mammalian cells by ionizing radiation are mainly localized to proteins. *Radiat Res* 160 (1): 95–102.
4. Waldren, C. A., D. B. Vannais, and A. M. Ueno. 2004. A role for long-lived radicals (LLR) in radiation-induced mutation and persistent chromosomal instability: Counteraction by ascorbate and RibCys but not DMSO. *Mutat Res* 551 (1–2): 255–265.
5. Abate, A., G. Yang, P. A. Dennery, S. Oberle, and H. Schroder. 2000. Synergistic inhibition of cyclooxygenase-2 expression by vitamin E and aspirin. *Free Radic Biol Med* 29 (11): 1135–1142.
6. Fedorocko, P., A. Egyed, and A. Vacek. 2002. Irradiation induces increased production of haemopoietic and proinflammatory cytokines in the mouse lung. *Int J Radiat Biol* 78 (4): 305–313.
7. Mizutani, N., Y. Fujikura, Y. H. Wang, M. Tamechika, N. Tokuda, T. Sawada, and T. Fukumoto. 2002. Inflammatory and anti-inflammatory cytokines regulate the recovery from sublethal x irradiation in rat thymus. *Radiat Res* 157 (3): 281–289.
8. Popp, W., U. Plappert, W. U. Muller, B. Rehn, J. Schneider, A. Braun, P. C. Bauer, et al. 2000. Biomarkers of genetic damage and inflammation in blood and bronchoalveolar lavage fluid among former German uranium miners: A pilot study. *Radiat Environ Biophys* 39 (4): 275–282.
9. Bond, V. P. 1969. Radiation mortality in different species. In *Comparative Cellular and Species Radiosensitivity*, ed. V. P. Bond and T. Sagahara, 5. Tokyo: Igaku Shoin.
10. Bond, V. P., T. M. Fliedner, and J. O. Aychambeau. 1965. *Mammalian Radiation Lethality*. New York, NY: Academic Press.
11. Demidchik, Y. E., V. A. Saenko, and S. Yamashita. 2007. Childhood thyroid cancer in Belarus, Russia, and Ukraine after Chernobyl and at present. *Arq Bras Endocrinol Metabol* 51 (5): 748–762.
12. Neglia, J. P., L. L. Robison, M. Stovall, Y. Liu, R. J. Packer, S. Hammond, Y. Yasui, et al. 2006. New primary neoplasms of the central nervous system in survivors of childhood cancer: A report from the Childhood Cancer Survivor Study. *J Natl Cancer Inst* 98 (21): 1528–1537.
13. Henderson, T. O., J. Whitton, M. Stovall, A. C. Mertens, P. Mitby, D. Friedman, L. C. Strong, et al. 2007. Secondary sarcomas in childhood cancer survivors: A report from the Childhood Cancer Survivor Study. *J Natl Cancer Inst* 99 (4): 300–308.
14. Meadows, A. T., D. L. Friedman, J. P. Neglia, A. C. Mertens, S. S. Donaldson, M. Stovall, S. Hammond, Y. Yasui, and P. D. Inskip. 2009. Second neoplasms in survivors of childhood cancer: Findings from the Childhood Cancer Survivor Study cohort. *J Clin Oncol* 27 (14): 2356–2362.
15. Bartal, A. H., Y. Cohen, and E. Robinson. 1980. Malignant melanoma arising at tattoo sites used for radiotherapy field marking. *Br J Radiol* 53 (633): 913–914.

16. Stillman, R. J., J. S. Schinfeld, I. Schiff, R. D. Gelber, J. Greenberger, M. Larson, N. Jaffe, and F. P. Li. 1981. Ovarian failure in long-term survivors of childhood malignancy. *Am J Obstet Gynecol* 139 (1): 62–66.
17. Sherins, R. J., C. L. Olweny, and J. L. Ziegler. 1978. Gynecomastia and gonadal dysfunction in adolescent boys treated with combination chemotherapy for Hodgkin's disease. *N Engl J Med* 299 (1): 12–16.
18. Rubin, P., and G. Casarett. 1968. *Clinical Radiation Pathology*. Philadelphia, PA: W. B. Saunders.
19. Thomson, J. 1962. *Radiation Protection in Mammals*. New York, NY: Reinhold.
20. Weiss, J. F., and M. R. Landauer. 2009. History and development of radiation-protective agents. *Int J Radiat Biol* 85 (7): 539–573.
21. Capizzi, R. L., and W. Oster. 2000. Chemoprotective and radioprotective effects of amifostine: An update of clinical trials. *Int J Hematol* 72 (4): 425–435.
22. Allalunis-Turner, M. J., T. L. Walden Jr., and C. Sawich. 1989. Induction of marrow hypoxia by radioprotective agents. *Radiat Res* 118 (3): 581–586.
23. Anne, P. R. 2002. Phase II trial of subcutaneous amifostine in patients undergoing radiation therapy for head and neck cancer. *Semin Oncol* 29 (6 Suppl 19): 80–83.
24. Weiss, J. F., and M. R. Landauer. 2003. Protection against ionizing radiation by antioxidant nutrients and phytochemicals. *Toxicology* 189 (1–2): 1–20.
25. Borek, C., A. Ong, H. Mason, L. Donahue, and J. E. Biaglow. 1986. Selenium and vitamin E inhibit radiogenic and chemically induced transformation in vitro via different mechanisms. *Proc Natl Acad Sci U S A* 83 (5): 1490–1494.
26. Radner, B. S., and A. R. Kennedy. 1986. Suppression of x-ray induced transformation by vitamin E in mouse C3H/10T1/2 cells. *Cancer Lett* 32 (1): 25–32.
27. Kennedy, A. R., and N. I. Krinsky. 1994. Effects of retinoids, beta-carotene, and canthaxanthin on UV- and x-ray–induced transformation of C3H10T1/2 cells in vitro. *Nutr Cancer* 22 (3): 219–232.
28. Ushakova, T., H. Melkonyan, L. Nikonova, V. Afanasyev, A. I. Gaziev, N. Mudrik, R. Bradbury, and V. Gogvadze. 1999. Modification of gene expression by dietary antioxidants in radiation-induced apoptosis of mice splenocytes. *Free Radic Biol Med* 26 (7–8): 887–891.
29. Konopacka, M., M. Widel, and J. Rzeszowska-Wolny. 1998. Modifying effect of vitamins C, E and beta-carotene against gamma-ray-induced DNA damage in mouse cells. *Mutat Res* 417 (2–3): 85–94.
30. Gaziev, A. I., A. Podlutsky, B. M. Panfilov, and R. Bradbury. 1995. Dietary supplements of antioxidants reduce hprt mutant frequency in splenocytes of aging mice. *Mutat Res* 338 (1–6): 77–86.
31. Kumar, B., M. N. Jha, W. C. Cole, J. S. Bedford, and K. N. Prasad. 2002. D-alpha-Tocopheryl succinate (vitamin E) enhances radiation-induced chromosomal damage levels in human cancer cells, but reduces it in normal cells. *J Am Coll Nutr* 21 (4): 339–343.
32. O'Connor, M. K., J. F. Malone, M. Moriarty, and S. Mulgrew. 1977. A radioprotective effect of vitamin C observed in Chinese hamster ovary cells. *Br J Radiol* 50 (596): 587–591.
33. Weiss, J. F., and M. R. Landauer. 2000. Radioprotection by antioxidants. *Ann N Y Acad Sci* 899, 44–60.
34. Konopacka, M., and J. Rzeszowska-Wolny. 2001. Antioxidant vitamins C, E and beta-carotene reduce DNA damage before as well as after gamma-ray irradiation of human lymphocytes in vitro. *Mutat Res* 491 (1–2): 1–7.
35. Wu, W., L. Abraham, J. Ogony, R. Matthews, G. Goldstein, and N. Ercal. 2008. Effects of *N*-acetylcysteine amide (NACA): a thiol antioxidant on radiation-induced cytotoxicity in Chinese hamster ovary cells. *Life Sci* 82 (21–22): 1122–1130.
36. Langberg, M., C. Rotem, E. Fenig, R. Koren, and A. Ravid. 2009. Vitamin D protects keratinocytes from deleterious effects of ionizing radiation. *Br J Dermatol* 160 (1): 151–161.
37. Kennedy, A. R., Z. Zhou, J. J. Donahue, and J. H. Ware. 2006. Protection against adverse biological effects induced by space radiation by the Bowman–Birk inhibitor and antioxidants. *Radiat Res* 166 (2): 327–332.
38. Kennedy, A. R., J. H. Ware, J. Guan, J. J. Donahue, J. E. Biaglow, Z. Zhou, J. Stewart, M. Vazquez, and X. S. Wan. 2004. Selenomethionine protects against adverse biological effects induced by space radiation. *Free Radic Biol Med* 36 (2): 259–266.
39. de Moraes Ramos, F. M., F. Schonlau, P. D. Novaes, F. R. Manzi, F. N. Boscolo, and S. M. de Almeida. 2006. Pycnogenol protects against ionizing radiation as shown in the intestinal mucosa of rats exposed to X-rays. *Phytother Res* 20 (8): 676–679.
40. Kumar, K. S., V. Srinivasan, R. Toles, L. Jobe, and T. M. Seed. 2002. Nutritional approaches to radioprotection: Vitamin E. *Mil Med* 167 (2 Suppl): 57–59.
41. Manda, K., M. Ueno, T. Moritake, and K. Anzai. 2007. Alpha-lipoic acid attenuates x-irradiation–induced oxidative stress in mice. *Cell Biol Toxicol* 23 (2): 129–137.

42. Mansour, H. H., H. F. Hafez, N. M. Fahmy, and N. Hanafi. 2008. Protective effect of *N*-acetylcysteine against radiation induced DNA damage and hepatic toxicity in rats. *Biochem Pharmacol* 75 (3): 773–780.
43. Mutlu-Turkoglu, U., Y. Erbil, S. Oztezcan, V. Olgac, G. Toker, and M. Uysal. 2000. The effect of selenium and/or vitamin E treatments on radiation-induced intestinal injury in rats. *Life Sci* 66 (20): 1905–1913.
44. Satyamitra, M., P. U. Devi, H. Murase, and V. T. Kagiya. 2001. In vivo radioprotection by alpha-TMG: Preliminary studies. *Mutat Res* 479 (1–2): 53–61.
45. Shirazi, A., G. Ghobadi, and M. Ghazi-Khansari. 2007. A radiobiological review on melatonin: A novel radioprotector. *J Radiat Res (Tokyo)* 48 (4): 263–272.
46. Sridharan, S., and C. S. Shyamaladevi. 2002. Protective effect of *N*-acetylcysteine against gamma ray induced damages in rats—Biochemical evaluations. *Indian J Exp Biol* 40 (2): 181–186.
47. Srinivasan, M., A. R. Sudheer, K. R. Pillai, P. R. Kumar, P. R. Sudhakaran, and V. Menon. 2007. Lycopene as a natural protector against gamma-radiation induced DNA damage, lipid peroxidation and antioxidant status in primary culture of isolated rat hepatocytes in vitro. *Biochim Biophys Acta* 1770 (4): 659–665.
48. Harapanhalli, R. S., V. Yaghmai, D. Giuliani, R. W. Howell, and D. V. Rao. 1996. Antioxidant effects of vitamin C in mice following x-irradiation. *Res Commun Mol Pathol Pharmacol* 94 (3): 271–287.
49. Narra, V. R., R. S. Harapanhalli, R. W. Howell, K. S. Sastry, and D. V. Rao. 1994. Vitamins as radioprotectors in vivo. I. Protection by vitamin C against internal radionuclides in mouse testes: Implications to the mechanism of damage caused by the Auger effect. *Radiat Res* 137 (3): 394–399.
50. Ramakrishnan, N., W. W. Wolfe, and G. N. Catravas. 1992. Radioprotection of hematopoietic tissues in mice by lipoic acid. *Radiat Res* 130 (3): 360–365.
51. Karslioglu, I., M. V. Ertekin, I. Kocer, S. Taysi, O. Sezen, A. Gepdiremen, and E. Balci. 2004. Protective role of intramuscularly administered vitamin E on the levels of lipid peroxidation and the activities of antioxidant enzymes in the lens of rats made cataractous with gamma-irradiation. *Eur J Ophthalmol* 14 (6): 478–485.
52. Kocer, I., S. Taysi, M. V. Ertekin, I. Karslioglu, A. Gepdiremen, O. Sezen, and K. Serifoglu. 2007. The effect of L-carnitine in the prevention of ionizing radiation-induced cataracts: A rat model. *Graefes Arch Clin Exp Ophthalmol* 245 (4): 588–594.
53. Sezen, O., M. V. Ertekin, B. Demircan, I. Karslioglu, F. Erdogan, I. Kocer, I. Calik, and A. Gepdiremen. 2008. Vitamin E and L-carnitine, separately or in combination, in the prevention of radiation-induced brain and retinal damages. *Neurosurg Rev* 31 (2): 205–213; discussion 213.
54. Altas, E., M. V. Ertekin, C. Gundogdu, and E. Demirci. 2006. L-Carnitine reduces cochlear damage induced by gamma irradiation in Guinea pigs. *Ann Clin Lab Sci* 36 (3): 312–318.
55. Ramos, F. M., M. L. Pontual, S. M. de Almeida, F. N. Boscolo, C. P. Tabchoury, and P. D. Novaes. 2006. Evaluation of radioprotective effect of vitamin E in salivary dysfunction in irradiated rats. *Arch Oral Biol* 51 (2): 96–101.
56. Liu, Y., H. Zhang, L. Zhang, Q. Zhou, X. Wang, J. Long, T. Dong, and W. Zhao. 2007. Antioxidant *N*-acetylcysteine attenuates the acute liver injury caused by x-ray in mice. *Eur J Pharmacol* 575 (1–3): 142–148.
57. Vijayalaxmi, R., R. J. Reiter, D. X. Tan, T. S. Herman, and C. R. Thomas Jr. 2004. Melatonin as a radioprotective agent: A review. *Int J Radiat Oncol Biol Phys* 59 (3): 639–653.
58. Erol, F. S., C. Topsakal, M. F. Ozveren, M. Kaplan, N. Ilhan, I. H. Ozercan, and O. G. Yildiz. 2004. Protective effects of melatonin and vitamin E in brain damage due to gamma radiation: An experimental study. *Neurosurg Rev* 27 (1): 65–69.
59. Guan, J., J. Stewart, J. H. Ware, Z. Zhou, J. J. Donahue, and A. R. Kennedy. 2006. Effects of dietary supplements on the space radiation-induced reduction in total antioxidant status in CBA mice. *Radiat Res* 165 (4): 373–378.
60. Manda, K., M. Ueno, and K. Anzai. 2008. Memory impairment, oxidative damage and apoptosis induced by space radiation: Ameliorative potential of alpha-lipoic acid. *Behav Brain Res* 187 (2): 387–395.
61. Goel, H. C., J. Prasad, S. Singh, R. K. Sagar, I. P., Kumar, and A. K. Sinha. 2002. Radioprotection by a herbal preparation of *Hippophae rhamnoides*, RH-3, against whole body lethal irradiation in mice. *Phytomedicine* 9 (1): 15–25.
62. Gupta, M. L., S. Tyagi, S. J. Flora, P. K. Agrawala, P. Choudhary, S. C. Puri, A. Sharma, et al. 2007. Protective efficacy of semi purified fraction of high altitude podophyllum hexandrum rhizomes in lethally irradiated Swiss albino mice. *Cell Mol Biol (Noisy-le-grand)* 53 (5): 29–41.
63. Lee, T. K., R. M. Johnke, R. R. Allison, K. F. O'Brien, and L. J. Dobbs Jr. 2005. Radioprotective potential of ginseng. *Mutagenesis* 20 (4): 237–243.

64. Shimoi, K., S. Masuda, B. Shen, M. Furugori, and N. Kinae. 1996. Radioprotective effects of antioxidative plant flavonoids in mice. *Mutat Res* 350 (1): 153–161.
65. Goyal, P. K., and P. Gehlot. 2009. Radioprotective effects of *Aloe vera* leaf extract on Swiss albino mice against whole-body gamma irradiation. *J Environ Pathol Toxicol Oncol* 28 (1): 53–61.
66. Blumenthal, R. D., W. Lew, A. Reising, D. Soyne, L. Osorio, Z. Ying, and D. M. Goldenberg. 2000. Antioxidant vitamins reduce normal tissue toxicity induced by radio-immunotherapy. *Int J Cancer* 86 (2): 276–280.
67. Greenberger, J. S., and M. W. Epperly. 2007. Review. Antioxidant gene therapeutic approaches to normal tissue radioprotection and tumor radiosensitization. *In Vivo* 21 (2): 141–146.
68. Maliev, V. P., D. Popov, J. A. Jones, and R. C. Casey. 2007. Mechanisms of action of anti-radiation vaccine in reducing the biological impact of high-dose gamma-irradiation. *J Adv Space Res* 40 (4): 586–590.
69. McConnell, K. W., J. T. Muenzer, K. C. Chang, C. G. Davis, J. E. McDunn, C. M. Coopersmith, C. A. Hilliard, R. S. Hotchkiss, P. W. Grigsby, and C. R. Hunt. 2007. Anti-apoptotic peptides protect against radiation-induced cell death. *Biochem Biophys Res Commun* 355 (2): 501–507.
70. Stickney, D. R., C. Dowding, A. Garsd, C. Ahlem, M. Whitnall, M. McKeon, C. Reading, and J. Frincke. 2006. 5-Androstenediol stimulates multilineage hematopoiesis in rhesus monkeys with radiation-induced myelosuppression. *Int Immunopharmacol* 6 (11): 1706–1713.
71. Mills, E. E. 1988. The modifying effect of beta-carotene on radiation and chemotherapy induced oral mucositis. *Br J Cancer* 57 (4): 416–417.
72. Jaakkola, K., P. Lahteenmaki, J. Laakso, E. Harju, H. Tykka, and K. Mahlberg. 1992. Treatment with antioxidant and other nutrients in combination with chemotherapy and irradiation in patients with small-cell lung cancer. *Anticancer Res* 12 (3): 599–606.
73. Lamson, D. W., and M. S. Brignall. 1999. Antioxidants in cancer therapy; their actions and interactions with oncologic therapies. *Altern Med Rev* 4 (5): 304–329.
74. Sminia, P., A. H. van der Kracht, W. M. Frederiks, and W. Jansen. 1996. Hyperthermia, radiation carcinogenesis and the protective potential of vitamin A and *N*-acetylcysteine. *J Cancer Res Clin Oncol* 122 (6): 343–350.
75. Korkina, L. G., I. B. Afanas'ef, and A. T. Diplock. 1993. Antioxidant therapy in children affected by irradiation from the Chernobyl nuclear accident. *Biochem Soc Trans* 21 (Pt 3) (3): 314S.
76. Ben-Amotz, A., S. Yatziv, M. Sela, S. Greenberg, B. Rachmilevich, M. Shwarzman, and Z. Weshler. 1998. Effect of natural beta-carotene supplementation in children exposed to radiation from the Chernobyl accident. *Radiat Environ Biophys* 37 (3): 187–193.
77. Krinsky, N. I. 1989. Antioxidant functions of carotenoids. *Free Radic Biol Med* 7 (6): 617–635.
78. Hazuka, M. B., J. Edwards-Prasad, F. Newman, J. J. Kinzie, and K. N. Prasad. 1990. Beta-carotene induces morphological differentiation and decreases adenylate cyclase activity in melanoma cells in culture. *J Am Coll Nutr* 9 (2): 143–149.
79. Zhang, L. X., R. V. Cooney, and J. S. Bertram. 1992. Carotenoids up-regulate connexin43 gene expression independent of their provitamin A or antioxidant properties. *Cancer Res* 52 (20): 5707–5712.
80. Carter, C. A., M. Pogribny, A. Davidson, C. D. Jackson, L. J. McGarrity, and S. M. Morris. 1996. Effects of retinoic acid on cell differentiation and reversion toward normal in human endometrial adenocarcinoma (RL95-2) cells. *Anticancer Res* 16 (1): 17–24.
81. Meyskens, Jr., F. L. 1995. Role of vitamin A and its derivatives in the treatment of human cancer. In *Nutrients in Cancer Prevention and Treatment*, ed. K. N. Prasad, L. Santamaria, and R. M. Williams, 349–362. Totowa, NJ: Humana Press.
82. Vile, G. F., and C. C. Winterbourn. 1988. Inhibition of adriamycin-promoted microsomal lipid peroxidation by beta-carotene, alpha-tocopherol and retinol at high and low oxygen partial pressures. *FEBS Lett* 238 (2): 353–356.
83. McCay, P. B. 1985. Vitamin E: Interactions with free radicals and ascorbate. *Annu Rev Nutr* 5, 323–340.
84. Prasad, K. N., B. Kumar, X. D. Yan, A. J. Hanson, and W. C. Cole. 2003. alpha-Tocopheryl succinate, the most effective form of vitamin E for adjuvant cancer treatment: A review. *J Am Coll Nutr* 22 (2): 108–117.
85. Schwartz, J. L. 1995. Molecular and biochemical control of tumor growth following treatment with carotenoids or tocopherols. In *Nutrients in Cancer Prevention and Treatment*, ed. K. N. Prasad, L. Santamaria, and R. M. Williams, 287–316. Totowa, NJ: Humana Press.
86. Prasad, K. N., and J. Edwards-Prasad. 1992. Vitamin E and cancer prevention: Recent advances and future potentials. *J Am Coll Nutr* 11 (5): 487–500.

87. Witschi, A., S. Reddy, B. Stofer, and B. H. Lauterburg. 1992. The systemic availability of oral glutathione. *Eur J Clin Pharmacol* 43 (6): 667–669.
88. Niki, E. 1997. Mechanisms and dynamics of antioxidant action of ubiquinol. *Mol Aspects Med* 18 (Suppl): S63–S70.
89. Hiramatsu, M., R. D. Velasco, D. S. Wilson, and L. Packer. 1991. Ubiquinone protects against loss of tocopherol in rat liver microsomes and mitochondrial membranes. *Res Commun Chem Pathol Pharmacol* 72 (2): 231–241.
90. Devaraj, S., and I. Jialal. 2000. Alpha tocopherol supplementation decreases serum C-reactive protein and monocyte interleukin-6 levels in normal volunteers and type 2 diabetic patients. *Free Radic Biol Med* 29 (8): 790–792.
91. Guenechea, G., B. Albella, J. A. Bueren, G. Maganto, P. Tuduri, A. Guerrero, J. P. Pivel, and A. Real. 1997. AM218, a new polyanionic polysaccharide, induces radioprotection in mice when administered shortly before irradiation. *Int J Radiat Biol* 71 (1): 101–108.
92. Patchen, M. L., T. J. MacVittie, B. D. Solberg, M. M. D'Alesandro, and I. Brook. 1992. Radioprotection by polysaccharides alone and in combination with aminothiols. *Adv Space Res* 12 (2–3): 233–248.
93. Ross, W. M., and J. Peeke. 1986. Radioprotection conferred by dextran sulfate given before irradiation in mice. *Exp Hematol* 14 (2): 147–155.
94. Waselenko, J. K., T. J. MacVittie, W. F. Blakely, N. Pesik, A. L. Wiley, W. E. Dickerson, H. Tsu, et al. 2004. Medical management of the acute radiation syndrome: Recommendations of the Strategic National Stockpile Radiation Working Group. *Ann Intern Med* 140 (12): 1037–1051.
95. Coleman, C. N., C. Hrdina, J. L. Bader, A. Norwood, R. Hayhurst, J. Forsha, K. Yeskey, and A. Knebel. 2009. Medical response to a radiologic/nuclear event: Integrated plan from the Office of the Assistant Secretary for Preparedness and Response, Department of Health and Human Services. *Ann Emerg Med* 53 (2): 213–222.
96. Naidu, N. V., and O. S. Reddi. 1967. Effect of post-treatment with erythropoietin(s) on survival and erythropoietic recovery in irradiated mice. *Nature* 214 (5094): 1223–1224.
97. Vittorio, P. V., J. F. Whitfield, and R. H. Rixon. 1971. The radioprotective and therapeutic effects of imidazole and erythropoietin on the erythropoiesis and survival of irradiated mice. *Radiat Res* 47 (1): 191–198.
98. Ebel, J. P., G. Beck, G. Keith, H. Langendorff, and M. Langendorff. 1969. Study of the therapeutic effect on irradiated mice of substances contained in RNA preparations. *Int J Radiat Biol Relat Stud Phys Chem Med* 16 (3): 201–209.
99. Gudkov, S. V., I. N. Shtarkman, V. S. Smirnova, A. V. Chernikov, and V. I. Bruskov. 2006. Guanosine and inosine display antioxidant activity, protect DNA in vitro from oxidative damage induced by reactive oxygen species, and serve as radioprotectors in mice. *Radiat Res* 165 (5): 538–545.
100. Gudkov, S. V., O. Y. Gudkova, A. V. Chernikov, and V. I. Bruskov. 2009. Protection of mice against X-ray injuries by the post-irradiation administration of guanosine and inosine. *Int J Radiat Biol* 85 (2): 116–125.
101. Haydont, V., O. Gilliot, S. Rivera, C. Bourgier, A. Francois, J. Aigueperse, J. Bourhis, and M. C. Vozenin-Brotons. 2007. Successful mitigation of delayed intestinal radiation injury using pravastatin is not associated with acute injury improvement or tumor protection. *Int J Radiat Oncol Biol Phys* 68 (5): 1471–1482.
102. Holler, V., V. Buard, M. H. Gaugler, O. Guipaud, C. Baudelin, A. Sache, R. Perez Mdel, et al. 2009. Pravastatin limits radiation-induced vascular dysfunction in the skin. *J Invest Dermatol* 129 (5): 1280–1291.
103. Van der Meeren, A., M. H. Gaugler, M. A. Mouthon, C. Squiban, and P. Gourmelon. 1999. Interleukin 4 promotes survival of lethally irradiated mice in the absence of hematopoietic efficacy. *Radiat Res* 152 (6): 629–636.
104. Kawashima, R., Y. I. Kawamura, R. Kato, N. Mizutani, N. Toyama-Sorimachi, and T. Dohi. 2006. IL-13 receptor alpha2 promotes epithelial cell regeneration from radiation-induced small intestinal injury in mice. *Gastroenterology* 131 (1): 130–141.
105. Talmadge, J. E., H. Tribble, R. Pennington, O. Bowersox, M. A. Schneider, P. Castelli, P. L. Black, and F. Abe. 1989. Protective, restorative, and therapeutic properties of recombinant colony-stimulating factors. *Blood* 73 (8): 2093–2103.
106. Cui, Y. F., H. Yang, Q. L. Luo, B. Dong, X. L. Liu, H. Xu, B. Z. Mao, and D. W. Wang. 2004. Radioprotection of recombinant human interleukin-3 and granulocyte-macrophage colony-stimulating factor on peripheral lymphocytes of rhesus monkey irradiated by 3.0 Gy gamma-rays. *Zhongguo Wei Zhong Bing Ji Jiu Yi Xue* 16 (1): 22–25.

107. Okunieff, P., M. Mester, J. Wang, T. Maddox, X. Gong, D. Tang, M. Coffee, and I. Ding. 1998. In vivo radioprotective effects of angiogenic growth factors on the small bowel of C3H mice. *Radiat Res* 150 (2): 204–211.
108. Coeur, A., R. Rinaldi, and C. Raynfeld. 1962. Thyroid effects of the absorption of therapeutic doses of iodine compounds in the rat. *Therapie* 17, 621–627.
109. Ryu, T., N. Hosaka, T. Miyake, W. Cui, T. Nishida, T. Takaki, M. Li, K. Kawamoto, and S. Ikehara. 2008. Transplantation of newborn thymus plus hematopoietic stem cells can rescue supralethally irradiated mice. *Bone Marrow Transplant* 41 (7): 659–666.
110. Perry, A. R., and A. F. Iglar. 1990. The accident at Chernobyl: Radiation doses and effects. *Radiol Technol* 61 (4): 290–294.
111. Carder, T. A. 1993. *Handling of Radiation Accident Patients by Paramedical and Hospital Personnel*, 2nd ed. Boca Raton, FL: CRC Press.
112. Blakely, J. 1968. *The Care of Radiation Casualties*. Springfield, IL: Charles C Thomas.
113. Baranov, A., R. P. Gale, A. Guskova, E. Piatkin, G. Selidovkin, L. Muravyova, R. E. Champlin, N. Danilova, L. Yevseeva, and L. Petrosyan. 1989. Bone marrow transplantation after the Chernobyl nuclear accident. *N Engl J Med* 321 (4): 205–212.

17 Micronutrients in Prevention and Improvement of the Standard Therapy in Arthritis

INTRODUCTION

The term arthritis is derived from the Greek word *arthro* meaning joint, and it refers to inflammation; and thus it is called joint inflammation. This is one of the major health concerns throughout the world including the United States. There are several forms of arthritis. Rheumatoid arthritis (RA) and osteoarthritis (OA) are the commonest forms of arthritis. The analysis of the published results suggests that increased oxidative stress and inflammation play a central role in the initiation and progression of arthritis. Low-dose methotrexate (MTX) therapy is considered a gold standard for the treatment of RA. Recently developed anticytokine therapy, primarily with antitumor necrosis factor-alpha (anti-TNF-alpha) have been useful in improving the symptoms and reducing the progression of RA. The combination of MTX and anticytokine therapy yields better results than those produced by the individual agents. It should be pointed out that most current treatment strategies have focused on reducing inflammation; however, the significance of reducing oxidative damage has not drawn any significant attention either in prevention or treatment of arthritis. Therefore, no efforts have been made to evaluate the efficacy of the combination of anti-inflammation agents and antioxidants in patients with RA or OA. Since antioxidants reduce oxidative stress, and to a lesser degree, reduce inflammation, the combination of anti-inflammatory agents and multiple antioxidants may improve the current management of arthritic lesions.

This chapter describes briefly the incidence, cost, major types of arthritis (RA, OA, and childhood arthritis) and their symptoms, role of oxidative stress and inflammation, and current treatments. In addition, this chapter discusses the scientific rational and evidence in support of using multiple micronutrients including dietary and endogenous antioxidants in prevention and improvement of the standard therapy in patients with RA.

INCIDENCE AND COST

In 2008, the Centers for Disease Control and Prevention (CDC) has reported that based on 2003–2005 data from the National Health Interview Survey, about 46 million adults in the United States have self-reported or doctor-diagnosed arthritis, and about 19 million of them have arthritis-attributable activity limitation. Although arthritis remains a major health concern for all racial/ethnic groups, the disabling effects of arthritis (arthritis-attributable activity limitations, work limitations, and severe pain) affect racial/ethnic minorities more severely. A 2007 CDC study estimated that about 294,000 children under the age of 18 years in the United States suffer from juvenile rheumatoid arthritis (JRA).

The CDC has reported that in 2003, the total cost of arthritis and other rheumatic conditions in the United States was approximately $128 billion. This represented 1.2% of the 2003 U.S. gross domestic product. About $80.8 billion were from the direct cost (i.e., medical expenses) and about $47.0 billion were from the indirect cost (i.e., lost earnings).

TYPES OF ARTHRITIS

There are 100 different forms of arthritis that affect the joint, the tissue surrounding the joint, and other connective tissues. Arthritis, in general, involves the breakdown of the cartilage that protects the joint, allowing for smooth movements. Cartilage also absorbs shock when pressure is placed on the joints such as experienced during walking, running, or playing sports. The major causes include autoimmune disease, injury to the bones, general wear and tear on joints during aging, and bacterial or viral infection. The most common ones are RA, OA, and JRA. Some characteristic features of each of them are briefly described below.

RHEUMATOID ARTHRITIS

RA is considered an inflammatory disease and typically occurs in joints on both sides of the body such as hands, wrists, or knees. This symmetry generally helps to distinguish RA from other types of arthritis (WebMD). The primary symptoms include joint pain and swelling, reduced ability to move the joint, stiffness, especially in the morning or after sitting for long periods, warmth around a joint, redness of the skin around a joint, and fatigue. RA affects people differently. In most individuals, the joint symptoms develop gradually over several years; however, in some cases, it may progress rapidly, while in others, it may persist for a limited period and then enter a period of remission. This disease is more common in women than in men, but men are affected more severely than women. It generally appears in middle age or old age.

RA is characterized by the presence of inflammatory immune cells into the joints and joint-lining tissue (synovium). These inflammatory cells release reactive oxygen species (ROS), proinflammatory cytokines, prostaglandins, adhesion molecules, and compliment proteins, all of which are toxic to cells. This can cause joint irritation, wearing down of cartilage, swelling, and production of excessive amounts of joint fluid within the joint. The progression of damage to the cartilage can cause narrowing of the space between the bones and eventually may rub against each other leading to severe pain. In addition, the excessive proliferation and migration of synoviocytes play an important role in the pathophysiology of RA.

OSTEOARTHRITIS

OA is a degenerative joint disease and is the most common form of arthritis. It is characterized by focal and progressive loss of hyaline cartilage of joints. The pathological changes include narrowing of the space between the bones, osteophytes, and bone sclerosis. The major symptoms include pain, swelling, and stiffness. The incidence of OA in women is higher than in men. It generally occurs after the age of 50 years. The most common sites are knee, hip, and hand.

Chondrocytes are the only cell type present in mature cartilage, and their death may contribute to the metabolic and structural changes in cartilage of patients with OA. Increased apoptotic cell death was found in the lesion areas compared to that in nonlesioned areas of the cartilage from some patients with OA, whereas apoptotic cells are rarely seen in normal cartilage.[1] Chondrocyte apoptosis appears to be correlated with the age and severity of the disease.[2] In addition to apoptotic cells, cartilage also contained necrotic materials formed from dead cells. Since cartilage does not have phagocytes because of its avascular nature, dead cells are not removed and, thus, form membrane-enclosed structures resembling matrix vesicles.[3] These structures may contribute to matrix mineralization or degradation in OA.

The risk factors include excess body mass, joint injury (sports, work, or trauma), excessive mechanical stress, heavy lifting, knee bending and repetitive motions, structural abnormal alignment, and muscle weakness. In addition, age and genetics are important risk factors for developing OA.

JUVENILE RHEUMATOID ARTHRITIS

JRA is the most common childhood arthritis. This is considered an autoimmune disease in which immune cells attack healthy cells of the joint causing inflammatory reactions that release toxic chemical species, which cause progressive damage to the joints and their surrounding tissues causing redness, swelling, pain, and stiffness. Some children with JRA outgrow the illness. As a matter of fact, the symptoms of JRA disappear in about 50% of affected children. JRA may cause chronic fever and anemia, and can affect the heart, lungs, eyes, and nervous system. These arthritic episodes may last for several weeks, and then may recur with less severe symptoms. This disease can impair bone development and weaken fine motor skills. The incidence of JRA in girls is higher than in boys. Transient JRA may follow certain infections.

EVIDENCE FOR THE ROLE OF OXIDATIVE STRESS

There are numerous articles that have been published supporting the role of increased oxidative stress in the initiation and progression of[4-8] arthritis in humans. Animal studies also confirmed the role of oxidative stress in the etiology of arthritis.[9-11] Only arbitrarily selected recent references have been used in this section.

In a clinical study involving 25 patients with RA and 26 healthy control subjects, it was observed that the levels of DNA damage in the peripheral lymphocytes and plasma total antioxidant status and total oxidative status were elevated in patients with RA compared to healthy controls. In a clinical study involving 20 patients with RA and 16 healthy control subjects, it was found that the levels of thiobarbituric acid reactive substances (TBARS), lipid hydroperoxide, conjugated diene, protein oxidation (carbonyl), and DNA adduct (8-hydroxyguanosine) were significantly higher, whereas the levels of glutathione, and activities of glutathione peroxidase and CuZn SOD in the blood were lowered compared to healthy controls. Furthermore, the levels of TBARS, lipid hydroperoxide, conjugated diene, carbonyl, and 8-hydroxyguanosine were significantly higher, and catalase activity lowered in the synovial fluid of RA patients compared to healthy subjects.[12] In another clinical study, the production rates of ROS of neutrophils and monocytes from patients with RA were compared with normal healthy subjects, and non-rheumatic disease and correlated with the plasma levels of tumor necrosis factor-alpha (TNF-alpha), C-reactive protein (CRP), and the sedimentation rates of erythrocytes. A 2- to 8-fold increase in the production of superoxide by the phagocytes from RA patients was observed, when compared to healthy subjects or patients with non-rheumatic disease.[5] The enhanced NADPH oxidase–dependent superoxide generation correlated well with the elevated plasma levels of TNF-alpha. There was no such correlation with the plasma levels of CRP or the sedimentation rates of erythrocytes. Removal of circulating TNF-alpha by the dialysis of patient blood and inhibition of NADPH oxidase activity by prednisolone treatment normalized the elevated levels of ROS production to the levels of control subjects and correlated with the clinical improvements.[5] This study suggests that both increased oxidative stress and inflammation play a central role in the progression of RA. The leukocyte but not neutrophil mitochondria from the patients with RA produced 5-fold more ROS than those obtained from control subjects, and this correlated well with the increased plasma levels of TNF-alpha.[13] This study suggests that mitochondrial defects are also associated with RA. In a clinical study involving 30 patients with rheumatoid, 15 patients with OA, and 15 patients with systemic lupus erythematosus (SLE), it was observed that the levels of 3-nitrotyrosine in synovial fluid and sera of patients with RA and OA were elevated compared to SLE.[14] The levels of 3-nitrotyrosine also correlated with the disease activity. High levels of nitrated type III collagen was found in synovial tissues of the patients with RA and knee OA compared to healthy controls. In addition, the serum levels of nitrated type III collagen was elevated in patients with OA 1.5-fold more than in healthy control subjects.[15] In patients with OA, the erythrocyte levels of MDA and activities of SOD, glutathione peroxidase, and plasma glutathione-S-transferase activity increased, whereas the erythrocyte levels of glutathione and ascorbic acid and plasma vitamin E decreased compared to those in healthy control subjects.[16] Macrophages and T cells from RA patients produced more NO than that produced by these cells obtained from healthy subjects. TNF-alpha also increased production of NO in T cells obtained from RA patients. Overproduction of NO may contribute to the T-cell dysfunction that is commonly found in the inflamed joint.[17] The synovial fluid neutrophils from RA patients are activated to produce increased amounts of ROS within the cells.[18] It has been reported that aldehydic products, primarily the 4-hydroxy-2-alkenals, form adducts with proteins that make them highly immunogenic, which can induce pathogenic antibodies in RA.[19]

The analysis of several studies in a review has shown that increased oxidative stress plays a central role in pathophysiology of OA.[20] Among reactive aldehydes, 4-hydroxynonenal (HNE) is considered the most reactive species, and like ROS, HNE can induce various biological effects including apoptosis. Antioxidants such as N-acetylcysteine (NAC) and overexpression of glutathione-S-transferase A4-4 reduced HNE production and inhibited apoptosis in several cells. The levels of HNE were higher in synovial fluid of patients with OA than those found in healthy subjects.[21] It has been demonstrated that HNE can induce transcriptional and posttranscriptional modifications of type II collagen and matrix metalloproteinase-13 (MMP-13), resulting in extracellular matrix in cartilage from patients with OA.[21]

EVIDENCE FOR THE ROLE OF INFLAMMATION

RA is considered a chronic inflammatory disease. During the active phase of the disease, the plasma levels of proinflammatory cytokines, interleukin-6 (IL-6), interleukin-1beta (IL-1beta), tumor necrosis factor-alpha (TNF-alpha), and active-phase proteins are elevated.[22,23] Arachidonic acid metabolites, such as leukotrienes B4 (LTB4), play an important role in the pathogenesis of RA. The levels of LTB4 were low in the cultured media of RA synovial fibroblast (RASF), but the major LTB4 receptor (BLT2) was expressed in RASF. The addition of LTB4 markedly increased expression of TNF-alpha and IL-1beta at the mRNA and protein levels, suggesting that LTB4 contribute to the damage associated with RA via increasing the levels of proinflammatory cytokines.[24] In addition to leukocytes, RASF produced a number of inflammatory mediators that recruit, retain, and activate immune cells and resident parenchymal cells in the joints in order to promote tissue destruction.

Several studies have reported the presence of an increased number of mast cells in the synovial tissues and fluids of patients with RA and at the sites of cartilage damage.[25] Activated mast cells have been found in a significant number of specimens obtained from patients with RA. Activated mast cells release potent mediators, including histamine, heparin, proteinases, leukotrienes, and multifunctional cytokines such as TNF-alpha, IL-6, and IL-1beta that contribute to tissue destruction in the joints. It has been reported that the serum levels of TNF-alpha, soluble TNF-alpha receptors (sTNF-Rp55 and sTNF-R p75), but not TNF-beta, are good markers of RA.[26] The increased expression of IL-23 gene was found in all samples of synovial membranes, whereas the expression of IL-17A was found only in subset of synovial membranes. Both IL-23 and IL-17A colocalized in the synovial membranes. These results were interpreted to suggest that IL-17, by itself, may not be important in the pathogenesis of RA, but it may amplify the inflammatory responses.[27] Activation of mast cells in RA synovial explants released increased amounts of PGE2 that contributes to the pathogenesis of RA.[28] RA is also associated with increased arterial stiffness. It has been reported that elevated plasma levels of osteopontin, a cytokine, contribute to the arterial stiffness in RA patients.[29] Both cathepsin K and S proteins were present in synovium from patients with RA and OA. Cathepsin-K protein was present in synovium fibroblasts and stromal multinucleated giant cells and, to a lesser degree, in CD68+ macrophage-like-synoviocytes. In contrast to cathepsin-K, cathepsin-S expression was primarily located in CD68+ macrophage-like synoviocytes, endothelial cells of blood vessels.[30] Both Il-1beta and TNF-alpha increased cathepsin-K expression in RA- and

OA-derived synovial fibroblasts. It appears that both cathepsin-K and -S participate in the degradation of cartilage in RA and OA.

In an animal model of RA, it was demonstrated that TNF-alpha plays an important role in joint swelling, whereas IL-1beta plays a significant role in degeneration of cartilage.[31] Overexpression of IL-18 increased both joint inflammation and cartilage destruction in mice. Overexpression of IL-18 gene in IL-1-deficient mice induced joint inflammation without any cartilage damage; however, in vitro study suggested that IL-18-induced cartilage damage was dependent upon the presence of IL-1beta. On the other hand, overexpression of IL-18 in TNF-deficient mice showed that TNF-alpha was partly responsible for IL-18-induced joint swelling and influx of inflammatory cells, but that it has no role in IL-18-induced cartilage damage.[32] Toll-like receptors (TLRs) may contribute to the pathogenesis of AR. The presence of endogenous ligand for TLR has been found in the joints of RA patients. It has been reported that IL-1beta-induced local joint inflammation, cartilage proteoglycan depletion, and bone degeneration are dependent on TLR4 activation. On the other hand, TNF-alpha-induced RA pathology was less dependent upon TLR4 or TLR-2. Furthermore, IL-1beta-induced expression of cathepsin-K, a marker of osteoclast activity, was dependent on TLR4 activation.[33] A review of several studies indicates that autoantigen recognition by specific T cell is important to the development of rheumatoid sinovitis.[34] The involvement of T cells in the pathogenesis of RA is supported by the fact that numerous T-cell carrying activation markers were found in RA synovium. These T cells appear to participate in the complex network of cell- and mediator-driven biochemical events that cause joint destruction. The transgenic k/BxN mice develop an inflammatory joint disease with many features characteristic of RA. This model is based on a T-cell receptor transgene, KRN that recognizes both the foreign antigen, bovine RNase, and the ubiquitously expressed self antigen, glucose-6-phosphate isomerase (GPI). Using this model, it has been demonstrated that autoimmune response initiates at the levels of both adaptive and innate immune systems.[35]

Proinflammatory cytokines such as IL-1beta appears to be involved in the pathogenesis of OA through the production of catabolic enzymes and inflammatory mediators. Induction of heme oxygenase (HO-1) appears to exert anti-inflammatory effects. Induction of HO-1 by cobalt protoporphyrin IX increased the viability of primary culture of chondrocytes by inhibiting apoptosis, oxidative stress, and reducing the production of prostaglandin E_2.[36] In addition to proinflammatory cytokines, MMPs and other catabolic factors contribute to the pathogenesis of cartilage damage in OA. Proinflammatory cytokines such as IL-1 beta down-regulated H0-1, whereas IL-10 up-regulated HO-1 in OA chondrocytes.[37] Activation of HO-1 significantly reduced IL-1beta-induced damage to cartilage. It also inhibited MMP activity and expression of collagenases MMP-1 and MMP-13 at protein and mRNA levels.[37]

Elevated levels of PGE2 play a significant role in the pathogenesis of arthritis. The levels of protein and mRNA of an inducible microsomal prostaglandin synthase-1 (mPGES-1) were higher in OA cartilage compared to normal cartilage. IL-1beta treatment induced expression of mPGEs-1 mRNA in a dose-dependent manner in chondrocytes.[38] Treatment with TNF-alpha or IL-17 up-regulated expression of mPGEs-1 protein and exhibited synergistic effects on the above criteria in combination with IL-1beta in chondrocytes in cultures.[38]

ROLE OF ANTIOXIDANTS IN ARTHRITIS

ANIMAL STUDIES

In collagen-induced arthritis in rats, it was observed that intradermal administration of a low molecular weight mimetic of SOD improved clinical symptoms and degenerative changes in the joint and paw, and reduced the levels of nitrotyrosine (a marker of peroxynitrite formation) and DNA damage.[39] Similar results were obtained with Cu,ZN-SOD in collagen-induced arthritis in rats.[40] In collagen-induced arthritis in mice, it was found that depletion of vitamin from the diet induced increased expressions of joint tissue TNF-alpha and IL-1beta, and increased levels of circulating macrophage chemoattractant protein-1, nitric oxide, and PGE2. However, supplementation with vitamin E or quercetin restored these markers to control levels.[41] In an experimental rabbit inflammatory arthritis model (intra-articular injection of lipopolysaccharide), the effects of intra-articular injection of resveratrol, a polyphenolic compound, found in grape skin and red wine, on the cartilage and synovium, was investigated. The results showed that resveratrol protect cartilage against the development of chemical-induced inflammatory arthritis.[42] In a rat model of adjuvant arthritis, it was demonstrated that the levels of markers of oxidative damage and inflammation increased; however, administration of L-carnitine and alpha-lipoic acid reduced markers of oxidative damage and inflammation.[43] In a mice model of arthritis, supplementation with epigallocatechin-3-gallate improved clinical symptoms and reduced histological scores of arthritis.[44] In collagen-induced arthritis in mice, supplementation with alpha-lipoic acid reduced the incidence of arthritis and prevented bone erosion.[45] It also decreased the levels of ROS in lymphocytes obtained from inguinal lymph nodes, and the levels of TNF-alpha, IL-1beta, and IL-6 in the paws. These studies suggested that supplementation with alpha-lipoic acid may be useful as an adjunctive therapy for RA.

HUMAN STUDIES

A review of 20 randomized clinical trials in which the effects of individual antioxidants such as vitamins A, C, and E or selenium or their combination in the treatment of inflammatory arthritis and OA were evaluated and revealed inconsistent results.[46,47] Most of these studies were of poor quality with respect to selection of number, types, and doses of antioxidants, and treatment periods. Therefore, no conclusion with respect to efficacy of antioxidant supplements to improve the symptoms in patients with AR or OA can be drawn from these studies. In the Women's Health Study involving 39,144 subjects without RA, supplementation with 600 IU of vitamin E alone taken every other day was not associated with a significant reduction in the risk of developing RA.[48] In an open pilot study involving eight nonsmoking female patients with RA who received a nonsteroidal anti-inflammatory drug (NSAID) and/or second line of medication, the efficacy of antioxidant-enriched spread on the severity of RA was determined. The results showed that antioxidant supplementation decreased the number of swollen and painful joints and improved general health and decreased the Disease Activity Score from 28 to 1.6.[49] In randomized, double-blind placebo-controlled trials involving 20 patients with RA, the effects of supplementation with quercetin plus vitamin C or alpha-lipoic acid for a period of 4 weeks on the levels of biomarkers of proinflammatory cytokines and symptoms of the disease were evaluated. The results showed that antioxidant supplementation did not change the levels of inflammation markers or disease severity.[50] Despite contradictory results with individual antioxidants, some studies continue to suggest that a diet rich in antioxidants and omega-3 fatty acids with or without standard medications may improve the efficacy of therapy.[22,51,52] The therapeutic benefit of alpha-lipoic acid via down-regulation of NF-kappaB has been demonstrated in animal models of RA. Using cultures of fibroblast-like synovial cells from patients with RA, it was demonstrated that TNF-alpha-induced activation of NF-kappaB pathway was inhibited by pretreatment with alpha-lipoic acid.[53]

Treatment of synoviocyte cells (obtained from patients with RA) in culture with resveratrol inhibited proliferation of synoviocytes and induced apoptosis by activation of caspase-3.[54] In a rat model of RA (induced by streptococcal cell wall), administration of turmeric inhibited joint inflammation and periarticular joint destruction and prevented activation of NF-kappaB and decreased the levels of markers of inflammation.[55]

Treatment of bovine disc cells in culture with beta-fibroblastic growth factor (bFGF) or IL-1 increased the production of MMP-13 that was attenuated by the treatment with resveratrol; therefore, it was concluded that resveratrol treatment may slow the progression of intervertebral disc degeneration.[56] Resveratrol treatment of RA fibroblast-like synoviocytes induced apoptosis by activating caspase-8 that releases mitochondrial cytochrome.[57]

The pineal neurohormone melatonin enhances the function of immune cells through its specific receptors. In addition, it exhibits antioxidant activity; therefore, it has been tested in several chronic diseases yielding inconsistent results. The nocturnal plasma concentration of melatonin in patients with RA was higher than in healthy control subjects. In addition, melatonin was found in the synovial fluid of RA patients, and synovial macrophages express specific binding sites. These studies suggested that melatonin may promote progression of RA.[58] In a clinical study involving 20 patients with JRA and 20 health age and sex-matched controls, the serum levels of melatonin were elevated compared to controls, suggesting that melatonin may play a promoting role in JRA.[59] In contrast to these studies, melatonin treatment reduced proliferation of primary cultured human fibroblast-like synoviocytes through the activation of p21 and P27 mediated by phosphorylation of extracellular signal-regulated protein kinase (ERK).[60]

Treatment of RA synovial fibroblasts in culture with epigallocatechin-3-gallate suppressed TNF-alpha-induced production of MMP-1 and MMP-3 that play a significant role in destruction of cartilage and bone in RA joint.[61]

Animal studies have shown that 1alpha,25-dihydroxyvitamin D3 (vitamin D_3), the biologically active form of vitamin D, up-regulated MMPs that play a major role in the degeneration of cartilage in the joints. It has been found that vitamin D_3 is produced in the synovial fluid of arthritic joints, and vitamin D_3 receptors are located in RA synovial tissues and at the sites of cartilage damage.[62] Vitamin D_3 treatment of monolayer cultures of RA synovial fibroblasts did not affect the basal production of MPP or PGE2; however, it suppressed the production of MPP and PGE2 in IL-1beta–stimulated RA synovial fibroblasts. In contrast, vitamin D_3 treatment of monolayer cultures of human articular chondrocytes stimulated the basal production of MMP-1 and MMP-3, and it had no effect on IL-1beta-stimulated production of MMP-1 or PGE2. These differences in response of RA synovial fibroblasts and chondrocytes to vitamin D_3 make it difficult to recommend high doses of vitamin D in the management of RA.

CURRENT PREVENTION STRATEGIES

At present, there are no adequate preventive strategies to reduce the risk of RA or OA in normal population; therefore, a biological strategy that is based on scientific-based rationale and evidence is needed.

CURRENT TREATMENT STRATEGIES

The current treatment strategies involve multiple agents including low-dose MTX, anticytokines, and NSAIDs, individually or in combination. Supplementation with antioxidants has produced inconsistent results. Complimentary and alternative medicine approaches have been also adopted by the patients with RA in order to reduce pain associated with RA.

Low-Dose MTX

MTX, a folate inhibitor, initially was used for the treatment of cancer. Low-dose MTX is considered a gold standard for the treatment of RA and has been in use for the past 3 decades.[63–67] MTX is an immunosuppressive drug, which causes apoptosis via increased oxidative damage to proliferating cells in the joints of the patients with active RA. MTX has one of the best efficacy and toxicity ratios. It improves signs and symptoms of RA and physical function, and inhibits radiographic progression of cartilage damage, but to a smaller degree, compared to anti-TNF therapy. The proposed mechanisms of action include inhibition of T-cell proliferation, inhibition of transmethylation reactions required for the prevention of T-cell toxicity, interference with glutathione metabolism leading to alterations in recruitment of monocytes and other cells to the inflamed joints, and promotion of the release of the endogenous anti-inflammatory mediator adenosine. One case of an acute erythroleukemia was observed during low-dose MTX therapy. In spite of this rare case of cancer, low-dose MTX remains the first choice for the initial treatment of RA.

ANTICYTOKINES THERAPY

Over the past decade, the discovery of anticytokine inhibitors, primarily TNF-alpha inhibitors, has revolutionized the treatment of RA. However, severe side effects that include allergy, tuberculosis, opportunistic infections, demyelination, and cancer occur in some individuals. In a clinical study involving 29 patients with active RA and 25 healthy controls, it was observed that anti-TNF-alpha therapy rapidly decreased the influx of leukocytes into inflamed joints, but did not impair neutrophil chemotaxis and production of ROS.[68] In a clinical study with 55 RA patients who were unresponsive to conventional doses (3 mg/kg of body weight) of anti-TNF-alpha (infliximab), the effects of doses and frequency of infliximab infusions were evaluated. The results showed that changing the frequency of infliximab infusions in the active RA group was more effective than increasing the dose of infliximab for improving the clinical outcomes.[69] The antioxidant capacity of HDL-cholesterol decreased in patients with RA. Anti-TNF therapy with infliximab improved antioxidant capacity after 6 months of therapy that may explain the protective effect of anti-TNF therapy on cardiovascular morbidity in RA.[70] Angiogenesis is an important factor in the remodeling of bone components in both normal and pathological condition. The angiopoitin (Ang) family of growth factors regulates angiogenesis. Ang-1 appears to stabilize new blood vessels by recruiting mesenchymal cells and promoting their differentiation into vascular smooth muscle. The osetoblasts obtained from patients with RA, OA, and healthy subjects spontaneously secreted significant amounts of Ang-1. Stimulation with TNF-alpha or interferon gamma (IFN-gamma) had no significant effect on Ang-1 secretion; however, the combination of TNF-alpha and IFN-gamma caused dose- and time-dependent decrease in Ang-1 secretion.[71] Thus, overproduction of these cytokines may interfere with the remodeling of bone components in patients with RA or OA by decreasing the secretion of Ang-1. Treatment with anti-TNF-alpha therapy with infliximab reduces the levels of some adhesion molecules that are elevated in patients with active RA.[72]

Extensive clinical studies have been performed on disease-modifying antirheumatic drugs (DMARDs), also called Biologics, which include abatacept, adalimumab, anakinra, etanercept, infliximab, and rituximab in patients with RA. Among these, adalimumab, etanercept, and infliximab are TNF-alpha inhibitors, whereas anakinra is an IL-1 receptor antagonist. A detailed review on the relative efficacy and toxicity of these Biologics reported that anakinra was less effective than others and that etanercept caused fewer withdrawals due to toxicity than infliximab, anakinra, and adalimumab.[73] Certolizumab pegol is a PEGylated humanized Fab monoclonal antibody that neutralizes both membrane-bound and soluble TNF-alpha. In a randomized, double-blind, placebo-controlled trial involving 982 RA patients with an inadequate response to MTX alone, the efficacy of certolizumab pegol, in combination with MTX, was determined. The results showed that treatment with certolizumab pegol, in combination with MTX, improved signs and symptoms of RA, inhibited the progression of structural joint damage, and improved physical function compared to control patients receiving placebo in combination with MTX.[74,75] This TNF-alpha inhibitor alone or in combination with MTX was generally well tolerated. The most common reported adverse event was infection.[75,76] The combination of adalimumab in combination with MTX was superior to either adalimumab alone or MTX alone in improving signs and symptoms of RA, inhibiting radiographic progression of disease, and exhibited disease remission.[77] The beneficial effects of TNF-alpha inhibitors in combination with MTX were similar in older and younger patients with RA.[78]

In a randomized and placebo-controlled clinical trial involving 359 patients with active RA in whom the response to MTX was inadequate, the efficacy of tocilizumab, a humanized anti-IL-6 receptor antibody, alone or in combination with MTX in patients with RA, was evaluated. The results showed that a 20% improvement on the criterion of American College of Rheumatology score (ACR20 response) was observed in 61% to 63% of patients receiving tocilizumab alone, and in 63–74% patients receiving both tocilizumab and MTX. Tocilizumab was mostly well tolerated, and the safety profiles were similar to those of other Biologics.[79] In a clinical study involving 499 RA patients with inadequate response to one or more TNF-alpha inhibitors, the efficacy of tocilizumab in combination with MTX was evaluated. The results showed that a 20% improvement in ACR score was observed in about 30% to 50% of patients receiving tocilizumab in combination with MTX, depending upon the dose of tocilizumab; however, only 10% of control subjects receiving placebo showed such an improvement.[80] Similar beneficial effects of tocilizumab in combination with MTX were observed in another clinical study in which RA patients had an inadequate response to MTX.[81]

Toxicity of Standard Therapy

The common adverse effects of combined therapy with MTX and anticytokine therapy included increased incidence of infection, gastrointestinal symptoms, rash, and headache. Several cases of cancer have been reported in patients receiving etanercept, a TNF-alpha inhibitor.[82] The rate of tuberculosis in non-white patients with RA receiving anti-TNF-alpha was 6-fold higher than white patients with RA and the patients receiving infliximab or adalimumab had a 3- to 4-fold higher rate of tuberculosis than those receiving etanercept.[83] In addition, non-tuberculosis mycobacterial infections were observed in patients receiving TNF-alpha inhibitors with or without MTX or prednisone.[84]

Glucosamine and Chondroitin

In a clinical study involving 46 patients with OA and 22 patients with RA, supplementation with glucosamine sulfate, chondroitin sulfate, and quercetin together for a period of 3 months showed a significant improvement in pain symptoms, daily physical activities (walking and climbing up and down stairs), and visual analogue scale. It also altered the synovial fluid properties. These effects of supplementation were not observed in patients with OA.[85] In a randomized, double-blind, placebo-controlled trial, the Glucosamine/Chondroitin Arthritis Intervention Trial (GAIT), 1583 OA patients received daily 1500 mg of glucosamine, 1200 mg of chondroitin sulfate individually or in combination, 200 mg of celecoxib or placebo for a period of 24 weeks. Up to 4000 mg of acetaminophen was allowed as rescue analgesia. The patients were stratified according to the intensity of knee pain yielding 1229 patients with mild pain and 354 patients with moderate to severe pain. The primary end point was a 20% decrease in knee pain from baseline data. The results showed that overall, the treatment with glucosamine and chondroitin sulfate was not significantly better compared to the placebo in reducing knee pain by 20%. However, in patients with moderate to severe knee pain, the above treatment decreased the knee pain by about 25%.[86] The response rate in the celecoxib group was 10% higher than in placebo group, whereas in the group receiving both glucosamine and chondroitin sulfate, it was about 6.5% higher than in the placebo group. The above clinical study was extended to evaluate the effect of glucosamine and chondroitin sulfate, alone or in combination, celecoxib, and placebo on progressive loss of joint space and width (JSW) in 572 patients with knee OA who satisfied radiographic criteria [Kellgren/Lawrence grade 2 (K/L grade 2) or KL grade 3]. At the end of the observation period of 24 months, there was no significant difference in all treated groups compared to the placebo group. However, in KL grade 2 group, a trend toward improvement of JSW was observed relative to the placebo group.[87] It has been reported that glucosamine sulfate is more effective than glucosamine chloride.[88] In a randomized, double-blind, placebo-controlled trial involving 622 patients with knee OA, the effect of glucosamine sulfate on changes in JSW was evaluated in 309 patients receiving daily 400 mg of glucosamine sulfate and 313 patients receiving a placebo for 2 years. The results showed that a significant reduction in minimum JSW loss occurred in the supplemented group compared to the placebo group. The percentage of patients with radiographic progression of JSW was significantly reduced in the supplemented group compared to the placebo group. In addition, the knee pain was significantly improved in the supplemented group compared to the placebo group.[89] In a clinical study involving 89 patients with knee OA, supplementation with glucosamine chloride and chondroitin sulfate with or without exercise did not improve physical function, pain, or mobility after 1 month of treatment.[90]

NONSTEROIDAL ANTI-INFLAMMATORY DRUGS

Chronic pain from arthritis remains one of the major problems that can cause disability and poor quality of life. Despite increased concerns of long-term toxicity of NSAIDs, especially cyclooxygenase-2 inhibitors, these drugs remains one of the viable options for managing the pain associated with RA.[91]

COMPLEMENTARY MEDICINE

The patients with RA also utilized complementary and alternative medicine approaches to improve the symptoms of the disease. These include nutritional supplements, touch therapy, mind–body therapy, Reiki, acupuncture, herbal medicine, pulsed electromagnetic field, homeopathy, Ayurveda, and yoga.[92–94] A well-designed clinical study on any of the above complementary and alternative approaches has not been performed. The varying degrees of reduction in joint pain have been reported by the patients with RA.

In a clinical study involving 89 patients (90% female), supplementation with rose-hip powder (5 g/day) for a period of 6 months did not improve the pain intensity compared to the placebo group; it improved the physician global evaluation of disease activity.[95] Although L-carnitine and alpha-lipoic acid reduced MTX-induced oxidative damage in animal models,[96,97] it remains uncertain whether the antioxidants will have similar effects without interfering with the efficacy of MTX treatment in patients with RA or OA.

In a rat model of RA, supplementation with MTX and probiotic bacteria [Colinfant (COL)] significantly inhibited inflammation and destructive arthritis-associated changes.[98]

PROPOSED MICRONUTRIENT STRATEGIES FOR PREVENTION IN HIGH-RISK POPULATIONS

The high-risk populations include older individuals and persons with a family history of RA or OA. At present, there are no strategies to reduce the risk of AR or OA. Most studies with individual antioxidants have been performed with respect to the treatment of RA. There are substantial amounts of data that support the hypothesis that increased oxidative stress and inflammation plays a central role in the initiation and progression of RA. Since antioxidants at high doses can reduce oxidative stress as well as inflammation, they appear to be one of the rational choices for reducing the risk of AR. In addition, the modifications in the diet and lifestyle may also be very important in reducing the risk of RA.

PROBLEMS OF USING A SINGLE AGENT

The use of a single antioxidant in all clinical studies in high-risk populations of several chronic diseases has produced inconsistent results. This issue has been discussed in detail in Chapter 3. The high-risk populations for chronic diseases including RA generally have elevated internal oxidative environments. The individual antioxidant in the presence of a high internal oxidative environment is oxidized and then acts as a pro-oxidant. This reaction may increase the risk of chronic diseases. Therefore, I recommend the use of multiple micronutrients including dietary and endogenous antioxidants, B vitamins, and certain minerals for reducing the incidence of RA. Additional rationales for using multiple micronutrients are described below.

RATIONALE FOR USING MULTIPLE MICRONUTRIENTS

Because of the potential for increased levels of oxidative stress and inflammation in high-risk populations for RA, an oral supplementation with appropriate multiple micronutrients appears to be one of the rational choices for reducing the risk of RA. Experimental designs of most clinical studies in patients with RA have utilized only one or two antioxidants for improving the symptoms of the disease. These designs are not suitable for determining the efficacy of micronutrients in reducing the incidence of RA or improved treatment of the disease when combined with the standard therapy. This is due to the fact that their mechanisms of action and distribution at cellular and organ levels differ, their cellular and organ environments (oxygenation, aqueous and lipid components) differ, and their affinity for various types of free radicals differs. For example, beta-carotene (BC) is more effective in quenching oxygen radicals than most other antioxidants.[99] BC can perform certain biological functions that cannot be produced by its metabolite vitamin A, and vice versa.[100,101] It has been reported that BC treatment enhances the expression of the connexin gene, which codes for a gap junction protein in mammalian fibroblasts in culture, whereas vitamin A treatment does not produce such an effect.[101] Vitamin A can induce differentiation in certain normal and cancer cells, whereas BC and other carotenoids do not.[102,103] Thus, BC and vitamin A have, in part, different biological functions.

The gradient of oxygen pressure varies within cells. Some antioxidants, such as vitamin E, are more effective as quenchers of free radicals in reduced oxygen pressure, whereas BC and vitamin A are more effective in higher atmospheric pressures.[104] Vitamin C is necessary to protect cellular components in aqueous environments, whereas carotenoids and vitamins A and E protect cellular components in lipid environments. Vitamin C also plays an important role in maintaining cellular levels of vitamin E by recycling vitamin E radical (oxidized) to the reduced (antioxidant) form.[105] Also, oxidative DNA damage produced by high levels of vitamin C could be protected by vitamin E. Oxidized forms of vitamins C and E can also act as radicals; therefore, excessive amounts of any one of these forms, when used as a single agent, could be harmful over a long period of time.

The form of vitamin E used is also important in any clinical trial. It has been established that D-alpha-tocopheryl succinate (alpha-TS) is the most effective form of vitamin E both in vitro and in vivo.[106,107] This form of vitamin E is more soluble than alpha-tocopherol and enters cells more readily. Therefore, it is expected to cross the blood–brain barrier in greater amounts than alpha-tocopherol. However, this has not yet been demonstrated in animals or humans. We have reported that an oral ingestion of alpha-TS (800 IU/day) in humans increased plasma levels of not only alpha-tocopherol, but also alpha-TS, suggesting that a portion of alpha-TS can be absorbed from the intestinal tract before hydrolysis.[108] This observation is important because the conventional assumption based on the rodent studies has been that esterified forms of vitamin E such as alpha-TS, alpha-tocopheryl nicotinate, or alpha-tocopheryl acetate can be absorbed from the intestinal tract only after they are hydrolyzed to alpha-tocopherol. Our preliminary data showed that this assumption may not be true for the absorption of alpha-TS in humans.

Glutathione is effective in catabolizing H_2O_2 and anions. However, oral supplementation with glutathione failed to significantly increase plasma levels of glutathione in human subjects,[109] suggesting that this tripeptide is completely hydrolyzed in the GI tract. Therefore, I propose to utilize NAC and alpha-lipoic acid that increase the cellular levels of glutathione by different mechanisms in a multiple micronutrient preparation. In addition, R-alpha-lipoic acid and acetyl-L-carnitine together promoted mitochondrial biogenesis in murine adipocytes in culture; however, no effect was observed when these antioxidants were used individually.[110] These types of studies further emphasized the value of using more than one antioxidant in any clinical or laboratory studies involving RA or OA.

Other endogenous antioxidants, coenzyme Q_{10}, may also have some potential value in prevention and improved treatment of RA or OA. Since coenzyme Q_{10} is needed for the generation of ATP by mitochondria, it is essential to add this antioxidant in a multiple micronutrient preparation in order to enchance the function of mitochondria. A study has shown that Ubiquinol (coenzyme

Q_{10}) scavenges peroxy radicals faster than alpha-tocopherol,[111] and like vitamin C, can regenerate vitamin E in a redox cycle.[112] However, it is a weaker antioxidant than alpha-tocopherol. Coenzyme Q_{10} administration has been shown to improve clinical symptoms in patients with mitochondrial encephalomyopathies.[113]

Selenium is a cofactor of glutathione peroxidase, and Se-glutathione peroxidase increases the intracellular level of glutathione that is a powerful antioxidant. There may be some other mechanisms of action of selenium. Therefore, selenium and coenzyme Q_{10} should be added to a multiple micronutrient preparation for prevention and improved treatment of RA and OA.

Certain B vitamins have produced some beneficial effects in patients with diabetes. Therefore, in addition to dietary and endogenous antioxidants, all B vitamins that are necessary for general health should be added to a multiple micronutrient preparation for reducing the incidence or improved treatment of RA and OA combination with the standard therapy.

RECOMMENDED MICRONUTRIENT SUPPLEMENT FOR HIGH-RISK POPULATIONS

The high-risk populations include individuals with a family history of RA and those who are older. They provide an excellent opportunity to study the efficacy of multiple micronutrients on reducing the incidence of RA. A formulation of multiple micronutrients may include vitamin A (retinyl palmitate), vitamin E (both D-alpha-tocopherol and D-TS), natural mixed carotenoids, vitamin C (calcium ascorbate), coenzyme Q_{10}, R-alpha-lipoic acid, NAC, L-carnitine, vitamin D, all B vitamins, omega-3 fatty acids, selenium, zinc, and chromium. No iron, copper, or manganese would be included because these trace minerals are known to interact with vitamin C to produce free radicals. In addition, these trace minerals are absorbed from the intestinal tract more in the presence of antioxidants than in their absence that could result in increased body stores of free forms of these minerals. Increased iron stores have been linked to increased risk of several chronic diseases.[114] Omega-3 fatty acids are included because they are known to have anti-inflammation effects. Antioxidants from herbs, fruits, and vegetables were not included because they do not produce any unique biological effects that cannot be produced by antioxidants and omega-3 fatty acids present in the micronutrient preparation.

The recommended micronutrient supplements should be taken orally and divided into two doses, half in the morning and the other half in the evening with meal. This is because the biological half-lives of micronutrients are highly variable, which can create high levels of fluctuations in the tissue levels of micronutrients. A 2-fold difference in the levels of certain micronutrients such as alpha-TS can cause a marked difference in the expression of gene profiles (our unpublished data). In order to maintain relatively consistent levels of micronutrients in the body, the proposed micronutrients should be taken twice a day.

The efficacy of this formulation in high-risk populations should be tested by well-designed clinical studies. In the meanwhile, the proposed micronutrient recommendations may be adopted by the individuals who are at high risk for developing RA in consultation with their physicians or health professionals. It is expected that the proposed recommendations would reduce the incidence of RA in these populations.

RECOMMENDED MICRONUTRIENT SUPPLEMENT IN COMBINATION WITH STANDARD THERAPY FOR RA PATIENTS

Increased oxidative stress and inflammation contribute to the development and progression of RA. The current treatment with MTX and anticytokine medications produced beneficial effects in patients with RA; however, significant adverse side effects of these treatments include infections such as non-tuberculosis and tuberculosis bacteria, gastrointestinal symptoms, rash, headache, and cancer. Therefore, additional approaches should be developed in order to enhance the efficacy of current therapy in RA patients. The addition of a multiple micronutrient preparation such as that described in the previous paragraph of prevention may improve the efficacy of standard therapy. The efficacy of this micronutrient preparation in combination with standard therapy should be tested by well-designed clinical studies in RA patients. In the meanwhile, the proposed micronutrient recommendations may be adopted by the RA patients who are receiving standard therapy in consultation with their physicians or health professionals. It is expected that the proposed micronutrient recommendations would enhance the efficacy of standard therapy by increasing its response rates and decreasing its toxicity.

DIET AND LIFESTYLE RECOMMENDATIONS FOR HIGH-RISK POPULATIONS AND RA PATIENTS

A balanced diet is very necessary in addition to supplementation with multiple micronutrients for the prevention and improved treatment of RA. I recommend a balanced diet containing low-fat foods and plenty of fruits and vegetables. Lifestyle recommendations include daily moderate exercise, reduced stress, no tobacco smoking, and maintaining normal weight.

CONCLUSIONS

RA is considered an inflammatory disease and typically occurs in joints on both sides of the body such as hands, wrists, or knees. OA is a degenerative joint disease and is the most common form of arthritis. This disease affects a large number of people throughout the world including the United States. Increased oxidative stress and inflammation are the major biological processes associated with the initiation and progression of RA. At present, there are no effective preventive strategies to reduce the risk of RA. Low-dose MTX therapy is considered a gold standard for the initial treatment of RA or OA. Anticytokine therapy, especially TNF-alpha inhibitors, has been useful in improving the symptoms and reducing the progression of RA. The combination of MTX and anticytokine therapy has produced better results than either agent alone. Nevertheless, the current treatments are not considered optimal, and they produce severe side effects in some individuals. Therefore, an additional approach is needed to increase the efficacy of the current treatment. I have proposed that supplementation with a multiple micronutrient preparation, together with modifications in the diet and lifestyle, may reduce the risk of RA, and improve the efficacy of standard therapy. This proposal should be tested by well-designed clinical studies in patients with RA and OA. In the meanwhile, the proposed recommendations of supplementation with a multiple micronutrient preparation together with modifications in the diet and lifestyle may be adopted by the RA patients who are receiving standard therapy in consultation with their physicians or health professionals. It is expected that the proposed recommendations would reduce the incidence of RA and improve the efficacy of standard therapy by increasing its response rates and decreasing its toxicity.

REFERENCES

1. Kim, H. A., Y. J. Lee, S. C. Seong, K. W. Choe, and Y. W. Song. 2000 Apoptotic chondrocyte death in human osteoarthritis. *J Rheumatol* 27 (2): 455–462.
2. Mistry, D., Y. Oue, M. G. Chambers, M. V. Kayser, and R. M. Mason. 2004. Chondrocyte death during murine osteoarthritis. *Osteoarthritis Cartilage* 12 (2): 131–141.
3. Hashimoto, S., R. L. Ochs, S. Komiya, and M. Lotz. 1998. Linkage of chondrocyte apoptosis and cartilage degradation in human osteoarthritis. *Arthritis Rheum* 41 (9): 1632–1638.
4. Altindag, O., M. Karakoc, A. Kocyigit, H. Celik, and N. Soran. 2007. Increased DNA damage and oxidative stress in patients with rheumatoid arthritis. *Clin Biochem* 40 (3–4): 167–171.
5. Miesel, R., R. Hartung, and H. Kroeger. 1996. Priming of NADPH oxidase by tumor necrosis factor alpha in patients with inflammatory and autoimmune rheumatic diseases. *Inflammation* 20 (4): 427–438.

6. Mirshafiey, A., and M. Mohsenzadegan. 2008. The role of reactive oxygen species in immunopathogenesis of rheumatoid arthritis. *Iran J Allergy Asthma Immunol* 7 (4): 195–202.
7. Bauerova, K., and A. Bezek. 2004. Role of reactive oxygen and nitrogen species in etiopathogenesis of rheumatoid arthritis. *Gen Physiol Biophys* 18: 15–20.
8. Hitchon, C. A., and H. S. El-Gabalawy. 2004. Oxidation in rheumatoid arthritis. *Arthritis Res Ther* 6 (6): 265–278.
9. Nemirovskiy, O. V., M. R. Radabaugh, P. Aggarwal, C. L. Funckes-Shippy, S. J. Mnich, D. M. Meyer, T. Sunyer, R. W. Mathews, and T. P. Misko. 2009. Plasma 3-nitrotyrosine is a biomarker in animal models of arthritis: Pharmacological dissection of iNOS' role in disease. *Nitric Oxide* 20 (3): 150–156.
10. Strosova, M., I. Tomaskova, S. Ponist, K. Bauerova, J. Karlovska, C. M. Spickett, and L. Horakova. 2008. Oxidative impairment of plasma and skeletal muscle sarcoplasmic reticulum in rats with adjuvant arthritis—Effects of pyridoindole antioxidants. *Neuro Endocrinol Lett* 29 (5): 706–711.
11. Strosova, M., J. Karlovska, C. M. Spickett, Z. Orszagova, S. Ponist, K. Bauerova, D. Mihalova, and L. Horakova. 2009. Modulation of SERCA in the chronic phase of adjuvant arthritis as a possible adaptation mechanism of redox imbalance. *Free Radic Res* 43 (9): 852–864.
12. Seven, A., S. Guzel, A. Aslan, and V. Hamuryudan. 2008. Lipid, protein, DNA oxidation and antioxidant status in rheumatoid arthritis. *Clin Biochem* 41 (7–8): 538–543.
13. Miesel, R., M. P. Murphy, and H. Kroger. 1996. Enhanced mitochondrial radical production in patients which rheumatoid arthritis correlates with elevated levels of tumor necrosis factor alpha in plasma. *Free Radic Res* 25 (2): 161–169.
14. Khan, F., and A. A. Siddiqui. 2006. Prevalence of anti-3-nitrotyrosine antibodies in the joint synovial fluid of patients with rheumatoid arthritis, osteoarthritis and systemic lupus erythematosus. *Clin Chim Acta* 370 (1–2): 100–107.
15. Richardot, P., N. Charni-Ben Tabassi, L. Toh, H. Marotte, A. C. Bay-Jensen, P. Miossec, and P. Garnero. 2009. Nitrated type III collagen as a biological marker of nitric oxide-mediated synovial tissue metabolism in osteoarthritis. *Osteoarthritis Cartilage* 17 (10): 1362–1367.
16. Surapaneni, K. M., and G. Venkataramana. 2007. Status of lipid peroxidation, glutathione, ascorbic acid, vitamin E and antioxidant enzymes in patients with osteoarthritis. *Indian J Med Sci* 61 (1): 9–14.
17. Nagy, G., J. M. Clark, E. Buzas, C. Gorman, M. Pasztoi, A. Koncz, A. Falus, and A. P. Cope. 2008. Nitric oxide production of T lymphocytes is increased in rheumatoid arthritis. *Immunol Lett* 118 (1): 55–58.
18. Cedergren, J., T. Forslund, T. Sundqvist, and T. Skogh. 2007. Intracellular oxidative activation in synovial fluid neutrophils from patients with rheumatoid arthritis but not from other arthritis patients. *J Rheumatol* 34 (11): 2162–2170.
19. Kurien, B. T., and R. H. Scofield. 2008. Autoimmunity and oxidatively modified autoantigens. *Autoimmun Rev* 7 (7): 567–573.
20. Vaillancourt, F., H. Fahmi, Q. Shi, P. Lavigne, P. Ranger, J. C. Fernandes, and M. Benderdour. 2008. 4-Hydroxynonenal induces apoptosis in human osteoarthritic chondrocytes: The protective role of glutathione-S-transferase. *Arthritis Res Ther* 10 (5): R107.
21. Morquette, B., Q. Shi, P. Lavigne, P. Ranger, J. C. Fernandes, and M. Benderdour. 2006. Production of lipid peroxidation products in osteoarthritic tissues: New evidence linking 4-hydroxynonenal to cartilage degradation. *Arthritis Rheum* 54 (1): 271–281.
22. Miggiano, G. A., and L. Gagliardi. 2005. Diet, nutrition and rheumatoid arthritis. *Clin Ther* 156 (3): 115–123.
23. Taylor, P. C., and M. Feldmann. 2009. Anti-TNF biologic agents: Still the therapy of choice for rheumatoid arthritis. *Nat Rev Rheumatol* 5 (10): 578–582.
24. Xu, S., H. Lu, J. Lin, Z. Chen, and D. Jiang. 2009. Regulation of TNFalpha and IL1beta in rheumatoid arthritis synovial fibroblasts by leukotriene B4. *Rheumatol Int* in press.
25. Woolley, D. E., and L. C. Tetlow. 2000. Mast cell activation and its relation to proinflammatory cytokine production in the rheumatoid lesion. *Arthritis Res* 2 (1): 65–74.
26. Robak, T., A. Gladalska, and H. Stepien. 1998. The tumour necrosis factor family of receptors/ligands in the serum of patients with rheumatoid arthritis. *Eur Cytokine Netw* 9 (2): 145–154.
27. Stamp, L. K., A. Easson, L. Pettersson, J. Highton, and P. Hessian. 2009. A monocyte derived interleukin (IL)-23 is an important determinant of synovial IL-17a expression in rheumatoid arthritis. *J Rheumatol* 36 (11): 2403–2408.
28. Tetlow, L. C., N. Harper, T. Dunningham, M. A. Morris, H. Bertfield, and D. E. Woolley. 1998. Effects of induced mast cell activation on prostaglandin E and metalloproteinase production by rheumatoid synovial tissue in vitro. *Ann Rheum Dis* 57 (1): 25–32.

29. Bazzichi, L., L. Ghiadoni, A. Rossi, M. Bernardini, M. Lanza, F. De Feo, C. Giacomelli, I. Mencaroni, et al. 2009. Osteopontin is associated with increased arterial stiffness in rheumatoid arthritis. *Mol Med* 15 (11–12): 402–406.
30. Hou, W. S., W. Li, G. Keyszer, E. Weber, R. Levy, M. J. Klein, E. M. Gravallese, S. R. Goldring, and D. Bromme. 2002. Comparison of cathepsins K and S expression within the rheumatoid and osteoarthritic synovium. *Arthritis Rheum* 46 (3): 663–674.
31. van den Berg, W. B., L. A. Joosten, and F. A. van de Loo. 1999. TNF alpha and IL-1 beta are separate targets in chronic arthritis. *Clin Exp Rheumatol* 17 (6 Suppl 18): S105–S114.
32. Joosten, L. A., R. L. Smeets, M. I. Koenders, L. A. van den Bersselaar, M. M. Helsen, B. Oppers-Walgreen, E. Lubberts, Y. Iwakura, F. A. van de Loo, and W. B. van den Berg. 2004. Interleukin-18 promotes joint inflammation and induces interleukin-1-driven cartilage destruction. *Am J Pathol* 165 (3): 959–967.
33. Abdollahi-Roodsaz, S., L. A. Joosten, M. I. Koenders, B. T. van den Brand, F. A. van de Loo, and W. B. van den Berg. 2009. Local interleukin-1-driven joint pathology is dependent on toll-like receptor 4 activation. *Am J Pathol* 175 (5): 2004–2013.
34. Fournier, C. 2005. Where do T cells stand in rheumatoid arthritis? *Jt Bone Spine* 72 (6): 527–532.
35. Mandik-Nayak, L., and P. M. Allen. 2005. Initiation of an autoimmune response: Insights from a transgenic model of rheumatoid arthritis. *Immunol Res* 32 (1–3): 5–13.
36. Megias, J., M. I. Guillen, V. Clerigues, A. I. Rojo, A. Cuadrado, M. A. Castejon, F. Gomar, and M. J. Alcaraz. 2009. Heme oxygenase-1 induction modulates microsomal prostaglandin E synthase-1 expression and prostaglandin E(2) production in osteoarthritic chondrocytes. *Biochem Pharmacol* 77 (12): 1806–1813.
37. Guillen, M., J. Megias, F. Gomar, and M. Alcaraz. 2008 Heme oxygenase-1 regulates catabolic and anabolic processes in osteoarthritic chondrocytes. *J Pathol* 214 (4): 515–522.
38. Li, X., H. Afif, S. Cheng, J. Martel-Pelletier, J. P. Pelletier, P. Ranger, and H. Fahmi. 2005. Expression and regulation of microsomal prostaglandin E synthase-1 in human osteoarthritic cartilage and chondrocytes. *J Rheumatol* 32 (5): 887–895.
39. Salvemini, D., E. Mazzon, L. Dugo, I. Serraino, A. De Sarro, A. P. Caputi, and S. Cuzzocrea. 2001. Amelioration of joint disease in a rat model of collagen-induced arthritis by M40403, a superoxide dismutase mimetic. *Arthritis Rheum* 44 (12): 2909–2021.
40. Garcia-Gonzalez, A., M. Lotz, and J. L. Ochoa. Anti-inflammatory activity of superoxide dismutase obtained from *Debaryomyces hansenii* on type II collagen induced arthritis in rats. *Rev Invest Clin* 61 (3): 212–220.
41. Choi, E. J., S. C. Bae, R. Yu, J. Youn, and M. K. Sung. 2009. Dietary vitamin E and quercetin modulate inflammatory responses of collagen-induced arthritis in mice. *J Med Food* 12 (4): 770–775.
42. Elmali, N., O. Baysal, A. Harma, I. Esenkaya, and B. Mizrak. 2007. Effects of resveratrol in inflammatory arthritis. *Inflammation* 30 (1–2): 1–6.
43. Tastekin, N., N. Aydogdu, D. Dokmeci, U. Usta, M. Birtane, H. Erbas, and M. Ture. 2007. Protective effects of l-carnitine and alpha-lipoic acid in rats with adjuvant arthritis. *Pharmacol Res* 56 (4): 303–310.
44. Morinobu, A., W. Biao, S. Tanaka, M. Horiuchi, L. Jun, G. Tsuji, Y. Sakai, M. Kurosaka, and S. Kumagai. 2008. (−)-Epigallocatechin-3-gallate suppresses osteoclast differentiation and ameliorates experimental arthritis in mice. *Arthritis Rheum* 58 (7): 2012–2018.
45. Lee, E. Y., C. K. Lee, K. U. Lee, J. Y. Park, K. J. Cho, Y. S. Cho, H. R. Lee, S. H. Moon, H. B. Moon, and B. Yoo. 2007. Alpha-lipoic acid suppresses the development of collagen-induced arthritis and protects against bone destruction in mice. *Rheumatol Int* 27 (3): 225–233.
46. Canter, P. H., B. Wider, and E. Ernst. 2007. The antioxidant vitamins A, C, E and selenium in the treatment of arthritis: A systematic review of randomized clinical trials. *Rheumatology (Oxford)* 46 (8): 1223–1233.
47. Pattison, D. J., and P. G. Winyard. 2008. Dietary antioxidants in inflammatory arthritis: Do they have any role in etiology or therapy? *Nat Clin Pract Rheumatol* 4 (11): 590–596.
48. Karlson, E. W., N. A. Shadick, N. R. Cook, J. E. Buring, and I. M. Lee. 2008. Vitamin E in the primary prevention of rheumatoid arthritis: The Women's Health Study. *Arthritis Rheum* 59 (11): 1589–1595.
49. van Vugt, R. M., P. J. Rijken, A. G. Rietveld, A. C. van Vugt, and B. A. Dijkmans. 2008. Antioxidant intervention in rheumatoid arthritis: Results of an open pilot study. *Clin Rheumatol* 27 (6): 771–775.
50. Bae, S. C., W. J. Jung, E. J. Lee, R. Yu, and M. K. Sung. 2009. Effects of antioxidant supplements intervention on the level of plasma inflammatory molecules and disease severity of rheumatoid arthritis patients. *J Am Coll Nutr* 28 (1): 56–62.

51. Darlington, L. G., and T. W. Stone. 2001. Antioxidants and fatty acids in the amelioration of rheumatoid arthritis and related disorders. *Br J Nutr* 85 (3): 251–269.
52. Rennie, K. L., J. Hughes, R. Lang, and S. A. Jebb. 2003. Nutritional management of rheumatoid arthritis: A review of the evidence. *J Hum Nutr Diet* 16 (2): 97–109.
53. Lee, C. K., E. Y. Lee, Y. G. Kim, S. H. Mun, H. B. Moon, and B. Yoo. 2008. Alpha-lipoic acid inhibits TNF-alpha induced NF-kappa B activation through blocking of MEKK1-MKK4-IKK signaling cascades. *Int Immunopharmacol* 8 (2): 362–370.
54. Tang, L. L., J. S. Gao, X. R. Chen, and X. Xie. 2006. Inhibitory effect of resveratrol on the proliferation of synoviocytes in rheumatoid arthritis and its mechanism in vitro. *Zhong Nan Da Xue Xue Bao Yi Xue Ban* 31 (4): 528–533.
55. Funk, J. L., J. B. Frye, J. N. Oyarzo, N. Kuscuoglu, J. Wilson, G. McCaffrey, G. Stafford, et al. 2006. Efficacy and mechanism of action of turmeric supplements in the treatment of experimental arthritis. *Arthritis Rheum* 54 (11): 3452–3464.
56. Li, X., F. M. Phillips, H. S. An, M. Ellman, E. J. Thonar, W. Wu, D. Park, and H. J. Im. 2008. The action of resveratrol, a phytoestrogen found in grapes, on the intervertebral disc. *Spine (Phila Pa 1976)* 33 (24): 2586–2595.
57. Byun, H. S., J. K. Song, Y. R. Kim, L. Piao, M. Won, K. A. Park, B. L. Choi, et al. 2008. Caspase-8 has an essential role in resveratrol-induced apoptosis of rheumatoid fibroblast-like synoviocytes. *Rheumatology (Oxford)* 47 (3): 301–308.
58. Maestroni, G. J., A. Sulli, C. Pizzorni, B. Villaggio, and M. Cutolo. 2002. Melatonin in rheumatoid arthritis: Synovial macrophages show melatonin receptors. *Ann N Y Acad Sci* 966, 271–275.
59. El-Awady, H. M., A. S. El-Wakkad, M. T. Saleh, S. I. Muhammad, and E. M. Ghaniema. 2007. Serum melatonin in juvenile rheumatoid arthritis: Correlation with disease activity. *Pak J Biol Sci* 10 (9): 1471–1476.
60. Nah, S. S., H. J. Won, H. J. Park, E. Ha, J. H. Chung, H. Y. Cho, and H. H. Baik. 2009. Melatonin inhibits human fibroblast-like synoviocyte proliferation via extracellular signal-regulated protein kinase/P21(CIP1)/P27(KIP1) pathways. *J Pineal Res* 47 (1): 70–74.
61. Yun, H. J., W. H. Yoo, M. K. Han, Y. R. Lee, J. S. Kim, and S. I. Lee. 2008. Epigallocatechin-3-gallate suppresses TNF-alpha -induced production of MMP-1 and -3 in rheumatoid arthritis synovial fibroblasts. *Rheumatol Int* 29 (1): 23–29.
62. Tetlow, L. C., and D. E. Woolley. 1999. The effects of 1 alpha,25-dihydroxyvitamin D(3) on matrix metalloproteinase and prostaglandin E(2) production by cells of the rheumatoid lesion. *Arthritis Res* 1 (1): 63–70.
63. Herman, S., N. Zurgil, P. Langevitz, M. Ehrenfeld, and M. Deutsch. 2008. Methotrexate selectively modulates TH1/TH2 balance in active rheumatoid arthritis patients. *Clin Exp Rheumatol* 26 (2): 317–323.
64. Cronstein, B. N. 2005. Low-dose methotrexate: A mainstay in the treatment of rheumatoid arthritis. *Pharmacol Rev* 57 (2): 163–172.
65. Fiehn, C. 2009. Methotrexate in rheumatology. *Z Rheumatol* 68 (9): 747–756.
66. Swierkot, J., and J. Szechinski. 2006. Methotrexate in rheumatoid arthritis. *Pharmacol Rep* 58 (4): 473–492.
67. Braun, J., and R. Rau. 2009. An update on methotrexate. *Curr Opin Rheumatol* 21 (3): 216–223.
68. den Broeder, A. A., G. J. Wanten, W. J. Oyen, T. Naber, P. L. van Riel, and P. Barrera. 2003. Neutrophil migration and production of reactive oxygen species during treatment with a fully human anti-tumor necrosis factor-alpha monoclonal antibody in patients with rheumatoid arthritis. *J Rheumatol* 30 (2): 232–237.
69. Edrees, A. F., S. N. Misra, and N. I. Abdou. 2005. Anti-tumor necrosis factor (TNF) therapy in rheumatoid arthritis: Correlation of TNF-alpha serum level with clinical response and benefit from changing dose or frequency of infliximab infusions. *Clin Exp Rheumatol* 23 (4): 469–474.
70. Popa, C., L. J. van Tits, P. Barrera, H. L. Lemmers, F. H. van den Hoogen, P. L. van Riel, T. R. Radstake, M. G. Netea, M, Roest, and A. F. Stalenhoef. 2009. Anti-inflammatory therapy with tumour necrosis factor alpha inhibitors improves high-density lipoprotein cholesterol antioxidative capacity in rheumatoid arthritis patients. *Ann Rheum Dis* 68 (6): 868–872.
71. Kasama, T., T. Isozaki, T. Odai, M. Matsunawa, K. Wakabayashi, H. T. Takeuchi, S. Matsukura, M. Adachi, M. Tezuka, and K. Kobayashi. 2007. Expression of angiopoietin-1 in osteoblasts and its inhibition by tumor necrosis factor-alpha and interferon-gamma. *Transl Res* 149 (5): 265–273.

72. Gonzalez-Gay, M. A., M. T. Garcia-Unzueta, J. M. De Matias, C. Gonzalez-Juanatey, C. Garcia-Porrua, A. Sanchez-Andrade, J. Martin, and J. Llorca. 2006. Influence of anti-TNF-alpha infliximab therapy on adhesion molecules associated with atherogenesis in patients with rheumatoid arthritis. *Clin Exp Rheumatol* 24 (4): 373–379.
73. Singh, J. A., R. Christensen, G. A. Wells, M. E. Suarez-Almazor, R. Buchbinder, M. A. Lopez-Olivo, E. Tanjong Ghogomu, and P. Tugwell. 2009. Biologics for rheumatoid arthritis: An overview of Cochrane reviews. *Cochrane Database Syst Rev* (4): CD007848.
74. Keystone, E., D. Heijde, D. Mason Jr., R. Landewe, R. V. Vollenhoven, B. Combe, P. Emery, et al. 2008. Certolizumab pegol plus methotrexate is significantly more effective than placebo plus methotrexate in active rheumatoid arthritis: Findings of a fifty-two-week, phase III, multicenter, randomized, double-blind, placebo-controlled, parallel-group study. *Arthritis Rheum* 58 (11): 3319–3329.
75. Smolen, J., R. B. Landewe, P. Mease, J. Brzezicki, D. Mason, K. Luijtens, R. F. van Vollenhoven, et al. 2009. Efficacy and safety of certolizumab pegol plus methotrexate in active rheumatoid arthritis: The RAPID 2 study. A randomised controlled trial. *Ann Rheum Dis* 68 (6): 797–804.
76. Duggan, S. T., and S. J. Keam. 2009. Certolizumab pegol: In rheumatoid arthritis. *BioDrugs* 23 (6): 407–417.
77. Breedveld, F. C., M. H. Weisman, A. F. Kavanaugh, S. B. Cohen, K. Pavelka, R. van Vollenhoven, J. Sharp, J. L. Perez, and G. T. Spencer-Green. 2006. The PREMIER study: A multicenter, randomized, double-blind clinical trial of combination therapy with adalimumab plus methotrexate versus methotrexate alone or adalimumab alone in patients with early, aggressive rheumatoid arthritis who had not had previous methotrexate treatment. *Arthritis Rheum* 54 (1): 26–37.
78. Koller, M. D., D. Aletaha, J. Funovits, A. Pangan, D. Baker, and J. S. Smolen. 2009. Response of elderly patients with rheumatoid arthritis to methotrexate or TNF inhibitors compared with younger patients. *Rheumatology (Oxford)* 48(12): 1575–1580.
79. Maini, R. N., P. C. Taylor, J. Szechinski, K. Pavelka, J. Broll, G. Balint, P. Emery, et al. 2006. Double-blind randomized controlled clinical trial of the interleukin-6 receptor antagonist, tocilizumab, in European patients with rheumatoid arthritis who had an incomplete response to methotrexate. *Arthritis Rheum* 54 (9): 2817–2829.
80. Emery, P., E. Keystone, H. P. Tony, A. Cantagrel, R. van Vollenhoven, A. Sanchez, E. Alecock, J. Lee, and J. Kremer. 2008. IL-6 receptor inhibition with tocilizumab improves treatment outcomes in patients with rheumatoid arthritis refractory to anti-tumour necrosis factor biologicals: Results from a 24-week multicentre randomised placebo-controlled trial. *Ann Rheum Dis* 67 (11): 1516–1523.
81. Nishimoto, N., N. Miyasaka, K. Yamamoto, S. Kawai, T. Takeuchi, J. Azuma, and T. Kishimoto. 2009. Study of active controlled tocilizumab monotherapy for rheumatoid arthritis patients with an inadequate response to methotrexate (SATORI): Significant reduction in disease activity and serum vascular endothelial growth factor by IL-6 receptor inhibition therapy. *Mod Rheumatol* 19 (1): 12–19.
82. Rousseau, A., R. Taberne, F. Siberchicot, J. C. Fricain, and N. Zwetyenga. 2009. TNF-alpha inhibitor etanercept and oral cavity carcinoma. *Rev Stomatol Chir Maxillofac* 110 (5): 306–308.
83. Dixon, W. G., K. L. Hyrich, K. D. Watson, M. Lunt, J. Galloway, A. Ustianowski, and D. P. Symmons. 2009. Drug-specific risk of tuberculosis in patients with rheumatoid arthritis treated with anti-TNF therapy: Results from the British Society for Rheumatology Biologics Register (BSRBR). *Ann Rheum Dis* 69 (3): 522–528.
84. Winthrop, K. L., E. Chang, S. Yamashita, M. F. Iademarco, and P. A. LoBue. 2009. Nontuberculous mycobacteria infections and anti-tumor necrosis factor-alpha therapy. *Emerg Infect Dis* 15 (10): 1556–1561.
85. Matsuno, H., H. Nakamura, K. Katayama, S. Hayashi, S. Kano, K. Yudoh, and Y. Kiso. 2009. Effects of an oral administration of glucosamine-chondroitin-quercetin glucoside on the synovial fluid properties in patients with osteoarthritis and rheumatoid arthritis. *Biosci Biotechnol Biochem* 73 (2): 288–292.
86. Clegg, D. O., D. J. Reda, C. L. Harris, M. A. Klein, J. R. O'Dell, M. M. Hooper, J. D. Bradley, et al. 2006. Glucosamine, chondroitin sulfate, and the two in combination for painful knee osteoarthritis. *N Engl J Med* 354 (8): 795–808.
87. Sawitzke, A. D., H. Shi, M. F. Finco, D. D. Dunlop, C. O. Bingham 3rd, C. L. Harris, N. G. Singer, et al. 2008. The effect of glucosamine and/or chondroitin sulfate on the progression of knee osteoarthritis: A report from the glucosamine/chondroitin arthritis intervention trial. *Arthritis Rheum* 58 (10): 3183–3191.
88. Bruyere, O., and J. Y. Reginster. 2007. Glucosamine and chondroitin sulfate as therapeutic agents for knee and hip osteoarthritis. *Drugs Aging* 24 (7): 573–580.

89. Kahan, A., D. Uebelhart, F. De Vathaire, P. D. Delmas, and J. Y. Reginster. 2009. Long-term effects of chondroitins 4 and 6 sulfate on knee osteoarthritis: The study on osteoarthritis progression prevention, a two-year, randomized, double-blind, placebo-controlled trial. *Arthritis Rheum* 60 (2): 524–533.
90. Messier, S. P., S. Mihalko, R. F. Loeser, C. Legault, J. Jolla, J. Pfruender, B. Prosser, A. Adrian, and J. D. Williamson. 2007. Glucosamine/chondroitin combined with exercise for the treatment of knee osteoarthritis: A preliminary study. *Osteoarthritis Cartilage* 15 (11): 1256–1266.
91. Ross, E. 2009. Update on the management of pain in arthritis and the use of cyclooxygenase-2 inhibitors. *Curr Pain Headache Rep* 13 (6): 455–459.
92. Efthimiou, P., and M. Kukar. 2009. Complementary and alternative medicine use in rheumatoid arthritis: Proposed mechanism of action and efficacy of commonly used modalities, *Rheumatol Int* 30 (5): 571–586.
93. Chandrashekara, S., T. Anilkumar, and S. Jamuna. 2002. Complementary and alternative drug therapy in arthritis. *J Assoc Physicians India* 50, 225–227.
94. Zaman, T., S. Agarwal, and R. Handa. 2007. Complementary and alternative medicine use in rheumatoid arthritis: An audit of patients visiting a tertiary care centre. *Natl Med J India* 20 (5): 236–239.
95. Willich, S. N., K. Rossnagel, S. Roll, A. Wagner, O. Mune, J. Erlendson, A. Kharazmi, H. Sorensen, and K. Winther. 2009. Rose hip herbal remedy in patients with rheumatoid arthritis—A randomised controlled trial. *Phytomedicine* 17 (2): 87–93.
96. Sener, G., E. Eksioglu-Demiralp, M. Cetiner, F. Ercan, S. Sirvanci, N. Gedik, and B. C. Yegen. 2006. l-Carnitine ameliorates methotrexate-induced oxidative organ injury and inhibits leukocyte death. *Cell Biol Toxicol* 22 (1): 47–60.
97. Dadhania, V. P., D. N. Tripathi, A. Vikram, P. Ramarao, and G. B. Jena. 2009. Intervention of alpha-lipoic acid ameliorates methotrexate-induced oxidative stress and genotoxicity: A study in rat intestine. *Chem Biol Interact* 183 (1): 85–97.
98. Rovensky, J. S., M. Uteseny, J. Bauerova, and K. Jurcovicova. 2009. Treatment of adjuvant-induced arthritis with the combination of methotrexate and probiotic bacteria *Escherichia coli* O83 (Colinfant). *Folia Microbiol* 54, 359–363.
99. Krinsky, N. I. 1989. Antioxidant functions of carotenoids. *Free Radic Biol Med* 7 (6): 617–635.
100. Hazuka, M. B., J. Edwards-Prasad, F. Newman, J. J. Kinzie, and K. N. Prasad. 1990. Beta-carotene induces morphological differentiation and decreases adenylate cyclase activity in melanoma cells in culture. *J Am Coll Nutr* 9 (2): 143–149.
101. Zhang, L. X., R. V. Cooney, and J. S. Bertram. 1992. Carotenoids up-regulate connexin43 gene expression independent of their provitamin A or antioxidant properties. *Cancer Res* 52 (20): 5707–5712.
102. Carter, C. A., M. Pogribny, A. Davidson, C. D. Jackson, L. J. McGarrity, and S. M. Morris. 1996. Effects of retinoic acid on cell differentiation and reversion toward normal in human endometrial adenocarcinoma (RL95-2) cells. *Anticancer Res* 16 (1): 17–24.
103. Meyskens, Jr., F. L. 1995. Role of vitamin A and its derivatives in the treatment of human cancer. In *Nutrients in Cancer Prevention and Treatment*, ed. K. N. Prasad, L. Santamaria, and R. M. Williams, 349–362. Totowa, NJ: Humana Press.
104. Vile, G. F., and C. C. Winterbourn. 1988. Inhibition of adriamycin-promoted microsomal lipid peroxidation by beta-carotene, alpha-tocopherol and retinol at high and low oxygen partial pressures. *FEBS Lett* 238 (2): 353–356.
105. McCay, P. B. 1985. Vitamin E: Interactions with free radicals and ascorbate. *Annu Rev Nutr* 5, 323–340.
106. Prasad, K. N., B. Kumar, X. D. Yan, A. J. Hanson, and W. C. Cole. 2003. Alpha-tocopheryl succinate, the most effective form of vitamin E for adjuvant cancer treatment: A review. *J Am Coll Nutr* 22 (2): 108–117.
107. Schwartz, J. L. 1995. Molecular and biochemical control of tumor growth following treatment with carotenoids or tocopherols. In *Nutrients in Cancer Prevention and Treatment*, ed. K. N. Prasad, L. Santamaria, and R. M. Williams, 287–316. Totowa, NJ: Humana Press.
108. Prasad, K. N., and J. Edwards-Prasad. 1992. Vitamin E and cancer prevention: Recent advances and future potentials. *J Am Coll Nutr* 11 (5): 487–500.
109. Witschi, A., S. Reddy, B. Stofer, and B. H. Lauterburg. 1992. The systemic availability of oral glutathione. *Eur J Clin Pharmacol* 43 (6): 667–669.
110. Shen, W., K. Liu, C. Tian, L. Yang, X. Li, J. Ren, L. Packer, C. W. Cotman, and J. Liu. 2008. *R*-alpha-Lipoic acid and acetyl-l-carnitine complementarily promote mitochondrial biogenesis in murine 3T3-L1 adipocytes. *Diabetologia* 51 (1): 165–174.
111. Niki, E. 1997. Mechanisms and dynamics of antioxidant action of ubiquinol. *Mol Aspects Med* 18 (Suppl): S63–S70.

112. Hiramatsu, M., R. D. Velasco, D. S. Wilson, and L. Packer. 1991. Ubiquinone protects against loss of tocopherol in rat liver microsomes and mitochondrial membranes. *Res Commun Chem Pathol Pharmacol* 72 (2): 231–241.
113. Chen, R. S., C. C. Huang, and N. S. Chu. 1997. Coenzyme Q10 treatment in mitochondrial encephalomyopathies. Short-term double-blind, crossover study. *Eur Neurol* 37 (4): 212–218.
114. Olanow, C. W., and G. W. Arendash. 1994. Metals and free radicals in neurodegeneration. *Curr Opin Neurol* 7 (6): 548–558.

18 Myths and Misconceptions about Antioxidants and Health

INTRODUCTION

In recent years, many popular magazines, prestigious newspapers, internationally respected scientific journals, and books have described new advances in research into the function of antioxidants and their potential role in optimal health, disease prevention, and treatment. Unfortunately, many of these reports have produced contradictory claims regarding the usefulness of antioxidants in human health or disease prevention. As a result, a number of myths and misconceptions concerning the value of antioxidants exist among most physicians and other health professionals. This has created confusion in the minds of consumers, although most continue to take supplemental nutrition with or without the knowledge of their doctors. This chapter attempts to clarify some of the myths and misconceptions regarding the value of antioxidants in health and disease that exist at this time.

MISCONCEPTION 1

Misconception: The more supplementary micronutrients, including antioxidants, you take, the better you will feel.

Fact: This belief can be dangerous. Consuming excessive quantities of certain micronutrients may cause severe damage. For instance, taking large amounts of vitamin A (25,000 IU or more per day over a long period) may lead to liver and skin toxicity. Vitamin A at doses of 10,000 IU or more per day can increase the risk of birth defects in pregnant women. Excessive intakes of selenium, such as 500 µg or more per day over a long period, can cause cataracts, an eye disease in which the lens becomes opaque. Taking excessive quantities of vitamin B_6—50 mg or more per day over an extended period—can induce peripheral neuropathy, or numbness in the extremities, a condition that is reversible upon discontinuation.

MISCONCEPTION 2

Misconception: A balanced diet is sufficient for maintaining optimal health and disease prevention.

Fact: The concept of a balanced diet is very general. A balanced diet alone may not be adequate for optimal health and disease prevention. Trying to obtain the optimal levels of dietary and endogenous (made in the body) antioxidants at the appropriate times through a balanced diet only may not be possible or practical. In addition, all the food we consume on a daily basis contains both protective and toxic substances. In order to maximize the intake of protective substances, supplementary micronutrients, including antioxidants, are important.

MISCONCEPTION 3

Misconception: Most supplementary micronutrients, including antioxidants, pass out of the body in the urine and feces, so why take them?

Fact: This myth has no scientific justification. The intestines absorb about 10% of most orally ingested antioxidants. Consuming high doses of antioxidants, therefore, can lead to increased levels of these nutrients and their products in the urine and feces. The presence of excessive amounts of antioxidants in the intestinal tract may be beneficial, however, even if they are not totally absorbed into the blood stream.

Increased amounts of vitamins C and E (alpha-tocopherol) are needed in the stomach to lower the levels of nitrosamine, a potent cancer-causing agent that is formed from nitrite-containing foods such as bacon, sausage, hot dogs, or cured meats. Increased levels of toxic substances such as mutagens (chemicals that change genetic activity) are formed during digestion, and absorption of these toxic chemicals can have adverse effects over a long period. Supplementation with vitamins C, E, or in combination reduced the levels of these toxic substances in the feces. For these reasons, higher than normal amounts of antioxidants in the feces or urine should not be considered wasteful, since they have beneficial effects in the body even without being completely absorbed.

MISCONCEPTION 4

Misconception: All antioxidants have only one function: scavenging of free radicals.

Fact: This belief is incorrect. In addition to scavenging free radicals, antioxidants cause changes in gene expression, cell signaling proteins, and translocation of certain proteins from one part of the cell to another within the same cell. They also reduce inflammation and stimulate immune function.

MISCONCEPTION 5

Misconception: Antioxidants affect both normal and cancer cells in the same manner.

Fact: Normal cells and cancer cells respond to antioxidants in a different manner. High doses of antioxidants kill the cancer cells and reduce their growth without affecting the survival or growth of normal cells.

MISCONCEPTION 6

Misconception: All fat-soluble antioxidants are toxic to humans.

Fact: Only vitamins A and D, and mineral selenium, when taken at high doses over a long period or during pregnancy, have been shown to be potentially toxic. The safety window for vitamin A and selenium is very narrow.

MISCONCEPTION 7

Misconception: Supplemental beta-carotene and vitamin E are harmful to your health.

Fact: This is totally incorrect. This myth is based on a specific clinical study in which administering beta-carotene or vitamin E alone in male heavy smokers led to the observation of adverse health effects. Such results could have been predicted before the start of the study; heavy smokers have high oxidative environments in their bodies. When beta-carotene or vitamin E was administered individually, it was oxidized to become free radicals. This caused the increased risk of diseases. No such effects have been observed when beta-carotene or vitamin E is present in multiple vitamin preparations.

MISCONCEPTION 8

Misconception: All forms of vitamin E have the same function.

Fact: This statement is incorrect. Vitamin E in the form of D-alpha-tocopheryl succinate is the most potent form of vitamin E for killing cancer cells and offering radiation protection and protection against chemical toxicity.

MISCONCEPTION 9

Misconception: Natural and synthetic antioxidants have similar effects.

Fact: This belief is not true. Natural beta-carotene can reduce the formation of radiation-induced cancer, whereas synthetic beta-carotene cannot. Also, cells prefer to use natural vitamin E rather than the synthetic version.

MISCONCEPTION 10

Misconception: Supplementary vitamin C causes kidney stones.

Fact: This has not been observed in normal adults. If the urine becomes acidic, some of the waste products in the kidneys may solidify and form stones, but this biological phenomenon usually occurs if there is an imbalance in body chemistry, such as if acidic solutions cannot be neutralized in the blood. The body normally neutralizes any acidic solution it takes in. In certain specific disease conditions in which one's body has lost this capacity, one should not take vitamin C in large amounts.

The link between vitamin C intake and kidney stones is derived from two observations: (1) a person taking vitamin C at high doses sometimes shows increased excretion of oxalic acid in the urine and (2) many people who have kidney stones also have higher than normal levels of oxalic acid in the urine. These two separate observations have been interpreted to mean that high doses of vitamin C can heighten the risk of kidney stones. These observations may be unrelated; however, there are no published data to support the conclusion that high doses of vitamin C produce kidney stones in healthy people. Millions of people around the world consume high doses of vitamin C, but no increase in the risk of kidney stones has been reported in any region of the world.

MISCONCEPTION 11

Misconception: Taking multiple antioxidants once a day is sufficient for optimal health or disease prevention.

Fact: This belief may not be true. If you take multiple vitamins containing antioxidants in the morning, half of them are removed from your body by the evening, and another half by the next morning. This creates a high degree of fluctuation in the levels of antioxidants in the body. Our cells are very sensitive to the amounts of antioxidants present in the body. They are all the time trying to readjust their genetic activity to maintain cellular function, creating a stress on them over a long period. Taking antioxidant micronutrients orally twice a day (morning and evening), however, will achieve a more constant level of these nutrients in the body.

MISCONCEPTION 12

Misconception: The addition of trace minerals, such as iron, copper, and manganese, to antioxidant preparations containing vitamin C is good for your health.

Fact: It is well established that vitamin C in combination with iron, copper, or manganese generates excessive amounts of free radicals that can damage cells. In addition, the absorption of these minerals in the presence of antioxidants is enhanced markedly in the intestinal tract, which can then increase the body's storage of these minerals. Heightened free iron storage in the body has been associated with many chronic diseases, such as heart disease, cancer, and neurological diseases. Increased copper storage in the body has been associated with an increased risk of Alzheimer's disease.

MISCONCEPTION 13

Misconception: Frozen fruit and vegetable juices or antioxidant-supplemented water or fruit and vegetable juices are maintained when stored in the refrigerator.

Fact: Frozen fruit or vegetable juices may provide some antioxidants to your body, provided you drink them within a few hours of preparation. When they are stored in a cold place and exposed to light and/or air, however, antioxidants—particularly vitamin C—in solution rapidly deteriorate. After about 24 h, more than 50% of vitamin C is lost. Antioxidant-rich fruit or vegetable juices in cartons or opaque glass or plastic may have more antioxidants than those in clear plastic or glass containers. Repeated opening and closing of the bottles diminishes antioxidant levels as well.

MISCONCEPTION 14

Misconception: It is not possible for antioxidants to protect against damage produced by exposure to radiation, toxic chemicals, and pathogenic viruses and bacteria.

Fact: This myth is incorrect. Among known pharmacological agents and drugs, antioxidants are the only group of nutrients that can neutralize free radicals, decrease acute and chronic inflammation, and stimulate immune function. Radiation, such as X-rays, gamma rays, and certain toxic chemicals, such as mustard gas and chlorine gas, share some mechanisms of damage that include excessive amounts of free radicals and acute inflammation. Immune status of the individual is a determining factor in infection with the harmful viruses or bacteria. An optimal functioning immune system will reduce the risk of infection, whereas an impaired immune system will allow the infection to occur.

MISCONCEPTION 15

Misconception: Antioxidants cannot be useful in reducing the risk of most chronic diseases in humans.

Fact: This belief may not be true. In most chronic diseases—such as heart disease, cancer, diabetes, and neurological diseases such as Alzheimer's and Parkinson's disease—increased oxidative damage and chronic inflammation appear to play an important role in the initiation and progression of these diseases. Therefore, reducing these biological events (in combination with standard therapy) may be useful in preventing and treating these diseases.

MISCONCEPTION 16

Misconception: If you take supplementary micronutrients that include antioxidants, you do not have to worry about a balanced diet or a modification in lifestyle.

Fact: Supplementary micronutrients, a healthy diet (one that is low fat and high fiber) and lifestyle modification (meaning no tobacco smoking or consumption, regular exercise, increased consumption of fruits and vegetables, meditation, and so on) are equally important for optimal health and disease prevention.

At this time, many misconceptions exist regarding the value of antioxidant micronutrients in health and in disease prevention and treatment. A few have been discussed in this chapter. Putting these misconceptions to rest is a challenge for researchers, physicians, other health professionals, and educators. Improving the health of the general population depends upon the success of educating health professionals and others about these misconceptions.

Removing these misconceptions is equally important in order to promote the correct utilization of antioxidant micronutrient supplements for optimal health and disease prevention.

CONCLUSIONS

I hope the myths and misconceptions discussed in this chapter may further clarify the potential useful role of micronutrients, especially antioxidants in health and disease. The recommendations of micronutrients for maintaining good health and improving the current management of diseases presented in previous chapters may provide valuable guidelines as to why, when, and how to use micronutrients.

19 Dietary Reference Intakes of Selected Micronutrients

INTRODUCTION

The changes in the nutritional guidelines have evolved significantly since World War II due to a rapid expansion of knowledge in nutrition and health. The nutritional guidelines referred to as Recommended Dietary Allowances (RDAs) were first established in 1941. The Food and Nutrition Board of the United States subsequently revised them every 5–10 years.

DRI (DIETARY REFERENCE INTAKES)

RDA refers to the value of the daily dietary intake level of a nutrient considered sufficient to meet the requirements of 97–98% of healthy individuals of different ages and gender. Because of rapid growth of research on the role of nutrients in human health, the Food and Nutrition Board of the Institute of Medicine of the United States in collaboration with Health Canada, updated the values of RDAs and renamed them as Dietary Reference Intakes (DRIs) in 1998. Since then, the DRI values are used by both the United States of America and Canada. The DRA values of selected nutrients are listed in Tables 19.1 to 19.21. The DRI values are not currently used in nutrition labeling, but the RDA values of nutrients continue to be used for this purpose. The DRI values for carotenoids, alpha-lipoic acid, *N*-acetylcysteine, coenzyme Q_{10}, and L-carnitine have not been determined.

ADEQUATE INTAKE (AI)

AI refers to the value of a nutrient for which no RDA has been established, but the value established may be sufficient for everyone in the demographic group.

TOLERABLE UPPER INTAKE LEVEL (UL)

This is the maximum level of daily nutrient intake that is likely to pose no risk of adverse health effects. The Tolerable Upper Intake Level (UL) value represents the total intake of a nutrient from food, water, and supplements.

RDA, AI, or UL values of nutrients are expected to be adequate for individuals for normal growth and survival; however, values of micronutrients needed for prevention or improved management of human diseases are not known at this time. The data on doses obtained from the use of a single micronutrient in prevention or treatment of human diseases should not be extrapolated to the doses of the same micronutrient present in a multiple micronutrient preparation. In general, whenever a single micronutrient is used in the laboratory or clinical studies, high doses of a micronutrient are needed to observe any biological effects. Low doses of the same micronutrient may be needed when used in combination with multiple micronutrients for the same effects.

DRI VALUES FOR ANTIOXIDANTS, VITAMINS, MICRONUTRIENTS, AND MINERALS

The DRI values for antioxidants (Tables 19.1–19.3), vitamins (Tables 19.4–19.11), micronutrients (Table 19.12), and minerals (Tables 19.13–19.21) are given below.

TABLE 19.1
DRIs for Vitamin A

Age	RDA/AI* (μg/day)	UL (μg/day)
Infants		
0–6 months	400*	600
7–12 months	500*	600
Children		
1–3 years	300	600
4–8 years	400	900
Males		
9–13 years	600	1700
14–18 years	900	2800
19 years and over	900	3000
Females		
9–13 years	600	1700
14–18 years	700	2800
19 years and over	700	3000
Pregnancy		
≤18 years	750	2800
19–50 years	770	3000
Lactation		
≤18 years	1200	2800
19–50 years	1300	3000

Note: Values are adapted and summarized from the table of Dietary Reference Intakes (DRIs) published by www.nap.edu. RDA, Recommended Dietary Allowance; AI*, Adequate Intakes; UL, Tolerable Upper Intake Value. 1 μg retinol = 1 μg retinol activity equivalent (RAE); 1 IU (international unit) retinol = 0.3 μg retinol; and 2 μg beta-carotene = 1 μg of retinol.

TABLE 19.2
DRIs for Vitamin C

Age	RDA/AI* (mg/day)	UL (mg/day)
Infants		
0–6 months	40*	ND
7–12 months	50*	ND
Children		
1–3 years	15	400
4–8 years	25	650
Males		
9–13 years	45	1200
14–18 years	75	1800
19 years and over	90	2000
Females		
9–13 years	45	1200
14–18 years	65	1800
19 years and over	75	2000

Note: Values are adapted and summarized from the DRI tables published by www.nap.edu. ND, not determined.

TABLE 19.3
DRIs for Vitamin E

Age	RDA/AI* (mg/day)	UL (mg/day)
Infants		
0–6 months	4*	ND
7–12 months	5*	ND
Children		
1–3 years	6	200
4–8 years	7	300
Males		
9–13 years	11	600
14–18 years	15	800
19 years and over	15	1000
Females		
9–13 years	11	600
14–18 years	15	800
19 years and over	15	1000
Pregnancy		
≤18 years	15	800
19–50 years	15	1000
Lactation		
≤18 years	19	800
19–50 years	19	1000

Note: Values are adapted and summarized from the DRI tables published by www.nap.edu. 1 IU vitamin E = 0.66 mg of D-alpha-tocopherol and 0.45 mg DL-alpha-tocopherol.

TABLE 19.4
DRIs for Vitamin D

Age	RDA/AI* (µg/day)	UL (µg/day)
Infants		
0–12 months	5*	25
Children		
1–8 years	5*	50
Males		
9–50 years	5*	50
50–70 years	10*	50
>70 years	15*	50
Females		
9–50 years	5*	50
50–70 years	10*	50
>70 years	15*	50
Pregnancy		
≤18–50 years	5*	50
Lactation		
≤18–50 years	5*	50

Note: Values are adapted and summarized from the DRI tables published by www.nap.edu. 1 µg cholecalciferol = 40 IU vitamin D.

TABLE 19.5
DRIs for Vitamin B$_1$ (Thiamin)

Age	RDA/AI* (mg/day)	UL (mg/day)
Infants		
0–6 months	0.2*	ND
7–12 months	0.3*	ND
Children		
1–3 years	0.5	ND
4–8 years	0.6	ND
Males		
9–13 years	0.9	ND
14 years and over	1.2	ND
Females		
9–13 years	0.9	ND
14–18 years	1.0	ND
19 years and over	1.1	ND
Pregnancy		
≤18–50 years	1.4	ND
Lactation		
≤18–50 years	1.4	ND

Note: Values are adapted and summarized from the DRI tables of published by www.nap.edu.

Dietary Reference Intakes of Selected Micronutrients

TABLE 19.6
DRIs for Vitamin B_2

Age	RDA/AI* (mg/day)	UL (mg/day)
Infants		
0–6 months	0.3*	ND
7–12 months	0.4*	ND
Children		
1–3 years	0.5	ND
4–8 years	0.6	ND
Males		
9–13 years	0.9	ND
14 years and over	1.3	ND
Females		
9–13 years	0.9	ND
14–18 years	1.0	ND
19 years and over	1.1	ND
Pregnancy		
≤18–50 years	1.4	ND
Lactation		
≤18–50 years	1.6	ND

Note: Values are adapted and summarized from the DRI tables published by www.nap.edu.

TABLE 19.7
DRIs for Vitamin B_6

Age	RDA/AI* (mg/day)	UL (mg/day)
Infants		
0–6 months	0.1*	ND
7–12 months	0.3*	ND
Children		
1–3 years	0.5	30
4–8 years	0.6	40
Males		
9–13 years	1.0	60
14–50 years	1.3	80
50–70 years and over	1.7	100
Females		
9–13 years	1.0	60
14–18 years	1.2	80
19–30 years	1.3	100
50 years and over	1.5	100
Pregnancy		
≤18 years	1.9	80
19–50 years	1.9	100
Lactation		
≤18 years	2.0	80
19–50 years	2.0	100

Note: Values are adapted and summarized from the DRI tables published by www.nap.edu.

TABLE 19.8
DRIs for Vitamin B$_{12}$

Age	RDA/AI* (μg/day)	UL (μg/day)
Infants		
0–6 months	0.4*	ND
7–12 months	0.5*	ND
Children		
1–3 years	0.9	ND
4–8 years	1.2	ND
Males		
9–13 years	1.8	ND
14 years and over	2.4	ND
Females		
9–13 years	1.8	ND
14 years and over	2.4	ND
Pregnancy		
≤18–50 years	2.6	ND
Lactation		
≤18–50 years	2.8	ND

Note: Values are adapted and summarized from the DRI tables published by www.nap.edu.

TABLE 19.9
DRIs for Pantothenic Acid

Age	RDA/AI* (mg/day)	UL (mg/day)
Infants		
0–6 months	1.7*	ND
7–12 months	1.8*	ND
Children		
1–3 years	2*	ND
4–8 years	2*	ND
Males		
9–13 years	4*	ND
14 years and over	5*	ND
Females		
9–13 years	4*	ND
14 years and over	5*	ND
Pregnancy		
≤18–50 years	6*	ND
Lactation		
≤18–50 years	7*	ND

Note: Values are adapted and summarized from the DRI tables published by www.nap.edu.

Dietary Reference Intakes of Selected Micronutrients

TABLE 19.10
DRIs for Niacin

Age	RDA/AI* (mg/day)	UL (mg/day)
Infants		
0–6 months	2.0*	ND
7–12 months	0.4*	ND
Children		
1–3 years	6.0	10
4–8 years	8.0	15
Males		
9–13 years	12	20
14–50 years	16	30
50–70 years and over	16	35
Females		
9–13 years	12	20
14–18 years	14	30
19 years and over	14	35
Pregnancy		
≤18 years	18	30
19–50 years	18	35
Lactation		
≤18 years	17	30
19–50 years	17	35

Note: Values are adapted and summarized from the DRI tables published by www.nap.edu.

TABLE 19.11
DRIs for Folate

Age	RDA/AI* (µg/day)	UL (µg/day)
Infants		
0–6 months	65*	ND
7–12 months	80*	ND
Children		
1–3 years	150	300
4–8 years	200	400
Males		
9–13 years	300	600
14–50 years	400	800
19 years and over	400	1000
Females		
9–13 years	300	600
14–18 years	400	800
19 years and over	400	1000
Pregnancy		
≤18 years	600	800
19–50 years	600	1000
Lactation		
≤18 years	500	800
19–50 years	500	1000

Note: Values are adapted and summarized from the DRI tables published by www.nap.edu.

TABLE 19.12
DRIs for Biotin

Age	RDA/AI* (µg/day)	UL (µg/day)
Infants		
0–6 months	0.5*	ND
7–12 months	0.6*	ND
Children		
1–3 years	8*	ND
4–8 years	12*	ND
Males		
9–13 years	20	ND
14–50 years	25	ND
19 years and over	30	ND
Females		
9–13 years	20	ND
14–18 years	25	ND
19 years and over	30	ND
Pregnancy		
≤18 years	30*	ND
19–50 years	30*	ND
Lactation		
≤18 years	35*	ND
19–50 years	35*	ND

Note: Values are adapted and summarized from the DRI tables published by www.nap.edu.

TABLE 19.13
DRIs for Calcium

Age	RDA/AI* (µg/day)	UL (µg/day)
Infants		
0–6 months	210*	ND
7–12 months	270*	ND
Children		
1–3 years	500*	2500
4–8 years	800*	2500
Males		
9–18 years	1300*	2500
19–50 years	1000*	2500
51 years and over	1200*	2500
Females		
9–18 years	1300*	2500
19–50 years	1000*	2500
51 years and over	1200*	2500
Pregnancy		
≤18 years	1300	2500
19–50 years	1000	2500
Lactation		
≤18 years	1300	2500
19–50 years	1000	2500

Note: Values are adapted and summarized from the DRI tables published by www.nap.edu.

TABLE 19.14
DRIs for Magnesium

Age	RDA/AI* (mg/day)	UL (mg/day)
Infants		
0–6 months	30*	ND
7–12 months	75*	ND
Children		
1–3 years	80	65
4–8 years	130	110
Males		
9–13 years	240	350
14–18 years	410	350
19–30 years	400	350
31 years and over	420	350
Females		
9–13 years	240	350
14–18 years	360	350
31 years and over	320	350
Pregnancy		
≤18 years	400	350
19–30 years	350	350
31–50 years	360	350
Lactation		
≤18 years	360	350
31–50 years	320	350

Note: Values are adapted and summarized from the DRI tables published by www.nap.edu.

TABLE 19.15
DRIs for Manganese

Age	RDA/AI* (mg/day)	UL (mg/day)
Infants		
0–6 months	0.003*	ND
7–12 months	0.6*	ND
Children		
1–3 years	1.2*	2
4–8 years	1.5*	3
Males		
9–13 years	1.9*	6
14–18 years	2.2*	9
19 years and over	2.3*	11
Females		
9–13 years	1.6*	6
14–18 years	1.6*	9
19 years and over	1.8*	11
Pregnancy		
≤18 years	2.0*	9
19–50 years	2.0*	11
Lactation		
≤18 years	2.6*	9
19–50 years	2.6*	11

Note: Values are adapted and summarized from the DRI tables published by www.nap.edu.

TABLE 19.16
DRIs for Chromium

Age	RDA/AI* (μg/day)	UL (μg/day)
Infants		
0–6 months	0.2*	ND
7–12 months	5.5*	ND
Children		
1–3 years	11*	ND
4–8 years	15*	ND
Males		
9–13 years	25*	ND
14–50 years	35*	ND
51 years and over	30*	ND
Females		
9–13 years	21*	ND
14–18 years	24*	ND
19–50 years	25*	ND
Pregnancy		
≤18 years	29*	ND
19–50 years	30*	ND
Lactation		
≤18 years	44*	ND
19–50 years	45*	ND

Note: Values are adapted and summarized from the DRI tables published by www.nap.edu.

TABLE 19.17
DRIs for Copper

Age	RDA/AI* (μg/day)	UL (μg/day)
Infants		
0–6 months	200*	ND
7–12 months	220*	ND
Children		
1–3 years	340	1,000
4–8 years	440	3,000
Males		
9–13 years	700	5,000
14–18 years	890	8,000
19 years and over	900	10,000
Females		
9–13 years	700	5,000
14–18 years	890	8,000
19 years and over	900	10,000
Pregnancy		
≤18 years	1000	8,000
19–50 years	1000	10,000
Lactation		
≤18 years	1300	8,000
19–50 years	1300	10,000

Note: Values are adapted and summarized from the DRI tables published by www.nap.edu.

TABLE 19.18
DRIs for Iron

Age	RDA/AI* (mg/day)	UL (mg/day)
Infants		
0–6 months	0.27*	40
7–12 months	11	40
Children		
1–3 years	7	40
4–8 years	10	40
Males		
9–13 years	8	40
14–18 years	11	45
19 years and over	8	45
Females		
9–13 years	8	40
14–18 years	15	45
19–50	18	45
51 years and over	8	45
Pregnancy		
≤18–50 years	27	45
Lactation		
≤18 years	10	45
19–50 years	9	45

Note: Values are adapted and summarized from the DRI tables published by www.nap.edu.

TABLE 19.19
DRIs for Selenium

Age	RDA/AI* (μg/day)	UL (μg/day)
Infants		
0–6 months	15*	45
7–12 months	20*	60
Children		
1–3 years	20	90
4–8 years	30	150
Males		
9–13 years	40	280
14 years and over	55	400
Females		
9–13 years	40	280
14 years and over	55	400
Pregnancy		
≤18–50 years	60	400
Lactation		
≤18–50 years	70	400

Note: Values are adapted and summarized from the DRI tables published by www.nap.edu.

TABLE 19.20
DRIs for Phosphorus

Age	RDA/AI* (mg/day)	UL (mg/day)
Infants		
0–6 months	100*	ND
7–12 months	275*	ND
Children		
1–3 years	460	3000
4–8 years	500	3000
Males		
9–18 years	1250	4000
19–70 years	700	4000
>70 years	700	3000
Females		
9–18 years	1250	4000
19–70 years	700	4000
>70 years	700	3000
Pregnancy		
≤18 years	1250	3500
19–50 years	700	3500
Lactation		
≤18 years	1250	4000
19–50 years	700	4000

Note: Values are adapted and summarized from the DRI tables published by www.nap.edu.

TABLE 19.21
DRIs for Zinc

Age	RDA/AI* (mg/day)	UL (mg/day)
Infants		
0–6 months	2*	4
7–12 months	3	5
Children		
1–3 years	3	7
4–8 years	5	12
Males		
9–13 years	8	23
14–18 years	11	34
19 years and over	11	40
Females		
9–13 years	8	23
14–18 years	9	34
19 years and over	8	40
Pregnancy		
≤18 years	12	34
19–50 years	11	40
Lactation		
≤18 years	13	34
19–50 years	12	40

Note: Values are adapted and summarized from the DRI tables published by www.nap.edu.

CONCLUSIONS

The initial nutritional guidelines, RDAs, have been replaced by DRIs and are currently used by the United States and Canada. The DRI values of nutrients are sufficient for the growth and development of 97–98% of healthy individuals. The DRI values for carotenoids, alpha-lipoic acid, N-acetylcysteine, coenzyme Q_{10}, and L-carnitine have not been determined. The optimal values needed for prevention or improved management of human diseases are not known. Studies are in progress to establish these values.

Index

A

AA metabolites, 18
acetyl-L-carnitine, and aging, 44
acquired immunity, 19
acute inflammation, 17
AD (Alzheimer's disease)
    acetylcholinesterase inhibitors, rationale for using, 183
    and aging, 35
    alpha-lipoic acid, 177
    beta-amyloid
        cholesterol-induced generation of, 172–173
        mediation of neurotoxic effects through free radicals, 172
    antioxidant laboratory and clinical studies, 176–177
    B vitamins, 179
    caffeine, 180
    beta-carotene, 178
    clinical studies, vitamin E, 10, 27
    coenzyme Q10, 177
    cost, 168
    current treatments, 176
    diet and lifestyle recommendations, 184
    etiology, 168
    familial AD
        and NSAIDs, 175
        mutated genes' mediation of effects through increased production of beta-amyloid, 174
    Ginkgo biloba, 180
    green tea epigallocatechin-3-gallate (EGCG), 180
    idiopathic AD
        and NSAIDs, 175
        genetic defects in, 173–174
    incidence, 23, 167–168
    increased levels of markers of chronic inflammation, 174–176
    KGDHC (alpha-ketoglutarate dehydrogenase complex), 41
    melatonin, 7, 177–178
    and mitochondrial dysfunction, 38
    multiple micronutrients, rationale for, 180–182
    neuroglobin (Ngb), 176
    neuropathology, 168
    nicotinamide, 178
    nicotinamide adenine dinucleotide (NAD+), 178
    nicotinamide adenine dinucleotide dehydrogenase (NADH), 178
    NSAIDs
        in idiopathic AD, 175
        rationale for, 182
    omega-3 fatty acids, 180
    oxidative stress, and chronic inflammation in high-risk populations, 24
    oxidative stress–induced mitochondrial damage, 171–172
    proteasome inhibition induced neurodegeneration, 173
    recommended micronutrients/NSAIDs combinations for prevention of AD in high-risk populations, 183
    with standard therapy in patients with dementia, 183–184
    resveratrol, 179–180
    serum levels of dietary antioxidants, 179
    single nutrient problems, 180–181
    vitamin A, 178
    vitamin C, 179
    vitamin E, 178–179
adaptive immunity, 20
adaptive responses, of antioxidant enzymes, 40
aging
    chronic inflammation during, 39
    dietary recommendations, 46
    in humans, 35–36, 47
    influence on immune function, 39
    lifestyle-related recommendations, 46–47
    and mitochondrial dysfunction, 37–38
    and oxidative stress, 36–39
    rationale for not using single dietary antioxidant, 45
    rationale for recommending multiple micronutrients, 45–46
    recommended micronutrients for adults and children, 46
    See also healthy aging
AI (adequate intake), 343
alcohol, and cancer, 107
ALEs (advanced lipoxidation end products), and aging, 37
alpha-tocopheryl succinate (alpha-TS)
    and cancer prevention, 110–111
    effects of therapeutic doses on gene expression profiles in cancer cells, 140
    effects of therapeutic doses on growth of cancer and normal cells, 136
AMD (age-related macular degeneration), 41, 44
AMTP (active micronutrient treatment protocol), 156
antioxidant enzymes, and aging, 40–41
antioxidants, 11
    absorption, 6
    as affecting normal and cancer cells the same, 340
    biology, 24–25
    controversies, 8
    cooking, 5–6
    defense systems in humans, 7–8
    definitions, 7
    discovery, 1–2
    distribution in the body, 3–5
    evolution, 1, 14
    functions, 6, 8
    misuse in clinical studies, 8–10, 23
    as only scavenging free radicals, 340
    single *vs* multiple, 25
    solubility, 3
    storage, 5
    as toxic, 340

arthritis, 319, 331
  cost, 319
  diet and lifestyle recommendations, 331
  incidence, 319
  inflammation, 322–323
  oxidative stress, 321–322
  preventive strategies, 325
  role of antioxidants, 323–325
  treatment strategies, 325
    anticytokines therapy, 326–327
    complementary medicines, 328
    glucosamine and chondroitin, 327–328
    low-dose MTX, 325–326
    micronutrient strategies
      for prevention in high-risk populations, 328, 330
      problems of using a single agent, 328
      rationale for using multiple micronutrients, 329–330
    NSAIDs, 328
    recommended micronutrient supplement
      for combination with standard therapy, 330–331
      for prevention in high-risk populations, 330
    toxicity of standard therapy, 327
  types, 320–321
ascorbic acid, 4
  See also vitamin C
aspirin resistance, CAD (coronary artery disease), 57, 69
AT (ataxia telangiectasia), 111
ATBC study (Alpha-Tocopherol, Beta-Carotene Cancer Prevention study), 60–61

B

B cells (B lymphocytes), 19, 20
B vitamins
  AD (Alzheimer's disease), 179
  CAD (coronary artery disease), 66
  combination with multiple antioxidants, 25
  Dietary Reference Intake (DRI), 346–348
  discovery, 2
balanced diets, misconceptions, 339, 342
Bhattacharya, Sharmila, 120
biologics, 326
biotin, Dietary Reference Intake (DRI), 350
bone marrow syndrome, 298–299

C

CAD (coronary artery disease), 55, 69–70
  aspirin resistance, 57, 69
  clinical studies
    dietary antioxidants
      with cholesterol-lowering drugs, 63–64
      producing adverse or no effects, 60–62
    endogenous antioxidants
      with cholesterol-lowering drugs, 63
      producing beneficial or no effects, 62–63
    intervention human studies, 58
      with B vitamins, 66
    vitamin C
      alone, producing beneficial effects, 60
      with cholesterol-lowering drugs, 64
    vitamin E, 26–27, 57–58
      with cholesterol-lowering drugs, 63–64
      alone, producing beneficial effects, 59–60
  consequences of increased oxidative stress and chronic inflammation, 56–57
  cost, 56
  dietary recommendations, 69
  dose schedule importance, 68
  incidence, 23, 55
  lifestyle-related recommendations, 69
  multiple micronutrients
    proposed preparation, 68
    scientific rationale for using, 67–68, 69
  omega-3 fatty acids, 65–66
  oxidative stress and chronic inflammation in high-risk populations, 24
  resveratrol, 65
  risk factors, 56
  role of antioxidants, 57–58
caffeine
  AD (Alzheimer's disease), 180
  and cancer, 108
calcium, Dietary Reference Intake (DRI), 350
cancer
  carcinogens, 106
    diet-related, 108–109
    environment-related, 108
    lifestyle-related, 106–108
  clinical studies
    beta-carotene, 26
    multiple dietary antioxidants, 28–29, 150–151
    vitamin E, 26
  cost, 104
  diet and lifestyle recommendations, 157
  diet-related protective agents, 109
  experimental therapies
    effects of therapeutic doses of individual antioxidants
      cellular vaccine, 156
      gene therapy, 156
      hyperthermia, 154–155
      sodium butyrate and interferon-alpha2b, 155
  incidence, 23, 103–104, 133
  mortality, 104, 133
  oncologists' recommendations on antioxidants use, 135–136
  oxidative stress and chronic inflammation in high-risk populations, 24
  preventive and therapeutic dose ranges of antioxidants, 133–134
  preventive doses of antioxidants, effects on growth of cancer cells, 141
  proposed micronutrient protocols
    AMTP (active micronutrient treatment protocol), 156
    for after completion of standard therapy, 157
  proposed stages of human carcinogenesis, 104–106
  recommended micronutrients for reducing the risk and progression of chronic diseases, 30–31
  standard therapy, 133–134, 157–158
    rationale for not recommending antioxidant supplements, 152–154
    rational for using multiple micronutrients, 151–152
  therapeutic doses of individual antioxidants
    effects on chemotherapeutic agent-induced damage in cancer and normal cells

animal studies, 147
cell culture studies, 144–146
clinical studies, 147–149
effects on gene expression profiles in cancer cells, 140
effects on growth of cancer and normal cells, 136–140
effects on radiation-induced damage in cancer and normal cells
animal studies, 142–144
cell culture studies, 141–142
clinical studies, 144
mechanisms of enhancing efficacy of standard therapy, 150
treatment schedule, 140
tumor promoters, 106
cancer prevention
antioxidants
analysis of animals after treatment with, 110–112
analysis of cell cultures after treatment with, 110
analysis of epidemiologic studies, 112–114
analysis of intervention studies, 114
treatment with fat and fiber, 118–119
treatment with folate and B vitamins, 117–118
treatment with multiple dietary antioxidants, 116–117
treatment with NSAIDs, 119
treatment with single dietary antioxidant on heavy tobacco smokers, 114–115
treatment with single dietary antioxidant on other cancer risks, 115–116
treatment with vitamin D and calcium, 117
proposed strategies, 119, 123
for cancer-free high-risk individuals, 120, 121
for cancer-free normal individuals, 119–120
for cancer survivors, 121
rationale for using multiple micronutrients, 121–122
unique features of proposed micronutrient formulation, 122
relevant functions, 109–110
importance of, 103
beta-carotene
AD (Alzheimer's disease), 178
and cancer prevention, 110
clinical study with heavy tobacco users, 9–10, 26
conversion to vitamin A, 2
discovery, 2
distribution in the body, 3–4
as harmful to health, 340
natural *vs* synthetic, 25, 115–116, 341
preventive and therapeutic dose ranges for cancer, 134
sources and forms, 3
toxicity, 123, 293
See also ATBC study
carotenoids
and aging, 44
cooking, 5
discovery, 2
distribution in the body, 3–4
DRI values, 355
sources and forms, 3
storage, 5
Cartier, Jacques, 2

catalase, 40–41
cell phones, and cancer, 107
cerebral concussion, 250–251
CHAOS (Cambridge Heart Antioxidant Study), 59
Charlton, Clive, 205
chemokines, 18
chromium, Dietary Reference Intake (DRI), 352
chronic inflammation, 17
and antioxidants, 9
during aging, 39
increased levels of markers of, in AD, 174–176
PD (Parkinson's disease), 24, 203
clinical studies, 31
with fat and fiber, 29–30
misuse of antioxidants in, 8–10, 23
with multiple dietary antioxidants, cancer, 28–29, 150–151
recommended micronutrients combination, 30–31
with a single antioxidant, 26
reasons for inconsistent results, 27
using multiple micronutrients, 30
CMV (cytomegalovirus), 223
CNS (central nervous system) syndrome, 299
coenzyme Q10
AD (Alzheimer's disease), 177
and aging, 42–43
cooking, 6
diabetes mellitus, 85–86
distribution in the body, 4
DRI values, 355
effects of therapeutic doses
on chemotherapeutic agent-induced damage in cancer and normal cells, 148–149
on growth of cancer and normal cells, 140
functions, 7
preventive and therapeutic dose ranges for cancer, 134
sources and forms, 3
storage, 5
toxicity, 123, 293
coffee, and cancer, 108
complement proteins, 18
and innate immunity, 19
concussive injury *see* traumatic brain injury (TBI)
conductive hearing loss, 222
cooking, degradation of antioxidants, 5–6
copper, Dietary Reference Intake (DRI), 352
COX (cyclooxygenase), 18
Crane, Fredrick, 3
CT scans, 285, 287
Cu/Zn-SOD, 40–41
cytokines, 17–18

D

D-carnitine, 3
DALARA, 290
DATATOP (Deprenyl and Tocopherol Antioxidative Therapy of Parkinsonism), 27–28, 205–206
dehydroascorbic acid, 4
dementia, incidence, 23
dendritic cells, 19
diabetes mellitus, 77, 93–94
antioxidant mixtures, 86
antioxidants in combination with diabetic/cardiovascular drugs and/or insulin, 87

diabetes mellitus (*continued*)
  alpha-lipoic acid, 83
  aspirin, 90–91
  chromium, 87
  coenzyme Q10, 85–86
  complications, 79
  cost, 78
  diet and lifestyle recommendations, 93
  evidence for increased chronic inflammation, 80
  evidence for increased oxidative stress, 79–80
  folic acid and thiamine, 86–87
  incidence, 77–78
  L-carnitine, 84–85
  multiple micronutrients
    rationale for using, 91–92
    recommended supplement for prevention in high-risk populations, 92–93
    recommended supplement in combination with standard therapy in diabetic patients, 93
  NAC (*N*-acetylcysteine), 83–84
  omega-3 fatty acids, 88–89
  problems associated with using a single agent, 91
  treatments, 89–90
  types, 78–79
  vitamin A, 81
    and insulin, 86
  vitamin C, 81–82
  vitamin D, 82
  vitamin E, 82–83
dietary antioxidants, 41–42
dietary factors, and oxidative stress, 36–37
dihydrolipoic acid, and cancer prevention, 111
DL-tocopherol, 4
DRF (dose reduction factor), 298
DRI (dietary reference intakes), 343, 355

E

eicosanoids, 18
  See also AA metabolites
endogenous antioxidants, 41–42
endothelial adhesion molecules, 18
environmental stressors, and oxidative stress, 36
Evans, Herbert, 2

F

Fenton reaction, 15, 170
fish oil, vitamin E absorption, 43
flavonoids
  and aging, 44
  and cancer prevention, 113
  distribution in the body, 5
  functions, 7
folate, Dietary Reference Intake (DRI), 349
Folkers, Karl, 3
free radicals, 13
  formation from oxygen and nitrogen, 14–16, 169–170
  sources in normal brain, 168–169
  types, 14
freezing antioxidants, 341–342
Funk, Casimir, 2

G

gestational diabetes, 78
GI (gastrointestinal) syndrome, 299
Ginkgo biloba, AD (Alzheimer's disease), 180
glutamine, effects of therapeutic doses, on chemotherapeutic agent-induced damage in cancer and normal cells, 149
glutathione
  in AD and PD patients, 25
  and aging, 42, 44
  cooking, 6
  distribution in the body, 4
  functions, 7
  sources and forms, 3
  storage, 5
glutathione peroxidase, 40–41
Gomberg, Moses, 14
green tea epigallocatechin-3-gallate (EGCG), AD (Alzheimer's disease), 180
group A antioxidants, defense systems in humans, 7
group B antioxidants, defense systems in humans, 7
group C antioxidants, defense systems in humans, 8

H

HAART (highly active antiretroviral therapy), 269, 274–275, 277–278
Haber–Weiss reaction, 15, 170
HATS (HDL Atherosclerosis Treatment Study), 63–64
Hawkins, Sir Richard, 2
head injury *see* traumatic brain injury (TBI)
healthy aging, 35–36
hearing disorders, 221, 229–230
  agents or conditions causing, 223
  beneficial effects of antioxidants, 225–226
  cost, 222
  current prevention and treatment strategies, 223–224
  incidence, 221–222
  inflammation, 225
  measurement, 223
  multiple micronutrients
    micronutrient recommendation for prevention and improved treatment, 229
    rationale for using, 226–229
  oxidative stress, 225
  types, 222–223
helper T cells, 20
herbal antioxidants, avoidance for micronutrient supplementation, 31
high-fiber diet, and cancer, 28, 29, 116, 118
high LET radiation, 297
HIV/AIDS, 269, 278
  cost, 270
  current treatments, 274–275
  diet and lifestyle recommendations, 278
  history, 270
  incidence, 270
  inflammation, 271–272
  micronutrients
    evidence of reduction of progression of infection, 273–274
    rationale for using multiple micronutrients, 275–277

recommended formulation for improving efficacy
of antiviral therapy, 277–278
recommended formulation for primary and
secondary prevention, 277
role in combination with antiviral drugs, 275
oxidative stress, 271–272
prevention strategies
primary, 272
secondary, 273
role of immune function, 270
impairment from illicit drugs, 271
impairment from micronutrient deficiency, 270–271
HOCl (hypochlorous), 36
Hoffer, Michael, 242
HOPE (Heart Outcomes Prevention Evaluation), 26–27, 61–62
HPV (human papilloma virus), 105
human diets, compared to laboratory rodents, 109
hydroperoxy radical, 14
hydroxyl radical, 14–16

I

ICAM-1 (intracellular adhesion molecule-1), 18
immortalization of cells, in carcinogenesis, 105–106
immune system, 13, 18–19, 20
and aging, 39
See also acquired immunity; adaptive immunity; innate immunity
infection, free radicals to kill infective agents, 16
inflammation, 13, 16–17
and innate immunity, 19
products of inflammatory reactions, 17–18
types of inflammatory reactions, 17
innate immunity, 19–20
iNOS (inducible NOS), and CAD, 56
ionizing radiation, 297
bone marrow syndrome, 298–299
central nervous system (CNS) syndrome, 299
diagnostic doses, 285–286, 293
biochemical and genetic steps involved in radiation-induced carcinogenesis, 286
radiation protection
current recommendations, 290
evidence for a micronutrient strategy for biological protection, 290–291
recommended micronutrient preparations for biological protection, 291–293
risk of low-dose radiation-induced non-neoplastic diseases, 289–290
gastrointestinal (GI) syndrome, 299
high doses, 297–298, 311
damage caused, 298
late effects on cancer incidence, 300
late effects on the risk of non-neoplastic diseases, 300–301
to organs, 300
recommended multiple micronutrients
for combination with replacement therapy, 311
for radiation protection in humans, 310
interactions with chemical and biological carcinogens and tumor promoters, 287
radiation protection studies
with antioxidants in animal models, 302

with antioxidants in cell culture models, 301–302
with antioxidants in humans, 303
history, 301
with multiple antioxidants administered orally before and after irradiation in animals, 304
Drosophila melanogaster (fruit fly), 307
mice, 305–307
rabbits, 305
sheep, 304–305
scientific rationale for using multiple antioxidants, 303–304
with radiation therapeutic agents or procedures, 307–308
biological agents, 309–310
chemical agents, 308–309
risk estimate models of radiation-induced cancer, 287–289
iron, Dietary Reference Intake (DRI), 353

J

juvenile rheumatoid arthritis (JRA), 321

K

KGDHC (alpha-ketoglutarate dehydrogenase complex), in AD patients, 41
killer T cells, 20

L

L-carnitine
diabetes mellitus, 84–85
distribution in the body, 4
DRI values, 355
sources and forms, 3
LDL cholesterol, as "bad cholesterol", 56
leukocytes, and innate immunity, 20
alpha-linolenic acid (ALA), and cancer prevention, 113
Linxian General Population Nutrition Interventional Trial, 29, 116
lipid peroxidation, and aging, 37
alpha-lipoic acid, 4
AD (Alzheimer's disease), 177
and aging, 44
cooking, 6
diabetes mellitus, 83
DRI values, 355
effects of therapeutic doses
on chemotherapeutic agent-induced damage in cancer and normal cells, 148
on growth of cancer and normal cells, 140
functions, 7
preventive and therapeutic dose ranges for cancer, 134
storage, 5
toxicity, 123, 293
use in combination with dietary antioxidants, 25
low LET radiation, 297
lysosomal-mediated proteolytic activity, and aging, 38

M

macronutrients, 1
magnesium, Dietary Reference Intake (DRI), 351

manganese, Dietary Reference Intake (DRI), 351
McCollum, E.V., 1
melatonin
    AD (Alzheimer's disease), 7, 177–178
    and aging, 44
    distribution in the body, 5
    functions, 7
    storage, 5
Mellanby, Sir Edward, 2
Meniere's Disease (MD), 221, 222–223
    current prevention and treatment strategies, 224
    See also hearing disorders
meta-analyses, 10, 29
metabolic syndrome, 79
    evidence for increased oxidative stress, 80
micronutrients, 1
    as passing out of the body, 339–340
misconceptions about antioxidants and health, 339–342
mitochondria
    dysfunction and aging, 37–38
    incidental free radicals production, 16, 36
    oxidative stress and aging, 36
Mn-SOD, 40
MONICA (WHO/Multinational MONItoring of Trends and Determinants in Cardiovascular Disease) study, 57
more is better (misconception), 339
MTF-1 (metal-responsive transcriptional factor), and aging, 37
multiple dietary antioxidants
    clinical studies, cancer, 28–29, 150–151
    in aging, 44–45
multivitamins, 9
Myocardial Infarction and Vitamins Study, 86
myths about antioxidants and health, 339–342

N

NAC (N-acetylcysteine)
    and aging, 44
    and cancer prevention, 110–111, 114
    cooking, 6
    diabetes mellitus, 83–84
    distribution in the body, 4
    DRI values, 355
    effects of therapeutic doses
        on chemotherapeutic agent-induced damage in cancer and normal cells, 148
        on growth of cancer and normal cells, 139
    functions, 7
    storage, 5
    toxicity, 123, 293
    use in combination with dietary antioxidants, 25
NAD+ (nicotinamide adenine dinucleotide)
    AD (Alzheimer's disease), 178
    distribution in the body, 4–5
    functions, 7
NADH (reduced nicotinamide adenine dinucleotide)
    AD (Alzheimer's disease), 178
    cooking, 6
    distribution in the body, 4–5
    PD (Parkinson's disease), 206–207
    storage, 5
natural antioxidants, vs synthetic, 341

neuroglobin (Ngb), in AD, 176
niacin, Dietary Reference Intake (DRI), 349
nicotinamide, PD (Parkinson's disease), 205
night blindness, 1
nitrosylative stress, 15
NK (natural killer) cells, 19, 39

O

OA (osteoarthritis), 319, 320
omega-3 fatty acids, AD (Alzheimer's disease), 180
once-a-day doses of micronutrients, 30, 341
oxidation, and reduction, 16
oxidative damage, 9
oxidative stress, 13–14, 15, 20
    and aging, 36–39
    arthritis, 321–322
    hearing disorders, 225
    influence of environmental, dietary, metabolic, and lifestyle-related stress, 36–37
    levels in high-risk populations, 24
    PD (Parkinson's disease), 24, 201–203
    PTSD (posttraumatic stress disorder), 224, 237
    sources of, 36
oxygen pressure, and antioxidant effectiveness, 25

P

PAMARA, 290
pantothenic acid, Dietary Reference Intake (DRI), 348
PD (Parkinson's disease), 197
    and aging, 35
    animal model studies, 204–205
    antioxidant enzymes, 41
    chronic inflammation, 24, 203
    clinical studies, vitamin E, 10, 27–28
    cost, 198
    current treatments, 210
    diet and lifestyle recommendations, 211
    DJ-1 gene, 199–200
    etiology, 198
    genetics, 199
    human studies, 205–207
    in vitro studies, 204
    incidence, 23, 198
    mitochondrial dysfunction, 38, 203–204
    multiple antioxidants, rationale for, 207–208
    NADH (reduced nicotinamide adenine dinucleotide), 206–207
    neuropathology, 198–199
    NSAID, rationale for using, 209
    oxidative stress, 24, 201–203
    PTEN-induced putative kinase 1, 200
    recommended micronutrients/NSAIDs combinations
        for prevention of PD in high-risk populations, 209
        for reducing rate of progression in early-stage patients, 209
        in combination with standard therapy, 210–211
    single antioxidant problems, 207
    symptoms, 199
    alpha-synuclein gene, 200–201
peroxyl radical, 15–16
peroxynitrite, 15, 36, 170
    and vascular aging, 38

phagocytes, as source of free radicals, 36
phagocytosis, 20
phosphorus, Dietary Reference Intake (DRI), 354
Polyp-Prevention Trial, 29–30, 118
polyphenols
    cooking, 6
    distribution in the body, 5
    storage, 5
    See also flavonoids
prediabetes, 78–79
programmed cell death, 35
proteasome activity, and aging, 38
PTSD (posttraumatic stress disorder), 235, 243
    biochemical events, 236–237
    chronic inflammation, 237–238
    cost, 236
    diet and lifestyle recommendations, 243
    incidence, 235–236
    micronutrients
        problems of using a single micronutrient, 240
        rationale for recommending multiple micronutrients, 240–242
        rationale for using, 239–240
        recommended micronutrients for combination with standard therapy, 243
        recommended micronutrients for reducing the risk in high-risk populations, 242–243
    oxidative stress, 224, 237
    release of glutamate, 238
    standard therapy, 238
    symptoms, 236
Purina Chow, antioxidant levels in, 112

R

RA (rheumatoid arthritis), 319, 320
radiation syndrome, 298
RDAs (Recommended Dietary Allowances), 343, 355
reactive nitrogen species (RNS), formation, 15–16
reactive oxygen species (ROS), formation, 14–15
recommended micronutrient combinations
    AD (Alzheimer's disease)
        for prevention of AD in high-risk populations, 183
        with standard therapy in patients with dementia, 183–184
    for adults and children, to reduce rate of aging, 46
    for biological protection against low doses of radiation, 291–293
    CAD (coronary artery disease), proposed multiple micronutrient preparation, 68
    for clinical studies, 30–31
    for diabetic patients, 93
    for reducing risk and progression of chronic disease, cancer, 30–31
    for prevention and improved treatment of hearing disorders, 229
    for prevention of cancer in cancer-free high-risk individuals, 120, 121
    for prevention of cancer in cancer-free normal individuals, 119–120
    for prevention of diabetes in high-risk populations, 92–93
    PD (Parkinson's disease)
        in combination with standard therapy, 210–211
        for prevention of PD in high-risk populations, 209
        for reducing rate of progression in early-stage patients, 209
reduction, 16
refrigerating antioxidants, 341–342
resveratrol
    AD (Alzheimer's disease), 179–180
    CAD (coronary artery disease), 65
retinoic acid, 4–5
retinol activity equivalent (RAE), 2
retinyl acetate, 4
retinyl palmitate, 4
rickets, 2

S

sarcopenia, 38
scurvy, 2
SELECT (Selenium and Vitamin E Cancer Prevention Trial), 29, 111, 116
selenium
    Dietary Reference Intake (DRI), 353
    effects of therapeutic doses
        on chemotherapeutic agent-induced damage in cancer and normal cells, 149
        on growth of cancer and normal cells, 138–139
    role in antioxidants defense systems in humans, 7
    supplementation in combination with antioxidants, 25
    toxicity, 123, 293
sensorineural hearing loss, 222
Sevak, 150
smoking
    and cancer, 107–108
    and oxidative stress, 37
SSHL (sudden sensorineural hearing loss)
    current prevention and treatment strategies, 224
    incidence, 222
Strategic National Stockpile Radiation Working Group, 307–308
synthetic antioxidants, vs natural, 341
Szent-Gyorgyi, Albert, 2

T

T cells (T lymphocytes), 19, 20
    See also helper T cells; killer T cells
γδ T cells, 20
telomere, and aging, 38–39
thiamine deficiency, 87
    See also vitamin B1 (Thiamin), Dietary Reference Intake (DRI)
tinnitus, 222
TNF-alpha, and aging, 39
tocopherol, 2
Alpha-Tocopherol, Beta-Carotene Cancer Prevention Study, 115
alpha-tocopheryl acetate (alpha-TA), 4–5
alpha-tocopheryl succinate (alpha-TS), 4–5, 134
alpha-tocopheryl
    distribution in the body, 4
    storage, 5
    See also ATBC study
Tolerable Upper Intake Level (UL), 343
trace minerals, and antioxidant preparations, 341

traumatic brain injury (TBI), 249, 260–261
  biochemical events, 251
  causes, 249–250
  cost, 250
  diet and lifestyle recommendations, 260
  glutamate release, 254–255
    reduction of, by antioxidants, 256–257
  incidence, 250
  inflammation, 253–254
  matrix metalloproteinases, 255
  mitochondrial dysfunction, 252–253
  oxidative stress, 251–252
  risk of PTSD, 251
  symptoms and consequences, 250
    concussive injury, 250–251
  treatments, 255
    with antioxidants, 256
      problems using a single agent, 257
      rationale for using multiple micronutrients, 257–259
      recommended micronutrients for combination with standard therapy for penetrating head injury, 260
      recommended micronutrients for reducing late adverse effects in high-risk populations, 259–260
    sports-related concussive injury, 255
type 1 diabetes, 78
  evidence for increased oxidative stress, 79–80
type 2 diabetes, 78
  evidence for increased oxidative stress, 80
  omega-3 fatty acids, 88

U

UL (Tolerable Upper Intake Level), 343
UPDRS (Unified Parkinson Disease Rating Score), 206

V

vascular aging, and mitochondrial dysfunction, 38
VCAM-1 (vascular adhesion molecule-1), 18
VITAL (VITamins And Lifestyle) cohort study, 113
vitamin A
  AD (Alzheimer's disease), 178
  cooking, 5
  diabetes mellitus, 81
    and insulin, 86
  Dietary Reference Intake (DRI), 344
  discovery, 1
  distribution in the body, 4
  effects of therapeutic doses on growth of cancer and normal cells, 138
  functions, 6
  preventive and therapeutic dose ranges for cancer, 134
  sources and forms, 2
  storage, 5
  toxicity, 123, 293
vitamin B1 (thiamin)
  Dietary Reference Intake (DRI), 346
  See also thiamine deficiency
vitamin B12, Dietary Reference Intake (DRI), 348

vitamin B2, Dietary Reference Intake (DRI), 347
vitamin B6
  Dietary Reference Intake (DRI), 347
  toxicity, 123
vitamin C
  AD (Alzheimer's disease), 179
  and aging, 42
  and cancer prevention, 111–112
  as causing kidney stones, 341
  cancer cell growth, 25
  clinical studies
    CAD (coronary artery disease)
      alone, producing beneficial effects, 60
      with cholesterol-lowering drugs, 64
    diabetes mellitus, 81–82
  Dietary Reference Intake (DRI), 345
  discovery, 2
  distribution in the body, 4
  effects of therapeutic doses on growth of cancer and normal cells, 137–138
  functions, 6
  and iron, copper, manganese, 46
  preventive and therapeutic dose ranges for cancer, 134
  sources and forms, 3
  storage, 5
  toxicity, 123, 293
vitamin D
  combination with multiple antioxidants, 25
  diabetes mellitus, 82
  Dietary Reference Intake (DRI), 346
  discovery, 2
  functions, 6
vitamin E
  AD (Alzheimer's disease), 178–179
  and aging, 42, 43
  all forms as having the same function, 340
  and cancer prevention, 110–111, 115
  clinical studies
    AD (Alzheimer's disease), 10, 27
    CAD (coronary artery disease), 26–27, 57–58
      alone, producing beneficial effects, 59–60
      with cholesterol-lowering drugs, 63–64
    cancer, 26
    PD (Parkinson's disease), 10, 27–28
  cooking, 5
  diabetes mellitus, 82–83
  Dietary Reference Intake (DRI), 345
  discovery, 2
  distribution in the body, 4
  effects of therapeutic doses
    on chemotherapeutic agent-induced damage in cancer and normal cells, 149
    on growth of cancer and normal cells, 136–137
  functions, 6
  as harmful to health, 340
  natural *vs* synthetic, 25, 341
  preventive and therapeutic dose ranges for cancer, 134
  sources and forms, 3
  storage, 5
  toxicity, 123, 293
vitamines, 2

Index

W

WAVE trial (Women's Angiographic Vitamin and Estrogen trial), 62
Wheat Bran Fiber Trial, 117
WHI (Women's Health Initiative), 113
WHI Dietary Modification Trial, 118
Whistler, Daniel, 2
Windaus, A., 2

Women's Antioxidant Cardiovascular Study, 82–83
Women's Antioxidants and Folic Acid Cardiovascular Study, 87
Women's Health Initiative Dietary Modification Trial, 29

Z

zinc, Dietary Reference Intake (DRI), 354
zycose, 87

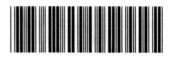